Therapy of Hematopoietic Neoplasia

HEMATOLOGY

Series Editors

Kenneth M. Brinkhous, M.D.
Department of Pathology
University of North Carolina
School of Medicine
Chapel Hill, North Carolina

Sanford A. Stass, M.D.
Hematopathology Program
The University of Texas System Cancer Center
M. D. Anderson Hospital and Tumor Institute
Houston, Texas

Volume 1 Prostaglandins and Leukotrienes: Blood and Vascular Cell Function, *Jonathan M. Gerrard*

Volume 2 Hematopoietic Stem Cells, *edited by David W. Golde and Fumimaro Takaku*

Volume 3 Bone Marrow Transplantation: Biological Mechanisms and Clinical Practice, *edited by Dirk W. van Bekkum and Bob Löwenberg*

Volume 4 Myelofibrosis: Pathophysiology and Clinical Management, *edited by S. M. Lewis*

Volume 5 Plasma Fibronectin: Structure and Function, *edited by Jan McDonagh*

Volume 6 The Acute Leukemias: Biologic, Diagnostic, and Therapeutic Determinants, *edited by Sanford A. Stass*

Volume 7 Hemostasis and Animal Venoms, *edited by Hubert Pirkle and Francis S. Markland, Jr.*

Volume 8 Hematopoiesis: Long-Term Effects of Chemotherapy and Radiation, *edited by Nydia G. Testa and Robert Peter Gale*

Volume 9 Coagulation and Bleeding Disorders, *edited by Theodore S. Zimmerman and Zaverio M. Ruggeri*

Volume 10 Disorders of the Spleen, *edited by Carl Pochedly, Richard H. Sills, and Allen D. Schwartz*

Volume 11 Red Blood Cell Membranes: Structure, Function, Clinical Implications, *edited by Peter Agre and John C. Parker*

Volume 12 Graft-vs.-Host Disease: Immunology, Pathophysiology, and Treatment, *edited by Steven J. Burakoff, H. Joachim Deeg, James Ferrara, and Kerry Atkinson*

Volume 13 Chronic Myelogenous Leukemia: Molecular Approaches to Research and Therapy, *edited by Albert B. Deisseroth and Ralph B. Arlinghaus*

Volume 14 Therapy of Hematopoietic Neoplasia, *edited by Emil J Freireich and Hagop Kantarjian*

Additional Volumes in Preparation

Biological Response Modifiers in the Treatment of Hematopoietic Neoplasia, *edited by Jordan Gutterman, Moshe Talpaz, and Razelle Kurzrock*

Therapy of Hematopoietic Neoplasia

edited by
Emil J Freireich
Hagop Kantarjian

University of Texas
M.D. Anderson Cancer Center
Houston, Texas

Marcel Dekker, Inc. New York • Basel • Hong Kong

ISBN: 0–8247–8455–3

This book is printed on acid-free paper

MARCEL DEKKER, INC.
207 Madison Avenue, New York, New York 10016

Current printing (last digit):
10 9 8 7 6 5 4 3 2 1

PRINTED IN THE UNITED STATES OF AMERICA

Series Introduction

For most of this century, hematology has followed a pattern of major scientific discoveries, improved understanding of disease, and rapid application of new knowledge in the clinic. The rate of advance continues at an accelerating pace, so that all but the most zealous have difficulty in keeping up with the literature in even a limited area of specialized interest. As the explosive development of knowledge continues apace, it is a continuing challenge to keep abreast of significant new developments as they impact on clinical and laboratory hematology. The Hematology series is designed to help in this respect, by providing up-to-date and expert presentations on important subject areas in our field. It is hoped that these works, both individually and collectively, will become important volumes for updating information and for reference for the clinician, investigator, teacher, and student, and in this manner contribute to the advancement of hematology.

This volume on therapy of the hematopoietic malignancies is the fourteenth in the Hematology series. It deals with one of the monumental accomplishments of modern medicine, the development of effective and often curative therapies in the management of these neoplastic disorders. Many landmarks stand out, with Hodgkin's disease being the first of the disorders to be controlled by radiation therapy and cured by chemotherapy. In the last decade there has been a virtual revolution in the biological understanding of these malignancies, with the new knowledge determining in large measure the development of new treatment regimens of many types. The demonstration in 1979 that treatment of acute myelogenous leukemia in remission by bone marrow transplantation, with long-lasting and disease-free survival, gave impetus to perfecting this mode of therapy, leading to its wide usage today in many of the hematopoietic malignancies. Developments in molecular biology have resulted in the availability of new recombinant products as interferon-alpha, erythropoietin, and other biological response modifiers. The use of the polymerase chain reaction is a major new tool in detecting minimal residual disease. A complete list of the many new applications would be a long one indeed. Clinical trials in specialized institutional settings and through interinstitutional study groups with a common clinical protocol have proven to be an effective method of advancing this complex field of investigation. The fruits of using and combining these multiple therapeutic approaches, both old and new, are evident throughout this book.

This volume provides comprehensive coverage of the current status of both conventional and investigative therapy of the hematopoietic malignancies. Concepts based on the state of the art in basic and clinical science and practice are emphasized by the authors of the various chapters in developing rationales for specific treatment regimens for the different malignancies. This makes for a lively and readable presentation that should be appealing to many readers. The volume provides the practicing hematologist-oncologist with treatment outlines that have been well tested and should thus be a valuable reference source. This work has been developed under the able leadership of a pioneer and authority in the field, Emil J Freireich, with coeditor Hagop Kantarjian.

Kenneth M. Brinkhous
Series Coeditor

Preface

Publications relating to medical diagnoses usually use the format of etiology, pathophysiology, diagnosis, and end with treatment. This stems from the paradigm that predicts that understanding of the basic science aspect of disease will lead ultimately to effective prevention and/or curative treatment. In reality the fundamental skill which the physician brings to the sick patient is his or her ability to control and/or cure the disease process in the affected host, and most of the basic knowledge about disease subserves the primary objective of controlling existing disease. Although physicians play many other roles in society including those of public health and administration, the fundamental role of the physician in a complex social order is to effectively tend to the sick. It is for this reason that this book is devoted entirely to treatment as the primary discipline, and other basic aspects of medicine that influence treatment choices are covered in association with the fundamental science of therapy.

Therapeutics is often confused with pharmacology and other laboratory disciplines. However, therapeutics are fundamental to all of the medical specialties. In the case of malignant diseases, surgery is currently the dominant modality of curative treatment. Radiation therapy adds an additional dimension for regional control of disease. The major residual therapeutic challenge for cancer is the treatment of metastatic or systemic cancer. Virtually all of the mortality and most of the morbidity associated with cancer diagnoses result from systemic forms of malignancy. The hematological malignancies are dominantly systemic from the outset of their biology and from the earliest possible diagnosis. Local and regional therapy plays a primary role in only a small minority of these patients, and beginning in 1942, with the discovery of nitrogen mustard for the treatment of lymphoma, the development of treatment strategies for systemic disease has been dominantly pioneered by observations made in the hematological malignancies. Thus the therapeutic science in the hematological malignancies plays a leadership role in the development of our knowledge about the control of systemic cancer.

Over the last 50 years of basic clinical research, therapy has reached the level where curative treatment is achievable for a majority of patients with these malignancies. The consequence of these fundamental advances in our ability to control the hematological malignancies is that the treatment has revealed enormous heterogeneity in these diagnoses. It is now clear that responsiveness to a given treatment is more fundamentally linked to the underlying biology of the tumor and not to a probability type of outcome which gives all patients equal likelihood of responding to any given treatment. This perception has led to a therapeutic strategy that is progressively more objective, more scientific, and therefore more specific for the individual patient. It is the purpose of this book to update our knowledge about the science of therapeutics in the subset of malignant diseases that are called the hematological malignancies, that is, those tumors arising in the myeloid and lymphoid organs of the host. The contributors to this volume are each not only experienced in the therapeutic science, but have each made substantial contributions to our existing knowledge of the disease and are therefore expert. It is the hope of the editors that this volume will represent a state of the art for this basic science and will serve as a backbone for understanding future developments in therapeutics.

Emil J Freireich
Hagop Kantarjian

Contents

Contributors

Zalman A. Arlin, M.D. Department of Hematology, New York Medical College, Valhalla, New York

Bart Barlogie, M.D.* Department of Hematology, University of Texas M. D. Anderson Cancer Center, Houston, Texas

Miloslav Beran, M.D. Department of Hematology, Leukemia Section, University of Texas M. D. Anderson Cancer Center, Houston, Texas

Gerald P. Bodey, M.D. Departments of Medicine and Medical Specialties, and Section of Infectious Diseases, University of Texas M. D. Anderson Cancer Center, Houston, Texas

Fernando Cabanillas, M.D. Department of Hematology, University of Texas M. D. Anderson Cancer Center, Houston, Texas

Elihu H. Estey, M.D. Department of Hematology, University of Texas M. D. Anderson Cancer Center, Houston, Texas

Emil J Freireich, M.D. D.Sc.(Hon) Adult Leukemia Research Program, Department of Hematology, University of Texas M. D. Anderson Cancer Center, Houston, Texas

Fredrick B. Hagemeister, M.D. Department of Hematology, University of Texas M. D. Anderson Cancer Center, Houston, Texas

Hagop Kantarjian, M.D. Departments of Medicine and Hematology, University of Texas M. D. Anderson Cancer Center, Houston, Texas

*Present Address: University of Arkansas for Medical Sciences, Arkansas Cancer Research Center, Little Rock, Arkansas

Michael J. Keating, M.D. B.S. Department of Hematology, University of Texas M. D. Anderson Cancer Center, Houston, Texas

Nancy Khardori, M.D. Section of Infectious Diseases, Department of Medical Specialties, University of Texas M. D. Anderson Cancer Center, Houston, Texas

Kenneth McCredie, M.D. Ch.B. Department of Hematology, University of Texas M. D. Anderson Cancer Center, Houston, Texas

Jorge R. Quesada, M.D. OnCol, Center for I.V. Therapies and Cancer Therapeutics, Houston, Texas

Moshe Talpaz, M.D. Department of Hematology, University of Texas M. D. Anderson Cancer Center, Houston, Texas

Ralph Wallerstein, Jr. Department of Hematology, University of Texas M. D. Anderson Cancer Center, Houston, Texas

1

Therapy for Acute Myelogenous Leukemia

Elihu H. Estey and Emil J Freireich

University of Texas
M. D. Anderson Cancer Center
Houston, Texas

In 1961, Freireich et al. reported that patients with acute leukemia who responded to chemotherapy lived longer than patients who failed to respond (1). The time spent "in remission" completely accounted for the difference in survival. The authors noted that "it is possible that patients . . . can be divided into those with mild disease (responders) and those with severe disease ('nonresponders')," and that this might account for the difference. However response to one drug did not predict response to a second and once a patient was a nonresponder survival was similarly brief, regardless of previous response. In short, "the patient is exposed to a high risk of death when active disease is present, and this risk is sharply reduced when hematologic improvement occurs." The most beneficial response in patients with either acute myelogenous leukemia (AML) acute lymphocytic leukemia (ALL), was one in which bone marrow and blood reverted to normal characteristics, providing the impetus to obtain and maintain such a response, commonly known as a complete remission (CR).

Subsequently, studies of the Cancer and Leukemia Group Group B (CALGB) indicated that patients who received one dose of 6-mercaptopurine (6-MP) in prednisone-induced CR were more likely to remain in CR than patients who received placebo (2). At times, patients given placebo obtained a second remission following administration of 6-MP. Addition of the time spent in these second remissions to the time spent in first remission to yield an "adjusted placebo curve" indicated that this curve approached but did not equal that of patients given 6-MP immediately after steroid-induced CR. This suggested that it would be easier to discover whether drugs, such as 6-MP, or therapeutic strategies were effective by utilizing them in patients in remission, rather than in patients in relapse. These results form the basis for administering both remission-induction therapy and some form of remission-maintenance therapy to patients with AML and for the assumption that both forms of therapy are appropriate targets for therapeutic research.

CONVENTIONAL THERAPY: 3 + 7 FOLLOWED BY LOWER-DOSE MAINTENANCE

Since the 1970s the standards of comparison for such research have been programs that use combinations of anthracyclines (usually daunorubicin, 45–60 mg/m^2 daily for 3 days) and cytarabine (cytosine arabinoside; ara-C) (usually 100–200 mg/m^2 daily for 7–10 days by continuous infusion), with or without 6-thioguanine (6-TG) for induction, and lower doses of one or more of these drugs, given monthly for 1–5 years, for maintenance. These programs are, themselves, probably quite similar, as illustrated by studies formally comparing daunorubicin 45 mg/m^2 daily for 3 days combined with either ara-C 100 mg/m^2 daily for 7 days (3 + 7), ara-C in the same dose for 10 days (3 + 10), or ara-C in the same dose for 7 days plus 6-TG 100 mg/m^2 every 12 hours for 7 days (TAD) (3). Given these similarities, Preisler et al. examined the frequency of long-term remission in all 760 patients with previously untreated AML who entered CR while receiving one of three different CALGB protocols operative between 1974 and 1979, each of which used 3 + 7 or a comparable variant for induction of remission and a 5-day courses of ara-C, 100 mg/m^2 daily, given monthly or bimonthly for remission maintenance (4). At least 6 years have elapsed since the entry of each patient to the study. The many patients and the relatively long follow-up time permitted a detailed analysis of the curative potential of conventional therapy in patients with untreated AML. One-half the patients relapsed within 1.1 years. The last recurrence occurred at the beginning of the ninth year of remission, with no recurrence yet occurring among the 34 patients at risk after that time. Of the patients, 16.4% (about 8% of all initially treated patients, among whom the CR rate was 45%) were projected by a life table analysis to be in remission after 8 years [standard error (SE) 1.6%]. The authors considered three different models to fit their data: one in which the relapse rate was constant; one in which a fraction of patients were considered cured, with the relapse rate constant in the remainder; and one in which the relapse rate declined with time, without assumptions about curability. The final model provided the best fit with a recurrence rate of ≥50% during the first 1 to 1.5 years of CR, declining to 10%/year by years 4 to 5 of CR, and approaching 1%/year by year 7 of CR. Resolution of the issue of curability would require follow-up of more patients in

CR at ≥7 years than was possible, even in this large study, indicating that the question of curability is moot, given the limitations of conventional therapy. Nonetheless, the decline in the recurrence rate with time is of not only practical importance, but may also indicate that different mechanisms may underlie relapse at different times, a point to which we will return.

Are there groups of patients with substantially better outcomes following conventional therapy than those outlined in the foregoing? The leukemia cell karyotype is extremely useful in predicting the curability of AML after administration of conventional therapy (5–7). The most favorable karyotypes are INV[16], del[16q], t(15;17), and t(8;21), with perhaps close to half the patients with INV[16], del[16q], or t(8;21) likely to be cured following conventional therapy. However fewer than 15% of patients with AML have INV[16], del[16q], t(15;17), or t(8;21)(5). Furthermore, although patients can be cured after a first relapse, the likelihood of this is only about half the likelihood of cure following initial diagnosis (8). Once a second, third, or additional relapse occurs, cure is practically impossible with current therapy (8).

A NEED FOR PROLONGED MAINTENANCE THERAPY?

Efforts to improve results have focused on the use of higher doses of ara-C, the use of new agents, and the use of bone marrow transplantation. Another issue that has received attention is the necessity for prolonged monthly maintenance therapy as described earlier. The CALGB investigators administered ara-C (100 mg/m^2 q12h SC for 5 days) plus 6-TG (months 1 and 5), vincristine and prednisone (months 2,4,5, and 8), or daunorubicin (45 mg/m^2 days 1 and 2, months 3 and 7) to 372 patients with AML brought into initial CR with 3 + 7 or comparable variants (668 patients, none with secondary leukemia, e.g., AML arising after chemotherapy for another malignancy, received induction therapy)(3). After the eighth month of this rotating maintenance therapy, 151 of the 224 patients still in CR were randomly assigned either to continue this therapy for a total of 3 years or to discontinue therapy. With all patients followed for at least 1 year after randomization, and most followed for at least 2 years after this time, 48 of the 77 patients assigned to stop maintenance therapy after 8 months relapsed (median CR duration 45 weeks after randomization), compared with 46 of the 74 assigned to continue maintenance therapy (median CR duration 71 weeks after randomization). Life table analysis projected that 35–40% in each group would be in CR at 3 years. Remission durations were similar in the 151 patients who participated in the randomized trial and the 73 who did not. The data suggest that prolongation of typical maintenance therapy beyond 8 months may delay disease recurrence, but will not affect the frequency of long-term remission. If this is correct, it would support the hypothesis, referred to in the foregoing, that different mechanisms may underlie recurrences at different times.

Early relapses might result from the (final) divisions of "nonclonogenic" blasts (i.e., those with limited self-renewal capacities, which constitute the vast majority of blasts) (9). Reduction in the number of these cells would result in a CR. Because conventional maintenance and induction therapies are quite similar, use of maintenance therapy would further retard the growth of nonclonogenic blasts, resulting in some prolongation of remission, unless the nonclonogenic cells became resistant to therapy. On the other hand, long-term remission would require control of clonogenic cells that given the frequency of long-term remission, have only a very limited sensitivity to conventional maintenance and induction therapy. Because late relapses are usually quite sensitive to chemotherapy, these would still reflect a high nonclonogenic/clonogenic blast ratio, with the former perhaps retaining sensitivity to chemotherapy because of relatively recent derivation (late relapse) from the latter. If different mechanisms do underlie relapses at different times, a new drug or strategy could conceivably affect one portion of a remission duration curve, rather than another, pointing out a possible need to separately analyze the different components of these curves.

Other studies have also addressed the need for prolonged maintenance therapy in previously untreated patients. The Swiss Group for Clinical Cancer Research gave 162 patients, under aged 65 in whom platelet support was possible (not thought to be alloimmunized), three to four courses of 3 + 7 (three courses if a major infection had occurred), one to two for induction (CR rate 72%), and the remainder for "consolidation" (10). After the final course of TAD, 74 patients were assigned to receive either maintenance therapy or no therapy (the 43 unassigned patients had either relapsed, received an allogenic transplant, or been considered protocol violations). Maintenance consisted of ara-C, 100 mg/m^2 SC every 12 hours for 5 days combined alternately, every 8 weeks, with 6-TG (weeks 1,15,29, etc.) or vincristine–prednisone (weeks 8,22,36, etc.) for 2 years. All patients received maintenance during the study's first year; thereafter, allocation was random. The median observation time was 44 months. Remission duration (and survival) curves had identical shapes in the group that received consolidation and in the group that received maintenance plus consolidation. Median remission duration was 18 months in both groups with 5/48 patients in the maintenance group in CR at a time beyond the last relapse occurring in the group versus 1/26 similarly in CR in the no maintenance group. The authors concluded that "conventional maintenance group . . . given after early consolidation . . . does not prolong duration of remission. . . ." Champlin et al., at UCLA, reached a similar conclusion after giving 95 consecutive patients TAD, with 46 of the 59 responders than receiving 5-azacytidine, 150 mg/m^2 daily for 5 days by continuous infusion, and doxorubicin (Adriamycin), 45–60 mg/m^2 on days 4 and 5, and 25 of the 46 subsequently received another course of TAD (the 13 who did not receive consolidation received instead an allogenic transplant) (11). Patients received no additional therapy. The median CR duration in the 46 patients given consolidation was 14 months, with 12 patients still in CR for 1–5 years (about two-thirds for at least 4 years), and 26% were projected to be in CR at 5 years. The authors noted that these results were similar to those they had previously observed after administration of the same induction therapy, followed by two courses of consolidation and 2.5 years of monthly maintenance therapy (they specified neither the consolidation nor the maintenance). Investigators at St. Bartholomew's Hospital (St. Barts) in London gave "short-term" therapy, generally consisting, of courses of 3 + 7 variants to patients under aged 60 (12). They planned to give six such courses with as short an intercycle time as possible. The median remission duration (the CR rate was 63%) was 1 year, with 37% of the 118 patients entering CR projected to be in CR at 5 years (median follow-up time, 3.5 years, three-fourths were followed 2 years or more). The interval between courses 1 and 2 (less than 5 weeks versus 5 weeks or more) was generally without influence on remission duration. Furthermore, patients who received only the first three cycles (generally because of debilitation) had remissions equivalent to patients who received all six cycles. These investigators concluded that the results of short-term therapy were in "marked improvement" to previous St. Bart's results. Finally, Italian investigators failed to find differences in disease-free survival among newly diagnosed patients who, after receiving 3 + 7 followed by four courses of TAD, were randomly assigned to discontinue therapy or to receive ara-C, 100 mg/m^2 daily for 5 days for 18 months plus 6-TG or etoposide 100 mg/m^2 daily for 3 days (13).

In contrast with these results, Buechner et al., in Germany, treated 334 patients with "TAD 9" (9 days of ara-C with daunorubicin, given on days, 3,4, and 5) and then randomly allocated 155 of the 204 responding patients to receive one TAD consolidation, followed either by no maintenance or by monthly maintenance courses combining ara-C (100 mg/m^2 q12h for 5 days) with daunorubicin (months 1,5, . . .), 6-TG (months 2,4,6,8 . . .), or cyclophosphamide (months 3,7 . . .) given for 3 years (14). Follow-up time was 1 year or longer in about half the patients. The use of the log-rank test to compare remission duration in the two groups indicated that recurrence was much less likely ($p=0.003$) in patients who received maintenance. The necessity for *some* form of postremission therapy is apparent from an Eastern Cooperative Oncology Group (ECOG) study. Of 191 patients, 126 entered CR following the TAD regimen. The investigators randomly assigned 77 of these 126 to receive either no further therapy, maintenance therapy (6-TG for 4 days, ara-C, 60 mg/m^2 on day 5 SC) weekly for 2 years, or consolidation therapy (see later discussion) (15). Of the 26 patients assigned "no-therapy" none remain in remission, only 1 had a remission duration longer than 1 year (17 months) and the median remission duration was only 4 months. In contrast, 4 of the 25 patients assigned to the maintenance regimen remain in remission from 11 to 27 months, with a median remission duration of 8 months. Both the log-rank and Peto–Peto Wilcoxon tests indicated superiority of the maintenance group's remission duration curve. The second CR rate was similar in both groups.

In summary, studies from CALGB (3), UCLA (11), Switzerland (10), the United Kingdom (12), and Italy (13) suggest that cure of patients with newly diagnosed AML occurs early during treatment, if it occurs at all, and that administration of more than three courses of chemotherapy is of no benefit, provided these courses are sufficient to produce a median CR duration longer than 1 year. In this context, the median CR duration was only 8 months in Buechner's patients who received consolidation without maintenance (versus 13 months in the patients who received both TAD and monthly maintenance) (14), and only 17% of the former were projected to be in CR at 2½ years. It is possible that the studies (10–13) that failed to demonstrate a benefit for prolonged maintenance therapy used "inadequate" maintenance. Details of myelosuppression during maintenance are rarely provided. A study of Dutcher and associates does provide these details (16). These investigators administered ara-C, 100 mg/m^2 every 12 hours, plus 6-TG to 86 patients entering CR after 3 + 7 (CR rate was 63%, none of the patients had had a previous hematological disorder). Treatment with ara-C plus 6-TG continued until marrow aplasia developed, and this scheme was pursued every 10 to 12 weeks for 3 years. One-third of the patients also received a splenectomy, and another third received neuraminidase-treated allogenic blasts; because the results in patients who received these therapies were similar to those in patients who received only "intensive" maintenance therapy, the authors considered all the patients (each of whom was followed for at least 5 years) as a single group, representative of the results of "intensive" maintenance therapy. Patients spent a mean of 14 days per course with fewer than 500 neutrophils/mm^2, infections occurred during 55% of the courses, and eight patients died while in CR. Fifty-five percent of the patients were alive and in CR at 1 year, and 23% were at 5 years. These results seem no better than those reported by the Swiss (10), UCLA (11), and UK (12) investigators who used much shorter durations of therapy. Nonetheless, although evidence would seem to indicate no need for more than three courses of therapy in most patients, there may be groups who would benefit from prolonged maintenance therapy. For example, Kantarjian and co-workers noted that patients with acute promyelocytic leukemia (APL) treated between 1973 and 1975 or 1980 and 1983, had longer remissions than patients treated between 1976 and 1978 or 1984 and 1985 (17); therapy continued for 18 months in each of the two former intervals and for 14 and 8 months in each of the two latter. The type of maintenance therapy also varied by period (discussed later), but, after adjustment for this variation, there was still evidence that the duration of maintenance influenced remission duration in patients with APL.

NEW DRUGS: AMSACRINE, IDARUBICIN, MITOXANTRONE, ETOPOSIDE

The debate over the proper duration of maintenance chemotherapy tends to obscure a more important debate: is any therapy *better* than three or four courses of 3 + 7 or a variant thereof? As mentioned earlier, attempts to improve the results of 3 + 7 have focused on use of new agents, higher doses, and marrow transplantation. Among the many agents tested, amsacrine, mitoxantrone, idarubicin, etoposide, all-*trans*-retinoic acid, and various colony-stimulating factors (CSFs) have either made their way into the treatment of newly diagnosed patients or seem of particular interest. As DNA-reactive drugs, amsacrine, mitoxantrone, and idarubicin have been compared with daunorubicin and with each other. Because these drugs all produce similar acute toxicities, comparisons should probably be made at doses that produce comparable degrees of toxicity. The difficulty in doing this is illustrated by a study of Berman and colleagues comparing conventional doses of ara-C with either idarubicin (12 mg/m^2 daily for 3 days) or daunorubicin (50 mg/m^2 daily for 3 days) in newly diagnosed patients under aged 60 (18). Forty-five evaluable patients were randomly assigned to receive idarubicin, of whom 3 died during induction and 36 entered CR, 27 in one course. Among the 41 patients assigned to the daunorubicin arm, 3 died and only 24 entered CR, 11 after only one course. Remissions were longer in idarubicin-treated patients (12 versus 8 months). However, only 1 daunorubicin-treated patient developed severe mucositis versus 5 idarubicin-treated patients. Thus, it is possible that the lesser antileukemia efficacy of daunorubicin reflected the use of a dose that was not equitoxic to the idarubicin dose.

Similarly, a Southwest Oncology Group (SWOG) study randomly assigned 232 patients with high-risk AML (in relapse or occurring after a prior malignancy) to induction with "high-dose" ara-C, high-dose ara-C plus amsacrine (100 mg/m^2 daily for 3 days), or high-dose ara-C plus mitoxantrone (10 mg/m^2 for 3 days) (19). The amsacrine group suffered a high early death rate, leading to termination of this arm of the study. However, again, the question of dose arises. Given the difficulties with this type of studies, it might be reasonable to assume that one of the daunorubicin, idarubicin, amsacrine, mitoxantrone set is superior to the others only when equitoxic doses are clearly used, or when separate studies, perhaps employing different doses, arrive at the same result and when the differences between drugs are large.

For amsacrine, an M. D. Anderson trial resulted in a 55% CR rate in 110 newly diagnosed patients given AMSA-OAP (amsacrine, 30 mg/m^2 daily for 7 days; conventional-dose ara-C, vincristine, and prednisone) versus a 46% CR rate in prognostically similar "pairmates" given AdOAP [doxorubicin (Adriamycin), 55 mg/m^2 for 1 day, and the same doses of ara-C, vincristine, and prednisone] during a previous study (20). The differences were greater (49%

versus 33%) in patients with a poorer pretreatment prognosis; these were primarily older patients.

A Memorial Sloan–Kettering trial produced a 70% CR rate in 46 newly diagnosed patients given amsacrine (190 mg/m^2 daily for 3 days) combined with conventional-dose ara-C and 6-TG, compared with 54% in patients assigned, by chance, to receive the same doses of cytanabine and 6-TG, but with daunorubicin (50 mg/m^2 daily for 3 days) (21). Again, differences were greater in patients over age 50. Two-thirds of the remissions occurred after one course in amsacrine-treated patients versus one-half in the daunorubicin group, and the log-rank test demonstrated longer remissions in the former. However, remissions were short in both groups (median 9.5 and 7.5 months), and death rates in patients over aged 50 were low in both groups (4/22 amsacrine, 2/13 daunorubicin) in comparison with those reported (30–40%) by others in larger trials (22). These facts raise questions about the adequacy of the sample size and, indeed, a large Southeastern Cancer Study Group (SEG) trial, using almost identical doses, resulted in 50 CRs in 121 patients over aged 50 given amsacrine plus ara-C (41%), compared with 71 in 146 patients (49%) given daunorubicin plus ara-C without differences in remission duration (23).

For idarubicin, in contrast, a "randomized" SEG trial in newly diagnosed patients over aged 50 produced a 72% CR rate in the idarubicin plus ara-C group, and a 59% rate in the daunorubicin plus ara-C group (doses similar to those of Berman et al., discussed previously), with an equal number of deaths in the two groups, perhaps indicating use of equitoxic doses (24). Remissions lasted longer, but not strikingly so, in the idarubicin group.

For mitoxantrone, Arlin and co-workers randomly assigned newly diagnosed patients without secondary leukemia or a prior hematological disorder to receive conventional-dose ara-C plus either mitoxantrone, 12 mg/m^2 daily for 3 days (98 patients), or daunorubicin, 45 mg/m^2 daily for 3 days (102 patients), followed in each group by two courses of lower-dose consolidation (Arlin Z, personal communication). As an illustration of potential difficulties even in "randomized" studies of this size, 26% and 6% of the mitoxantrone group had ECOG performance status scores of 0 and 4, respectively, compared with 17% and 11% in the daunorubicin group. The CR rates in patients under aged 60 were 80% mitoxantrone versus 69% daunorubicin and were 46% mitoxantrone versus 37% daunorubicin in older patients, with 89% of mitoxantrone-produced remissions occurring after one course, compared with 68% for daunorubicin, and with mitoxantrone-induced remissions lasting a median of 240 days versus 198 for daunorobucin. Twenty to twenty-five percent of the older patients died during induction in each group, suggesting that mitoxantrone may have more antileukemia activity at equitoxic doses. However, neither in this study nor in the idarubicin or amsacrine trials have differences been large, and none of the trials with presumably reasonable power to detect conventionally significant differences in remission duration have done so. As with cephalosporin antibiotics, there may be no single best DNA-reactive drug in AML.

Because etoposide produced remissions in 15–25% of patients with AML in relapse, Australian investigators randomly assigned 264 newly diagnosed patients to receive either etoposide (75 mg/m^2 daily for 7 days) plus 3 + 7 or 3 + 7 alone (25). Once in CR, patients received two further courses with 5 days of etoposide and ara-C. All patients then received a typical ara-C rotating maintenance scheme, as in CALGB studies. There was little difference in remission rates between the two groups, but patients under aged 55 who received etoposide had longer remissions, which were not due to the relative preponderance of low pretreatment blast counts in the etoposide group, and lived longer. The etoposide-treated patients had more diarrhea and spent more time during consolidation with low neutrophil and platelet counts. Thus, it is possible that an increase in the dose of ara-C might have produced results comparable with those observed after addition of etoposide. Indeed only about 40% of the responding patients under aged 55 treated with etoposide were projected to remain in CR at 4 years (median follow-up time was 40 months for all patients) and only 22% (±6% SE) of the younger etoposide-treated patients were projected to be alive at 4 years (which was no different from the 17±4% in 3 + 7 group). As we shall see later, comparable or better results have followed use of daunorubicin and ara-C by themselves.

HIGH-DOSE CYTARABINE AS THERAPY IN REMISSION

In addition to exploring new antileukemia agents, such as amsacrine, mitoxantrone, idarubicin, and etoposide, investigators have also focused on the use of higher doses of an older agent, ara-C. Ten years ago Rudnick et al. found that ara-C doses of 3 g/m^2 given over 2 hours and repeated at 12-hour intervals produced remissions in patients whose disease was unresponsive to conventional doses of 100–200 mg/m^2 daily for 5–7 days (26). Plunkett and associates found a basis for this phenomenon (27). Conventional ara-C doses produced plasma ara-C concentrations that were insufficient to form maximal amounts of intracellular araCTP, the active metabolite of ara-C. Rather, formation of maximal cellular araCTP concentrations required plasma ara-C concentrations obtained with ara-C infusions of at least 0.5–1.0 g/m^2 over 2 hours, although administration of doses above 0.5–1.0 g/m^2 did not yield further increases in araCTP concentrations, presumably because these higher doses resulted in ara-C concentrations that exceeded the ability of deoxycytidine kinase to phosphorylate ara-C.

Has the use of high-dose ara-C (3 g/m^2 at 12 hour intervals for 3–12 doses) improved the outcome of therapy beyond producing what are almost invariably brief remissions in patients failing to respond to lower doses, the original finding of Rudnick et al. (26)? To answer this question, Wolff and associates administered high-dose ara-C (3 g/m^2 over 1 hour every 12 hours for 12 doses) plus daunorubicin (30 mg/m^2 on the subsequent 3 days) to 87 patients in first CR (28). Induction therapy had consisted of 3 + 7, or a variant thereof, and the median interval from remission to beginning daunorubicin plus high-dose ara-C was 1 month (over 3 months in 5 of the 87), during which time 20 patients received another cycle of 3 + 7 or a variant thereof. Up to three courses of daunorubicin plus high-dose ara-C were planned, but only 1 patient could receive three courses, whereas 25 patients received two courses, and 61 one course. With a median follow-up time of 3-½ years, 35 of the 87 patients have had recurrence of disease and 6 have died. The probability of remaining in remission at 8 years is 50% [95% confidence intervals (CI), 37–60%]. Age gave the best prediction of duration of remission, with over 80% of patients under aged 25, 50% of those aged 26–45, and 20% of those over aged 45 predicted to remain in CR at 8 years. Most patients who could receive more than one course were younger. However, the number of courses received affected results only in older patients (those who received two courses had longer remissions), and if patients dying during treatment are excluded from analysis (these deaths occurred only during the first course), the number of courses received (one versus two) did not influence remission duration. Perhaps the better outcome in younger patients, at least partially, reflected the historic tendency for older patients to have prognostically unfavorable karyotypes (karyotypes were not determined in this study). At any rate, as the authors point out, the overall results are similar to those following allogeneic marrow transplantation during first CR.

ECOG studies have also examined the use of one course of high-dose ara-C, given at 3 g/m^2 every 12 hours for 12 doses. Unlike Wolff et al., the ECOG investigators combined the high-dose ara-C with amsacrine (100 mg/m^2 for 3 days), rather than daunorubicin. In an initial ECOG study, Cassileth et al. treated 35 patients induced into CR with TAD (29). A median of 29 days elapsed from remission to high-dose ara-C–amsacrine, and no therapy was given during this time. Patients received no further therapy after completing the high-dose ara-C–amsacrine regimen. Six of the 35 patients died during the high-dose ara-C–amsacrine trial, disease eventually recurred in 19, and 11 remain in remission for 17–44 months (median 26); the probability of being alive in CR is about 30% (95% CI, ±16%) at 36 months. Given this experience, the ECOG randomly assigned patients induced into CR with TAD (CR rate, 67%) to receive either one course of high-dose ara-C–amsacrine, as before, or 2 years of maintenance (4 days of TG weekly and ara-C 60 mg/m^2, given SC once weekly) (30). Patients aged 40 or younger, with a histocompatible sibling, were assigned to receive allogenic transplantations. With a 1.5-year median follow-up, the probability of being alive and in CR at 2 years was 32% (±11%, 2SE) in 82 patients given high-dose ara-C–amsacrine and 21% (± 10%) in 85 patients given maintenance (only patients under aged 60 were eligible for study, and high-dose ara-C–amsacrine was associated with a 16% death rate, primarily in older patients). In patients aged 40 or younger, probabilities were 14±16% in 22 patients given maintenance, 38±18% in patients given high-dose ara-C–amsacrine, and 50±15% in patients receiving an allogenic transplant (i.e., there was no difference by conventional statistical criteria in the outcome between transplant and high-dose ara-C, although both these approaches were, by these criteria, superior to maintenance, even though the maintenance employed would probably be considered inadequate by many investigators). Certainly, the results of Cassileth and associates (29, 30) appear inferior to those of Wolff et al. (28) and, although some of this inferiority reflects a higher death rate (16 versus 7%), some also reflects a higher relapse rate. Although Cassileth and co-workers' use of amsacrine, rather than daunorubicin, might be an explanation for the differences between their results and those of Wolff and associates, perhaps a more likely explanation is the differences in the criteria used to select patients for the two studies. It is interesting that both the Wolff study and studies of allogenic transplantation during first CR produce similarly "good" results, and that both raise similar questions of potential bias in patient selection.

Champlin et al. have also studied high-dose ara-C in patients brought into first CR with 3 + 7 or variants, but, unlike Wolff and associates and the ECOG investigators, they administered 8 rather than 12 doses (31). Upon entering CR, 49 patients received this high-dose ara-C regimen, together with daunorubicin, 45 mg/m^2 on the 3 subsequent days. Subsequently, patients received an additional course of 3 + 7. Twenty-seven patients remain alive and in CR, the majority for less than 2 years. The probabilities of being alive and in CR at 2 and 4 years are 50% and 30%, respectively. Comparable figures were 30% and 20% in previous patients, who, although receiving the identical induction regimen and also receiving two courses immediately upon entering CR (as described in the earlier reference to Champlin et al.; 11) did not receive high-dose ara-C. The remission duration curve was also superior (p. <0.01) in the group receiving high-dose ara-C. However, actual remission time ranged from zero to 4 years in the high-dose ara-C study compared with 4–8 years in the older study, leaving open the possibility that further observation might lessen the differences between the two studies.

In contrast with the foregoing, investigators for the CALGB set out to give four *courses* of high-dose ara-C once patients were in CR. After completion of the high-dose ara-C regimen, patients would receive four courses of conventional-dose ara-C plus daunorubicin (32). They conducted a Phase I trial in which successive groups of patients received either a 5-day continuous infusion at increasing doses (beginning at 250 mg/m^2) or 3 g/m^2 every 12 hours, with the number of doses increasing (beginning with three doses). They found that the optimal doses for future studies (i.e., the maximum doses that could be given repetitively for four courses) were 400 mg/m^2 by continuous infusion and 3 g/m^2 every 12 hours on days 1,3, and 5. The probability of remaining in remission was greater in patients who received five or more doses of ara-C, 3 g/m^2. However, as the authors point out, this was not a formally comparative study. Median follow-up time was less than 2 years. The CALGB is now conducting a Phase III study in which patients brought into CR with 3 + 7 are assigned at random to receive four courses of either (1) conventional-dose ara-C; or (2) ara-C, 400 mg/m^2 daily for 5 days by continuous infusion; or (3) ara-C, 3 g/m^2 every 12 hours on days 1,3, and 5, followed in each case by four courses of conventional dose ara-C and daunorubicin.

In contrast with the results of Wolff et al. (28), Champlin et al. (31), and Mayer et al. (32), but not Cassileth et al. (29, 30), Preisler and associates failed to find an advantage in adding high-dose ara-C to postremission therapy (33). They assigned 123 patients immediately upon entering CR to receive either two courses of amsacrine (90 mg/m^2 for 3 days) plus conventional dose ara-C, or two courses of ara-C, 3 g/m^2 every 12 hours for eight doses; in each group each course followed a course of 3 + 7 (patients were not randomly assigned to receive or not to receive high-dose ara-C, but were reportedly prognostically similar in the two groups). Remission duration curves were similarly shaped in the group that did and the group that did not receive high-dose ara-C, and there were no differences between the curves using conventional statistical criteria of significance. Follow-up time was also longer in the patients receiving conventional-dose ara-C. About 45% of all patients were projected to be in remission at 5 years, with 60% of those under aged 45 projected to be in remission at that time. These results (28–33) suggest that if postremission therapy is identical with induction therapy, there may be no advantage to the addition of high-dose ara-C. This point is illustrated in Table 1, in which studies are categorized according to the ara-C dose used for postremission therapy and the "intensity" of postremission therapy vis-à-vis induction therapy. "Conventional-dose" ara-C refers to doses in the range of 100–200 mg/m^2 for 5–7 days. If postremission therapy included therapy identical with that used for induction, the intensity of postremission therapy was considered equal to that of induction therapy; if high-dose ara-C was used the intensity was considered greater, otherwise it was considered less. The projected percentage of patients in CR was determined from remission duration curves provided in the literature cited; the percentage in CR at the longest follow-up was used, realizing that there may be wide confidence intervals about those particular percentages. Table 1 demonstrates that best results seem to have been in studies during which the intensity of postremission therapy was at least equal to that of induction therapy. Aside from the study of Wolff and colleagues, there is no evidence that therapy of greater intensity is advantageous. The debate over the need to include high-dose ara-C in postremission therapy is reminiscent of the debate over the need for prolonged maintenance therapy: in both cases, there may be no such need if postremission therapy includes at least some therapy identical with that used for induction. However, just as there may be a few patients who benefit from prolonged maintenance therapy (see page 6), there may be a few patients who benefit from use of high-dose ara-C.

SPECIFIC THERAPIES FOR SPECIFIC PATIENTS?

A hint of this latter possibility comes from an M. D. Anderson trial in which high-dose ara-C was given by continuous infusion as both induction and postremission therapy to 51/52 newly diagnosed patients under aged 50 (34). The rationale for a continuous infusion was Plunkett and co-workers' observation that, with the intermittent administration of high-dose ara-C (3 g/m^2 every 12 hours), cellular araCTP concentrations often fell below those needed to inhibit DNA synthesis in leukemia cells (35). Because there was a correlation (in patients whose disease failed to respond to conventional-dose ara-C) between duration of inhibition of DNA synthesis and response, it seemed desirable to avoid times when araCTP concentrations would be insufficient to inhibit leukemia cell DNA synthesis. For this purpose Plunkett and associates proposed a continuous ara-C infusion at a dose of 1.5–2.0 g/m^2 daily; administration of higher doses did not produce higher araCTP concentrations because of presumed saturation of deoxycytidine kinase (discussed earlier). A 4-day continuous infusion at a daily dose of 1.5 g/m^2 was tolerable and effective in patients whose disease had recurred, and this was the schedule used both for induction and for three "intensifications" in newly diagnosed patients. An intercalator was used only between the two intensifications: daunorubicin at 60 mg/m^2 once monthly for 3 months. One hundred twenty-five weeks have elapsed since entry of the 51st patient. In previous patients under aged 50 with newly diagnosed AML at M. D. Anderson the relapse rate declined sharply 125 weeks after initial treatment. Thus, the 16% 8/51 of patients in first CR ≥125 weeks after beginning treatment may represent a reasonable estimate of the long-term CR rate with continuous-infusion, high-dose ara-C. By comparison, 15% of 221 consecutive patients under aged 50 with newly diagnosed AML were in first CR 125 weeks after entry onto previous studies that used conventional doses of ara-C plus either doxorubicin or amsacrine. The distribution of karyotypes was similar in the patients treated with continuous-infusion high-dose ara-C and the patients treated with conventional doses combined with a DNA-reactive drug. Three of four continuous-infusion high-dose ara-C-treated patients with INV[16] or del [16q] are in first CR ≥125 weeks after initial treatment compared with 3/15 historical patients ($p=0.04$). However, 0/4 continuous-infusion high-dose ara-C-treated patients with t(15;17) are in CR at ≥125 weeks compared with 5/18 historical patients. No patients with abnormalities of chromosomes 5 or 7 (-5,5q–,-7, or

Table 1 Studies of Conventional and High-Dose ara-C in Newly Diagnosed Patients in First Remission

Study	ara-C dose	Patients	Follow-up	Projected % in CR at 2 yr	2.1–4.9 yr	5 yr	>5 yr	"Intensity" of postremission to induction
Preisler et al. (4)	Conventional	760[b]	≥6 yr (all)	35		20	16 (at 8 yr)	Less
Sauter et al. (10)	Conventional	74[c]	4.5 yr (med)	30–40	25 (at 3 y)	Unavailable		Equal (consol.)
Champlin et al. (11)	Conventional	46[b]	4 yr (med)	35		25	Unavailable	Less
Rohatiner et al. (12)	Conventional	118[d]	3.5 yr (med)	40		37	37 (at 7.5 yr)	Equal
Buechner et al. (14)	Conventional	71[b]	1 yr (med)	35	30 (at 3y)	Unavailable		Less
Dutcher et al. (16)	Conventional ("intensive maintenance")	86[e]	≥5 yr (all)	50		25	20 (at 10 yr)	Less
Preisler et al. (33)	Conventional	44[f]	3 yr (med)	50[k]	40 (at 4.5y[k])	Unavailable		Equal
Wolff et al. (28)	3 × 12[a] (1-3 courses)	87[g]	3.5 yr (med)	50		50	50 (at 8 yr)	Greater
Cassileth et al. (29)	3 × 12 (1 course)	35[h]	2 yr (med)	30	30 (at 3.5 yr)	Unavailable		Greater

Cassileth et al. (30)	3 × 12 (1 course)	28[i]	1.5 yr (med)	32	Unavailable		Greater
Champlin et al. (31)	3 × 8 (1 course)	49[b]	1.5 yr (med)	55	35–40 (at 3.5 yr)	Unavailable	Greater
Mayer et al. (32)	3 × 5–8 (4 courses)	62[j]	1.5 yr (med)	50	Unavailable		Greater
Preisler et al. (33)	3 × 8 (2 courses)	60[f]	2 yr (med)	50[k]	50 (at 3.5 y[k])	Unavailable	Greater

[a] g/m^2 per dose × number of doses.
[b] All patients eligible.
[c] Age <65 eligible.
[d] Age <60 eligible.
[e] Ineligible if antecedent hematological disorder.
[f] Age <70 eligible.
[g] Some referred in CR.
[h] Age <70; ineligible if antecedent hematological disorder, X-ray therapy, or chemotherapy for prior malignancy.
[i] Age <60, de novo AML.
[j] De novo AML.
[k] Results statistically similar.

7q–) are in CR at 125 weeks. Hence high-dose ara-C given by continuous infusion may produce overall long-term results similar to conventional anthracycline (or amsacrine) plus ara-C programs, but may be superior in patients with INV[16] or del[16q], worse in patients with t(15,17), and equally bad in patients with chromosome 5 or 7 abnormalities. In support of the value of high-dose, continuous-infusion ara-C in patients with INV[16] or del[16q] is the failure to detect parenchymal leukemic infiltrates (e.g., in the brain) after this treatment, whereas such cases were not uncommon when patients with 16q abnormalities received conventional-dose ara-C (36).

The concept that specific therapeutic strategies may be beneficial exclusively in certain subsets of patients is buttressed by observations in patients with promyelocytic leukemia. As noted earlier, Kantarjian and colleagues suggested that these patients, perhaps unlike the majority of patients, might benefit from prolonged maintenance therapy (17). These authors also noted that patients with promyelocytic leukemia who received methotrexate and 6-MP during remission had significantly higher 3-year remission rates than patients who did not (56% versus 30%, $p<0.01$), a finding that could not be accounted for by thc greater duration of postremission therapy in patients who received these drugs or by differences in their induction regimens. Ganem and co-workers have also noted longer remissions in patients with APL receiving 6-MP and mitoguazone (methyl-GAG) once in daunorubicin-induced CR (37). An agent that may be very useful in APL is all-*trans*-retinoic acid (ATRA). Castaigne and associates have found that ATRA, 45 mg/m^2 orally for 90 days, produced remissions in 14/22 patients with APL of whom only 1 had de novo APL. The CR rate was 10/11 in patients in first relapse (38). Strikingly, therapy was so well-tolerated that it was given largely on an outpatient basis: specifically there was no disseminated intravascular coagulopathy. This report confirms earlier Chinese studies. Interestingly, the Chinese report that ATRA is less successful in other subtypes of AML. If the phenomenon of specific therapies having effect in only specific subtypes is widespread, a problem will arise. Studies sufficiently large to include an adequate number of patients with different subtypes, some of which are relatively uncommon (e.g., only about 10% of newly diagnosed patients have either 16q abnormalities or APL), will require a long time to complete and, thereby, interfere with the conduct of other studies.

COLONY-STIMULATING FACTORS IN THE THERAPY OF ACUTE MYELOGENOUS LEUKEMIA

From the foregoing, there is an apparent need to improve the chemotherapy of AML. Hematopoietic growth factors (also known as colony-stimulating factors, or CSFs) have the potential to affect this improvement. Colony-stimulating factors could be used in three different ways in the treatment of AML. These correspond to their roles (1) as proliferative stimuli for normal multipotent "stem" cells, CFU-GEMM (*c*olony *f*orming *u*nit—*g*ranulocyte, *e*rythroid, *m*acrophage, *m*egakaryocyte), CFU-GM, and CFU-G and functional activators of the mature progeny of these cells; (2) as proliferative stimuli for leukemia stem cells (AML-CFU); and (3) as stimuli of differentiation of AML-CFU (39). Because they do not seem to favorably affect the balance between proliferation and differentiation, use of CSFs expressly for the last purpose is not currently considered particularly promising (40). As proliferative stimuli for normal stem cells, CSFs (e.g., GM-CSF or G-CSF) would be given after chemotherapy, in the expectation that chemotherapy had altered the balance between AML-CFU and normal stem cells, such that use of CSFs would result in the more rapid appearance of normal neutrophils. Accelerated recovery of neutrophils, particularly those with CSF-enhanced capabilities of chemotaxis, phagocytosis, superoxide production, and antibody-dependent cellular cytotoxicity (ADCC), might be useful in reducing the frequency of major or fatal infections, which are prone to occur in settings of profound neutropenia. This approach might be particularly useful in elderly or bedridden patients, who are prone to die of infection during remission induction.

At first glance, the therapeutic use of CSFs (e.g., IL-3, GM-CSF, or G-CSF) to stimulate proliferation of AML-CFUs appears paradoxical. However, it has been shown that in vitro exposure to GM-CSF of myeloblasts from patients with AML increases killing of these cells by ara-C (41). This occurs coincident with an increase in proliferation, although other mechanisms for enhanced cytotoxicity might also be operative. Use of CSFs before or simultaneous with administration of chemotherapeutic agents that predominantly kill proliferating cells (almost all drugs effective in AML are in this category) might thus overcome the resistance to chemotherapy that is usually responsible for therapeutic failure in AML. Overcoming resistance more quickly might also permit earlier appearance of normal neutrophils if, as widely believed, AML myeloblasts produce inhibitors of normal myelopoiesis. It is possible that use of CSFs to stimulate proliferation of AML-CFUs before or simultaneous with chemotherapy might make the chemotherapy less, rather than more effective. Furthermore, because the dose-response curves of AML-CFU and normal stem cells to CSFs appear similar (42), use of CSFs in this fashion might increase the sensitivity of normal stem cells to chemotherapy, producing long periods of myelosuppression with the attendant risk of infection. However, it has been reported that exposure of normal bone marrow mononuclear cells, on the one hand, and myeloblasts from patients with AML,on the other, to GM-CSF in conjunction with ara-C increased araCTP/dCTP ratios in the malignant more than in the normal cells (43). The expected result would be that a higher percentage of the cells killed by ara-C would be malignant, rather than normal. Table 2 outlines the main approaches to the use of CSFs plus chemotherapy in AML as discussed in the foregoing.

Table 2 Approaches to Use of CSFs Plus Chemotherapy in AML

Primary role of CSF	Timing of CSF administration	Target patient population	Benefits	Risks
Stimulate proliferation of normal CFU-GM, CFU-G; functional activation of mature progeny of these cells	After completion of chemotherapy	Elderly, poor performance	Reduction in rate of fatal infection	Regrowth leukemia after chemotherapy
Stimulate proliferation of AML-CFU; other cytotoxic effects	Before or simultaneous with chemotherapy	As above plus patients with karyotypes associated with high relapse rate	As above plus overcome resistance to chemotherapy	Increased leukemic resistance; increased sensitivity normal progenitors to chemotherapy

Johns Hopkins trials using "timed-sequential chemotherapy" are relevant to consideration of the use of CSFs to stimulate blast cell proliferation before chemotherapy (44, 45). These trials have employed a 2-day continuous ara-C infusion (total dose 2–6 g/m^2) together with daunorubicin, 45 mg/m^2 given on each of these 2 days as well as the subsequent day; the resultant death of myeloblasts triggers release of humoral-stimulating factors that induce dormant cells to enter the cell cycle. Maximal concentrations of humoral-stimulating factors occur 8–10 days after initiation of initial chemotherapy and, at this time, a second infusion of chemotherapy is given. Although the exact nature of these humoral-stimulating factors has not been elucidated, they might include interleukin-3 (IL-3), GM-CSF, and others. In trials of timed-sequential chemotherapy between 1975 and 1978, 59 patients received ara-C, 2 g/m^2 over 48 hours (days 1–2), and daunorubicin, 45 mg/m^2 on days 1, 2, and 3, with an identical ara-C infusion given beginning on day 8 or day 10. Patients were not excluded on the basis of presence of a secondary leukemia, age, or such. The 34 patients entering CR received no further therapy. Four remain in first remission at 5–9 years (44). These results might be contrasted with those of Cassileth and co-workers for the ECOG (described earlier) in which none of 26 patients who entered CR after TAD and who then received no further therapy had a remission lasting more than 17 months (15). Median remission durations in the two studies were not dissimilar (4 months ECOG, 8 months Hopkins). These results suggest that, although mechanisms of resistance other than the presence of dormant cells underlie relapse in *most* cases, there may be patients who benefit from recruitment of such dormant cells.

In subsequent trials, the Hopkins investigators have attempted to give a second cycle of timed-sequential therapy beginning 9–10 weeks after the first (45). A study conducted between 1980 and 1982 enrolled 75 patients, of whom 27 (all in CR) were judged able to tolerate a second course. As might be expected, these were primarily younger patients (median age 36). The probability of being alive and in CR at 8.5 years in patients under aged 55 who received a second cycle is about 45%, with follow-up time ≥6 years on all patients still in remission. More recently, the Hopkins investigators have modified the details of timed-sequential therapy to enable more patients to receive a course in remission. Although these modifications have succeeded, the overall results have remained the same. Thus, it appears that long-term results with two cycles of timed-sequential chemotherapy are similar to those of Wolff et al. and to those following allogenic transplantation during first CR, with all results obtaining in patients probably selected on similar grounds of age, performance status, and such. If an analogy can be drawn between timed-sequential chemotherapy and pretreatment with CSFs, the expectation might be that the overall long-term results of CSF pretreatment will be no better than those obtainable with currently available therapy. It is possible that results will be better in certain subgroups (if this can be determined with statistical validity) who might be particularly sensitive to a particular CSF. Of course, different subgroups might be sensitive to different CSFs or combinations of CSFs. That this is possible is suggested by the great variation in the ability of different CSFs to stimulate proliferation of leukemia cells explanted from different patients (40, 46). This result could reflect the suspected derivation of AML-CFU from CFU-GM in some patients, from CFU-GEMM in others, and from multipotent stem cells in still others (47). A possible direction of future research might involve administration of different CSFs to different patients, based on in vitro patterns of proliferation in response to CSFs. This might be more fruitful than a uniform approach (e.g., GM-CSF or timed-sequential chemotherapy).

The two earliest trials of CSFs in AML employed GM-CSF. One was conducted at the University of Texas M. D. Anderson Cancer Center (48) and the other at the University of Munster in Germany (49). In both, GM-CSF administration followed completion of chemotherapy (i.e., GM-CSF was used in role (1), described on page 17). Estey et al. at M. D. Anderson treated 12 newly diagnosed patients at high risk of early death during induction, as judged by a multivariate model. Chemotherapy consisted of ara-C, 6.0 g/m^2 over 96 hours by continuous IV infusion. Thereafter, GM-CSF (the recombinant, *Escherichia coli*-derived, nonglycosylated product, supplied by the Schering–Plough Corp.) 120 $\mu g/m^2$ daily by continuous IV infusion began 2 days after completion of ara-C and continued until the neutrophil count was $\geq 1000/\mu L$. Rates of fatal infection (42%), pneumonia or sepsis (83%), and CR (50%) did not differ significantly ($p < 0.05$) from those observed following administration of the identical chemotherapy without GM-CSF to 53 historical controls with newly diagnosed AML at similarly high risk of early death. There were no significant differences between the GM-CSF-treated and the historical groups in the time required to reach neutrophil counts of 500 or $1000/\mu L$ after administration of chemotherapy. Four patients died of infection before they could have benefited from the earliest recovery of neutrophil count observed in patients who entered CR. Growth of leukemia following GM-CSF administration was observed in only one of the eight patients who survived long enough for response to induction therapy to be fully evaluated; this patient was the only one treated for promyelocytic leukemia. In the German study Buechner et al. treated 23 patients with GM-CSF 250 $\mu g/m^2$ daily by continuous IV infusion beginning 4 days after completion of chemotherapy (TAD-9 in 15 newly diagnosed patients over aged 65 and 1 patient in late relapse, and high-dose ara-C plus mitoxantrone, so-called S-HAM, in patients in earlier relapse) provided the marrow was aplastic. Neutrophil recovery occurred a median of 5 days earlier in patients who received TAD-9 followed by GM-CSF than in patients who previously received TAD-9 without GM-CSF ($p=0.006$) and occurred a median of 9 days earlier in patients who received GM-CSF after S-HAM than in previous patients treated with

S-HAM alone (p=0.005). Comparisons of infection rates or CR rates between patients who did or did not receive GM-CSF were not provided. Regrowth of leukemia occurred in three patients, disappearing in one after discontinuation of GM-CSF. Hence, both the M. D. Anderson and German trials suggest that regrowth of leukemia following administration of GM-CSF upon completion of chemotherapy probably occurs no more frequently than expected if GM-CSF were not administered (except perhaps in patients with promyelocytic leukemia). It remains possible that a deleterious effect resulting from administration of GM-CSF after completion of chemotherapy will be detected only as briefer durations of remission; no shortening of remission duration was reported in the German study, however. Both the M. D. Anderson and German studies apparently failed to detect any improvement in infection or remission rates, although as mentioned, the German study (which was twice the size of the M. D. Anderson trial) did detect a shortening of the period of neutropenia. The infrequent regrowth of leukemia seen in both studies suggests that it might be safe to undertake larger randomized studies to definitively define the role of GM-CSF when administered after completion of chemotherapy.

Less is known about administration of GM-CSF before chemotherapy (i.e., the use of GM-CSF in role (2), described on page 17). Muhm et al. in Austria gave 12 patients GM-CSF 250 $\mu g/m^2$ (*E. coli* product) for 1–2 days before chemotherapy (50). Ten CRs resulted, and neutrophil recovery was accelerated by a mean of 4 days in responding patients. Cell cycle analysis done in 4 patients demonstrated an increase in the percentage of cells in S phase in all 4, indicating the feasibility of using CSF pretreatment to stimulate proliferation in vivo. Although the magnitude of the increases were not impressive, it is possible that impressive increases occurred in clonogenic cells, but could not be detected because measurements were done in bulk (i.e., in both clonogenic and nonclonogenic cells). In another trial, a group at the Dana–Farber Institute in Boston is giving patients in relapse GM-CSF before high-dose ara-C, and a similar trial is planned at Johns Hopkins. Finally, a group at Memorial Hospital in New York City is administering a G-CSF before conventional-dose ara-C in patients in relapse or newly diagnosed patients with AML thought to be secondary to a prior malignancy. Results from these studies are all quite preliminary.

HISTOCOMPATIBILITY ANTIGEN-IDENTICAL ALLOGENEIC MARROW TRANSPLANTATION

The role of allogeneic bone marrow transplantation in AML remains a source of discussion. Investigators at the Fred Hutchinson Center in Seattle have summarized their experience in 363 patients who received transplants between 1973 and 1986 (51). Two hundred and thirty-one of the patients received a transplant in first remission, 54 in untreated first relapse, 29 in "resistant first relapse" (i.e., after failing reinduction therapy), and 49 in second remission. The median age of patients in each of the four groups was about 25 years (range 1–53). All patients received cyclophosphamide (CY) 60 mg/kg IV on 2 consecutive days, followed by total body irradiation (TBI). Donors and recipients were histocompatibility locus antigen (HLA)-identical siblings. A variety of immunosuppressive therapies were used to prevent graft-versus-host disease (GvHD). The probability of *disease recurrence* within 10 years of transplantation was about 25% (95% CI, 18–32%) in patients in first remission, and 36% (16–45%), 56% (30–81%), and 37% (17–57%) for patients in untreated first relapse, resistant first relapse, and second remission, respectively. Thus, statistically, the risk of relapse relative to the risk for patients receiving transplants during first remission was higher only for patients treated in resistant first relapse. The increased risk of relapse in this group was present only for the first 100 days after transplantation. The probabilities of 10-year *survival* were about 48% (95% CI, 42–55%) in patients in first remission, and 28% (12–43%), 24% (9–40%), and 31% (18–45%) in patients in untreated first relapse, resistant first relapse, and second remission, respectively. Thus, results were statistically better only in patients receiving transplants during first remission. Specifically, they were no better in patients who received transplants during second remission than in those during first relapse.

The Seattle survival data are remarkably similar to data from the International Bone Marrow Transplant Registry (IBMTR) (52). The IMBTR found that following the use of various preparative regimens the probability of 4-year survival was 45% (95% CI, 38–52%) for 447 patients receiving transplants during first remission versus 27% (14–40%) for 114 patients receiving them during second remission, and 21% (13–29%) for 178 patients with more advanced disease who received BMT. Thus, again, there appeared to be little improvement when transplantation was done during second remission, compared with when it was done during relapse. The probability of relapse within 4 years of transplantation was about 25% for patients in first CR, a result again similar to the Seattle result. The shapes of survival and disease recurrence curves from Seattle and from the IBMTR were quite similar and showed that the vast majority of deaths or relapses occurred within 2 years of transplantation.

Accordingly, results from studies in which close to 700 patients received transplants during first remission indicate that allogeneic marrow transplantation almost certainly reduces the risk of relapse. It is possible that the superiority of transplantation here reflects a "lead-time bias." That is, if transplantation is performed only several months after remission is achieved, patients who would have relapsed during these months will be excluded from analysis. Neither the Seattle nor the IBMTR reports present detailed information on timing of transplantation during first remission. Nonetheless, it seems unlikely that the differences in relapse probabilities [25% transplant versus 50% for the most favorable chemotherapy series, e.g., Wolff et al.(29) or Preisler et al. (33)] entirely reflect this type of bias.

The situation becomes murkier when survival becomes the endpoint. Here, results following allogeneic transplantation during first remission or following the most favorable chemotherapy series are quite similar (e.g., 50% long-term survival). It should be pointed out, however, that these types of outcomes are more frequently reported following transplantation than chemotherapy and that chemotherapy series also may not be entirely free of bias.

The uncertainty about the relative advantages of allogeneic transplantation during first remission has spawned three major single-hospital studies. At UCLA, Champlin and co-workers assigned 67 consecutive patients in CR after receiving TAD to allogeneic transplantation if they were under age 45 and had an HLA-identical sibling as a donor and to chemotherapy if they did not meet these two criteria (53). Cyclophosphamide (CY) plus total body irradiation (TBI) was the preparative transplant regimen. Chemotherapy consisted of one course of 5-azacytidine plus doxorubicin and one additional course of TAD. Only 1 patient assigned to transplantation failed to receive a transplant, and this patient was analyzed with the transplantation group. The probability of remaining in remission at 5 years was 30% in the chemotherapy group compared with 60% in the transplant group; several statistical tests, some weighing early and late events equally, and some late events more heavily, favored the transplant group. However, the same tests did not favor either group when survival became the endpoint, although the probability of 5-year survival was higher in the transplant group (27 versus 40%), and surviving patients in this group had been followed somewhat longer than patients in the chemotherapy group. This study is open to criticism because the authors failed to specify the total number of patients treated with TAD at diagnosis. This failure raises the possibility that, although the time from remission to either transplantation or continued chemotherapy was similar (medians of 50 and 32 days, respectively), patients were referred to UCLA once in CR expressly to receive a transplant, with all the bias thereby implied.

An M. D. Anderson study is not open to this specific criticism (54). The 109 patients participating in this study were brought into CR at M. D. Anderson, were under aged 40, and had a low probability, as identified by a multivariate model, of continued CR. Sixty-nine patients without an HLA-identical sibling donor received continued chemotherapy; 40 patients had a donor, of whom 23 actually received a transplant. Median follow-up time was about 3 years in the 40 patients assigned to transplant and the 69 patients who received chemotherapy. Comparison of results in the two groups indicated a lower relapse rate (log rank $p < 0.01$) in the transplant group, regardless of diagnosis (AML or ALL), but longer survival (by conventional statistical criteria) after transplantation only in patients with ALL. This study is open to criticism because of changing eligibility criteria and the use of an unorthodox transplant preparative regimen (piperazinedione plus TBI).

In Seattle, between 1977 and 1982, Appelbaum and associates assigned 90 patients under age 50 induced into CR with TAD (the CR rate was 81%) to receive an allogenic transplant if an HLA-identical donor was available (44 patients) or to receive continued chemotherapy containing two courses of TAD identical with the induction regimen (46 patients) (55). Eleven of the 44 patients assigned to transplant did not receive a transplant, but instead, received continued chemotherapy (10 of the 11 refused a transplant and 1 was excluded). The 33 patients in the transplantation arm received a transplant within 4 months of attaining CR. Five of the 33 were in relapse at the time of transplant. The investigators did not consider these 5 as failures at the time of transplantation. Three of the 46 patients assigned chemotherapy would not have been offered transplantation, even if they had matched siblings and, hence, were not included in the chemotherapy group, and the patient excluded from transplantation was also excluded from analysis. This left three groups for analysis: 43 patients receiving chemotherapy because they lacked a donor, 10 patients receiving chemotherapy because they declined transplantation (these patients had the worst outcomes), and 33 patients receiving a transplant. When the latter two groups were combined into a single "transplant group" the probability of being alive and in remission at 5 years was higher ($p < 0.06$) in this group than in the chemotherapy group (the same was true when patients declining transplantation were excluded from analysis or were combined with the chemotherapy group). Three patients whose disease recurred after receiving chemotherapy remain alive (2 having been salvaged with mismatched or autologous transplant). The probabilities of 5-year *survival* were 40% in the transplant plus the decline-transplant group and 30% in the chemotherapy group, a difference that did not reach statistical significance ($p=0.25$). This study is open to criticism because, although all patients were entered at diagnosis (unlike, probably, the UCLA study; 53) some were specifically referred for transplantation because they had an HLA-identical sibling. Also it is unclear how the 5 patients in relapse at time of transplantation were analyzed. Finally, mention should again be made of the aforementioned ECOG study assigning patients in CR to receive maintenance (likely to be judged inadequate by many), consolidation (one course of ara-C 3 g/m^2 every 12 hours for 12 doses plus amsacrine) or, if aged 40 or less with an HLA-identical donor, an allogenic transplant (31). To date, the probability of being alive and in CR at 2 years in patients aged 40 and less is $38 \pm 15\%$ in the consolidation group and $50 \pm 15\%$ in the transplant group.

A few conclusions emerge from these comparative studies in patients in first CR. First it will be difficult to demonstrate a clear advantage in survival for a group receiving a transplant (if such an advantage exists, as trends suggest) unless many more patients are entered into a single study than have yet been entered. Second, because this larger study will have to encompass many hospitals, it too will likely be as open to question as the aforementioned single-hospital studies. Third, in all the studies, patients in the chemotherapy group lacked an

HLA-identical sibling donor (or if they had one were either unwilling or judged unable to receive a transplant). Hence, none of the studies have addressed the possibility that patients in first remission who have a donor might receive a transplant only at time of relapse. Fourth, none of the studies have formally analyzed whether *some* patients with HLA-identical sibling donors might better be served by a transplant during first remission, whereas *others* might do better with continued chemotherapy. We will consider these last two points.

The possibility of delaying transplantation until first relapse arises from the following: Assume chemotherapy cures 30–40% of patients in first remission (see Table 1) and allogeneic transplantation in untreated first relapse cures 30% (the Seattle result) (52). Given these rates, the cure rate with a strategy that reserves transplantation for patients in first relapse following chemotherapy should result in a cure rate of at least 50% [30% + (30%) (70%)]. This result is comparable with that following allogenic transplantation during first remission. Delaying transplantation until necessary would produce considerable logistic and financial advantages. Note, however, that this strategy assumes that every patient whose disease is in first relapse can receive a transplant within a short time, and that adverse effects that might occur during chemotherapy in first CR do not preclude transplantation at first relapse. Note also that the Seattle and IBMTR results suggest that a delay should not encompass an attempt to transplant during second remission, rather than first relapse (52–55).

The prognosis in patients whose disease recurs after transplantation was recently described (56). Among 95 such patients, median survival was about 3 months, and only 4 are alive (all 4 are 4–5 years after recurrence). Thirty-three of these 95 were not treated, whereas 13 received a second transplant (2 of the latter are alive). Median disease-free survival was 6 months in patients who initially received transplants during remission, 6 months in patients who initially received transplants during relapse, 7.5 months in patients whose disease recurred ≥100 days after transplantation, and less than 1 month in patients whose disease recurred <100 days after transplant.

If characteristics that identify patients who will have a favorable outcome after transplantation differ from characteristics that identify patients who will have a favorable outcome after chemotherapy, it might be possible to rationally assign patients to receive one treatment or the other. Age is an obvious characteristic here. Seattle studies indicate that age is the most powerful predictor of survival after transplantation during first CR, with 80% of patients under age 10 alive and likely cured (n=20) versus 65% aged 11–20 (n=52), 42% aged 21–30 (n=89), 40% aged 31–40 (n=44), and 40% aged >40 (up to aged 53, n=22) (57). Studies at Johns Hopkins and Memorial Sloan–Kettering Cancer Center have found similar effects of age on survival (58), although McGlave and associates, in Minneapolis, also using CY+TBI found similar disease-free survival rates in patients aged 10–20 (59%; 95% CI, 41–77%, n=30), 20–30 (59%, 33–85%, n=15), and 30–45 (57%, 31–83%, n=14); no patients over aged 45 received a transplant (59). Many chemotherapy studies indicate that age does not predict outcome once patients are in CR. Hence, it might seem reasonable to assign all patients under aged 20 to receive an HLA-identical sibling transplant. However, as noted earlier, Wolff et al. found that long-term remissions occurred in over 80% of patients aged 7–25 (7 was the age of the youngest patient) versus 50% of those aged 26–45 (28). On the basis of these results, it could be argued that patients under age 25 might receive chemotherapy with an advantage equal to that of transplantation.

Tallman et al. have undertaken the most sophisticated attempt to identify factors that might be associated with a relatively favorable outcome following chemotherapy vis-a-vis transplantation during first CR and vice versa (60). The transplant group for the analysis was derived from Seattle studies and the chemotherapy group from SWOG studies, which produced a relatively low 5-year survival rate of 23 ± 3% for patients in first CR (contrast with Table 1). Tallman et al. used mathematically defined "interaction terms," large values for which independently identified patients at relatively high risk after transplantation (or relatively low risk following chemotherapy). Interaction terms with large values for survival included older age, male sex, achievement of CR after one course of induction therapy, and the absence of circulating blast cells. To test whether these interaction terms could be profitably used to assign patients, they divided patients receiving chemotherapy into one of three groups, depending on whether values for the interaction term were in the top, middle, or bottom third of the group; the same was done for patients who had received transplants. There was little difference in survival according to group among chemotherapy patients, but patients in the bottom third transplant group did much worse than in the other two transplant groups: their survival approximated that of the chemotherapy groups. This suggested that chemotherapy might be the preferred option for patients with interaction values in the bottom third of the transplant group.

The search for prognostic factors that might identify patients more likely to benefit from chemotherapy than transplantation or vice versa is likely to continue. Because leukemia cell karyotype is a prime variable influencing survival in chemotherapy-treated patients in CR (5–7), it will be particularly important to determine if the same is true in patients receiving transplantation during first CR. However, a few findings suggest that prognostic factors for a poor outcome following chemotherapy, such as monosomes or deletions of chromosomes 5 or 7, will do the same following transplant. The IBMTR has found that the major factor influencing leukemia-free survival in patients receiving transplants during second CR (as in patients receiving chemotherapy during second CR) is the length of the first CR (61); the latter is primarily influenced by karyotype. Both the IBMTR and McGlave and associates have noted that relapses after transplantation during first CR are more common in patients who have high white cell counts at diagnosis or FAB subtypes M4 or M5 (59,61). The unfavorable effects of a high presenting white cell count and subtypes M4 and M5 have also been noted in patients treated with chemotherapy (e.g., Ref. 62).

Newer Approaches

Only 30% of patients will have an HLA-identical sibling. Attempts to widen the donor pool have used donors who, although related to the recipient, are not HLA-identical. Seattle investigators have defined the tolerable limits of HLA disparity between related donors and recipients by performing transplantation in 281 patients with hematological malignancies and varying degrees of donor–recipient HLA incompatibility (63). Twenty-nine of the 281 patients were phenotypically identical, 119 were incompatible for one locus, and the remaining 133 were incompatible for two or three loci. The relative risk of severe acute GvHD increased 2.16-fold for each incompatible locus ($p < 0.0001$). However, the occurrence of GvHD conveyed a lower risk of relapse. The survival of one–locus-mismatched transplants approximated that of HLA-identical sibling transplants because a lower relapse rate balanced an increased rate of GVHD (although it is not clear if this was true specifically for patients with AML and if it was true in all stages of the disease, e.g., first relapse, second relapse). The survival of patients with a greater number of mismatches was much poorer.

Both the Seattle group (64) and investigators at the Medical College of Wisconsin (65) have demonstrated the feasibility of performing allogeneic transplantation using unrelated donors. In Seattle, 23 patients with leukemia and 7 with severe aplastic anemia received such transplants. Twenty-seven of the 30 were HLA-A, B, DR matched and MLC nonreactive. All patients with leukemia "engrafted." Eleven were alive and in remission 1 month to 3 years after transplantation, whereas 5 died with acute GVHD. The death rate from acute GVHD decreased when cyclosporine was added to methotrexate for GVHD prophylaxis. Studies are in progress to define the maximum tolerable degree of HLA incompatibility between an unrelated donor and a recipient. Depending on the results it is possible that donors could be identified for most patients.

Nonetheless, there will likely still be a substantial number of patients without a potential donor. Furthermore, patients over age 50 tend to have unfavorable outcomes following allogeneic transplantation. These facts underlie much of the continued interest in autologous transplantation. This technique has been most frequently employed in Europe, where the probability of 3-year disease-free survival has been reported to be close to 50% (58). However, the applicability of these results are in doubt, given that patients often received transplants only after several months in remission, raising the issue of lead-time bias, in addition to other questions about patient selection procedures. The Seattle group has reported less favorable outcomes following autologous transplantation in 13 patients in first remission whose remission duration at the time of transplantation ranged from 1–13 months (median, 3) (66). Methotrexate, with or without human leukocyte interferon, was used after transplantation to eliminate transfused leukemia cells or leukemia cells remaining after CY+TBI. Engraftment was delayed in comparison with engraftment following syngeneic marrow transplantation in patients with AML, some of whom also received methotrexate or interferon posttransplant. Two patients died within 4 months of transplantation, 8 had recurrence of disease within a year of transplantation, and 3 remained alive and in remission 26–50 months after transplantation. The authors stressed that these results were not superior to those expected following use of conventional chemotherapy.

Attempts to improve results after autologous transplantation have focused on the use of "purging" residual leukemia cells in the stored marrow (58). This can be done by incubating the marrow with 4-hydroperoxycyclophosphamide (4-HC) or mafosfamide (both of which in solution become 4-hydroxycyclophosphamide, an early metabolite of cyclophosphamide), or with monoclonal antibodies or immunotoxins. It is also possible to isolate normal stem cell progenitors after growth of autologous marrow in culture and then to expand these normal cells in long-term culture before infusion into patients. The largest number of patients infused with purged marrow has been reported from Johns Hopkins (58). The investigators used 4-HC as the purging agent and treated 17 "high-risk" patients in first remission, and 59 and 12 patients in second and third remission, respectively. With a median follow-up of about 2 years, the disease-free survival was 47% for patients in first remission and 28% for those in second or third remission. The probability of relapse was 46% for those in first remission and 64% and 55% for those in second and third remission, respectively. Although some details are unclear (e.g., the time to which these percentages refer), the relapse rate seems similar to that following syngeneic transplantation and the disease-free survival rate similar to that following allogeneic transplantation.

The different results obtained following syngeneic transplantation, on the one hand, and allogeneic transplantation, on the other, have helped lead to an appreciation of the "graft-versus-leukemia phenomenon" (GvL). Gale and Champlin compared the probability of disease recurrence in 392 patients who received a transplant in first remission from an HLA-identical sibling with the probability in 31 patients also in first remission whose donor was an identical twin (67). Both groups received transplantation at the same hospitals and had been observed for comparable lengths of time (median 2–3 years). The probability of relapse was threefold higher in the group that received transplants from HLA-identical siblings. Graft-vs-host disease is very rare in recipients of transplants from identical twins, compared with recipients of transplants from HLA-identical siblings. Accordingly, GvHD prophylaxis is rarely administered following syngeneic transplantation. The increased relapse rate in recipients of twin transplants could have resulted from the omission of GvHD prophylaxis, from the deaths of recipients of HLA-identical sibling transplants before relapse could be observed, or from a combination of a genetic susceptibility to development of AML in the donor and exposure to an environmental abnormality in the recipient. These possibilities appear less likely, however, than an antileukemia effect produced by transplantation of allogeneic bone marrow cells—so called GvL.

Other evidence also suggests the existence of the GvL phenomenon. Data from Seattle indicate that patients who develop "clinical extensive" chronic GvHD after allogenic transplantation during first CR have a relapse rate about half that of patients in whom this complication does not develop (51). This beneficial effect is countered by an increase in mortality from infections and other complications. As noted earlier, the same is true in the setting of one–locus-mismatched transplants.

Because a significant part of the antileukemia effect that follows allogeneic transplantation may be due to the GvL phenomonen, rather than the use of high doses of chemotherapy, with or without radiation, it might be worthwhile to produce GvL in patients undergoing autologous transplantation or in those who are receiving or have completed chemotherapy. This assumes that it will be possible to separate the effects of GvL from those of GvHD. Attempts to nonspecifically induce GvHD and, thereby, it was hoped GvL, in recipients of allogeneic transplants by using unusually short courses of methotrexate or adding donor buffy coat cells have increased death rates from GvHD and had no effect on disease recurrence (68). However, other approaches to induce GvL [e.g., expansion of the NK cell pool possibly through the use of IL-2 or the induction of autologous GvHD (69)] may be more fruitful.

ACKNOWLEDGMENT

The authors thank Latressie Bogan for skilled secretarial assistance.

REFERENCES

1. Freireich E, Gehan E, Sulman D, et al: The effect of chemotherapy on acute leukemia in the human. *J Chronic Dis* 1961; 14:593–608.
2. Freireich E, Gehan E, Frei E, et al: The effect of 6-mercaptopurine on the duration of steroid-induced remissions in acute leukemia: A model for evaluation of other potentially useful therapy. *Blood* 1963; 21:699–716.
3. Preisler H, Davis R, Kirshner J, et al: Comparison of three remission induction regimens and two postinduction strategies for the treatment of acute nonlymphocytic leukemia: A Cancer and Leukemia Group B study. *Blood* 1987; 69:1441–1449.
4. Preisler H, Anderson K, Rai K, et al: The frequency of long-term remission in

patients with acute myelogenous leukaemia treated with conventional maintenance chemotherapy: A study of 760 patients with a minimal follow-up time of 6 years. *Br J Haematol* 1989; 71:189–194.
5. Sixth International Workshop in Chromosomes in Leukemia: The clinical significance of karyotype in acute myelogenous leukemia. *Cancer Genet Cytogenet* 1989; 40:203–216.
6. Schiffer C, Lee E, Tomiyasu T, et al: Prognostic impact of cytogenetic abnormalities in patients with de novo acute nonlymphocytic leukemia. *Blood* 1989; 73:263–270.
7. Keating M, Cork A, Broach Y, et al: Toward a clinically relevant cytogenetic classification of acute myelogenous leukemia. *Leuk Res* 1987; 11:119–133.
8. Keating M, Kantarjian H, Smith T, et al: Response to salvage therapy and survival after relapse in acute myelogenous leukemia. *J Clin Oncol* 1989; 7:1071–1080.
9. Griffin J, Loewenberg B: Clonogenic cells in acute myeloblastic leukemia. *Blood* 1986; 68:1185–1195.
10. Sauter C, Fopp M, Imbach P, et al: Acute myelogenous leukaemia: Maintenance chemotherapy after early consolidation treatment does not prolong survival. *Lancet* 1984; 1:379–382.
11. Champlin R, Gale R, Elashoff R, et al: Prolonged survival in acute myelogenous leukaemia without maintenance chemotherapy. *Lancet* 1984; 1:894–896.
12. Rohatiner A, Gregory W, Bassan R, et al: Short-term therapy for acute myelogenous leukemia. *J Clin Oncol* 1988; 6:218–226.
13. Mandelli F: Presented at the UCLA Symposium on Molecular and Cellular Biology, Acute Myelogenous Leukemia. Lake Lanier, GA, 30 November 1989.
14. Buechner T, Urbanitz D, Hiddemann W, et al: Intensified induction and consolidation with or without maintenance chemotherapy for acute myeloid leukemia (AML): Two multicenter studies of the German AML Cooperative Group. *J Clin Oncol* 1985; 3:1583–1589.
15. Cassileth P, Harrington D, Hines J, et al: Maintenance chemotherapy prolongs remission duration in adult acute nonlymphocytic leukemia. *J Clin Oncol* 1988; 6:583–587.
16. Dutcher J, Wiernik P, Markus S, et al: Intensive maintenance therapy improves survival in adult acute nonlymphocytic leukemia: An eight-year follow-up. *Leukemia* 1988; 2:413–419.
17. Kantarjian H, Keating M, Walters R, et al: Role of maintenance chemotherapy in acute promyelocytic leukemia. *Cancer* 1987; 59:1258–1263.
18. Berman E, Raymond V, Gee T, et al: Idarubicin in acute leukemia: Results of studies at Memorial Sloan–Kettering Cancer Center. *Semin Oncol* 1989; 16(suppl 2):30–34.
19. Karanes C, Kopecky K, Durie B, Grever M: Increased risk of early death with high-dose ara-C (HDAC) and m-AMSA compared to HDAC alone or HDAC and mitoxantrone. *Proc Am Soc Clin Oncol* 1989; 8:201.
20. Keating M, Gehan E, Smith T, et al: A strategy for evaluation of new treatments in untreated patients: Application to a clinical trial of AMSA for acute leukemia. *J Clin Oncol* 1987; 5:710–721.
21. Berman E, Arlin Z, Gaynor J, et al: Comparative trial of cytarabine and thioguanine

in combination with amsacrine or daunorubicin in patients with untreated acute nonlymphocytic leukemia: Results of the L-16M protocol. *Leukemia* 1989; 3:115–121.

22. Keating M, McCredie K, Benjamin R, et al: Treatment of patients over 50 years of age with acute myelogenous leukemia with a combination of rubidazone and cytosine arabinoside, vincristine, and prednisone (ROAP) *Blood* 1981; 58:584–591.
23. Vogler W, Stein R, Winton E, Raney M: A randomized trial of induction and maintenance in acute myelogenous leukemia (AML) in patients over the age of 50. *Proc Am Soc Clin Oncol* 1987; 6:149.
24. Vogler W: Presented at the UCLA Symposium on Molecular and Cellular Biology: Acute myelogenous leukemia. Lake Lanier, GA., 30 November 1989.
25. Bishop J, Lowenthal R, Joshua D, et al: Etoposide in acute nonlymphoycytic leukemia. *Blood* 1990; 75:27–32.
26. Rudnick S, Cadman E, Capizzi R, et al: High-dose cytosine arabinoside in refractory acute leukemia. *Cancer* 1979; 44:1189–1193.
27. Plunkett W, Liliemark J, Adams T, et al: Saturation of 1-β-D-arabinofuranosylcytosine-5'-triphosphate accumulation in leukemia cells during high-dose 1-β-D-arabinofuranosylcytosine therapy. *Cancer Res* 1987; 47:3005–3011.
28. Wolff S, Herzig R, Fay J, et al: High-dose cytarabine and daunorubicin as consolidation therapy for acute myeloid leukemia in first remission: Long-term follow-up and results. *J Clin Oncol* 1989; 7:1260–1267.
29. Cassileth P, Begg C, Silber R, et al: Prolonged unmaintained remission after intensive consolidation therapy in adult acute nonlymphocytic leukemia. *Cancer Treat Rep* 1987; 71:137–140.
30. Cassileth P, McGlave P, Harrington D, et al: Comparison of post remission therapy in AML: Maintenance versus intensive consolidation therapy versus allogeneic bone marrow transplantation. *Proc Am Soc Clin Oncol* 1989; 8:197.
31. Champlin R, Ho W, Winston D, et al: Treatment of adults with acute myelogenous leukemia: Prospective evaluation of high-dose cytarabine in consolidation chemotherapy and with bone marrow transplantation. *Semin Oncol* 1987; 14(suppl 1):1–6.
32. Mayer R, Schiffer C, Peterson B, et al: Intensive postremission therapy in adults with acute nonlymphocytic leukemia using various dose schedules of ara-C: A progress report from the CALGB. *Semin Oncol* 1987; 14(suppl 1):25–31.
33. Preisler H, Raza A, Early A, et al: Intensive remission consolidation therapy in the treatment of acute nonlymphocytic leukemia. *J Clin Oncol* 1987; 5:722–730.
34. Estey E, Keating M, Plunkett W, et al: Continuous infusion high-dose cytosine arabinoside without anthracyclines as induction and intensification therapy in adults under age 50 with newly diagnosed acute myelogenous leukemia. *Semin Oncol* 1987; 14(suppl 1):58–63.
35. Plunkett W, Iacoboni S, Estey E, et al: Pharmacologically-directed ara-C therapy for refractory leukemia. *Semin Oncol* 1985; 12(suppl 3):20–30.
36. Holmes R, Keating M, Cork A, et al: A unique pattern of central nervous system leukemia in acute myelomonocytic leukemia associated with inv(16)(p13q22). *Blood* 1985; 65:1071–1078.

37. Ganem G, Fischer J, Marty M, et al: Prognostic factors in acute promyelocytic leukemia (APL): A retrospective study of 101 patients treated by DNR containing remission induction regimen. *Blood* 1983; 62:171a.
38. Castaigne S, Chomienne C, Ballerini P, et al: All-*trans*-retinoic acid: A novel differentiation therapy for acute promyelocytic leukemia. *Blood* 1989; 74(suppl 1):117a.
39. Morstyn G, Burgess A: Hemopoietic growth factors: A review. *Cancer Res* 1988; 48:5624–5637.
40. Loewenberg B, Salem M, Delwel R: Effects of recombinant multi-CSF, GM-CSF, G-CSF and M-CSF on the proliferation and maturation of human AML in vitro. *Blood Cells* 1988; 14:539–549.
41. Cannistra S, Groshek P, Griffin J: Granulocyte–macrophage colony-stimulating factor enhances the cytotoxic effects of cytosine arabinoside in acute myeloblastic leukemia and in the myeloid blast crisis phase of chronic myeloid leukemia. *Leukemia* 1989; 3:328–334.
42. Begley C, Metcalf D, Nicola N: Primary human myeloid leukemia cells: Comparative responsiveness to proliferative stimulation by GM-CSF or G-CSF and membrane expression of CSF receptors. *Leukemia* 1987; 1:1–8.
43. Bhalla K, Birkhofer M, Arlin Z, et al: Effect of recombinant GM-CSF on the metabolism of cytosine arabinoside in normal and leukemic human bone marrow cells. *Leukemia* 1988; 2:810–813.
44. Vaughan W, Karp J, Burke P: Two-cycle timed-sequential chemotherapy for adult acute nonlymphocytic leukemia. *Blood* 1984; 64:975–980.
45. Geller R, Burke P, Karp J, et al: A two-step timed sequential treatment for acute myelocytic leukemia. *Blood* 1989; 74:1499–1506.
46. Vellenga E, Young D, Wagner K, et al: The effects of GM-CSF and G-CSF in promoting growth of clonogenic cells in acute myeloblastic leukemia. *Blood* 1987; 69:1771–1776.
47. Keinaenen M, Griffin J, Bloomfield M, et al: Clonal chromosomal abnormalities showing multiple-cell-lineage involvement in acute myeloid leukemia. *N Engl J Med* 1988; 318:1153–1158.
48. Estey E, Dixon D, Kantarjian H, et al: Treatment of poor-prognosis newly-diagnosed AML with ara-C and recombinant human GM-CSF. *Blood* (1990).
49. Buechner T, Hiddemann W, Koenigsmann M, et al: Hematologic and therapeutic effects of recombinant human GM-CSF following chemotherapy (CT) in patients with acute leukemias at higher age or after relapse. *Blood* 1989; 74(suppl 1):271a.
50. Muhm M, Andreeff M, Geissler K, et al: RhGM-CSF in combination with chemotherapy—a new strategy in the therapy of acute myeloid leukemia. *Blood* 1989; 74(suppl 1):117a.
51. Clift R, Buckner C, Thomas E, et al: The treatment of acute non-lymphoblastic leukemia by allogeneic marrow transplantation. *Bone Marrow Transplant* 1987; 2:243–258.
52. Champlin R, Advisory Committee of the International Bone Marrow Transplant Registry: Bone marrow transplantation for acute leukemia: A preliminary report from the International Bone Marrow Transplant Registry. *Transplant Proc* 1987; 19:2626–2628.

53. Champlin R, Ho W, Gale R, et al: Treatment of acute myelogenous leukemia: A prospective controlled trial of bone marrow transplantation versus consolidation chemotherapy. *Ann Intern Med* 1985; 102:285–291.
54. Zander A, Keating M, Dicke K, et al: A comparison of marrow transplantation with chemotherapy for adults with acute leukemia of poor prognosis in first complete remission. *J Clin Oncol* 1988; 6:1548–1557.
55. Appelbaum F, Fisher L, Thomas E, Seattle Marrow Transplant Team: Chemotherapy v marrow transplantation for adults with acute nonlymphocytic leukemia: A five-year follow-up. *Blood* 1988; 72:179–184.
56. Mortimer J, Blinder M, Schulman S, et al: Relapse of acute leukemia after marrow transplantation: Natural history and results of subsequent therapy. *J Clin Oncol* 1989; 7:50–57.
57. Buckner C, Sanders J, Appelbaum F: Allogeneic marrow transplantation for acute non-lymphoblastic leukemia: First remission versus after first relapse. *Bone Marrow Transplant* 1989; 4(suppl 1):244–246.
58. Santos G: Marrow transplantation in acute nonlymphocytic leukemia. *Blood* 1989; 74:901–908.
59. McGlave P, Haake R, Bostrom B, et al: Allogeneic bone marrow transplantation for acute nonlymphocytic leukemia in first remission. *Blood* 1988; 72:1512–1517.
60. Tallman M, Kopecky K, Amos D, et al: Analysis of prognostic factors for the outcome of marrow transplantation or further chemotherapy for patients with acute nonlymphocytic leukemia in first remission. *J Clin Oncol* 1989; 7:326–337.
61. Gale R: Presented at the UCLA Symposium on Cellular and Molecular Biology: Acute Myelogenous Leukemia, Lake Lanier, GA, 30 November 1989.
62. Weinstein H, Mayer R, Rosenthal D, et al: Chemotherapy for acute myelogenous leukemia in children and adults: VAPA update. *Blood* 1983; 62:315–319.
63. Anasetti C, Beatty P, Sanders J, et al: Graft-versus-host reaction, relapse and survival after HLA-nonidentical marrow transplants for malignancy [abstr]. *Exp Hematol* 1988; 16:495.
64. Beatty P, Hansen J, Anasetti C, et al: Marrow transplantation from unrelated donors [abstr]. *Exp Hematol* 1988; 16:470.
65. Ash RC, Casper J, Menitove J, et al: Successful allogeneic marrow transplant utilizing HLA-closely matched unrelated donors [abstr]. *Exp Hematol* 1988; 16:470.
66. Stewart P, Buckner C, Bensinger W, et al: Autologous marrow transplantation in patients with acute nonlymphocytic leukemia in first remission. *Exp Hematol* 1985; 13:267–272.
67. Gale R, Champlin R: How does bone-marrow transplantation cure leukaemia? *Lancet* 1984; 2:28–30.
68. Sullivan K, Storb R, Buckner C, et al: Graft-versus-host disease as adoptive immunotherapy in patients with advanced hematologic neoplasms. *N Engl J Med* 1989; 320:828–834.
69. Jones R, Vogelsang G, Hess A, et al: Induction of graft-versus-host disease following autologous bone marrow transplantation. *Lancet* 1989; 1:754–757.

2

Treatment of Myelodysplastic Syndromes

Miloslav Beran

University of Texas
M. D. Anderson Cancer Center
Houston, Texas

DEFINITION

On the basis of our current understanding, *myelodysplastic syndromes* (MDS) represent a highly heterogeneous group of diseases (or various stages of the same disease). The dominant feature is an ineffective hematopoiesis involving, to various degrees, one or all hematopoietic lineages. The resulting anemia, thrombocytopenia, neutropenia, or combinations thereof are the result of a disjunction between the proliferation and differentiation of hematopoietic progenitor cells, either multipotent or committed to a particular cell lineage. In contrast with myeloproliferative disorders (MPD), the predominant defect in MDS is in the differentiation process. The well-defined marrow dysplastic changes and architectural disorganization represent, along with the peripheral cytopenia(s), the cornerstones for MDS diagnosis (1–3). *Chronic myelomonocytic* leukemia (CMML) is a special subcategory of MDS with shared dysplastic (erythroid, megakaryocytic) and proliferative (granulocytic–monocytic) features (4–6). It resembles Philadelphia chromosome (Ph)-negative chronic myelogenous leukemia and thus bears similarities to both MDS and MPD (7).

The concept of MDS evolved gradually, over the past several decades, to encompass entities previously identified by deficient production of mature blood cells. Initial attention was drawn to the deficient erythropoiesis, manifested by anemia unrelated to nutritional deficiencies and characterized by certain morphological features. It was then recognized that other hemopoietic lineages may be affected in association with, or before the development of, anemia and may be manifest as peripheral neutropenia or thrombocytopenia. These conditions were often found to precede the development of overt acute leukemia; hence, their designation as *preleukemic* syndromes. Other terms have included smoldering leukemia, oligoblastic leukemia, and low infiltrate leukemia. This has created confusion in the classification of MDS and in the attempts to study the disease biology and treatment results. Terms referring to the preleukemic nature of MDS are unfortunate and should be avoided, since they are applied only retrospectively and since only a fraction of patients with MDS develop acute leukemia.

CLASSIFICATION

Given the heterogeneity of MDS conditions, a simple and universally accepted classification will help in studying the natural history of these disorders, their biology, and their response and outcome with different therapeutic maneuvers.

In 1982, the French–American–British (FAB) Working Group published their joint proposal for the classification of MDS (Table 1) (1,2). This expanded our knowledge of the natural history of MDS, of the risk of leukemic development within morphological categories, and of the response of subcategories to therapeutic manipulations. Suggested modification of the original FAB classification was recently presented in a proposal for morphologic, immunologic, and cytogenetic (MIC) classification of myelodysplastic disorders (3). The new proposal recognizes the heterogeneity within each FAB category, and seeks to further evaluate the prognostic significance and therapeutic implications of various phenotypic and genotypic (cytogenetic) subsets of MDS.

Although the FAB classification of MDS represented a major advance in our knowledge, it has been criticized for the lack of more "biological" criteria. Since MDS are clonal disorders of the hematopoietic stem cells (8–11), karyotypic abnormalities are expected to be present in analogy with other clonal diseases such as acute and chronic leukemias. Indeed, abnormal karyotypes are found in 50–60% of patients with primary MDS (1,3,12–16), and in 60–80% of those with secondary MDS (sMDS) (16). Karyotypic abnormalities in MDS were reported by several studies to have important prognostic importance. Clonal evolution generally represents an ominous sign for response to therapy and survival (17–20). In combination with the FAB classification, karyotypic analysis represents a powerful prognostic tool, and it may be useful for predicting responses to therapy and possibly for treatment individualization.

GENERAL MANAGEMENT

The heterogeneity of the natural history of MDS determines the decision on initial management (21–27). In general, the intensity of treatment is best determined by (1) the aggressiveness of the disease and (2) the patient's age. After

Table 1 FAB Criteria for Classification of MDS

MDS type	% Blasts: Bone marrow	% Blasts: Blood	% Ringed sideroblasts[a]	Dyspoiesis	Monocytes blood ($\times 10^3/\mu L$)
Refractory anemia (RA), refractory cytopenia (RC)	<5	<1	<15	+ to ++	<1
Refractory anemia with ringed sideroblasts (RARS)	<5	<1	<15	± to +	<1
Refractory anemia with excess of blasts (RAEB)	5–20	<5	Variable	++ to +++	<1
RAEB in transformation (RAEBT)	20–30	>5	Variable	++ to +++	
	or <20 with Auer rods	or with Auer rods	<1		
Chronic myelomonocytic leukemia (CMML)[b]	1–20	?	Variable	++	≥1

[a]Percentage of total marrow nucleated cells.
[b]CMML in transformation (CMML-T) with marrow blasts 21–30%, a category not included in FAB classification.

establishing the diagnosis and identifying the prognostic factors, an observation period is appropriate to obtain information on a probable clinical course. When possible, supportive care, such as transfusions of blood products, should be withheld, particularly in young healthy patients who are considered to be candidates for allogeneic bone marrow transplantation (BMT). In these patients, histocompatibility antigen (HLA) typing of siblings and family members should be performed as soon as possible, particularly if the MDS is secondary to chemoradiotherapy or associated with pancytopenia or cytogenetic abnormalities. Patients should have a thorough medical and cardiopulmonary evaluation, and treatment for unrelated disorders should be optimized. The initial management with red blood cell (RBC) transfusions should be conservative; the goal is to keep them at a minimum while reducing symptoms related to anemia, particularly in elderly patients.

Platelet transfusions are indicated only with evidence of bleeding, and they should not be guided by the degree of thrombocytopenia, since the correlation between platelet counts and bleeding tendency is poor. Thrombocytopenia is, however, a major poor prognosis sign in most prognostic models (21–27) and strongly suggests the need for therapeutic intervention. Although the presence or development of neutropenia signals a more aggressive disease and the need for treatment, the long-term use of prophylactic antibiotics is controversial. Leukocyte transfusions alone have no place in the therapy of MDS. A major risk in supportive care-only for MDS is the colonization of patients by potential pathogens, particularly by fungal species, which increases the risk of complications in patients subsequently treated with chemotherapy or BMT. *Candida* and *Aspergillus* species are major causes of early death among elderly patients treated with intensive chemotherapy. In this setting, prophylaxis with combinations of antibacterial (e.g., trimethoprim–sulfamethoxazole) and antifungal (e.g., ketoconazole, fluconazole) agents may be useful, as has been found in patients with acute leukemia and chemotherapy-associated neutropenia (28).

Patients with isolated anemia (e.g., RA and RARS) with a diploid karyotype represent the most benign category of MDS, and have a low risk for developing acute leukemia or life-threatening cytopenias (21–27). These patients should be managed with RBC transfusions only, unless trials with human erythropoietin prove to be superior. A possible exception are young patients ($<$50 years) with severe transfusion requirements (e.g., 2–4 units every month), for whom promising investigational approaches should be considered.

SPECIFIC THERAPIES

Glucocorticoids, Anabolic Steroids, and Vitamins

Although there have been occasional reports on the successful use of vitamins (B_6, B_{12}, folic acid) in "refractory" anemias, there is no convincing evidence for their activity in MDS. In patients responding to such treatment, the diagnosis of MDS must be questioned.

The value of glucocorticoids in MDS has been extensively studied by Bagby et al. (29), who noted hematological improvement in 10% of patients. In some patients, glucocorticoid effects in vivo correlated with their in vitro effect on the clonal growth of hematopoietic progenitor cells (29). The improvements, however, were transient. In a recent study (30), 47 patients with previously untreated RA, RARS, and RAEB received prednisone, 0.8–1.0 mg/kg, for 2–4 weeks. The hemoglobin normalized in 3 of 29 patients with RA or RAEB; only transient and minor platelet responses were seen. Given their numerous side effects, glucocorticoids may be hazardous in patients with MDS who already have a compromised immune system (31).

Anabolic steroids have been used with some success in the treatment of aplastic anemia and, occasionally, have been claimed to improve various MDS abnormalities. Some of the responses in MDS may have been due to past diagnostic difficulties in separating aplastic anemia from MDS. In two large studies, patients with RAEB or RAEBT treated with high doses of androgens showed no improvement in their hematological values (32,33).

Danazol, a new synthetic attenuated androgen (34), was originally reported to improve thrombocytopenia and anemia in patients with MDS (35–37). Several groups were unable to confirm these findings (38–40). Recently, Marini et al. (41) treated 16 consecutive patients with MDS (2 RA, 2 RARS, 6 RAEB, 1 RAEBT, and 5 CMML) with danazol, 200 mg orally three times daily for 12 consecutive weeks, and noted normalization of platelet counts in five of eight thrombocytopenic patients. No patient had a pretreatment platelet count below $40 \times 10^3/\mu L$, and the magnitude of the response was inversely related to the degree of initial thrombocytopenia. Small-scale studies with danazol suggest temporary improvements in thrombocytopenia and anemia in some patients. Unfortunately, an adequate follow-up to evaluate the duration of response is not available. In the absence of large trials, the use of danazol, like many other therapeutic modalities in MDS, remains controversial. The optimal dosage and duration of treatment as well as parameters necessary to identify patients likely to benefit from this treatment are unknown. For an adequate trial, 200 mg of danazol three times daily should probably be given for at least 12 weeks (41). Similarly, maintenance doses in responding patients are not established. There is no evidence that danazol suppresses the abnormal clone (41). Given the biological features of MDS, the use of danazol must be considered a temporary measure. Its true value should be tested in patients with platelet counts below $30 \times 10^3/\mu L$, if no other conservative treatment to alleviate a life-threatening thrombocytopenia is available. In the group of patients with "advanced" MDS (RAEB, RAEBT), and in chronic myelomonocytic leukemia (CMML), androgens, in fact, may accelerate disease progression (32). Because of the relative ineffectiveness of treatment with androgens in MDS, their indiscriminate use may delay the institution of effective treatments and, thereby, indirectly compromise patient outcome.

Vitamins D_3 Analogues

The active metabolite of vitamin D, 1,25-dihydroxyvitamin D_3 [1,25-$(OH)_2D_3$], influences proliferation and differentiation of various cell lineages (42). In some murine and human leukemia cell lines, 1,25-$(OH)_2D_3$ inhibits proliferation and induces differentiation in vitro (42–47). In contrast with retinoic acid, which induces maturation along the granulocytic pathway (42–47), vitamin D_3 analogues trigger maturation of leukemic cells (42–48) as well as granulocyte–macrophage colony-forming cell (GM-CFC) (48) into the monocyte–macrophage lineage. Leukemic cell lines of differentiated phenotype tend to be more responsive, whereas proliferation and differentiation of phenotypically immature blasts cell lines are not modulated (47,50). The in vitro effects of vitamin D_3 analogues on primary leukemic cells from patients with acute myelogenous leukemia (AML) are variable. Differentiation is observed in the cells of some patients, but only at relative high concentrations ($1–10 \times 10^{-7}$ M) of 1,25-$(OH)_2D_3$ (49–51). Such concentrations are far higher than the achievable plasma levels of $\sim 1 \times 10^{-10}$ M obtained with oral daily doses of 2 μg of vitamin D_3 (49). In addition to its in vitro effects, vitamin D_3, given to mice that have been injected with M1 leukemia cells, prolongs their survival (51).

Taken together, the differentiation and antiproliferative actions of 1,25-$(OH)_2D_3$ suggested its therapeutic potential and prompted clinical trials in patients with MDS. To date, the results with 1,25-$(OH)_2D_3$ have been rather disappointing. Mehta et al. (53) treated four patients with RAEB and two with AML following MDS with 1 μg orally daily for several months, without any signs of hematological or clinical benefits. Koeffler et al. (50) treated 18 MDS patients with 2 μg of 1,25-$(OH)_2D_3$ daily for at least 12 weeks. Minor and transient improvements of granulocyte and platelet counts were noted in 8 patients, but no sustained improvements in peripheral blood cells or in marrow blast infiltration were seen in any patient at the end of the trial period (50). Hypercalcemia was seen in half of the patients (53,54), which is the most serious side effect limiting dose escalation. By using a slightly higher dose, 2.5 μg of 1,25-$(OH)_2D_3$ daily for a minimum of 8 weeks (range 8–28 weeks), Richard et al. (54) treated eight patients without observing any beneficial effect.

Thus, currently available preparations of vitamin D_3 show no clinical benefits at maximally tolerated doses. Numerous D_3 analogues, currently studied in vitro (55), may circumvent toxicities and provide better therapeutic results.

It was proposed that 1,25-$(OH)_2D_3$ could be more efficaciously used in combination with other differentiation inducers or with low-dose chemotherapy. No substantial activity was reported in 37 patients treated with 1,25-$(OH)_2D_3$, 3 μg daily given for at least 8 weeks, following initial prednisone therapy (30).

Responses were observed only in patients with RA; increases in hemoglobin levels in 2 and granulocyte counts in 3 of 13 patients. No responses were seen in patients with RARS, RAEB, and RAEBT. These results suggest a possible benefit from high doses of vitamin D_3 in the RA subcategory of MDS. The duration of such responses is unknown, and experience with a larger number of patients is necessary.

Retinoids

Retinoids inhibit the process of carcinogenesis and prevent malignant progression in preneoplastic epithelial lesions (55). They also inhibit proliferation of established malignant cell lines and, in some instances, induce terminal differentiation of tumor cells in general (56), and leukemic cells in particular (57).

The rationale for their use in MDS was strengthened by findings that both all-*trans*- and 13-*cis*-retinoic acids induce terminal differentiation of some human myeloid leukemia cell lines in vitro (58–60) and inhibit proliferation of clonogeneic HL60 leukemic cells in cultures (61). The growth inhibition and differentiation into either granulocytic or monocytic cells after exposure to retinoids was commonly observed in leukemic cell lines with primarily more "mature" characteristics (HL60, A-937, TPH-1) (57,62). More "primitive" cell lines are not responsive to the differentiation-inducing action of retinoic acid, albeit some of them are sensitive to its growth inhibitory action (57,59,62,63). The mechanisms of action of retinoids are unknown, but studies with structurally modified retinoids suggest that the same structural characteristics are responsible for their differentiation-inducing and growth-modulating effects in normal and leukemic hematopoiesis (60).

Although retinoids induce differentiation (58,60) and growth inhibition (60,63) in leukemic cell lines in vitro, studies on fresh leukemic cells from patients with AML demonstrate such effects in only a small fraction, in particular, those with a "differentiated" morphology (57,62,64). Caution is warranted in clinical trials since 13-*cis*-retinoic acid may occasionally stimulate leukemic growth in vitro (61).

Several case reports documented the achievement of partial (PR) and complete (CR) remissions in patients with acute promyelocytic leukemia (APL) with 13-*cis*-retinoic acid (65–67). In a recent study of 24 patients with APL treated daily with 45–100 mg/m^2 of all-*trans*-retinoic acid, 23 achieved CR (68). Sixteen patients were previously untreated and, 8 were either "unresponsive" or "resistant" to chemotherapy. Patients achieved CR after daily treatment for between 20 and 119 days (68). These observations were confirmed by a French study using the same drug (70). The incidence of chemical and clinical disseminated intravascular coagulopathy was low in both studies. This suggests a potential role of all-*trans*-retinoic acid in the treatment of leukemias and possibly MDS. An additional rationale for the use of retinoids in MDS is their in vitro ability to enhance hematopoietic factor-dependent growth of granulocytic and erythroid colonies from normal human marrow cells (57,69). All-*trans*- and 13-*cis*-retinoic acids are equally potent stimulants of in vitro growth of committed myeloid progenitor cells (57) and inducers of differentiation of HL60 leukemic cells (58). Whether they have a comparable effect on malignant hematopoiesis in vivo is unknown.

Since the first report on the use of retinoic acid in MDS (71), considerable experience with 13-*cis*-retinoic acid has accumulated. The results from various studies are contradictory, and the value of 13-*cis*-retinoic acid in the treatment of MDS remains controversial (Table 2). Phase I–II studies, usually on a small number of patients, showed a variety of responses, including improvement of anemia, granulocytopenia, or thrombocytopenia in a minority of patients (71–76). Occasionally, a decrease in the marrow blast infiltration was noted (71). The heterogeneous dose schedules used make any conclusions difficult (see Table 2). Most responses were short-lived, even in patients continuing treatment.

The variations in the responses may be related to the dose and treatment duration. At least one study suggested that a significant response can be seen only in patients tolerating prolonged (4 months or more) treatment with high doses ($\geq$ 100 mg/m^2 per day) of 13-*cis*-retinoic acid (77). Of seven patients tolerating such regimen, two achieved a complete remission and five a partial remission. In one patient with RAEB, remission was associated with disappearance of the abnormal karyotype (78).

The encouraging results from early trials could not be confirmed in a larger, double-blind, placebo-controlled randomized study in which 68 patients were treated either with 100 mg/m^2 per day of 13-*cis*-retinoic acid for $\geq$ 6 months or placebo. No significant responses were observed, and survival was similar in the two groups (79). Disappointing results were also seen in a second randomized study in which 98 patients received either 20 mg/day of 13-*cis*-retinoic acid or no treatment (80). The interpretation of the results in this study is complicated by its design, calling for initial treatment of patients with $\geq$ 5% marrow blasts with cytarabine (10 mg/day for 12 weeks) before adding 13-*cis*-retinoic acid to the cytarabine regimen and continuing the treatment with both drugs. Overall survival in treated and control groups was no different after 2 years, with the exception of the group of nonsideroblastic RA in which a slightly better survival was observed in patients receiving 13-*cis*-retinoic acid ($p = 0.036$) (80).

Because of the large clinicopathological and biological heterogeneity on MDS, comparison of the results of 13-*cis*-retinoic acid are difficult. There is insufficient information to suggest that any one FAB or cytogenetic subtype of MDS is more likely to respond to retinoids. Possibly, more indolent stages (RA, RARS) respond more frequently to 13-*cis*-retinoic acid or tend to have improved survival (71,72,76). This may be important, since responses are observed only after several months of treatment. Thus, patients with indolent, slowly progressing MDS (RA, RARS) may be good candidates for 13-*cis*-retinoic acid therapy

Table 2 Phase I–II Trials of Oral 13-*cis* Retinoic Acid in MDS

Trial	FAB group	No. of patients	Treatment dose/schedule	Response
Gold et al. (71)	Total	17	20–125 mg/m^2 daily	5/15 (33%)
	RA	2	for ≥21 days	
	RAEB	11		
	CMML	4		
Greenberg et al. (72)	Total	18	1–3 mg/kg daily	3PR/18 (17%)
Hoffman et al. (73)	Total	4	80–120 mg/day	0/4 (0%)
Picozzi et al. (74)	Total	15	2.5–4.0 mg/kg daily for 6 wk	"Improvement" in 8 patients
Kerndrup et al. (75)	Total	8	20 mg/m^2 daily for 6–10 wk	"Improvement" in 4 patients
Leoni et al. (76)	Total	20	50–100 mg/day	
	RA/RARS	16	≥4 wk	Anemia improved in 12 patients, Granulocytopenia improved in 7 patients
	RAEB	2		0
	RAEBT	2		0
Besa et al. (77)	Total	24	100 mg/daily × >4 mo	2/7 CR, 5 PR
			50 mg daily × <4 mo	1/9 stable, 8/9 progression
		8	Placebo × 6 mo	6/8 stable 2/8 progression
Koeffler et al. (79)[a]	Total	68	100 mg/m^2 daily × 6 mo versus placebo	No responses; identical survival
Clark et al. (80)[a]	Total	98	20 mg/day ± ara-C versus no treatment	Improved survival in RA group??

[a]Randomized study; CR, complete remission; PR, partial remission.

(see Table 2). In other MDS categories, no single variable or combinations of variables, including cytogenetics, predicts the response (77). Additional large-scale studies would be necessary to identify subpopulations of MDS likely to respond.

The toxicity with this treatment is not negligible. High doses administered over prolonged periods are associated with hepatotoxicity, skin and mucous membrane dryness, myalgia, drowsiness, headache, and attention defects. In view of the remarkable responses and acceptable toxicity with all-*trans*-retinoic acid in APL, trials in MDS would be justified. Perhaps all-*trans*-retinoic acid is less toxic in vivo, and higher doses may be better tolerated.

Because retinoids induce differentiation of more mature monocytoid cell lines (60), the use of 13-*cis*-retinoic acid in patients with CMML (4–6) is appealing. CMML shares characteristics with MDS (trilineage dysplasia) and MPD (leukocytosis) (1–7). It is not known whether the monocytic component represents a response to the expansion of the malignant clone, or whether it is a major part of the malignant clone. The latter may be supported by recent studies showing a high frequency of mutated *ras* oncogene in patients with CMML (81). In contrast, malignant cells from Philadelphia chromosome-positive CML show a low frequency of *ras* mutation (81,82). These findings support the notion that CMML is a specific entity and, as such, should be treated differently. Retinoic acid has been used in a few patients with CMML, and the results are inconclusive (71–80). One patient with CMML had normalization of platelet counts repeatedly obtained after treatment with 13-*cis*-retinoic acid (47). In view of the poor prognosis of CMML, trials with 13-*cis*-retinoic acid or all-*trans*-retinoic acid, in combination with chemotherapy or other inducers of monocytic differentiation (e.g., interferon gamma) are worthwhile. In vitro studies in the HL60 cell line suggest that combinations of 13-*cis*-retinoic acid with tumor necrosis factor-alpha (TNF) or interferon gamma act synergistically as differentiation inducers (83,84). Neither such combinations nor combinations of retinoic acid with chemotherapeutic agents have yet been explored in clinical trials.

Interferons

Both the natural and recombinant forms of interferon alpha (IFN-α) and gamma (IFN-γ) have been used with varying success in hematological malignancies (85), including hairy cell leukemia, chronic myelogenous leukemia, and multiple myeloma (85–88). This prompted its use in MDS. In one study, fourteen patients with MDS (2 RA, 1 RARS, 9 RAEB, 2 CMML) were treated with recombinant IFN-α, 1.5–2.0 $\times$ 10^6 units/m^2 three times weekly for 2 weeks, every 4 weeks. No complete or partial remissions were reported. A transient improvement in platelet counts was noted in 5 patients and transient antileukemic effect in 1 patient with CMML (89). In 6 patients, the disease progressed during therapy (89). Similar results were reported by Galvani et al. (90) in eight patients treated with a more intensive regimen consisting of 3×10^6 units daily of interferon alpha-1 (Welferon) for up to 6 months: only one patient with RAEB had a partial response (90). A limited Phase II trial of IFN-α at our institution also failed to achieve lasting hematological benefits in five patients with MDS. Besides nonspecific side effects, IFN-α often results in an aggravation of neutropenia and thrombocytopenia, which limits its use in this group of disorders. Whether high doses of IFN-α, given along with platelet support and prophylactic antibiotics, would lead to a suppression of the MDS clone and restoration of normal hematopoiesis is unknown.

The ability of IFN-γ to induce functional maturation in some cell systems, along with its antiproliferative activity (83–85, 91–93), justified a trial of IFN-γ in MDS and smoldering AML. In an initial trial of purified, natural IFN-γ in four patients with smoldering AML or MDS, one complete cytogenetic remission was obtained in a patient with RAEB/AML (94). In another patient with smoldering AML and 46,XY,t(8;21) karyotype, IFN-γ resulted in a decrease in white blood cell counts and a shift toward the more mature cells, suggesting both antiproliferative and differentiation-inducing actions (94).

Given these results, 24 patients with MDS or smoldering leukemia were subsequently treated at our institution (Beran M, unpublished) with recombinant human IFN-γ (rHuIFN-γ, *E. coli* product). In 15 previously untreated MDS patients who received between 0.125 and 0.50 mg/m^2 intravenously or intramuscularly daily for at least 4 weeks, no hematological benefits were observed. The maximal tolerated dose of rHuIFN-γ in MDS patients appears to be 0.5 mg/m^2 daily. Aggravation of neutropenia and thrombocytopenia, along with fever, weight loss, and fatigue were the most serious problems. These results are consistent with the findings of Stone and associates, who observed no hematological responses among six patients treated with rHuIFN-γ for MDS or AML (95). These results are in contrast with those in myeloproliferative disorders, such as CML, for which rHuIFN-γ showed activity (97,98).

Among the nine patients treated for smoldering, previously untreated, or relapsing leukemia, one patient achieved a CR lasting 18 months and another had long-lasting reduction of the marrow leukemia infiltrate. As with natural IFN-γ, the onset of these responses was slow, and CR was obtained after IFN-γ was given intravenously at 0.25 mg/m^2 daily for at least 28 days. Both patients responding to rHuIFN-γ had hypo- or normocellular marrows, and blasts were undifferentiated by morphology and cytochemistry (Beran M et al., unpublished results).

Under these conditions, the responses to IFN-α and to IFN-γ in MDS are rare, at the expense of considerable toxicity owing to aggravation of an already existing thrombocytopenia and neutropenia. Their use for remission maintenance deserves further exploration, since low-intensity maintenance chemotherapy does not prevent relapse, and intensive consolidation therapy is poorly tolerated in elderly patients.

The use of combinations of interferons with other biological agents or chemotherapy has not been explored systematically. In a pilot study, a combination of INF-α with low-dose cytarabine (ara-C) and retinoic acid was reported to produce remissions (96). These results, however are no different from those obtained with ara-C alone (99). Although biological agents including interferons, retinoic acid, vitamin D analogues and, lately, hematopoietic growth factors have failed to consistently induce complete remissions, or at least a sustained multilineage hematological improvement in overt MDS, their value in maintaining remissions achieved by other approaches (e.g., chemotherapy or bone marrow transplantation) might be more promising.

Low-Dose Chemotherapy

Myelodysplastic syndromes affect preponderantly elderly patients, their median age, being 65–75 years (1,3,20–27,100). Only 5–10% of patients are younger than 50 years of age. The frequent presence of associated medical problems, poor performance status, and multiple organ dysfunctions, explain the cautious approach to chemotherapeutic intervention, despite the generally disappointing results with supportive care only.

A new surge in the search for innovative treatments sprung from two pertinent observations: (1) that MDS is a group of disorders with maturation arrest within one or more hematopoietic lineages, and (2) experimental observations that certain murine and human leukemic cell lines differentiate under the effect of numerous chemical compounds, including chemotherapeutic agents such as dactinomycin (actinomycin D), 6-mercaptopurine, 5-azacitidine, 6-thioguanine, doxorubicin, and, in particular, with one of the most potent antileukemic agents available, cytarabine (ara-C) (101–109). Most of the differentiation-inducing cytotoxic agents are inhibitors of DNA synthesis (106,108), and their ability to induce differentiation of leukemic cells in vitro is limited (101–108). Nonetheless, they may induce phenotypic changes consistent with maturation in primary leukemic cells (110–112). As with biological agents, induction of differentiation with cytotoxic agents occurs in leukemic cell lineages that have some degree of maturation. Although in vitro studies were performed in cell lines derived from AML the clinical applications occurred primarily in MDS, in which maturation arrest of the pathological clone is less pronounced than in AML (1–3, 113). Furthermore, because of the fewer therapeutic options in MDS, the possibility of exploiting induction of differentiation in vivo as a treatment modality was rapidly translated into clinical practice.

There were several appealing aspects to this approach. By inducing differentiation, the abnormal clone may generate mature cells which, although not functionally normal, still may contribute to an improvement in the abnormal functions of the hematopoietic system in MDS. Since, in experimental systems, an increased differentiation is often accompanied by a decreased size of the malignant precursor pool (108), it was also hoped that by shifting the balance toward differentiation, the malignant clone might slowly "differentiate out" and, eventually, be replaced by normal stem cells surviving in a quiescent state and capable of resuming a coordinated self-renewal and differentiation. Through this mechanism, a complete remission could be achieved, without a major aplasia and the life-threatening side effects that often result from standard or high-dose antileukemic treatment. The genuine cytotoxic effect of drugs used for the foregoing purpose was expected to be of minor importance at the low-dose protracted schedules used.

The first success with such treatment strategy using low-dose cytarabine (LD ara-C) was reported a decade ago in a patient with RAEB. An improvement of blood cell production, without observation of aplasia in bone marrow, which remained hypercellular and retained some degree of dysplasia, was interpreted as a possible consequence of induction of differentiation by ara-C, rather than suppression of the abnormal clone and partial restoration of normal hematopoiesis (114). Subsequently, several reports confirmed that hematological improvements (115–117) and objective complete remissions (118) can be obtained in patients with advanced MDS (RAEB, RAEBT). Variable degrees of myelosuppression and marrow aplasia were noted, but there was no direct evidence supporting induction of differentiation as a mechanism of action. In one study, cytogenetic abnormalities persisted in three MDS patients during the hematological improvement (117). These observations were followed by numerous reports on the use of LD ara-C (99,119–148). Pilot studies in MDS frequently sought to evaluate the mechanisms of action of LD ara-C (i.e., differentiation versus cytotoxicity).

The evaluation of the experience with LD ara-C is hampered by (1) the heterogeneity of MDS; (2) the diagnostic uncertainties in some reports; (3) the variations in the ara-C daily dose (5–30 mg/m^2), length of treatment (1 week to >30 days courses), mode of administration (subcutaneous, intravenous); and (4) the maintenance therapy.

Recently, two groups attempted to critically evaluate the published results on LD ara-C in MDS. The first (149) analyzed data on 129 patients with MDS entered on studies from 1979 through 1986. The authors concluded that the overall CR and PR rates were 24% and 27%, respectively. Although they considered the results "encouraging," it was noted that the duration of responses was brief (CR durations 5–9 months; PR duration 3–6 months) (149). The second study reviewed 53 publications reported between 1979 and 1986 on 170 patients with primary MDS (150) and was, to a large extent, based on the same reports as the first one (149). The reviewers concluded that CR and PR rates in primary

Table 3 Low-Dose Chemotherapy in Patients with MDS: Results of Single-Institution Trials Involving More Than 20 Patients

	Treatment dose/schedule		
	Powell et al. (147)	MDACC (146)	MDACC[b]
Patient characteristics	ara-C 10 mg/m^2 SC q12h × ≤42 days	ara-C 7.5mg/m^2 SC q12h × 21 days	ara-C 15 mg/m^2 IV over 24 hr qd × 14–21 days Daunorubicin 30 mg/m^2 IV, day 1 + 7
Patients elegible	40	25	29
Sex (male/female)	23/17	14/11	21/8
Median age (range; yr)	68(29–87)	64(42–99)	66(43–82)
≤50	NA	4	3
Diagnosis (%)			
RA with cytopenia	0	1(4)	3(11)
RAEB	28(70)	9(36)	14(48)
RAEBt	8(20)	15(60)	12(41)
CMML	4(10)	0	0

Early death (%)	4(11)	1(4)	3(11)[a]
Abnormal cytogenetics (%)	10/19 (53)	16/24 (66)	16/29 (55)
Previous therapy yes (%)	4/(10)	2(8)	9(34)
Secondary MDS %	?	6(24)	6(20)
CR (%)	9(24)	9(36)	14(48)
PR (%)	4(11)	2(8)	1(4)
CR duration: median (range) (mo)	9.8(2.4–17.9)	16(1.5–47+)	6.5(1–27)

[a]One in CR.
[b] Compiled unpublished data from M. D. Anderson Cancer Center and (99).
NA, data not available.

MDS were 16% and 25%, respectively. There was no clear-cut advantage for continuous infusion versus subcutaneous modes of administration (CR rates 15% versus 20%, respectively). However, only 15 patients had received intravenous treatment (150). The median CR duration, calculated from data available on only 17 patients, was 10 months, and the median survival was 15 months. No reliable information was obtained on the association between response and survival, but "little evidence was found that achieving a CR exerted a substantial influence on survival" (150). Both reviews concluded that, despite the many patients treated, the deficiencies in the designs of studies prevented any firm conclusions about the advantage of LD ara-C treatment over supportive care.

The major questions to be answered with LD ara-C in MDS are (1) the frequency of response, (2) the quality of response, (3) the duration of response, and (4) the impact on the survival or the natural course in various subcategories of MDS. Ideally, these questions should be answered in the context of the biology of the disease, aiming to identify patients likely to benefit from this treatment modality.

Two studies involving large numbers of patients from single institutions suggest the usefulness of LD ara-C in (1) patients with more aggressive types of MDS (RAEB, RAEBT), and (2) patients with fewer than 5% blasts out with pancytopenia (Table 3). In one study (147), 38 evaluable patients with MDS received 10 mg/m^2 of ara-C twice daily for up to 42 days (median 27, range 2–42 days): 24% achieved CR, and 11% had PR. The median duration of CR was 10 months (range 2.5–18 months). No correlation was found between response or CR duration and pretreatment characteristics. A significant difference in survival was found between responders and nonresponders. Interestingly, only a fraction of patients became aplastic with the treatment, and there was no significant correlation between the degree of reduction of marrow cellularity by chemotherapy and the ability to reach CR. These results are better than those reported in numerous smaller trials and are in agreement with our own experience in patients with "higher-risk" MDS. In our first study (see Table 3) (99,126), ara-C was given for 21 days every 6 weeks. The results are summarized in Table 3. Upon achieving CR or PR, patients were maintained with ara-C for 8 days every month for up to 1 year. Upon relapse, they were often retreated with a 21-day course of LD ara-C. Overall, CR was observed in nine patients (36%); the median duration was 16 months (range 1.5–47+ months). Two (8%) patients had a PR or a hematological improvement. All patients needed platelet support for severe thrombocytopenia. There was one treatment-related death of a cerebral hemorrhage. In agreement with the report of Powell et al. (147), we have observed a higher response rate compared with previously published data.

The quality of remissions, vis-a-vis the persistence of the MDS clone, was studied by (1) karyotypic analyses and (2) by invitro growth of granulocyte–macrophage progenitor cells (GM-CFC) before and after therapy. In all patients achieving CR, the bone marrow studies indicated suppression of the pathological clone, as detected either by disappearance of the cytogenetic marker or changes in the in vitro growth pattern of GM-CFC from abnormal to "normal." There was a correlation between the absence of cytogenic marker and normalization of in vitro growth of GM-CFC (99) (Table 4). This finding is important in patients with diploid karyotype who constituted the majority of patients achieving CR. All of the diploid patients had abnormal GM-CFC growth before treatment that normalized upon achieving CR. With one exception, all patients relapsed. Invariably, the relapse was associated with initial cytopenia and aggravation of bone marrow dysplasia, in vitro GM-CFC growth abnormalities, and reappearance of the same cytogenetic marker as seen before treatment (Beran, unpublished).

Because of the heterogeneity of MDS, we sought biological features that would be associated with response by analyzing response to LD ara-C in relation to the initial degree of anemia, thrombocytopenia, marrow blast infiltration, FAB classification, in vitro growth of GM-CFC, and bone marrow karyotype. In this group, karyotype was the only pretreatment feature associated with response (Table 5) ($p = 0.06$) (99).

All patients who achieving CR or PR had normalized blood counts and experienced a major improvement in their quality of life. The survival of patients achieving CR was significantly longer than that of those who failed treatment ($p < 0.003$) (Fig. 1). When the observed survival was compared with the expected survival of patients based on a multivariate–analysis-derived prognostic model, the observed survival was improved in responders (115 weeks versus expected 90 weeks), but not in nonresponders.

Eighty percent of patients achieved CR did so after one course of chemotherapy. This suggests that patients who fail after one course of LD ara-C may be given the option of early change of therapy. There is a significant dose–response relationship with LD ara-C. Twelve of the 13 patients achieving CR relapsed on maintenance LD ara-C regimen given for 8 days every month. Three of them (25%) were reinduced into CR with a 3-week ara-C treatment using identical daily doses. Thus, either the total dose of ara-C, or the exposure duration, are important for response.

Given these findings, we initiated a second trial of LD ara-C (15 mg/m^2 daily by continuous infusion for 2 weeks), given with daunorubicin 30 mg/m^2 intravenously on days 1 and 7 of each course. Eligible patients had either previously untreated MDS or had relapsed on the LD ara-C regimen. The results are summarized in Tables 3, 4 and 5. The study confirmed the dose–response relationship in MDS (Fig. 2): several patients who failed induction after 3 weeks of LD ara-C achieved a CR with the addition of daunorubicin. Two patients who failed induction with LD ara-C alone achieved CR and PR, respectively, with this induction, and four patients with RAEB or RAEBT, who relapsed on LD ara-C maintenance regimen were reinduced into CR with the combination of

Table 4 Suppression of the Pathological Clone of MDS in Remission as Measured by Cytogenetics and In Vitro Growth Pattern of Marrow GM–CFC[a]

		Before treatment		In complete remission	
Case	FAB	Cytogenetics	GM-CFC Growth pattern	Cytogenetics	GM-CSF Growth pattern
Low-dose-cytarabine					
1.	RAEB	46,XY	No growth	46,XY	Normal growth
2.	RAEBT	46,XX	No growth	46,XX	Normal growth
3.	RAEBT	46,XX	Excess clusters	46,XX	Normal growth
4.	RAEBT	46,XX	Excess clusters	46,XX	Normal growth
5.	RAEB	46,XY	No growth	46,XY	Normal growth
6.	RAEB	11q-	No growth	46,XY	Normal growth
7.	RAEB	+8	No growth	46,XY	Normal growth
8.	RAEBT	–7	Excess clusters	46,XX	Normal growth
Low-dose cytarabine plus daunorubicin					
1.	RAEB	46,XX	Excess clusters	46,XX	Normal growth
2.	RAEBT	+8	No growth	46,XY	Normal growth
3.	RAEBT	IM	No growth	46,XX	Normal growth
4.	RAEBT	IM	No growth	46,XX	Normal growth
5.	RAEBT	KI-5, –7	Excess clusters	Diploid 70%[b] –5, –7 30%	Normal growth[b]
6.	RAEB	5q-	Excess clusters	5q-[c]	Excess clusters[c]

[a]Results compiled from studies at our institution.
[b]Relapsed 1 month after study.
[c]In hematological CR, relapsed 2 months after study.

Table 5 Response to Low-Dose Chemotherapy by Pretreatment Karyotype in MDS

Karyotype	No. of evaluable patients	No. CR(%)	Median CR duration (range in mo)	Median survival (range in mo)
Low-dose ara-C				
Diploid	5	4(80)	10(17–69)	12.5(9.5–74+)
Karotypic abnormalities	20	6(30)	12.5(6–47)	8.0(3.0–51+)
Involving 5,7	11	1(9)		
Involving +8	3	1(33)		
Others	4	1(25)		
IM[a]	2	2(100)		
Total	25	9(36)	16.5(1.5–47+)	18(3–43+)
sMDS	5	2(40)		
Low-dose ara-C + daunorubicin				
Diploid	11	9(82)	6.5(0.5–29)	18(2–40)
Karyotypic abnormalities	17	7(41)	11.0(4–40)	14.0(2–40)
Involving 5,7	11	1(9)		
Involving +8	5	3(60)		
Others	1	0(0)		
IM	1	1(100)		
Total	29	13(44)	6.5(2–28)	16.5(2–48)

[a]insufficient metaphases

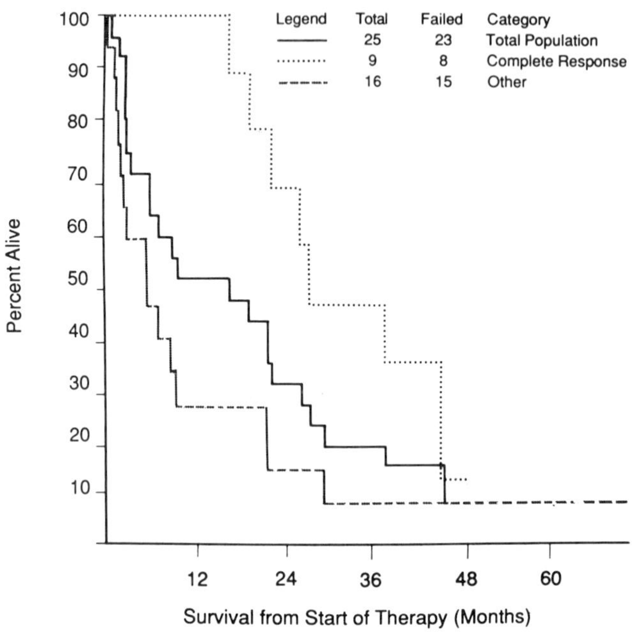

Figure 1 Survival in MDS patients treated with low-dose cytarabine (LD ara-C), overall, and by response.

daunorubicin and LD ara-C. The toxicities of the two regimens were similar. Thrombocytopenia and associated bleeding were the major risk factors and required extensive platelet support. With an opposite approach of attenuating a standard antileukemic regimen, Owens et al. (152) reported similar promising preliminary results in MDS.

The mechanism of action of LD ara-C in MDS remains debatable. Most evidence favors the suppression of the MDS clone (i.e., a cytotoxic effect, as a prerequisite for achievement of a durable CR; (see Table 4) (99,128,129,134). There is, however, convincing evidence in some patients, for in vivo differentiation of the leukemic or MDS clones, demonstrated by the premature chromosome condensation technique (153–155), which showed unequivocally aneuploid karyotypes in mature granulocytes. The extent to which ara-C can "differentiate out" the pathological clone and induce remission is undetermined, but it is not frequent (128,129,138).

Intensive Chemotherapy

In a retrospective analysis of the results of antileukemic chemotherapy in 20 patients with RAEB (13 patients) or CMML (7 patients), Armitage and co-

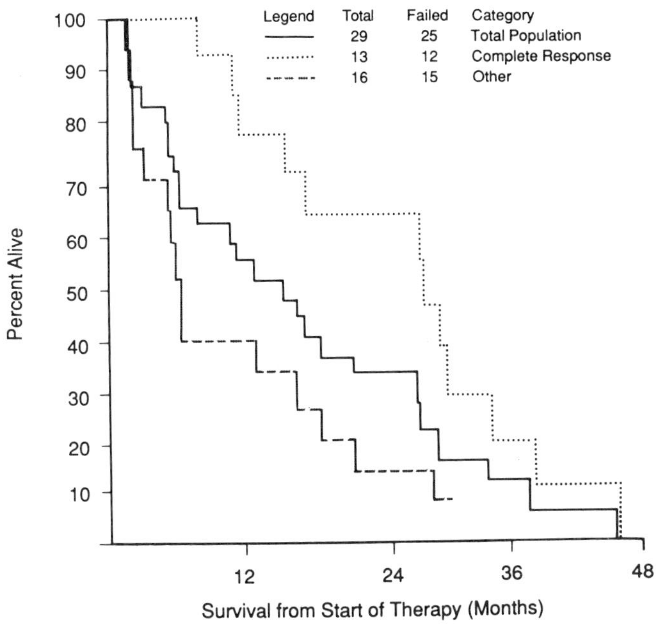

Figure 2 Survival of MDS patients treated with daunorubicin and low-dose cytarabine, overall, and by response.

workers (156) reported 3 CRs, all in patients with RAEB. The patients not responding to intensive chemotherapy had a shortened survival, compared with a group of untreated MDS patients. The authors suggested that a subgroup of young MDS patients, with no history of previous cytotoxic therapy, may benefit from intensive antileukemic therapy, but that most patients may have a worse prognosis with intensive chemotherapy. Subsequently, several investigators reported their results with intensive chemotherapy in MDS (157–165) (Table 6). Even though all are based on small numbers of patients, they yielded interesting data pertinent to the management of MDS.

Tricot et al. (160) treated nine patients with RAEB or RAEBT with a combination of daunorubicin and conventional-dose ara-C, or with high-dose ara-C. All five patients younger than 60 years achieved CR, compared with one of four patients older than 60 years. The karyotype in all responders was diploid or showed insufficient mitoses. Nonresponders tended to have abnormal karyotypes. Age, however, did not appear to be important in the study of Fenaux and associates (162), who treated 20 patients with MDS using zorubicin (Rubidazone), 200 mg/m^2 daily for 3–4 days, and ara-C, 200 mg/m^2 daily for 5–7 days. The CR rates were 41% in 12 patients younger than 50 years and 62% in 8 patients older than 50 years. The duration of CR tended to be longer in younger

Table 6 Intensive Chemotherapy in Myelodysplastic Syndromes: Summary of Published Results

Study (Ref.)	No. of patients	FAB category at the onset of treatment/ no. of patients	CR(%)	Fail(%)	Induction death (%)	CR Duration (mo)	Survival from onset of treatment (mo)
Armitage (156) et al.	13	RAEB/13	3(21)	8(61)	2(15)	14,34+,37+	31,35+,37+
Tricot (160) et al.	9	RAEB/3 RAEBT/6	6(66)		3(33)	8,11,12,12,12, 14+	NA
Fenaux (162) et al.	20	RAEB/2 RAEBT/16 CMML/2	10(50)	4(20)	6(30)	1+,2+,2.5,4,5,5, 9+,13,25+,28	2,2+,4,10,10+,11+ 14,18,26+,50
Preisler (161) et al.	6	NA	1(16)	2(32)	3(50)	NA	NA
Mertelsman (157) et al.	45	RAEB/31 CMML/14	14(45) 9(64)	NA NA	NA NA	8.4^b 6.2^b	9.0^b 11.4^b
Dohy (163) et al.	6	RAEB	2(33)	2(33)	2(33)	NA	NA
MDACC[a]	17	RAEB/2 RAEBt/14 CMMLt/1	9(53)	2(12)	6(35)	1+–20+	0.5–22+

[a]Unpublished data, compiled from results in patients treated at MD Anderson Cancer Center 1987–1989.
[b]Median; CR, complete remission; NA, data not available.

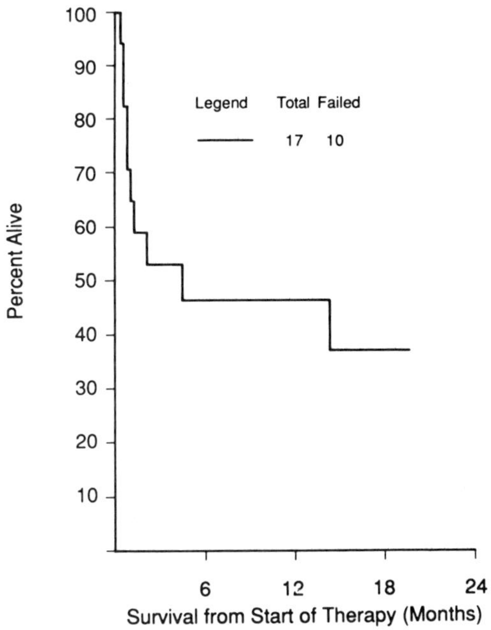

Figure 3 Survival of patients with MDS treated with intensive chemotherapy.

patients (162). The early death rate was similar in younger and older patients (4/12 and 3/8, respectively). Patients with a diploid karyotype had a higher frequency of response and a longer CR duration (162).

Since 1987, 17 patients with MDS have been treated with intensive chemotherapy by our group (Table 7, Fig 3). Fourteen patients had a diagnosis of RAEBT, 2 had RAEB, and 1 had CMML in transformation (CMML-T). Thirteen patients received high-dose ara-C, either alone or in combination with amsacrine. Nine patients achieved CR (70%), 7 of them after one course (see Table 7). Age and karyotype were the most important prognostic factors for both remission induction and survival. Only one CR of short duration (3 months) was achieved in 7 patients (14%) older than 60 years. The "poor prognosis" karyotypes were more frequently associated with advanced age. In patients younger than 50 years, diploid or favorable [t(8;21); t(15;17); inversion 16] karyotypes were associated with a CR rate of 80% (Fig. 4), which is comparable with the results of similar subsets of patients with de novo AML treated with intensive chemotherapy at our institution (see Table 7).

The results of other studies are shown in Table 6. In general, they strongly

Table 7 Results of Intensive Chemotherapy in Patients with MDS at M. D. Anderson Cancer Center[a]

Patient characteristics	No. patients	No. CR(%)	CR duration (wk)	Survival (wk)
Age, median (range)				
All; 44(24–76)	17	9(53)	3+–80+	1–85+
<50 yr; 40 (24–49)	10	8(80)	6 –80+	4–85+
≥50 yr; 70 (63–76)	7	1(14)	3+	1–10+
Karyotype[b]				
Favorable	3	3(100)	6,36,58	9,62,62
Intermediate	7	6(86)	3+,8,12+,67, 67+,80+	3,10+,18+, 25+,72+, 73, 85+
Poor	7	0(0)	0	1,2,2,3,4,5,19
FAB category				
RAEB	2	2(100)	6,67+	9,72+
RAB ET	14	7(50)	3+,8,12+, 36,58,67,67+	1,2,3,4,5,10+, 18+,19,25,62, 62+,73,73+, 85
CMMLT	1	0(0)	0	2

[a]Unpublished data, compiled from results in patients treated at M. D. Anderson Cancer Center 1987–1989.
[b]Favorable karyotype includes t:[15;17}, t:[8;21] and inversion 16; intermediate include diploid patients and insufficient metaphases; poor karyotype include all others.

suggest that intensive chemotherapy yields favorable results in younger patients with diploid or favorable karyotypes.

Bone Marrow Transplantation

An extremely poor prognosis is observed in patients with MDS characterized by unfavorable cytogenetic abnormalities (deletions or missing chromosomes 5, 7, or 21; trisomy 8; complex and unstable karyotypic abnormalities). In these patients, no long-term survival is achieved. The prognosis of patients with

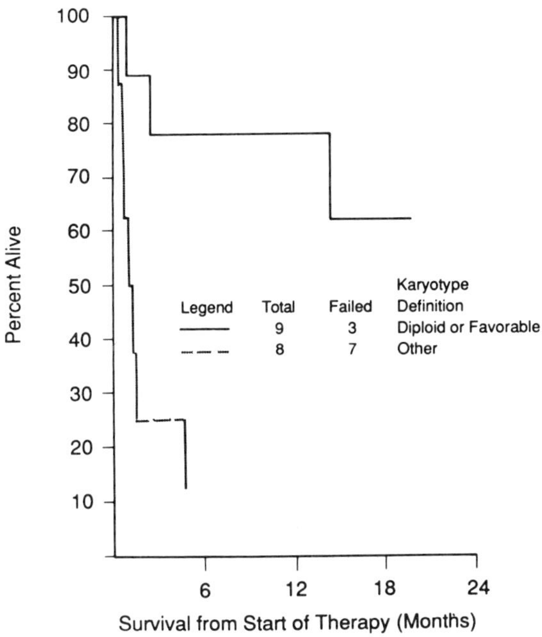

Figure 4 Survival of patients with MDS treated with intensive chemotherapy by karyotype. A favorable karyotype includes t(15;17), inversion 16, and t(8;21).

secondary MDS is also extremely poor. For them, alternative treatments with a curative potential are indicated.

Experience with syngeneic and allogeneic transplantation in MDS is limited (169–178) (Table 8). In 1984, Appelbaum et al. (169) first reported on ten patients with MDS treated with allogeneic bone marrow transplantation (BMT). Seven patients prepared with cyclophosphamide (CY) and total body irradiation (TBI) showed marrow engraftment, whereas three prepared with CY alone relapsed within 6 months after transplantation. This suggested that CY alone, although successfully used in aplastic anemia, was unable to eradicate the abnormal clone in MDS. Six of the seven patients conditioned with CY plus TBI were alive with no evidence of disease from 7 to 25 months after transplant. These results were encouraging, particularly in that seven of ten patients had cytogenetic abnormalities involving chromosomes 7 or 8.

Recently, a summary of the European experience (173,174) with allogeneic BMT in 31 patients with primary MDS confirmed the experience of Applebaum et al. (169,170). Allogeneic BMT in young patients with MDS in "preleukemic" phase was feasible, and the prognosis favorable, if performed before the de-

Table 8 Allogeneic Bone Marrow Transplantation in MDS

Study (Ref.)	No. of Patients	Median (range) (in yr)	Median time to transplant in months (range)	Conditioning regimen	Relapse No.	Relapse (mo)	DFS No.	DFS (mo)
Appelbaum et al. (169)	10	29(4–54)	6(2–50)	Cy or Cy +TBI	3		7	(12+–215+)
Forman et al. (176)	14	36(4–48)	4.5(3–48)	TBI+chemotherapy or chemotherapy	3		5	(30+–85+)
Belanger et al. (172)	8	34.5(3–35)	6.5(3–30)	BU +Cy Cy + TBI	1	(6.5)	5	(9+–35+)
Kolb et al. (175)	7	24(3–47)	12(3–37)	Cy + TBI Bu + Cy	1	(3)	4	(8+–37+)

DFS, disease-free survival; CY, cyclophosphamide; BU, busulfan; TBI, total body irradiation.

velopment of leukemia. The 2-year disease-free survivals among 10 patients with RAEBT and 12 patients with RAEB were 50% and 64%, respectively (173,174) (Table 9).

The updated results from the Seattle group on bone marrow transplantation in MDS confirmed their previous experience, with 40–50% of patients with MDS being long-term, disease-free survivors (178). Favorable prognostic factors for outcome of transplantation were (1) a younger patient age, (2) the presence of chromosomal abnormalities, (3) MDS subgroup of RA, (4) absence of marrow fibrosis (Table 10). In patients younger than 30 years, disease-free survival and overall survival were significantly better than in older patients. This was mainly due to a decreased incidence of nonmalignant death, rather than to relapse. No relapses were observed in RA patients or in patients with hypoplastic marrow and abnormal karyotype, whereas the probability of relapse was 45% in patients transplanted for RAEB or RAEBT. This may be related to the increased tumor burden in these categories. A high degree of fibrosis in MDS (grade 3–4) had a negative effect on outcome. The results in six patients with secondary MDS were similar to those in patients with primary MDS. In contrast with the results with both low-dose and intensive chemotherapy, the presence of clonal cytogenetic abnormality was paradoxically favorable. This appeared to be due to differences in nonrelapse deaths. Finally, patients with a shorter duration of the disease before transplant had slightly better survival, disease-free survival, and fewer nonrelapse deaths. Promising results were also reported in patients who received transplants with partially HLA-matched and unrelated-HLA-matched donor marrows: 6 of 14 such patients were alive, compared with 22 of 45 genotypically matched transplant patients (178).

Whether cytoreductive treatment with conventional chemotherapy should be attempted before transplantation remains to be determined. The severely compromised immunological status of MDS patients with defective monocyte–

Table 9 EGBMT Survey on Allogeneic Bone Marrow Transplantation for MDS

Disease	No. of patients	No. of transplant-related mortality	No. of relapses	2-yr disease-free survival
RAS	9	2	0	58
RAEB	12	2	3	64
RAEBT	10	2	2	50

MDS, myelodysplastic syndromes; EGBMT, European Group for Bone Marrow Transplantation; RAS, refractory anemia with ring sideroblasts; RAEB, refactory anemia with excess of blasts; RAEBT, RAEB in transformation.
Source: Ref. 173.

Table 10 Prognostic Factors in Allogenic Bone Marrow Transplantation in the MDS: Seattle Experience

		Relapse			Nonrelapse death		Disease-free survival (DFS)		
Disease variable	No. of patients	N	Time to relapse (mo)	Actuarial probality[a]	N	Actuarial probality[a] at 3 yr	N	Time (mo)	Probability at 3 yr[a]
MDS, ALL[b]	59	8	0.5–26	23(10–39)	23	43	28	12–215	45(35–59)
RA	17			0		47			53
RAEB	24			36		44			40
RAEBT	6			50		0			50
Primary	53			23(9–38)		43(29–57)			45(31–51)
Secondary	6			20(1–95)		37(13–98)			50(1–70)
Karyotype									
Diploid	15			33		67			11
Abnormal	6			20		31			57
Age (yr)									
<20	12			20		17			67
20–29	16			20		27			59
30–39	21			24		60			30
>40	10			36		65			30

[a]Percentage: 3-yr product-limit estimate; 95% CI in parentheses.
[b]Forty-seven patients with FAB classified MDS, 4 patients with myelofibrosis, and 6 patients with cytogenetic abnormality in aplastic bone marrow.
Source: Ref. 178.

granulocyte functions might increase their risk of death with severe myelosuppression when chemotherapy is attempted to reduce tumor burden before transplantation. This, and the extent of supportive–care-only before BMT, are critical problems to be clarified.

Another question relates to the categories of MDS for which patients should be treated by transplantation. The known natural history of MDS and experience with chemotherapy support the idea of giving transplants to otherwise eligible patients with a diagnosis of RAEB, RAEBT, and CMML, regardless of karyotype. Patients with RA, with or without neutropenia or thrombocytopenia, represent a more difficult category. Those with poor-prognosis karyotypes, and those with cytopenia-related complications should also be considered for transplantation. On the other hand, elderly patients with diploid RA or RARS may follow a relatively benign course for many years with conventional therapy.

Patients with secondary (therapy-related) MDS have a poor prognosis. Probably this is related to (1) the presence of a more aggressive malignant clone, evidenced by an increased frequency of abnormal karyotypes (15,179,180); (2) a high frequency of transformation into AML; and (3) a compromised normal marrow stem cell pool from previous chemotherapy. Since this patient population is often younger than patients with de novo MDS, all patients with secondary MDS eligible for allogeneic BMT should receive transplants as soon as possible after diagnosis, regardless of the karyotype or severity of the disease (178). Once the secondary MDS develops into an acute leukemia, transplantation results are poor compared with relapsed de novo AML (173,174). In patients with secondary AML in which allogenic BMT was performed in CR induced by polychemotherapy, the results are comparable with those in patients with de novo AML who received transplants during CR (173,174). This may be due to in vivo selection of patients with more sensitive disease by chemotherapy before transplantation.

Hematopoietic Growth Factors

Two questions are relevant to the use of hematopoietic growth factors in MDS: (1) Is the extent of the endogenous production of such factors decreased, in particular in the bone marrow microenvironment; and (2) is the response of stem cells and their progeny to these factors inherently abnormal and caused by lower sensitivity secondary to either receptor defects or defects in the signal transmission?

Genetically engineered human hematopoietic growth factors, such as granulocyte–macrophage colony-stimulating factor (rHuGM-CSF) (181), granulocyte colony-stimulating factor (rHuG-CSF) (182,183), interleukin-3 (rHuIL-3) (184), and erythropoietin (rHuEPO) (185), are now available for clinical use. This has offered opportunities to investigate the second question; namely, can lineage-related maturation defects and cell production be corrected by administration of factors known to exercise such effects on hematopoietic cells in vitro (186)? The in vivo approach is complex, since interactions between factors and cells can lead to induction of secondary factors. Although it is difficult to assess the in vivo mechanisms of action of growth factors, the endpoints are measurable in terms of cell lineage specificity and quantity and quality of produced mature cells.

rHuGM-CSF and rHuG-CSF

The in vivo effects of rHuGM-CSF in patients with MDS were initially reported by Vadhan-Raj et al. (187,188) and subsequently confirmed by other groups (189–192) (Table 11). The initial trials used rHuGM-CSF given intravenously daily, in various schedules over a limited time. The most characteristic feature of response of MDS patients to rhuGM-CSF was a rapid dose-dependent rise in the white blood cells (WBC). Although neutrophilia accounts for most of the leukocytosis, eosinophilia is common and, in some patients, the absolute numbers of monocytes and T and B lymphocytes increase as well (see Table 11) (187–196). The kinetic characteristics of the neutrophilic response suggest that several mechanisms might be involved. The initial rise is probably due to a shift in the marginated pool and a release of granulocytes from bone marrow compartment. Although a multilineage response to GM-CSF is occasionally observed, lasting and clinically significant increases in platelet counts or correction of anemia are uncommon (187–192, 194) (see Table 11). In fact, a decrease in platelet counts may be observed in some patients after intravenous or subcutaneous administration of rHuGM-CSF (194). Recurrence of immune thrombocytopenia has been associated with the administration of rHuGM-CSF (197). Thrombocytopenia, granulocytopenia, and the associated bleeding and infectious complications are the major causes of morbidity and mortality in MDS patients (197,198).

The ability of GM-CSF (187–192), and G-CSF (200,201,208) to increase granulocyte production could potentially control the infections in MDS. Besides stimulating proliferation of granulocyte, eosinophil, and monocyte precursors, and production of mature effector cells, GM-CSF also enhances various functions of mature neutrophils, monocytes, and eosinophils (202–206). This may be of importance in MDS patients with known granulocyte function defects (198–199, 209–211). In a murine bone marrow transplant model, mice injected with *Salmonella typhimurium* showed increased resistance to injections and prolonged survival when receiving intraperitoneal GM-CSF twice daily for 18 days (207). Whether the elevation of neutrophils and other white blood cells after administration of CSFs indeed reduces the incidence of infections is presently being addressed in several clinical trials.

Prospective randomized studies are necessary to evaluate the ability of GM-CSF or other CSFs to modify infectious complications in the course of MDS. A comparison of pretreatment frequency of infections with that during the treatment would provide an additional criterion. The overall impact of growth factor

Table 11 Phase I–II Trials of Human Granulocyte–Macrophage Colony-Stimulating Factor (HuGM-CSF) in Myelodysplastic Syndromes

	Houston (1987) (187)	Frankfurt (1989) (189)	Boston (1988) (190)	Seattle (1989) (192)
No. of patients	8	10	7	16
Median age (range)	66(39–79)		55(39–69)	59(17–80)
No. previously treated for MDS	4	1	4	7
FAB category				
RA	1	3	2	7
RARS	0	0	0	0
RAEB	3	5	4	8
RAEBT	4	0	—	1
CMML	0	2	0	0
rHuGM-CSF expressed in	Immunex yeast	Immunex yeast	Immunex yeast	*E. coli*
Treatment				
Dose ($\mu g/m^2/d$)	30–500	15–150	15–480	0.3–10 μg/kg
Schedule—daily for	14 days	7–14 days	7–14 days	10 days
Administration	24h IV	8h IV	Variable IV	Subcutaneous
No. Response				
WBC	8	10	6	10
Neutrophils	8		6	12
Eosinophils	7	6	0	12
Monocytes	8	7		10
Lymphocytes	8	10	0	4
Blasts	0	4	2	2
Platelets	3	0	0	2
Reticulocytes	8	0	7	3

therapy on morbidity, quality of life, rate of transformation to acute leukemia, and overall survival, needs careful evaluations.

An important question is whether or not growth factor therapy can accelerate the transformation to an acute leukemic phase in patients with MDS. Although the present knowledge is incomplete, it appears that patients with elevated marrow blast percentage (greater than 5 or 10%) and those with CMML have a higher incidence of growth factor therapy-associated increase of blasts, which often reverts to baseline levels with discontinuation of therapy. The leukemogenic promotion effect of growth factors, however, must be evaluated in carefully controlled clinical trials. GM-CSF appears to stimulate proliferation and differentiation of both normal and abnormal clones in MDS (212). In only one case a suppression of abnormal clone of GM-CSF have been reported (213).

The role of low-dose growth factor therapy (e.g., M G-CSF at 3–30 $\mu g/m^2$ daily) in patients with MDS requires evaluation. It is possible that a subset of patients with "mild" MDS, such as RA with a granulocyte count higher than 500/μL, may be ideal candidates for such relatively nontoxic therapy.

Side effects of GM-CSF, particularly bone discomfort or pain, are to some degree dose-dependent (187–191). The bone pain is usually localized to the spine, ribs, and pelvis, and can be severe after higher doses ($> 120\ \mu g/m^2$ per day). Flulike symptoms, with low-grade fever, myalgia, and occasionally rigors and chills, are common. Anorexia, weight loss, and nausea are also observed. Local erythematous skin reactions are common with subcutaneous therapy. (192).

The maximum tolerated dose with daily subcutaneous injection, was 10 μg/kg daily (192). At high doses, particularly after intravenous administration, fluid retention, pulmonary edema, and pericarditis are serious complications requiring discontinuation or dose adjustment of GM-CSF.

Erythropoietin

Anemia is often the first clinical symptom of MDS. In a subset of patients (RARS), it may remain the only clinical problem, the nature of which is not well understood. There is evidence suggesting a maturational defect in erythroid progenitor cells and, thus, a possible benefit from therapies with erythropoietin or other hematopoietic factors. Whether endogenous erythropoietin production and bioavailability in MDS is altered remains controversial. In recent studies in patients with MDS, plasma erythropoietin levels varied from slightly above normal to very high levels (214–216). Although they show a weak inverse relationship with hemoglobin concentration, the plasma erythropoietin levels do not always reflect the degree of anemia or total erythroid production (214).

Recombinant human erythropoietin (rHuEPO) has been successfully used to reverse anemia associated with renal failure. In transfusion-dependent patients with chronic renal failure, rHuEPO, given at 50–300 units/kg, three times weekly, increased hemoglobin levels in a dose-dependent fashion (217,218).

The response was comparable after intravenous or subcutaneous administration, and is maintained for the entire observation period (up to 1 year). No antibody response to rHuEPO was reported.

More recently, rHuEPO has been shown to raise the hematocrit in anemic patients with rheumatoid arthritis (219), and in those with acquired immune deficiency syndrome (AIDS) receiving zidovudine (AZT) (220,221). In the latter group, improvement of anemia and associated clinical symptoms was observed only in patients with low pretreatment endogenous erythropoietin level ($\leq$ 500 mU/mL); no response was seen in patients with initial high plasma levels ($>$ 500 mU/mL) (220,221).

Two recent preliminary reports suggest that rHuEPO may stimulate erythropoiesis in MDS. In three of eight patients with MDS, Hirashima et al. (222) reported improvement of anemia after intravenous injection of a total dose of 3000–24,000 units/day, three times weekly. In another study (223), two patients with RARS and one with RA and 5q– syndrome were treated with escalating doses of subcutaneous rHuEPO (40–270 units/kg per day), three times a week. Increases in reticulocyte counts, hemoglobin concentrations, and hematocrit levels were observed in both cases of RARS at a level of 120 units/kg and 240 units/kg, respectively; one of them became transfusion-independent (223). There were no increases in WBC or platelets, an observation compatible with the view that EPO acts mainly on committed erythroid precursors (186). Although preliminary, these studies suggest that some patients with MDS and anemia may benefit from rHuEPO, perhaps at higher dosages than those used in anemia of renal failure. Whether endogenous levels of EPO may predict for EPO response as seen in patients with anemia of chronic disease or in AIDS patients (220,221) is unknown. In one patient with RAEBT, the increase in hemoglobin concentration was associated with a decrease in the endogenous EPO level (222).

Given the remarkable safety of the use of rHuEPO at doses up to 150 units/kg three times weekly, EPO treatment should be investigated in patients with RA and RARS and anemia as an alternative to RBC transfusions. In these patients, chemotherapy is rarely effective and the associated risks unacceptable. Differentiation-inducing agents such as retinoids, vitamin D analogues, prednisone, and anabolic steroids have a low activity. Even though an increase in the EPO dose above 300 units/kg carries a substantial risk of hypertension in uremic patients, probably because of an increase in the peripheral resistance, similar problems may not occur in MDS patients. The dose escalation may be necessary, since the abnormal clone could be expected to display a decreased sensitivity to EPO. In patients with RAEB or RAEBT, treatment with EPO alone is probably not justified, in view of its anticipated effect on erythropoiesis only. In these patients, neutropenia and thrombocytopenia represent a far greater problem than anemia, and therapy must be directed toward the correction of the multilineage failure. Erythropoietin may prove beneficial in combination with other growth factors in a treatment-tailored approach to the individual clinical problem (i.e., EPO for anemia and G/GM-CSF for leukopenia).

Interleukin-3

Interleukin-3 (IL-3) is now available for clinical trials. In vitro studies provided evidence that the target of this molecule is a primitive progenitor cell, possibly of multilineage potential (186). This in contrast to granulocyte lineage-restricted progenitor cells responding to G-CSF and predominantly granulocyte–macrophage lineage-committed cells responding to GM-CSF. Thus, administration of IL-3 might stimulate progenitor cells capable of differentiation along granulocyte–monocyte, erythroid, and megakaryocytic pathways, and increase cell production along these pathways in MDS. Preliminary studies support, to some degree, this in vitro prediction. Ganser et al. (224) reported on 26 patients with progressive neoplasm, 7 of whom had bone marrow failure, treated with subcutaneous IL-3 at 30–500 $\mu g/m^2$ daily. An increase in platelet counts was seen in 5 of 8 patients with bone marrow failure; reticulocyte counts increased in 3, and neutrophil count in 8 of 8 evaluable patients. Kurzrock et al. (225) gave IL-3 (30–500 $\mu g/m^2$ IV) as a 4-hour infusion daily for 28 days to patients with bone marrow failure, including 7 patients with MDS. Neutrophil and eosinophil increases appear to be a common response, whereas durable increases in platelet counts and reticulocytes are rare. Multilineage responses were noted in two patients. Unlike with GM-CSF, the neutrophil responses were slow to develop, but persistent after IL-3 discontinuation. Side effects were dose-related, observed after both intravenous and subcutaneous administration, and similar to those described for GM-CSF. These preliminary results in patients with MDS are encouraging, but more extensive studies are needed to evaluate the nature and duration of responses.

Combinations of Hemotopoietic Growth Factors and Chemotherapy

Treatment of MDS with rHuGM-CSF alone increases neutrophil counts in most patients with MDS, but fails to improve platelet counts and alleviate anemia. Furthermore, in some patients with excess blasts ($> 10\%$) or monocytosis, an increase in the blast or monocytes percentages is seen with rHuGM-CSF administration, which is at times reversible after discontinuing of therapy or reducing the dose (187–196) (see Table 11). In a recent study, 22 patients were treated with GM-CSF 120 $\mu g/m^2$ daily by continuous infusion for 1–4 months. The marrow blast infiltrate doubled in 6/17 patients with RAEB or RAEBT, but in none of the patients with RA (194). Although this may have been due to the natural course of disease, GM-CSF may have stimulated the growth of an abnormal population. Thus, GM-CSF could trigger abnormal progenitors into the cell cycle and increase their sensitivity to chemotherapeutic agents, and at the same time stimulate differentiation and production of mature cells.

Combinations of GM-CSF and low-dose ara-C may test two possibilities: (1) whether GM-CSF might increase the sensitivity of the malignant clone to ara-C when given prior or concomitantly with the drug (leukemic sensitization), and

(2) whether to use GM-CSF after ara-C to hasten granulocytic recovery (supportive therapy). Preliminary results from two ongoing Phase II trials are available. Hoelzer et al. (226) reported on the concomitant use of rHuGM-CSF (250 $\mu g/m^2$ subcutaneously twice daily for 2 weeks, and ara-C, 20 mg/m^2 daily subcutaneously, given as one dose, 12 hours after GM-CSF for 2 weeks. Of nine patients with RAEB or RAEBT who completed three cycles of therapy, platelet counts improved in six patients, and the marrow blasts percentage decreased in eight patients. Increase in neutrophil counts was commonly observed. No effect on reticulocyte counts was seen, and information on remission status was not provided (226). In an ongoing EORTC study (227), patients with MDS and 10–30% marrow blasts received ara-C, 10 mg/m^2 subcutaneously twice daily for 2 weeks, and rHuGM-CSF (mammalian, glycosylated), 150 μg subcutaneously twice daily, either concomitantly with ara-C during the second week of ara-C treatment, or during the third week immediately after completion of ara-C treatment. Evaluation of 23 patients who received at least two courses showed response in 15 (65%). Eight patients achieved CR (34%) and PR was noted in 7 patients (31%). Only 1 patient progressed into AML (227). No information is available on differences between the two study arms. This information is important because, with concomitant administration, both sensitivity of progenitor cells to ara-C and their differentiation ability is influenced, whereas when GM-CSF is given *after* ara-C, it should predominantly effect recovery of hematopoiesis and differentiation.

REFERENCES

1. Bennett JM, Catovsky D, Daniel M-T, et al: Proposals for the classification of the myelodysplastic syndromes. *Br J Haematol* 1982; 57:189–199.
2. Bennett JM; Classification of the myelodysplastic syndromes. *Clin Haematol* 1986; 15:909–923.
3. Third MIC Cooperative Study Group: Recommendations for a morphologic, immunologic, and cytogenetic (MIC) working classification of primary and therapy-related myelodysplastic disorders. *Cancer Genet Cytogenet* 1988; 32:1–10.
4. Bernadou A, Zittoun R, Bilski-Pasquier G, Bousser J: Les leucemies myelomonocytaires subaigues. A propos de 27 observations. *Ann Med Interine (Paris)* 1972; 123:449–458.
5. Alessandrino EP, Orlandi E, Brusamolini E; et al: Chronic myelomonocytic leukemia: Clinical features, cytogenetics and prognosis in 30 consecutive cases. *Hematol Oncol* 1985; 3:147–155.
6. Solal-Celigny P, Dessaint B, Herrera JE, et al: Chronic myelomonocytic leukemia according to the FAB classification: Analysis of 35 cases. *Blood* 1984; 63:634–638.
7. Kantarjian HM, Shtalrid M, Kurzrock R, et al: Significance and correlations of molecular analysis results in patients with Philadelphia chromosome-negative

chronic myelogenous leukemia and chronic myelomonocytic leukemia. *Am J Med* 1988; 639–644.
8. Raskind AU, Tirumali WH, Jacobson R, et al: Evidence for multistep pathogenesis of a myelodysplastic syndrome. *Blood* 1984; 63:1318–23.
9. Hogge D, Shannon K, Kalousek D, et al: Juvenile myelodysplasia with monosomy 7:Evidence that the disease originates in a pluripotent stem cell. *Blood* 1986; 68 (suppl 1):200.
10. Fialkow PJ: Clonal and stem cell origin of blood cell neoplasms. In Lobne J, Gordon AS, Silber R, Muggia F (eds.): *Contemporary Hematology and Oncology* vol 1. New York, Plenum Press, 1988: 1–46.
11. Layton DM, Mufti GJ, Lyons J, et al: Loss of *ras* oncogene mutation in a myelodysplastic syndrome after low dose cytarabine therapy. *N Engl J Med* 1988; 2:1468–1469.
12. Second International Workshop on Chromosomes in Leukemia: Chromosomes in preleukemia. *Cancer Genet Cytogenet* 1980; 2:108–113.
13. Heim S, Mittelman F: Chromosome abnormalities in the myelodysplastic syndromes. *Haematol* 1986; 15:1003–1021.
14. Borgstrom GH: Cytogenetics of the myelodysplastic syndromes. *Scand J Haematol* 1986; 36(supp 45):74–77.
15. Horiike S, Misawa, Taniwaki M, 1986; et al: Chromosome abnormalities, karyotypic evolution and their prognostic implications in myelodysplastic syndromes. In, Uchino H, Takaku F, Yoshida Y, (eds): *Myelodysplastic Syndromes. Pathology and Treatment*. Amsterdam, Elsevier Science Publication, 1988, pp 49–66.
16. Bloomfield CD: Chromosome abnormalities in secondary myelodysplastic syndromes. *Scand J Haematol* 1986; 36(suppl 45):82–90.
17. Gleen LD, Sanger WG, Vaughan WP: Failure of karyotypic instability to predict clinical progression in patients with dysmyelopoietic syndromes. *Blood* 1986; 68(suppl 1):199.
18. Pierre RV: Cytogenetic studies in preleukemia: Studies before and after transition to acute leukemia in 17 subjects. *Blood Cells* 1975; 1:163–170.
19. Tomonaga M, Tomonaga Y, Kusano M, Ichimaru M: Sequential karyotypic evolutions and bone marrow aplasia preceding acute myelomonocytic transformations from myelodysplastic syndrome. *Br J Haematol* 1984; 58:53–60.
20. Benitez J, Carbonell J, Sanchez-Fayos F, Heimpel H: Karyotypic evolution in patients with myelodysplastic syndromes. *Cancer Genet Cytogenet* 1985; 16:157–67.
21. Jacobs RH, Cornbleet MD, Wardiman JW, et al: Prognostic implications of morphology and karyotype in primary myelodysplastic syndromes. *Blood* 1986; 67:1765–1772.
22. Coiffier B, Adeleine P, Gentilhomme D, et al: Myelodysplastic syndromes. A multiparametric study of prognostic factors in 336 patients. *Cancer* 1987; 60:3029–3032.
23. Maddox AM, Keating MJ, Smith TL, et al: Prognostic factors for survival of 194 patients with low infiltrate leukemia. *Leuk Res* 1986; 10:995–1006.
24. Mufti GJ, Stevens JR, Oscier DG, et al: Myelodysplastic syndromes: A scoring system with prognostic significance. *Br J Haematol* 1985; 59:425–433.

25. Tricot G, Vlientick R, Boogaerts MA, et al: Prognostic factors in the myelodysplastic syndromes: Importance of initial data on peripheral blood counts, bone marrow cytology, trephine biopsy and chromosomal analysis. *Br J Haematol* 1985; 60:19–32.
26. Yunis JJ, Lobell M, Arnesen MA, et al: Refined chromosome study helps define prognostic sub-groups in most patients with primary myelodysplastic syndrome and acute myelogenous leukemia. *Br J Haematol* 1988; 68:189–194.
27. Sanz GF, Sanz MA, Vallespi T, et al: Two regressions models and a scoring system for predicting survival and planning treatment in myelodysplastic syndromes: A multivariate analysis of prognostic factors in 370 patients. *Blood* 1989; 74:395–408.
28. Estey E, Maksynmiak A, Smith T, et al: Infection prophylaxis in acute leukemia. Comparative effectiveness of sulfamethoxazole and trimethoprim, ketoconazole, and a combination of the two. *Arch Intern Med* 1984; 144:1562–1568.
29. Bagby GC, Gabourel JD, Linman JW: Glucocorticoid therapy in the preleukemic syndrome (hemopoietic dysplasia). Identification of responsive patients using in vitro techniques. *Ann Intern Med* 1980; 92:55–58.
30. Yoshida Y, Oguma S, Yamazishi M, et al: Prednisone, 1-hydroxyvitamin D_3 and androgens in the management of patients with refractory anemias. In, Uchino H, Takaku F, Yoshida Y (eds): *Myelodysplastic Syndromes, Pathophysiology and Treatment*. Amsterdam, Excerpta Medica 1988, pp 189–202.
31. Dreyfus B: Preleukemic states. *Nouv Rev Fr Hematol* 1976; 17:33–55.
32. Najean Y, Pecking A: Refractory anemia with excess of myeloblasts in the marrow: A clinical trial of androgens in 90 patients. *Br J Haematol* 1977; 37:25–33.
33. Najean Y, Pecking A: Refractory anemia with excess of blast cells: Prognostic factors and effect of treatment with androgens and cytosine arabinoside. Results of a prospective trial in 58 patients. *Cancer* 1979; 44:1976–1982.
34. Madanes AE, Farber M: Danazol. *Ann Intern Med* 1985; 96:625–630.
35. Cines DB, Cassileth PA, Kiss JE: Danazol therapy in myelodysplasia. *Ann Intern Med* 1985; 103:58–60.
36. Adler TS, Oppenheimer TC, Nawabi I: Response to danazol in the treatment of refractory anemia associated with red cell aplasia and myelodysplastic syndromes [abstr]. *Blood* 1986; 68(suppl 1):52a.
37. Kornberg A, Yona R, Inklea S, Kaufman S: Danazol and myelodysplastic syndromes. *Ann Intern Med* 1986; 104:445–446.
38. Lippman SM, Durie GM, Garewal HS, et al: Efficiency of danazol in pure red cell aplasia. *Am J Hematol* 1986; 23:373–379.
39. Doll DC, Scott Ringeberg Q, Yarbro LW: Danazol therapy in acquired idiopathic sideroblastic anemia. *Acta Haematol* 1987; 77:170–171.
40. Buzaid AC, Garewal HS, Lippman SM, et al: Danozol in the treatment of myelodysplastic syndromes. *Eur J Haematol* 1987; 39:346–348.
41. Marini B, Bassan R, Barbui T: Therapeutic efficacy of danazol in myelodysplastic syndromes. *Eur J Cancer Clin Oncol* 1988; 24:1481–1489.
42. Abe E, Chisato M, Sakagami H, et al: Induction of monocytic differentiation and bone resorption by 1,25-dihydroxyvitamin D_{3*}. *Proc Natl Acad Sci USA* 1981; 78:4990.

43. Tanaka H, Abe E, Miyura C, et al: Differentiation of mouse myeloid leukemia cells induced by 1α,25-dihydroxyvitamin D_3. *Biochem J* 1982; 204:713.
44. Bar-Savit Z, Teitelbaum SL, Reitsma P, et al: 25-Dihydroxycholecalciferol and human myeloid leukemia cell line (HL-60). *Proc Natl Acad Sci USA* 1983; 80:5907.
45. Mangelsdorf SJ, Koeffler HP, Donalson CA, et al: 1,25-Dihydroxyvitamin D_3-induced differentiation in a human promyelocytic leukemia cell line (HL-60): Receptor-mediated maturation to macrophage-like cells. *J Cell Biol* 1984; 98:391.
46. McCarthy DM, San Miguel JP, Friake HC, et al: 1,25-Dihydroxyvitamin D_3 inhibits proliferation of human promyelocytic leukemia (HL-60) cells and induces monocyte–macrophage differentiation in HL-60 and normal human bone marrow cells. *Leuk Res* 1983; 7:51.
47. Paquette R, Koeffler HP: Retinoids and 1,25-dihydroxyvitamin D_3 role in myelodysplastic syndromes and leukemia. In, Uchino H, Takaku F, Yoshida Y, (eds): *Myelodysplastic Syndromes: Pathophysiology and Treatment*. Amsterdam, Excerpta Medica, 1988; pp 173–186.
48. Koeffler HP, Amatruda T, Ikekawa N, et al: Induction of macrophage differentiation of human normal and leukemic myeloid stem cells by 1,25-dihydroxyvitamin D_3 and its fluorinated analogues. *Cancer Res* 1984; 44:5624.
49. Munker R, Norman H, Koeffler HP: Vitamin D compounds. Effect on clonal proliferation and differentiation of human myeloid cells. *J Clin Invest* 1986; 78:424.
50. Koeffler HP, Hirji K, Itri L: 1,25-Dihydroxyvitamin D_3: In vivo and in vitro effects on human preleukemic and leukemic cells. *Cancer Treat Rep* 1985; 69:1399.
51. Irino S, Taoka T, Kubota Y, Tanaka T: In vitro and in vivo differentiation of leukemic cells induced by vitamin D_3. In, Uchino H, Takaku F, Yoshida Y (eds): *Myelodysplastic Syndromes, Pathophysiology and Treatment*. Amsterdam, Excerpta Medica, 1988, pp 139–150.
52. Honma Y, Hozumi M, Abe E, et al: 1α,25-Dihydroxyvitamin D_3 and 1α-hydroxyvitamin D_3 prolong survival time of mice incubated with myeloid leukemia cells. *Proc Natl Acad Sci USA* 1983; 80:201.
53. Mehta AB, Kumaran TO, Marsh GW: Treatment of advanced myelodysplastic syndrome with alfacalcidol. *Lancet* 1984; 2:761.
54. Richard C, Mazo E, Cuadrado MA, et al: Treatment of myelodysplastic syndrome with 1,25-dihydroxyvitamin D_3. *Am J Hematol* 1986; 23:175–178.
55. Truitt GA, Tamborini P, Stern LL, et al: Differentiation of HL60 cells induced by vitamin D derivatives: A comparison of chole- and ergocalciferols. In, Uchino H, Takaku F, Yoshida Y (eds): *Myelodysplastic Syndromes: Pathophysiology and Treatment*. Amsterdam, Excerpta Medica, 1988, pp 133–138.
56. Sporn MB, Roberts AB: Role of retinoids in differentiation and carcinogenesis. *Cancer Res* 1983; 43:3034–3038.
57. Koeffler HP, Amatruda TT III: The effect of retinoids on haemopoiesis—clinical and laboratory studies. In, *Retinoids, Differentiation and Disease. Ciba Found Symp* 1985; 113:252–267.
58. Breitman TR, Selonick SE, Collins SJ: Induction of differentiation of the human

promyelocytic leukemia cell line (HL 60) by retinoic acid. *Proc Natl Acad Sci USA* 1980; 77:2936.
59. Ferrero D, Gallo E, Lanfrancone L, Tarella C: Functional and phenotypic characterization of two HL 60 clones resistant to dimethylsulfoxide. *Exp Cell Res* 1983; 147:111.
60. Olsson IL, Breitman TR: Induction of differentiation of the human histocytic lymphoma cell line U-937 by retinoic acid and cyclic adenosine 3'-5'-monophosphate inducing agents. *Cancer Res* 1982; 42:3924.
61. Lawrence HJ, Conner K, Kelly MA, et al: *cis*-Retinoic acid stimulates the clonal growth of some myeloid leukemia cells in vitro. *Blood* 1987; 69:302–307.
62. Ferrero D, Pessano S, Pagliardi GL, Rovera G: Induction of differentiation of human leukemias: Surface changes probed with monoclonal antibodies. *Blood* 1983; 61:171.
63. Douer D, Koeffler HP: Retonoic acid. Inhibition of the clonal growth of human myeloid leukemic cells. *J Clin Invest* 1982; 69:277.
64. Breitman TR, Collins SJ, Keene BR: Terminal differentiation of human promyelocytic cells in primary cultures in response to retinoic acid. *Blood* 1981; 57:1000.
65. Flynn PJ, Miller WJ, Weisdorf DJ, et al: Retinoic acid treatment of acute promyelocytic leukemia: In vitro and in vivo observations. *Blood* 1983; 62:1211.
66. Nilsson B: Probable in vivo induction of differentiation by retinoic acid of promyelocytes in acute promyelocytic leukemia. *Br J Haematol* 1984; 57:365.
67. Fontana JD, Rodes JS, Druham JP: The role of *cis*-retinoic acid in the induction of remission of a patient with acute promyelocytic leukemia. *Cancer* 1986; 57:209.
68. Yu-Chen Y, Shu-rong C, Jin-ren C et al: Use of all-*trans*-retinoic acid in the treatment of acute promyelocytic leukemia. *Blood* 1988; 72:567–572.
69. Douer D, Koeffler HP: Retinoic acid enhances colony-stimulating factor-induced clonal growth of normal human myeloid progenitor cells in vitro. *Exp Cell Res* 1983; 147:111.
70. Chomienne C, Ballerin R, Balifrand N, et al: Retinoic acid therapy for promyelocytic leukemia. *Lancet* 1989; 1:746.
71. Gold EJ, Mertelsmann RH, Itri LM, et al: Phase I clinical trial of 13-*cis*-retinoic acid in myelodysplastic syndromes. *Cancer Treat Rep* 1983; 67:981–986.
72. Greenberg BR, Durie BG, Barnett TC, Meyskens FL Jr: Phase I–II study of 13-*cis*-retinoic acid in myelodysplastic syndrome. *Cancer Treat Rep* 1985; 69:1369–1374.
73. Hoffman SJ, Robinson WA: Use of differentiation-inducing agents in the myelodysplastic syndrome and acute nonlymphocytic leukemia. *Am J Hematol* 1988; 28:124–127.
74. Picozzi VJ, Swanson GF, Morgan R, et al: 13-*cis*-Retinoic acid treatment of myelodysplastic syndromes. *J Clin Oncol* 1986; 4:589–595.
75. Kerndrup G, Bendix-Fausen K, Pedersen B, et al: 13-*cis*-Retinoic acid treatment of myelodysplastic syndromes. *Leuk Res* 1987; 11:7–16.
76. Leoni F, Ciolli S, Longo G, et al: 13-*cis*-Retinoic acid treatment in patients with myelodysplastic syndrome. *Acta Haematol (Basel)* 1988; 80:8–12.
77. Besa EC, Hyzinski M, Nowell PC, Abrahm JL: High dose, prolonged 13-*cis*-

retinoic acid (RA) is required for clinical response in myelodysplastic syndrome (MDS). *Blood* 1985 66(suppl 1):194a.

78. Abrahm J, Besa EC, Hyzinski M, et al: Disappearance of cytogenetic abnormalities and clinical remission during therapy with 13-*cis*-retinoic acid in a patient with myelodysplastic syndrome: Inhibition of growth of the patient's malignant monocytoid clone. *Blood* 1986; 67:1323–1327.
79. Koeffler HP, Heitjan D, Mertelsmann R, et al: Randomized study of 13-*cis*-retinoic acid vs placebo in the myelodysplastic disorders. *Blood* 1987; 71:703–708.
80. Clark RE, Ismail SAD, Jacobs A, et al: A randomized trial of 13-*cis*-retinoic acid with or without cytosine arabinoside in patients with the myelodysplastic syndrome. *Br J Haematol* 1987; 66:77.
81. Hirch-Ginsburg C, LeMaistre A, Kantarjian H, et al: *ras* Mutations are rare events in Philadelphia-negative/BCR negative chronic myelogenous leukemia (CML) but prevalent in chronic myelomonocytic leukemia. (submitted).
82. Collins SJ, Howard M, Andrews DF, Rare occurrence of N-*ras* point mutations in Philadelphia chromosome positive chronic myeloid leukemia. *Blood* 1988; 73:1028.
83. Tobler A, Munker R, Heitjan D, Koeffler HP: In vitro interaction of recombinant tumor necrosis factor α and all-*trans*-retinoic acid with normal and leukemic hematopoietic cells. *Blood* 1987; 70:1940.
84. Hemmi H, Breitman TR: Combinations of recombinant human interferons and retinoic acid synergistically induce differentiation of the human promyelocytic leukemia cell line HL60. *Blood* 1987; 69:501.
85. Goldstein D, Laszlo J: Interferon therapy in cancer: From imagination to interferon. *Cancer Res* 1986; 46:4315.
86. Quesada JR, Reuben T, Manning JT, et al: alpha-Interferon for induction of remission in hairy cell leukemia. *N Engl J Med* 1984; 310:15–18.
87. Talpaz M, McCredie KB, Mavligit GM, Gutterman JU: Leukocyte interferon-induced myeloid cytoreduction in chronic myelogenous leukemia. *Blood* 1983; 62:689–692.
88. Talpaz M, Kantarjian HM, McCredit KB, et al: Hematologic remission and cytogenetic improvement induced by recombinant human interferon alpha A in chronic myelogenous leukemia. *N Engl J Med* 1988; 314:1065–1069.
89. Elias L, Hoffman R, Boswell S, et al: A trial of recombinant alpha$_2$-interferon in the myelodysplastic syndromes: I. Clinical results. *Leukemia* 1987; 1:105–107.
90. Galvani DW, Nethersell ABW, Conley JC: α-Interferon in myelodysplasia; clinical observations and effects on NK cells. *Leuk Res* 1988; 12:257–262.
91. Perussia P, Dayton ET, Fanning V, et al: Immune interferon and leucocyte conditioned medium induce normal and leukemic myeloid cells to differentiate along the monocytic pathway. *J Exp Med* 1983; 158:2058.
92. Rubin BY, Gupta SL: Differential efficacies of human type I and type II interferons as antiviral and antiproliferative agents. *Proc Natl Acad Sci USA* 1980; 77:5928–5932.
93. Dezy H, Lechleiter M, Martha CHH, et al: Effects of human recombinant alpha$_2$ and gamma-interferon on the growth of human cell lines from solid tumors and hematological malignancies. *J Interferon Res* 1985; 5:147–157.

94. Beran M, Andersson B, Kantarjian HM, et al: Hematologic response of four patients with smoldering acute myelogenous leukemia to partially pure gamma interferon. *Leukemia* 1987; 1:52–57.
95. Stone R, Spriggs AK, Griffin J, et al: A phase I–II trial of recombinant human interferon gamma (rIFNγ) for acute myelocytic leukemia (AML) and myelodysplastic syndromes (MDS). *Proc Am Soc Clin Oncol* 1989; 8:208.
96. Robert K, Hellstrom E, Einhorn S, Gahrton G et al.: Acute myelogenous leukemia of unfavorable prognosis treated with retinoic acid, vitamin D_3, alpha-interferon and low-doses of cytosine arabinoside. *Scand J Haematol* 1986; 34 (suppl 44):61–74.
97. Kurzrock R, Talpaz M, Kantarjian H, et al: Therapy of chronic myelogenous leukemia with recombinant interferon gamma. *Blood* 1987; 70:943–947.
98. Silver RT, Reich SD, Coleman M, et al: gamma Interferon (IFN) has activity in treating chronic myeloid leukemia (CML). *Blood* 1986; 68(suppl 1):232a.
99. Beran M, Keating MJ, McCredie KB: Biological features of myelodysplastic syndromes (MDS) predict for survival and therapy response. In, Uchino H, Takaku F, Yoshida Y (eds): *Myelodysplastic Syndromes, Pathophysiology and Treatment*. Amsterdam, Excerpta Medica, 1988, pp 155–172.
100. Foucar K, Langdon RM, Armitage JO, Myelodysplastic syndrome, a clinical and pathological analysis of 109 cases. *Cancer* 1985; 56:553–561.
101. Sachs L: The differentiation of myeloid leukemia cells. New possibilities for therapy. *Br J Haematol* 1978; 40:509–517.
102. Lotem J, Sachs L: Potential pre-screening for therapeutic agents that induce differentiation in human myeloid leukemia cells. *Int J Cancer* 1980; 25:561–564.
103. Papac RJ, Brown AE, Schwartz EL, et al: Differentiation of human promyelocytic leukemia cells in vitro by 6-thioguanine. *Cancer Lett* 1980; 10:33–38.
104. Takeda K, Minowada J, Leasure JA, et al: Comparison of the ability of various cytotoxic agents to induce differentiation of human myeloblastic leukemia cells in vitro. *Proc Am Assoc Cancer Res* 1982; 23:226.
105. Takeda K, Minowada T, Bloch A: Kinetics of appearance of differentiation associated characteristics in ML-1, a line of human myeloblast leukemia cells, after treatment with 12-*0*-tetradecanoylphorbol-13 acetate, dimethyl sulfoxide, or 1-β-arabinofuranosylcytosine. *Cancer Res* 1982; 42:5152–5158.
106. Griffin T, Munroe D, Kufe D: Induction of differentiation of human leukemia cells by inhibitors of DNA synthesis. *Exp Hematol* 1982; 10:774–781.
107. Koeffler D: Induction of differentiation of human acute myelogenous leukemia cells: Therapeutic implications. *Blood* 1983; 62:709–721.
108. Bloch A: Induced cell differentiation in cancer therapy. *Cancer Treat Rep* 1984; 68:199–205.
109. Rowley PT, Ohlsson-Wilhelm OM, Farley BA, et al: Inducers of erythroid differentiation in K 562 human leukemia cells. *Exp Hematol* 1981; 9:32–37.
110. Honma Y, Fumita Y, Kasukabe T, et al: Induction of differentiation of human non-lymphocytic leukemia cells in primary culture by inducers of differentiation of human myeloid leukemia cell line HL-60. *Eur J Cancer Clin Oncol* 1983; 19:251–261.
111. Hoelzer D, Ganser A, Anger B, et al: Low-dose ara-C in the treatment of acute leukemia: Cytotoxicity or differentiation induction: *Blut* 1984; 48:233–238.
112. Michalewiz R, Lotem J, Sachs L: Cell differentiation and therapeutic effect of low

doses of cytosine arabinsoide in human myeloid leukemia. *Leuk Res* 1980; 8:783–790.
113. Koeffler HP, Golde SW: Human preleukemia. *Ann Intern Med* 1980; 93:347–353.
114. Baccarani M, Tura S: Differentiation of myeloid leukemic cells: new possibilities for therapy. *Br J Haematol* 1979; 42:485–490.
115. Housset M, Daniel T, Degos L: Small doses of ara-C in the treatment of acute myeloid leukemia: Differentiation of myeloid leukemia cells. *Br J Haematol* 1982; 51:125–129.
116. Baccarani M, Zaccaria A, Bandini G, et al: Low dose arabinosyl cytosine for treatment of myelodysplastic syndromes and subacute myeloid leukemia. *Leuk Res* 1983; 7:539–545.
117. Wisch JS, Griffin JD, Kufe DW: Response of preleukemic syndromes to continuous infusion of low-dose cytarabine. *N Engl J Med* 1983; 309:1599–1602.
118. Castaigne S, Daniel M, Tilly H, et al: Does treatment with ara-C in low dosage cause differentiation of leukemic cells? *Blood* 1983; 62:85–86.
119. Cooperative group for the Study of Aplastic and Refractory Anemias: Refractory anemia with excess of blast cells: Prognostic factors and effect of treatment with androgens or cytosine arabinoside. Results of a prospective trial in 58 patients. *Cancer* 1979; 44:1976–1982.
120. Mufti GJ, Oscier DG, Hamblin TJ, Bell AJ: Low doses of cytarabine in the treatment of myelodysplastic syndrome and acute myeloid leukemia. *N Engl J Med* 1983; 309:1653–1654.
121. Jehn U, DeBock R, Haanen C: Clinical trial of low dose ara-C in the treatment of acute leukemia and myelodysplasia. *Blut* 1984; 48:255–261.
122. Solal-Celigny P, DeSaint B, Herrera A, et al: Chronic myelomonocytic leukemia according to FAB classification. *Blood* 1984; 63:634–638, 1984.
123. Schiff RD, Mertelsmann R, Andreeff M, et al: Low dose arabinosyl cytosine (LD ara-C) in hematologic malignancies and myelodysplastic syndromes (MDS). *Proc Am Soc Clin Oncol* 1984; 3:804.
124. Tricot G, DeBock R, Dekker AW, et al: Low dose cytosine arabinoside (ara-C) in myelodysplastic syndromes. *Br J Haematol* 1984; 58:231–240.
125. Weiss R, Lessin, Pierce L, et al: Low dose ara-C in treatment of refractory anemia with excess blasts (RAEB) and acute nonlymphocytic leukemia (ANLL). *Proc Am Soc Clin Oncol* 1984; 3:791.
126. Beran M, Andersson BS, Ayyar R, et al: Clinical response and mechanisms of action of low dose cytosine arabinoside (ara-C) in myelodysplastic syndromes (MDS) and myelogenous leukemias (AML, CMML). *Proc Am Soc Clin Oncol* 1985; 4:678.
127. Hoelzer D, Ganser A, Schneider W, Heimpel H: Low dose cytosine arabinoside in the treatment of acute nonlymphoblastic leukemia and myelodysplastic syndromes. *Semin Oncol* 1985; 12:208–211.
128. Hossfeld DK, Weh HJ, Kleeberg UR: Low-dose cytarabine: Chromosomal findings suggesting its cytostatic as well as differentiating effect. *Leuk Res* 1985; 9:329–330.
129. Tagawa M, Shibata T, Tomonaga M, et al: Low-dose cytosine arabinoside regimen induced a complete remission with normal karyotype in a case with hypoplas-

tic acute myeloid leukemia with no. 8 trisomy: In vitro and in vivo evidence for normal hematopoietic recovery. *Br J Haematol* 1985; 60:449–455.
130. Izumi Y, Sawada H, Okazaki T, et al: Favorable remission rate by repeating low dose ara-C treatment in ANLL and RAEB. *Br J Haematol* 1985; 73:71–74.
131. Roberts JD, Ershler WB, Tindle BH, Stewart JA: Low-dose cytosine arabinoside in the myelodysplastic syndromes and acute myelogenous leukemia. *Cancer* 1985; 56:1001–1005.
132. Winter JN, Variakojis D, Gaynor ER, et al: Low dose cytosine arabinoside (ara-C) therapy in the myelodysplastic syndromes and acute leukemia. *Cancer* 1985; 56:443–449.
133. Jacobs A, Clark RE, Smith SA, et al: A randomised clinical trial of retinoic acid and cytosine arabinoside in the treatment of myelodysplastic syndrome (MDS). *Blood* 1985; 66:690.
134. Spiers ASD, Chikkappa G, Lorch CA: Myelodysplastic syndrome: Cytogenetic changes before and after response to low-dose ara-C. *Blood* 1985; 66:607.
135. Kufe DW, Griffin JD, Spriggs DR: Cellular and clinical pharamacology of low-dose ara-C. *Semin Oncol* 1985; 12:200–207.
136. Tricot G, DeBock R, Dekker AW, et al: Low dose cytosine arabinoside in myelodysplastic syndrome. *Br J Haematol* 1984; 58:231–240.
137. Allessandrino EP, Orlandi E, Brusamolino E, et al: Low dose ara-C in acute leukemia after a myelodysplastic syndrome and in elderly leukemia. *Am J Hematol* 1985; 20:191–193.
138. Griffin JD, Spriggs D, Wish JS, Kufe DW: Treatment of preleukemic syndromes with continuous intravenous infusion of low dose cytarabine. *J Clin Oncol* 1985; 3:982–991.
139. Hoelzer D, Ganser A, Schneider W, Heimpel H: Low-dose cytosine arabinoside in the treatment of acute nonlymphoblastic leukemia and myelodysplastic syndromes. *Semin Oncol* 1985; 12(suppl):208–211.
140. Inbal A, Januszewicz E, Rabinowicz M, Shaklai M: A therapeutic trial with low-dose cytarabine in myelodysplastic syndromes and acute leukemia. *Acta Haematol* 1985; 73:71–74.
141. Jensen MK, Ahlbom F: Low dose cytosine arabinoside in the treatment of acute nonlymphocytic leukemia. *Scan J Haematol* 1985; 34:261–263.
142. Kreis W, Chaudhri F, Chan K, et al: Pharmacokinetics of low-dose 1-β-D-arabinofuranosylcytosine given by continuous intravenous infusion over twenty-one days. *Cancer Res* 1985; 45:6498–6501.
143. Tagawa M, Shibata J, Tomonaga M, et al: Low-dose cytosine arabinoside regimen induced a complete remission with normal karyotypes in a case with hypoplastic acute myeloid leukemia with no. 8 trisomy: In vitro. *Br J Haematol* 1985; 60:449–455.
144. Vincent PC, Young GAR, Buck M, Benson WJ: Low-dose cytarabine in acute nonlymphoblastic leukemia or myelodysplastic syndrome: *Aust NZ J Med* 1985; 15:10–15.
145. Weh HJ, Zschaber R, von Paleske A, Hossfeld DK: Treatment of acute myeloid leukemia and myelodysplastic syndrome by low dose cytosine arabinoside. *Hematol Blood Transfusion* 1985; 29:60–62.

146. Beran M, Estey EH, Keating MJ, et al: Initial response, remission duration, response to salvage chemotherapy and survival of patients with myelodysplastic syndromes (MDS) treated with chemotherapy of varying intensity. *Blood* 1988; 72 (suppl 1):189a.
147. Powell BL, Capizzi RL, Jackson DV, et al: Low dose ara-C for patients with myelodysplastic syndromes. *Leukemia* 1988; 2:153–156.
148. Kuryiama U: Effect of low dose ara-C regimen on myelodysplastic syndrome (MDS). *Gan To Kagaku Ryoho* 1988; 15:1198–1204.
149. Bolwell BJ, Cassileth PA, Gale PR: Low-dose cytosine arabinoside in myelodysplasia and acute myelogenous leukemia: A review. *Leukemia* 1987; 1:575–579.
150. Cheson BD, Tasperse DM, Simon R, Freidman MA: A critical appraisal of low-dose cytosine arabinoside in patients with acute non-lymphocytic leukemia and myelodysplastic syndrome. *J Clin Oncol* 1986; 4:1857–1864.
152. Owens MR, Bennett JM: Effectiveness of a attenuated chemotherapy in myelodysplastic syndromes: A preliminary report. *Med Pediatr Oncol* 1988; 16:107–110.
153. Hittelmann WN, Hawkins M, Doyle S, et al: Direct cytogenetic evidence of induced maturation of leukemic cells in vivo. *Proc Am Assoc Cancer Res* 1985; 26:718.
154. Hittelman WN, Agbor P, Petkovic I, et al: Detection of leukemic clone maturation in vivo by premature chromosome condensation. *Blood* 1988; 72:1950–1960.
155. Beran M, Hittelman W, Andersson B, McCredie KB: Induction of differentiation in human myeloid leukemia cells with cytosine arabinoside (ara-C). *Leuk Res* 1986; 10:1033–1039.
156. Armitage JO, Dick FR, Needleman SW, Burns CP: Effect of chemotherapy for the dysmyelopoietic syndrome. *Cancer Treat Rep* 1981; 65:601–605.
157. Mertelsman R, Thaler HT, To L, et al: Morphological classification, response to therapy and survival in 263 adult patients with acute non-lymphoblastic leukemia. *Blood* 1980; 56:773–781.
158. Keating MJ, McCredie KB, Benjamin RS, et al: Treatment of patients over 50 years of age with acute myelogenous leukemia by a combination of Rubidazone and cytosine arabinoside, vincristine and prednisone (ROAP). *Blood* 1981; 57:584–591.
159. Scoazec JY, Imbert M, Crofts M, et al: Myelodysplastic syndrome or acute myelogenous leukemia: A study of 28 cases presenting with borderline features. *Cancer* 1985; 55:2390–2394.
160. Tricot G, Boogaerts MA, et al: The role of aggressive chemotherapy in the treatment of myelodysplastic syndromes. *Br J Haematol* 1986; 63:477–483.
161. Preisler HD, Raza A, Barcos M, et al: High dose cytosine arabinoside in the treatment of preleukemia disorders. *Am J Haematol* 1986; 23:131–134.
162. Fenaux P, Lai JL, Joneb JP, et al: Aggressive chemotherapy in adult primary myelodysplastic syndromes. *Blut* 1988; 57:297–302.
163. Dohy K, Kyo T: Intensive chemotherapy of refractory anemia with excess of blasts. *Gan To Kagaku Ryoho* 1988; 4:1223–1228.
164. DeWitte T, Muus P, DePauw B, Haanen C: Intensive chemotherapy for patients with myelodysplastic syndromes and acute myelogenous leukemia younger than 65 years. *Bone Marrow Transplantation* 1989; 4(suppl 3):33–34.

165. Richard C, Iriondo A, Garijo J, et al: Therapy of advanced myelodysplastic syndrome with aggressive chemotherapy. *Oncology* 1989; 46:6–9.
166. Gajewski J, No NG, Nimer S, et al: Efficacy of intensive chemotherapy for acute myelogenous leukemia associated with a preleukemic syndrome. *J Clin Oncol* 1989; 7:1637–1645.
167. Kleinhauer E, et al: The preleukemic syndromes (hematopoietic dysplasia). *Eur J Pediatr* 1980; 133:5–10.
168. Cohen JR, Greger WP, Greenberg PL, Schrier SL: Subacute myeloid leukemia: A clinical review. *Am J Med* 1979; 66:959–966.
169. Appelbaum FR, Dahlberg S, Thomas ED, et al: Allogeneic marrow transplantation in the treatment of preleukemia. *Ann Intern Med* 1984; 100:689–693.
170. Appelbaum FR, Storb R, Ramberg R, et al: Treatment of preleukemic syndromes with marrow transplantation. *Blood* 1987; 69:92–96.
171. O'Donnell MR, Nademanee AP, Snyder DS, et al: Bone marrow transplantation for myelodysplastic and myeloproliferative syndromes. *J Clin Oncol* 1987; 5:1822–1826.
172. Belanger R, Gyger M, Perreault C, Bonny Y: Bone marrow transplantation for myelodysplastic syndromes. *Br J Haematol* 1988; 69:29–33.
173. DeWitte T, Zwaan F, Hermans J, et al: An EGBMT survey on allogeneic bone marrow transplantation for secondary leukemia and bad prognosis myelodysplastic syndromes. *Bone Marrow Transplantation* 1989; 4 (suppl 2):9.
174. DeWite T, Zwan F, Hermans J, et al: Allogeneic bone marrow transplantation for secondary leukemia and myelodysplastic syndromes. *Bone Marrow Transplantation* 1989; (suppl 3):38–39.
175. Kolb HJ, Holler E, Bender-Gotze E, et al: Myeloablative conditioning for bone marrow transplantation in myelodysplastic syndromes and paroxysmal nocturnal haemoglobinuria. *Bone Marrow Transplantation* 1989; 1:29–34.
176. Forman SJ, O'Donnell MR, Blume KG, Feinstein DI: Role of allogeneic bone marrow transplantation as primary therapy for chronic myelomonocytic leukemia. *Blut* 1987; 54:189–192.
177. Lutz P, Foll G, Albert A, et al: Role of allogeneic transplantation of bone marrow in juvenile chronic myelomonocytic leukemia. *Presse Med* 1988; 17:2113–6.
178. Appelbaum FR, Barral J, Storb R, et al: Bone marrow transplantation for patients with myelodysplasia. *Ann Intern Med* 1990; 112:590–597.
179. Levine EG, Bloomfield CD: Secondary myelodysplastic syndromes and leukemias. *Clin Haematol* 1986; 15:1037–1079.
180. Kantarjian HM, Keating MJ, Walters R, et al: Therapy-related leukemia and myelodysplastic syndromes: Clinical, cytogenetic, and prognostic features. *J Clin Oncol* 1986; 4:1748–1757.
181. Wong GG, Witek JS, Temple PA, et al: Human GM-CSF: Molecular cloning of the complementary DNA and purification of the recombinant proteins. *Science* 1985; 228:810–815.
182. Souza LM, Boon TC, Gabrilove J, et al: Recombinant human granulocyte colony stimulating factors: Effect on normal and leukemic myeloid cells. *Science* 1985; 232:61–65.
183. Nagata S, Tschuiya M, Asano S, et al: Molecular cloning and expression of cDNA for human granulocyte colony-stimulating factor. *Nature* 1986; 319:415–418.

184. Yang YC, Ciarletta AB, Temple PA, et al: Human IL-3 (multi-CSF): Identification by expression cloning of a novel hematopoietic growth factor related to murine IL-3. *Cell* 1986; 47:3–10.
185. Jacobs K, Shoemaker C, Rudersdorf R, et al: Isolation and characterization of genomic and c-DNA clones of human erythropoietin. *Nature* 1985; 313:806–810.
186. Seiff CA: Hematopoietic growth factors *J Clin Invest* 1989; 79:1549–1557.
187. Vadhan-Raj S, Keating M, LeMaistre A, et al: Effects of recombinant human granulocyte–macrophage colony stimulating factor in patients with myelodysplastic syndromes. *N Engl J Med* 1987; 317:1545–1552.
188. Vadhan-Raj S, Hittelman WN, LeMaistre A, et al: Treatment of myelodysplastic syndrome (MDS) with recombinant human granulocyte–macrophage colony stimulating factor (GM-CSF)—follow up. *Blood* 1988; 72 (supple 1):137a.
189. Hoelzer D, Ganser A, Volkers B, et al: In vitro and in vivo action of recombinant human GM-CSF (rhGM-CSF) in patients with myelodysplastic syndromes. *Blood Cells* 1988; 14:551–559.
190. Antin JH, Smith BR, Holmes W, Rosenthal DS: Phase I–II study of recombinant human granulocyte–macrophage, colony-stimulating factor in aplastic anemia and myelodysplastic syndrome. *Blood* 1988; 72:705–713.
191. Thompson J, Lee D, Rubin E, et al: Treatment of myelodysplastic syndrome (MDS) with subcutaneous (SC) recombinant granulocyte–macrophage colony stimulating factor (r-GM-CSF). *Blood* 1988; 72(suppl, 1):230a.
192. Thompson JA, Lee DJ, Kidd P, et al: Subcutaneous granulocyte–macrophage colony-stimulating factor in patients with myelodysplastic syndrome: Toxicity, pharmacokinetics, and hematological effect. *J Clin Oncol* 1989; 7:629–637.
193. Rifkin RM, Hersh EM, Hultquist KN, Salmon SE: Therapy of the myelodysplastic syndrome (MDS) with subcutaneously (SC) administered recombinant human granulocyte–macrophage colony-stimulating factor (GM-CSF). *Proc Am Assoc Clin Oncol* 1989; 8:178.
194. Estey E, Kurzrock R, Talpaz M, et al: Therapy of myelodysplastic syndromes (MDS) with GM-CSF. *Proc Am Assoc Clin Oncol* 1989; 8:200.
195. Schuster MW, Allen SL, Lichtman SM, et al: The efficacy of GM-CSF in the treatment of myelodysplastic syndrome and aplastic anemia. *Blood* 1989; 74:332a.
196. Sulecki M, Rosenfeld CS, Evans C, et al: Comparison of intravenous (IV) versus subcutaneous (SQ) Recombinant human granulocyte macrophage colony-stimulating factor (rHuGM-CSF) in myelodysplasia (MDS). *Blood* 1989; 74:155a.
197. Lieschike GJ, Mahler D, Cebon T, et al: Effects of bacterially synthesized recombinant human granulocyte–macrophage colony-stimulating factor in patients with advanced malignancy. *Ann Intern Med* 1989; 110:357–364.
198. Boogaerts MD, Nelissen V, Rodant V, et al: Blood neutrophilic function in primary myelodysplastic syndromes, *Br J Haematol* 1983; 55:217.
199. Ruutu P: Granulocyte function in myelodysplastic syndromes. *Scand J Haematol* 1986; 36 (suppl 45):66–70.
200. Negrin RS, Haeber DH, Nagler A, et al: Treatment of myelodysplastic syndromes with recombinant human granulocyte colony-stimulating factor. *Ann Intern Med* 1989; 110:976–984.
201. Negrin RS, Haeber DH, Nagler A, et al: Persistent improvement in neutrophil

counts and decreased incidence of infection in patients with myelodysplastic syndromes (MDS) chronically treated with recombinant human granulocyte colony stimulating factor (G-CSF); *Blood* 1989 74 (suppl 1): abstr 44.
202. Gasson JC, Weisbart RH, Kaufman SE, et al: Purified human granulocyte–macrophage stimulating factor: Direct action on neutrophils. *Science* 1984; 226:1339.
203. Weisbart RH, Golde DW, Clark SC, et al: Human granulocyte–macrophage colony stimulating factor is a neutrophic activator. *Nature* 1985; 314:316–363.
204. Grabstein KH, Urdal KL, Tushinski RJ: Induction of macrophage tumorocidal activity by granulocyte–macrophage colony-stimulating factor. *Science* 1986; 232:506.
205. Lopez AF, Williamson DJ, Gamble JR, et al: Recombinant human granulocyte–macrophage colony stimulating factor stimulates in vitro mature human neutrophil and eosinophil function surface expression and survival. *J Clin Invest* 1986; 78:1220–1228.
206. Weisbart RH, Kwan L, Golde DW, Gasson JC: Human GM-CSF primes neutrophils for enhanced oxidation metabolism in response to major physiological chemoattractants. *Blood* 1987; 69:18.
207. Riklis I, Fabian I: Enhanced resistance of bone marrow transplanted mice to bacterial infection induced by recombinant granulocyte/macrophage colony-stimulating factor. *Blood* 1989; 74(suppl 1):323a.
208. Negrin RS, Haeuber DH, Nagler A, et al: Maintenance treatment of myelodysplastic syndromes (MDS) with recombinant human granulocyte colony stimulating factor (G-CSF). *Exp Hematol* 1989; 17 (suppl 17):657.
209. Pasguali F, Bernasconi P, Casalone R, et al: Pathogenetic significance of "pure" monosomy 7 in myeloproliferative disorders. Analysis of 14 cases. *Hum Genet* 1982; 62:40–51.
210. Ruutu P, de la Chapelle A: Defective chemotaxis in monosomy 7. *Nature* 1977; 265:146–147.
211. Ruutu P, Ruutu T, Repo H, et al: Defective neutrophil migration in monosomy-7 *Blood* 1982; 58:739–745.
212. Hittelman WN, Tigaud J-D, Estey E, et al: Relative maturation of aneuploid and diploid elements in patients with myelodyplasia (MDS) treated with granulocyte–macrophage colony stimulating factor (GM-CSF), *Blood* 1988; 72 (suppl 1):121a.
213. Vadhan-Raj S, Broxmayer HE, Spitzer G, et al: Stimulation of nonclonal hematopoiesis and suppression of the neoplastic clone after treatment with recombinant granulocyte–macrophage colony stimulating factor in a patient with therapy-related myelodysplastic syndrome. *Blood* 1989; 74:1491–1498.
214. Bowen DT, Jacobs A, Coses MP, Lewis TC: Serum erythropoietin and erythropoiesis in patients with myelodysplastic syndromes. *Eur J Haematol* 1990; 44:30–32.
215. Jacobs A, Tanowska-Wieczarek A, Caro J, et al: Circulating erythropoietin in patients with myelodysplastic syndromes. *Br J Haematol* 1989; 73:36–39.
216. Vadhan-Raj S, Hittelman WN, Lepe Zuniga JL, et al: Regulation of endogenous erythropoietin levels in anemia associated with myelodysplastic syndrome. *Blood* 1990; 75:1749–1750.

217. Eschbach JW, Adamson JW: Correction of the anemia of hemodialysis (HD) patients with recombinant human erythropoietin (r-HuEPO): Results of a multicenter study. *Kidney Int* 1989; 33:189.
218. Eschbach JW, Egrie JC, Downing MR, et al: Correction of the anemia of end stage renal disease with recombinant human erythropoietin: Results of a combined phase I and II trial. *N Engl J Med* 1987; 316:73–78.
219. Means RT Jr, Olsen NJ, Krantz SB, et al: Treatment of the anemia of rheumatoid arthritis with recombinant erythropoietin: Clinical and in vitro studies. *Arthritis Rheum* 1989; 32:638–642.
220. Henry DH: Human recombinant erythropoietin in the treatment of severe anemia in patients with AIDS. *Im-Intern Med Specialists* 1989; 10:39–49.
221. Rudnick SA: Human recombinant erythropoietin (rHuEPO). A double blind, placebo controlled study in acquired immunodeficiency syndrome (AIDS) patients with anemia induced by disease and AZT. *Proc Am Soc Clin Oncol* 1989; 8:2.
222. Hirashima K, Bessho M, Susaki K, et al: Improvement of anemia by intravenous injection of recombinant erythropoietin in patients with myelodysplastic syndrome and aplastic anemia. *Exp Hematol* 1989; 17:657.
223. Isnard F, Baillou CL, Ghaffari S, et al: Stimulation of erythropoiesis in patients with refractory anemias by recombinant human erythropoietin. *Blood* 1989; 74(suppl 1):326a.
224. Ganser A, Lindemann A, Seipelt G, et al: Effect of recombinant human interleukin-3 (rhIL-3) in patients with bone marrow failure—a Phase I/II trial. *Blood* 1989; 74 (suppl 1):50a.
225. Kurzrock R, Talpaz M, Salewski E, Gutterman JU: Phase I study of recombinant human interleukin-3 in patients with bone marrow failure. *Blood* 1989; 74 (suppl 1): 154a.
226. Hoelzer D, Ganser A, Seipelt G, et al: Simultaneous treatment with recombinant human granulocyte–macrophage colony-stimulating factor (rhGM-CSF) and low-dose cytosine arabinoside (LD-arcC) in patients with myelodysplastic syndromes (MDS). *Blood* 1989; 74 (suppl 1):118a.
227. Gerhartz HH, Visani G, Delmer A. et al: Randomized Phase II study with GM-CSF and low-dose ara-C in patients with "high risk" myelodysplastic syndromes (MDS). *Blood* 1989; 74(suppl 1):119a.

3

Acute Lymphocytic Leukemia in Adults: Current Approaches and Future Directions

Zalmen A. Arlin

New York Medical College
Valhalla, New York

The last 20–25 years have witnessed dramatic improvement in the outlook for both children and adults with acute lymphoblastic leukemia (ALL), and the favorable outcome in patients with this disease seen in a single institution (1–4) has now been duplicated throughout the United States and the rest of the world (5–11). These achievements have come from the emergence of a better understanding of the disease and from the proper use of chemotherapy and appropriate timing of bone marrow transplantation. The approach to the therapy of ALL has served as a model for treating other leukemias and has encouraged investigators to aim for eradication of disseminated cancers by similar methods.

Consistently, the results in children have been superior to that achieved in adults, given comparable treatment (2). For a long time, the higher cure rate was thought to be due to the ability of younger patients to better tolerate the toxic effects of chemotherapy and, consequently, to the possibility of delivering curative treatment to a greater percentage of these patients. Although this, in part, may be true, recent studies favor the view that adults with ALL are more likely to have a disease that is intrinsically more resistant to conventional therapy (11). This may account for the gains seen in adults with "curable" ALL that have resulted from intensive chemotherapy, but have failed in patients with an unfavorable prognosis. Further progress may be limited by the inclusion, in treatment protocols for ALL, of groups of patients who, by virtue of their characteristics, cannot be cured with conventional chemotherapy.

DIAGNOSIS

The separation of acute lymphoblastic leukemia from acute myelogenous leukemia (AML) remains a critical first step in the selection of therapy and in the definition of prognosis. When the distinction was not made accurately, poor results were common (13). When accurate diagnostic methods were employed, a favorable outcome was more likely for patients with the diagnosis of ALL (4–11).

In recent years, we have come to recognize that the leukemic population should be fully characterized by morphological, histochemical, cytogenetic, and immunological methods. It is important to continue using traditional histochemical-staining methods to establish the best diagnosis, and then, to add to these, tests for the presence of terminal deoxynucleotidyl transferase (Tdt) (14), common ALL antigen (CALLA, CD10) (15,16), and other surface antigens including T1 (CD5), T11 (CD2), MY7 (CD17), and MY9 (CD33) (17–19). In the future, the presence of immunoglobulin gene rearrangement (20) or T-cell receptor rearrangement (21,22) may help resolve diagnostic dilemmas.

When the morphologic characteristics are consistent with a diagnosis of ALL, and histochemical reactions for myeloid leukemia are absent (e.g., the myeloperoxidase stain); when the Tdt is positive, and associated ALL antigens are present, the diagnosis is unequivocal, and this phenotype mandates therapy for ALL.

The appearance of inconsistency in this pattern (e.g., the presence of myeloid surface antigens (MY7, MY9)) (18,19) should not change the diagnosis or therapy. In some instances, application of traditional morphological and histochemical definitions may be confusing, since they may establish a diagnosis of either a "hybrid" leukemia (23,24), in which single cells express markers for both myeloid and lymphoid lineages, or a "biphenotypic" leukemia (25,26), in which the leukemic population is characterized by cells that express myeloid markers, as well as others with lymphoid markers.

Similarly, CD10 may also be absent in up to 15% of patients with ALL (15,16). Although this may have an important impact on prognosis, primary induction therapy should not be changed. On the other hand, certain karyotypes (12) may require a change in either induction or postinduction therapy. In the future, refinements in therapy may be required for different subsets, but it is now unclear how this should be modified, and the conventional approach requires that all patients should be treated with the current best induction therapy for ALL. Postinduction therapy, especially as it relates to the timing of a bone marrow transplant, may be influenced by cytogenetic results (see later discussion).

The therapy for these leukemias is now undergoing investigation, and appropriate therapy may ultimately be defined by other characteristics (e.g., cytogenetics). Although definitive therapy for these patients has not been fully established, it is especially important to separate the biphenotypic leukemias from

ALL, since, if included, their unfavorable prognosis may place a limitation on the percentage of patients with ALL who are curable. Failure to obtain an accurate diagnosis of ALL may result in inappropriate therapy for these groups, and an accurate diagnosis will offer the opportunity to optimize treatment in patients with potentially curable disease.

With this diagnostic approach, we can expect that up to 20% of adults with acute leukemia will have a diagnosis of ALL. Within this 20%, Tdt positivity will be found in virtually all of the pre-B- and T-cell ALLs and, where absent, the leukemia will usually have a B-cell phenotype. Most of the Tdt-positive cases are likely to have lymphocytes that do not stain positively with either Sudan black or peroxidase, and they will likely express antigenic determinants characteristic of pre-B or T cells. Myeloid antigens may be present in up to 30% or more of patients, but this should not affect the diagnosis. Cytogenetic evaluation is a crucial adjunct to traditional methods for establishing an accurate diagnosis of ALL.

This has become increasingly important for confirming the correct diagnosis, determining prognosis, and establishing curability. Certain karyotypes occur in ALL, such as t(l;14), t(10;14), t(8;14), and t(9;22) (12). Others are seen exclusively in AML [e.g., t(15;17), t (8;21), and t(9;11)]. Other karyotypes, such as t(4;11), may characterize a mixed lineage or biphenotypic leukemia (27,28).

Approximately 11–32% of patients who present with ALL will have the Philadelphia chromosome (Ph^1)(12,29), 5% will have the t(4;11), 6% will have the 8q24, and 7% will have 14q+. With conventional treatment, virtually none of these adult patients are curable. Since this group represents more than 30% of the total patient population, it may represent an upper limit on curability of patients with this disease.

Indeed, karyotype, more than any other parameter, has become the most important factor in establishing prognosis.

PROGNOSTIC FACTORS

The identification of patients with ALL in whom conventional treatment is likely to achieve cure, and those in whom it is unlikely, is based upon the critical assumption that variations in conventional therapy have not established a regimen that is clearly superior to others, and that success is not as dependent on variation in treatment as it is on the intrinsic character of the disease. This is not entirely true, since, for example, the T-cell phenotype is an unfavorable prognostic factor in children (17), and was also unfavorable in one of the large series in adults (7). On the other hand, the T-cell phenotype is a favorable factor in the two largest series, which are characterized by more intensive postinduction treatment (4,5). Keeping this in mind, it is possible to separate prognostic features into those that are *critical,* those that are *important,* and those that are *relevant,* but when unfavorable and present, do not preclude cure. In the first group, it is possible to identify only cytogenetics as a critical factor. In a recent review of 330 patients with newly diagnosed ALL, Bloomfield et al. (12) summarized the experience of the Third International Workshop on Chromosomes in Leukemia.

Although remission induction rates higher than 50% were seen in all cytogenetic subtypes, remission duration varied significantly among the subgroups. Thus, in patients with hyperdiploidy, the median remission duration was longer than 40 months, and in patients with hypodiploidy, the remission duration was a median of 8 months. Patients with translocations, such as with t(9:22) and t(4:11), had a median duration of remission of 8 and 4 months, respectively. Patients with abnormal 8q24 [most often t(8;14)], had remission duration of only 4 months. Differences were apparent in the younger and older aged groups. Thus, children with hyperdiploidy had a median remission duration of longer than 5 years, with more than 70% remaining in continuous complete remission, whereas children with t(4;11) and 8q24 had median remission durations of 3 and 4 months, respectively. Children with hyperdiploidy had a median duration of 14 months; those with the Ph^1 the median duration was 14 months; and those who were diploid with additional abnormalities, 17 months. Because of the overall poor results in the adults treated in these programs, no group was identified with long remission duration. The most favorable category in adults, as in children, had hyperdiploidy, but, in this series, had a median remission duration of only 14 months.

Failure to have identified patients with long-term survival probably reflects that none of the patients received optimal treatment for their ALL. But even in this series, none of the cytogenetic abnormalities that were unfavorable precluded successful remission induction.

Several of the subtypes had no long-term survivors. Thus, of 18 patients with t(4:11) there were no survivors. Similarly, all six children with the 8q24 abnormality died, and there were only two survivors of the ten adults with this abnormality. If we combine these two groups, we see that none of the 14 patients who died, survived more than 9 months. The two remaining patients are in the first complete remission at 33+ and 66+ months and, presumably, have achieved cure. The Ph^1 group is also at extreme risk with conventional chemotherapy (12,29). In one series (12), there were 29 patients with Ph^1, of which only 1 survives in her first complete remission. Of 9 children with Ph^1, 2 are alive in their first complete remission. In the other large series (30), consisting only of adults with Tdt + Ph^1 + acute leukemia, there were no long-term survivors among the 25 patients receiving conventional chemotherapy. The 1 long-term survivor underwent bone marrow transplantation after achieving remission of her acute leukemia. In these patients we do not have information on the position of the breakpoint in the breakpoint cluster region *(bcr)* of chromosome 22 (31–33). As a result, it is unknown whether the curable patients are more likely to have a breakpoint in the minor region of the *BCR* gene (31) as opposed to the one seen in CML (32).

For reasons that we still do not understand, the group with the translocations are at extreme risk. Although rare patients can be identified who survive, the vast majority have a disease that is associated with virtually no long-term survivors. Thus, conventional therapy does not seem to offer a solution for this group. Removal of patients with translocations from analysis of results of therapeutic trials is likely to confer a better-than-expected survival for that series (8). Alternatives, such as transplantation, for patients who achieve remission and who have a translocation may be, at present, the only valid therapeutic alternative available (34).

Other prognostic factors are also *important,* but unlike the case of cytogenetic translocations, they do not preclude cure. Gaynor (35) reviewed the clinical characteristics and outcome in 199 consecutive previously untreated adults with ALL who were treated with the L10 series of programs. The factors associated with relapse and "failure to cure" included, (1) white blood cell counts (WBC) $> 20 \times 10^9$/L, (2) non–T-cell ALL, (3) age > 60 years old, (4) Ph^1, and (5) more than 5 weeks to achieve remission. Gaynor then defined three separate groups bearing variable likelihoods of relapse. The most favorable group (with either none or one unfavorable characteristic) had a 61% chance of achieving long-term survival, the intermediate group (with patients who had a delayed response with one additional unfavorable characteristic), had a 43% chance, and the most unfavorable group (with patients who had at least two of the foregoing characteristics 1–4) had only a 20% chance of long-term survival. Thus, clinical characteristics may help define the character of the remissions that will be achieved and may help select alternative therapies to conventional treatment. However, unless alternate therapies are provided that are superior to that which is conventional, the latter treatment still offers a finite and best chance for cure, even in the most unfavorable group. It is also possible that refinements in chemotherapy may lead to an improved result in some of the patients with unfavorable features. This should be distinguished from the situation discussed in the foregoing relative to the translocations, for which the chance for survival is considerably less than 10%, and minor modifications are unlikely to achieve further improvement.

Therefore, in the Gaynor analysis, if we exclude patients with the Ph^1, it may be possible to improve the results achievable, since more effective antileukemic therapy during induction and consolidation could result in a better outcome for patients in whom a small improvement could result in disease eradication. It is probable that the greatest improvement will be seen in the favorable and intermediate groups, and to make progress in the most unfavorable group, a much greater innovation may be required.

The importance of the prognostic factors evaluated by Gaynor have also been confirmed by Hoelzer et al. (36). Thus, the high white blood cell (WBC) count, long interval to achieve CR, older-aged group, and non–T-cell phenotype, all are associated with poor prognosis.

In the series from Linker et al. (8), the T-cell phenotype had no influence. A possible explanation might be found in the exclusion of Ph^1 cases from the series. These patients are virtually only non-T and, therefore, only unfavorable cases are excluded with the exclusion of Ph^1. Removal of unfavorable non-T cases increases the percentage of favorable non-T cases in the series. In children, the T-cell phenotype has been associated with a poor prognosis (16) and both children and adults with CALLA (CD10)-positive disease are more likely to be long-term survivors (15,16). As indicated earlier, the T-cell phenotype in adults (4,5) is now recognized as a favorable feature.

A more recent, but not universally tested parameter, is the identification of myeloid antigen expression in patients with adult ALL (18,19). The study by Cancer and Leukemia Group B (CALGB) suggests that the presence of myeloid antigens may be *relevant* and unfavorable (18,19).

Issues raised by the presence of myeloid antigen expression for diagnosis have already been addressed and, in the future, it will be important to clearly define whether any of the patients who historically have been called ALL should be more properly placed in a different category. However, in terms of prognosis, the presence of myeloid antigen in ALL, although *relevant* and unfavorable, does not preclude cure. Thus, the remission rate of patients who possess myeloid antigen was only 35%, when compared with the 76% in those in whom it was absent (18,19). Remission duration does not appear to be affected by the presence of myeloid antigen, but survival is reduced if the antigen is detected. Within subgroups of B- and T-cell ALL, the presence of the myeloid antigen appears to be more crucial in those with B-cell disease. Thus, in remission induction rates, patients who have B-cell ALL and a myeloid phenotype also had a 29% remission rate versus 71% for ALL without a myeloid phenotype.

In T-cell disease, no significant difference was detected. Since remission duration does not seem to be influenced substantially by the presence of the antigen, we must conclude that patients with this phenotype who achieve remission probably have a reasonable expectation of cure, assuming that the other factors are not adverse.

Whether or not a different induction regimen that is more effective against myeloid cells, while still being effective against lymphoid cells, may be superior remains to be seen.

PRINCIPLES OF THERAPY

Historically, treatment for adults with ALL has followed the principles developed in children (37). This includes recognition of the need to treat systemic disease as well as to treat sanctuary sites (CNS and testes). Treatment of sanctuary sites required a recognition in adults that central nervous system is the primary sanctuary and that testicular relapse, although a problem in children, is not a major issue in this aged group. Reasons for this are not clear, but presumably relate to the changes that occur in puberty.

Systemic disease has been treated primarily using methods outlined by Skipper and Schabel in mouse leukemia. This program applied as "induction," "consolidation," and "maintenance" therapy successfully cured increasing numbers of children.

TREATMENT OF SYSTEMIC DISEASE

Treatment usually begins with combinations of vincristine, prednisone, and a third agent. In some programs, the third agent is doxorubicin (Adriamycin) (4), and in others, it is asparaginase. More recently, podophyllins alone or in combination with cytarabine (8,38,39) have been added effectively to this backbone of vincristine–prednisone, with success. But regardless of the regimen employed, remission rates of approximately 70–85% have been consistently obtained. In one of the programs with the most favorable results, aggressive administration of the three agents is required (4). Thus, up to 4 mg of vincristine are administered weekly in the L10 protocol and, similarly, no upper limit was placed on the amount of prednisone or doxorubicin that a large surface area requires (i.e., the concept of dose-intensity) (40,41). In some programs a fourth drug is added; thus, Hoelzer (5) and Linker (8) both add asparaginase to initial induction therapy and Memorial Hospital has tested the addition of an initial dose of cyclophosphamide. These modifications have not resulted in higher cure rates.

After achieving remission, patients then undergo *consolidation therapy*. This primarily consists of cell cycle-specific drugs, since early relapse was felt to be due to persistence of rapidly proliferating cells (3). After recovery from several cycles of consolidation, patients then receive an *eradication* schedule that includes cycle-specific and nonspecific drugs. The latter are employed to eradicate the out-of-cycle cycle or G_0 cells that are thought to be responsible for late relapse.

It is universally accepted that patients must receive intensive chemotherapy to achieve remission, but the role of consolidation in the development of curative therapy remains controversial. Some of the best results have been achieved with an intensive phase immediately after achieving remission (4–11).

Consolidation or postinduction treatment has also varied. At Memorial Hospital, this previously included six cycles of chemotherapy lasting 4–6 months. Because of the long periods of hospitalization that this required, a more recent modification now requires that patients receive only two cycles, with some increase in intensity of drug administration to increase the leukemia cytoreduction that might be compromised by reducing the number of cycles of treatment (42).

Linker (8) extended the period of consolidation to approximately 11 months, and in his regimen, he alternates cycles of either teniposide and cytarabine with doxorubicin–vincristine–prednisone. Hoelzer (5) called the first consolidation, the second induction regimen. Patients receive cytarabine, thioguanine, cyclophosphamide (not very different from that which Memorial had previously used) followed by vincristine–prednisone and an anthracycline and, then again, the same program with cyclophosphamide–vincristine and anthracycline before the initiation of maintenance therapy. This program has consolidation of approximately 3 months, which is comparable with the current Memorial program.

In at least one randomized trial, there was no clear-cut indication that favored the administration of intensive consolidation (43). The importance of consolidation, however, as in the case of AML, may reflect the efficiency of the induction therapy in achieving reduction in the leukemia burden. Thus, when the induction therapy is inadequate, consolidation therapy becomes critical. When induction has been more effective and greater reduction in total leukemia burden has occurred, consolidation becomes less important.

In the series from Belgium (43), the overall results of both arms, with and without intensive consolidation, were inferior to those achieved at Memorial Hospital (4). Conceptually, maintenance therapy is given to maintain the leukemia burden at a level that permits normal hematopoiesis. Remissions have been "maintained" most often with a combination of oral 6-mercaptopurine and methotrexate. The Memorial program added cycle-nonspecific therapy and more properly is designated an *eradication* schedule, since there is clear-cut intent to induce cure by the elimination of the last leukemic cell. For reasons that are not obvious, it would appear the mercaptopurine and methotrexate are also effective in achieving eradication in some patients. A possible explanation for the effectiveness of these agents may lie once again in the effectiveness of induction and consolidation therapy in achieving minimal residual disease. The duration of maintenance or eradication is arbitrary, but programs as short as 3 years, 2-½ years, and 2 years have been tested and found effective. Logic would have us believe that a shorter course of eradication therapy might be acceptable if eradication of all leukemic cells is achieved earlier.

Thus far, programs that have attempted to deliver shorter periods of maintenance therapy, have not proved effective. The most clear-cut example of this is the CALGB protocol in which therapy stopped after 7 months. Induction therapy consisted of 3 weekly injections of vincristine with daily prednisone and either three doses of mitoxantrone or daunorubicin (DNR) on days 1, 2, and 3. Following recovery of blood counts, the patients who had received DNR then received intrathecal and high-dose intravenous methotrexate with leucovorin (citrovorin factor) as prophylaxis against central nervous system leukemia; followed by two cycles of DNR, and then intensification with two cycles of daunorubicin, vincristine, prednisone; then continuous-infusion cytarabine, and finally mercaptopurine with asparaginase for 1 month. The patients who had achieved remission with mitoxantrone-based therapy received consolidation therapy with daunorubicin, vincristine, prednisone, followed by a repeat of the mitoxantrone, vincristine, prednisone regimen; cytarabine by continuous infusion, and then 1 month therapy of mercaptopurine and asparaginase. Neither of these programs was effective, and the high relapse rate seen in both arms led to early termination of this trial.

All the details of treatment actually given and the outcome have, as yet, not been fully reported. Although it is true that the absence of maintenance therapy may have contributed to the poor result, it is also probable that the unusual induction–consolidation program (which is so different from all the other effective therapies) was suboptimal and may have contributed to the poor outcome.

The entry criteria vary in the effective programs and, therefore, the results are not directly comparable. Thus, the Linker (8) program did not include people older than aged 50 and also did not have patients with the Ph^1 chromosome. The Hoelzer (5) program was all-inclusive, as was the Memorial program (4), although in the initial report from the latter center, the smaller than expected number of patients with the Ph^1 raises the possibility that some may have been inadvertently excluded and classed with blastic phase of chronic myelogenous leukemia (30). The median remission duration, survival, and the percentage of long-term survival are comparable. It would appear that the differences in the results of these various systemic chemotherapy programs may be a function of variability in the characteristics of the patients treated. Since the conceptual design was similar, this should not be surprising.

Treatment of sanctuary sites in children by aggressive therapy of the central nervous system (CNS) with either radiation therapy or intrathecal therapy has led to reduction in relapse rates (1,4,5). With the best therapy, CNS leukemia is an infrequent complication of the disease, occurring in approximately 8% of cases. Similarly, aggressive assessment of the testis by biopsy and subsequent radiation, if needed, has also reduced this as a cause for failure. In adults, as noted earlier, testicular relapse has not been an important cause of failure, and treatment of sanctuary sites has primarily been directed at prevention of CNS disease. In adults without specific therapy directed to the CNS, from the time of diagnosis the relapse rate can be as high as 20% (44). Historically, for prophylaxis, children have received up to 2400 cGy to the CNS. Although children may develop secondary cognitive disorders, this virtually never occurs in adults. Because of this, radiation therapy is considered useful in adults, and two of the larger groups (5,8) still employ this modality for prophylaxis. However, the administration of intensive intrathecal therapy with methotrexate is an equally effective approach (44).

In one of the earlier series, intrathecal therapy was limited to induction and consolidation phases, so that patients received no more than six to eight doses of treatment (2). However, in a subsequent trial, a more vigorous approach was employed, so that the patients received intrathecal methotrexate twice during the first, third, and fifth weeks of induction, then repeatedly during consolidation, and then, two additional doses were given at 11-week intervals during 3 years of maintenance (4). The rate of relapse, at least in this series, was no worse than that of radiation therapy. This has been confirmed by other trials using the same methodology. Another modification to this method is the use of an Ommaya reservoir (45) to deliver the methotrexate directly into the lateral ventricle. This serves to distribute the methotrexate more evenly throughout the cerebrospinal fluid (CSF) (46).

This is the method used especially for patients with high-risk ALL—those with the highest WBC counts (above 20×10^9/L). In the series most carefully studied (4), the risk of CNS relapse in the patients with the high count was equal to that of patients at low risk, suggesting an advantage for patients receiving methotrexate through the Ommaya reservoir. Whether this implies that patients who are at low risk might additionally benefit by having an Ommaya reservoir placed is unclear. Since the risk in these patients is so low, it is unlikely that this question will be answered. However, the ease of administration supports the use of the reservoir, which in some instances, has been left it in place for more than 10 years even after the reservoir was not required.

Other agents (e.g., systemic or intrathecal cytarabine) (47) have been employed for treating established CNS disease, and this may also be useful in prophylaxis. In children and adults, high-dose systemic methotrexate has also been employed as a means of prophylaxis. Intrathecal cytarabine should be used in patients sensitive to methotrexate.

Established CNS leukemia is usually treated with intrathecal methotrexate or cytarabine, or both agents, to clear the spinal fluid and with radiation therapy to clear meningeal disease. It has been reported that high-dose cytarabine is also effective in treating CNS disease (47). However, this requires the administration of 3 g/m^2 of cytarabine twice daily, and in older patients or in those who have received CNS radiation therapy, cerebral or cerebellar toxicity may limit its use.

BONE MARROW TRANSPLANTATION

Bone marrow transplantation (BMT) is an effective method of achieving long-term disease-free survival in adults with ALL. The great difficulty facing clinicians is selecting appropriate timing for the procedure. Bone marrow transplantation can cure the occasional patient with ALL in relapse (48–50). In some series, the cure rate is 10–15%, and if this number were representative of all trials, it would suggest that patients with ALL in relapse are not well-served by undergoing BMT as a routine at this phase of the disease. In at least one small series, 4/15 (26%) of patients achieved long-term survival after BMT while in relapse, and it is thus possible that with improved methods of cytoreduction, this can become a valid alternative (50). However, long-term survival is more commonly encountered after BMT of patients while in remission, and a favorable outcome has been reported if performed in patients in either first, second, or even third remission (49–52). As in AML, there appears to be an advantage in some series for doing the procedure at time of first remission (51,52). However, long-term survival of patients with ALL in first remission, who then undergo BMT, is not substantially higher than in patients who receive optimal chemotherapy without BMT (4,51).

Long-term disease-free survival of adults in second remission (51) in one series was 26 ± 6% and in another, 6 of 15 or 40% of patients more than 20 years old achieved long-term survival (50). The risk of relapse after BMT in second remission for a combined group of children and adults was 52 ± 8% and, in this series, was worse than the relapse rate that occurred in patients who received transplants in first remission, (30% ± 10%) (51). Similarly, in another trial, 16 of 27 adults with ALL receiving an allogeneic BMT in first CR were still in remission, with a median follow-up of 56 months (52). These trials support a BMT in first remission. However, if patients undergoing reinduction therapy for second CR were to receive treatment to which they were not even partially resistant, such as high-dose myelosuppressive therapy not previously used, and leukemic cytoreduction was equal to or greater than that achieved during the first CR, the higher relapse rate should not be anticipated.

In the Barrett series (51), adults who received BMT in first remission, had a higher mortality from transplant-related complications than did children. Relapse, as well as transplantation-related complications led to poor results for patients in second CR. Although the results in second CR are not as good as those for first CR, they are better than the results of chemotherapy alone for patients in second remission (53).

In the chemotherapy group, long-term survival is very infrequent and virtually not reported in most series. Results of the Dinsmore experience (50) therefore demonstrate a favorable outcome for patients with a transplant in second CR and support the continued use of chemotherapy as primary treatment of the disease. This supports the limitation of BMT to salvaging patients who have failed curative sublethal chemotherapy of ALL.

The foregoing comments apply only to patients with ALL who are curable with conventional treatment. As noted, patients with cytogenetic translocations can be treated effectively and achieve remission at approximately the same rate as that for standard ALL. However, apart from the occasional success that occurs in the youngest patients, long-term disease-free survival is rare. Recently Foreman et al. (34) reported success with BMT in a group of patients with t(9;22). In this series, 6 of 11 patients who received transplants during their first CR achieved long-term disease-free survival. A similar finding might also be true for the other translocations, and BMT is worthy of investigation in these groups.

Apart from selection of "remission status" in the timing of BMT, other factors are also important in predicting relapse.

In the Barrett series (51), the use of methotrexate together with steroids to prevent graft-versus-host disease (GVHD) was associated with the lowest probability of relapse (17 $\pm$ 14%), but when cyclosporine, cyclosporine with steroids, or a T-depleted BMT was used, a statistically significantly higher risk of relapse occurred (5.2 times greater, $p < 0.0003$). Patients without any evidence of GVHD had a risk of relapse 3.1 times higher than those with acute or chronic GVHD ($p < 0.0004$). This has also been seen in CML (54). Total elimination of all GVHD is associated with a higher relapse rate. This increased risk of relapse however, may be an acceptable risk in adults who are older and at higher risk for GVHD and death. To avoid problems of relapse, one might speculate that intensive therapy directed at reducing the leukemic burden to a minimum (55, 56), followed by the best GVH prophylaxis, even if it eliminates GVHD completely, may offer the best chance for long-term survival. In addition, manipulation of the NK cell system by interleukin-2 (57) in the post-BMT period may stimulate "immunotherapy" against the leukemia, without the harmful effects of GVHD.

It is self-evident that the majority of adults with ALL are not suitable for allogeneic BMT, either by virtue of advanced age (older than 50 years) or the absence of a suitable donor. For these patients, several options with autologous BMTs are available. Since transplantation of bone marrow harvested from patients with leukemia in remission may harbor significant numbers of clonogenic leukemic cells that may result in relapse, several methods for purging these residual leukemic cells have been developed. They include purging with (1) anti-CD9, anti-CD10 (CALLA), and complement (58, 59), (2) chemotherapeutic agents such as 4-hydroperoxycyclophosphamide (60, 61); and (3) a cocktail of several different monoclonal antibodies (62), as developed by the group in Minnesota.

A purging protocol with anti-CALLA monoclonal antibodies was developed at the Dana–Farber Cancer Center (58, 59). Bone marrow cells are incubated first with the antibody and then complement, and then cryopreserved. After the patient has received curative supralethal treatment, the marrow is then reinfused. The program was initially developed for children with relapsed ALL (58) and, more recently, has been applied to adults (59). In 11 adults who have undergone the procedure, all demonstrated engraftment, 3 patients died of infection and 1 died of acute myocardial infarction. Of the remaining patients, 2 relapsed at 4 and 6.8 months, respectively after BMT, and 5 patients remain in CR at 8+ to 56 months post-BMT. This very encouraging result demonstrates the availability of alternative effective therapy for a group of patients who historically have had very limited survival. As was proposed for allogeneic BMT, it supports the use of this methodology in patients who are in first remission and are at high risk of relapse. Currently, the data is probably good enough to warrant its incorporation into the primary treatment of patients with ALL in first CR who have the translocations. Success in this group might encourage its expansion into patients with high-risk disease, with low but definite cure rates. Yeager et al. have shown that autologous BMT following ex vivo marrow treatment with 4-hydroperoxycyclophosphamide (4-HC) (60, 61) is very effective in AML, but poor results in ALL have not encouraged widespread use of this procedure. Fifteen adults with ALL were treated in this manner. Recovery of bone marrow was consisent with granuloycytes recovering in a median of 26 days. Of the fifteen patients with ALL, 12 had hematological relapse in a median of 116 days, range 63–473 days, after BMT. Of the remaining 3, one had isolated CNS relapse at 283 days and another is in CR at 365 days. These data do not support the use of 4-HC as an effective purging agent in adults with ALL, and other methodologies using chemotherapy will have to be developed.

A third approach was developed in children, using a cocktail of monoclonal antibodies: BA-1, BA-2, BA-3, with complement (62). In this program, 23 patients in remission received high-dose chemotherapy followed by bone marrow treated with a combination of monoclonal antibodies consisting of BA-1, BA-2, BA-3, and rabbit complement. All 23 patients had engraftment and, of the 23 patients, 7 have remained disease free, from 6 to 32 months. The remaining patients have all relapsed, except 1 who died of infection. Since long-term survival is possible after reconstitution with bone marrow treated with these monoclonal antibodies, its applicability in adults warrants further evaluation.

These three programs with ABMT began with great expectations, and the trial in adults with anti-CD9 and CD-10 has proved worthy of more aggressive evaluation in high-risk patients, and the Minnesota programs should now also be explored in adults. Further testing of autologous programs that use innovative purging techniques will be required, since many patients do not have compatible donors and are at high risk for relapse. Although great efforts will still be required to improve purging methodologies, this would be more successful if the leukemia burden to be purged were minimal.

The introduction of therapies that during induction–consolidation result in more effective leukemic cytoreduction than in the past, is equally important for autologous BMT to become a reality. It is even possible that current purging techniques are adequate, in the context of minimal residual disease (63), but inadequate because of the use of less optimal induction–consolidation.

INNOVATIONS FOR THE FUTURE

The critical steps necessary for an increase in cure rate are (1) to develop accurate means of diagnosing ALL inpatients who are curable with chemotherapy, (2) to develop programs that will assure a cure in these patients, (3) to discover new programs with improved efficacy against ALL. Therefore, it may be helpful to be able to identify *minimal residual disease* (63), which will identify patients who have achieved sufficient leukemic cytoreduction with current conventional therapy and, accordingly, are suitable to receive curative therapy with either conventional chemotherapy or BMT.

Similarly, it will be important to identify those whose leukemic burden is excessive and, consequently, precludes cure. The latter will require an alternative. It is insufficient to simply suggest that those who cannot be cured by chemotherapy should receive BMT, since some of these patients (by virtue of an excess leukemia burden) may also not be curable by BMT, and performing an unnecessary procedure, with its inherent toxic effects, is not appropriate. For those who cannot be cured with chemotherapy and who also cannot be cured by BMT, it is worthwhile to reintroduce the concept of maintenance chemotherapy that aims to maintain the leukemia burden at a minimum for as long as possible, consistent with quality survival.

It is also important to test new concepts of therapy in the hope that increasing numbers of patients will be included in the group curable with chemotherapy. Thus, if we again examine prognostic factors and remove patients with *critical* unfavorable characteristics (cytogenetic translocations) (12), the average expected remission rate among the potentially curable patients (representing 70% of the total patient population) should be 75%. If all of these are cured, then 52.5% (75% × 70) would be the limit achievable with chemotherapy. However, this value is unrealistically high, since no current regimen that we have is able to cure all patients entering remission. With a higher CR rate we may reach a potential for cure in 65–70%. Since we currently cure only about 35% of the patients with this diagnosis and since in most analyses the translocations have not been removed, it suggests that, unless there is a major change in our treatment, we may be close to the theoretical limit achievable.

To achieve the maximum cure rate, it may be worthwhile to explore the approach developed at St. Jude for high-risk ALL (38, 39). Patients received teniposide and cytarabine at time of presentation before receiving vincristine–prednisone, and with this approach, they were able to demonstrate an increased cure rate over the results achievable with the conventional approach (starting treatment with vincristine–prednisone).

In this program, the application of effective myelosuppressive therapy before administration of vincristine–prednisone offers the potential for delivery of higher total doses of effective anti-ALL therapy than is possible with the previous approach (64). It should be remembered that administration of myelosuppressive therapy after patients have achieved remission is very toxic to the recovering normal hematopoietic stem cells. As a result, dose modification downward from the maximum is a characteristic of many programs. Administration of myelosuppressive therapy when the patient is myelosuppressed anyway because of the presence of leukemia offers the potential of delivering the maximum effective antileukemic dose.

An example of a second program that incorporates full doses of myelosuppressive therapy for induction therapy in patients with evidence of leukemia, is the combination of amsacrine with high-dose cytarabine (65, 66). Forty patients received amsacrine, 200 mg/m^2 intravenously daily for 3 days, with cytarabine, 3 g/m^2 over 3 hours once daily, for 5 days. In this series, there were 36 patients in relapse and 4 with primary refractory disease. There were 27 complete responders of the 36 patients in relapse, and there were 2 responders in the primary refractory cases. Thus, it was possible to demonstrate remission induction rates comparable with those achieved with vincristine–prednisone. In the patients who achieved remission, the median time to CR was 28 days, which was identical with that achieved with vincristine–prednisone.

A similar result has been reported by Hiddemann et al. (67) for the combination of mitoxantrone with high-dose cytarabine. Patients received cytarabine, 3 g/m^2 intravenously every 12 hours, with mitoxantrone 10 mg/m^2 daily for 4 or 5 doses. Of the 27 patients treated, there were 13 CRs, including 4 CRs in 8 patients with primary refractory disease and 9 responders in 16 patients who had a previous remission. Two patients, who were treated for relapse after a previous BMT, failed to achieve CR. At M. D. Anderson (68), 25 patients with refractory ALL received mitoxantrone, 5 mg/m^2 daily for 5 days, with cytarabine, 3 g/m^2 over 2 hours every 12 hours for 6 doses. Of these, 9 (36%) achieved CR; 3 died during induction (32%); and 8 had resistant disease. Complete remission was achieved in 3 of 11 (27%) of the patients in first relapse; 2 of 7 (28%) in second relapse; and 4 of 7 (57%) in third relapse or higher CR.

The demonstration that combinations of myelosuppressive agents are effective therapy in these programs supports a novel approach to treating primary untreated ALL (64). It may make more sense to administer effective myelosuppressive therapy to patients who are myelosuppressed at time of diagnosis because of the diagnosis of ALL, rather than to deliver it during consolidation. Then, after patients achieve remission, it should be appropriate to deliver nonmyelosuppressive (vincristine–prednisone-based) consolidation therapy as the first consolidation phase. Since it may be possible to start this consolidation therapy virtually simultaneously with achieving CR, there could also be less concern about recovery of residual leukemia during the "intertreatment" period. With the traditional approach, patients frequently are given a "rest" after CR is achieved.

Although repeated courses of consolidation may be undersirable, it may be appropriate to administer one or, at most, two additional courses of consolidation, since in some programs, intensive therapy is required for a high cure rate in some of the subsets of ALL (e.g., T-cell). Following this, it is appropriate to administer an eradication schedule that is consistent with a fairly normal lifestyle. A variation of the eradication schedule developed at Memorial Hospital could be considered, although others are also worthy of evaluation. Essentially, the programs could combine pulse doses of vincristine–prednisone with mercaptopurine–methotrexate and agents such as doxorubicin and cyclophosphamide to eradicate the out-of-cycle (G_0) cells.

This approach, at a minimum, would reduce toxicity and the number of hospitalizations that the previous programs necessitated. It would also test whether delivery of maximum doses of myelosuppressive therapy and full-dose vincristine–prednisone-based therapy would result in greater reduction in the leukemia burden. It is possible that this approach will achieve sufficient reduction of the leukemia burden that the eradication schedule would eliminate the remaining burden. Whether amsacrine, mitoxantrone, or a third agent is the essential ingredient for this approach, remains to be clarified. It will be necessary, in the future, to optimize therapy with these agents by "fine-tuning" the dose schedule and selection of second or third drugs for the combination.

The patients with Ph^1 plus ALL remain a great challenge. The amsacrine-based therapy described in the foregoing has proved ineffective in inducing remissions (none of 18 patients receiving this treatment achieved CR) (69). However, the majority of patients treated were Ph^1-positive and frequently possessed a breakpoint on chromosome 22 in the major breakpoint region of the *BCR* gene. Thus, many could have been more properly classed as blastic phase of chronic myelogenous leukemia. In the future, it may be important to rapidly identify patients who have the breakpoint in the minor region of the *BCR* gene. (This is becoming more available through the polymerase chain reaction). If additional studies show that patients who are bcr– and Ph+ respond to myelosuppressive therapy, it might be possible to test the hypothesis in this group as well. If this group is also not responsive to myelosuppressive therapy, we may have to accept the results of previous studies that support the use of vincristine–prednisone for induction therapy (12, 30).

This group could then benefit from an autologous BMT, since presumably, when these patients enter remission, they often have recovery of normal hematopoiesis. This contrasts with the situation in CML in which remission of blast crisis infrequently induces recovery of normal hematopoiesis. With this disease, an allogeneic BMT is the only logical therapeutic option.

CONCLUSION

Acute lymphocytic leukemia has served as a model for cure of neoplasia for the last several decades. Recently, several programs have begun to reflect the curability of this disease with long-term survival reaching 30–35%. Although the application of curative therapy is now possible worldwide, the last decade has not seen further improvement in the results in centers that have traditionally led the way in increasing cure rates.

Further progress will require (1) establishing an accurate diagnosis for the identification of patients who are curable by chemotherapy; (2) careful definition of prognostic subgroups so that alternatives can be developed for high-risk patients, in whom conventional chemotherapy offers only a limited chance of survival; (3) improvement in the effectiveness of chemotherapy by the introduction of newer agents and more effective scheduling of these agents; (4) allogeneic bone marrow transplantation in patients in second or subsequent remission with standard-risk ALL, and BMT for patients in first remission with unfavorable *critical* prognostic features; (5) improvement in the methodologies used in autologous BMT, such that increasing numbers of patients who are not curable with chemotherapy can be offered an effective alternate approach with an increasing expectation of cure.

ACKNOWLEDGMENTS

To Sanford J. Kempin for reviewing the manuscript and for his helpful suggestions; and to Hazel Amodio for her dedication in the preparation of the manuscript.

REFERENCES

1. Haghbin M, Murphy ML, Tan CC, et al: A long-term clinical follow-up of children with acute lymphoblastic leukemia treated with intensive chemotherapy regimens. *Cancer* 1980; 46:241.
2. Gee TS, Haghbin M, Dowling MD, et al: Acute lymphoblastic leukemia in adults and children. Differences in response with similar therapeutic regimens. *Cancer* 1976; 37:1256.
3. Arlin Z, Fried J, Clarkson B: Therapeutic role of cell kinetics in acute leukemia. *Clin Hematol* 1978; 7:339–36.
4. Schauer P, Arlin Z, Mertelsmann R, et al: Treatment of acute leukemia in adults: Results of the L-10 and L-10M protocols. *J Clin Oncol* 1983; 1:462–470.
5. Hoelzer D, Thiel E, Loffler H, et al: Intensified therapy in acute lymphoblastic and acute undifferentiated leukemia in adults. *Blood* 1984; 64:38–47.
6. Blacklock HA, Matthews JRD, Buchanan JG, et al: Improved survival from acute lymphoblastic leukemia in adolescents and adults. *Cancer* 1981: 43:1931.
7. Radford JE Jr, Burns CP, Jones MP, et al: Adult acute lymphoblastic leukemia: Results of the Iowa Hop-L protocol. *J Clin Oncol* 1989; 7:58–66.
8. Linker CA, Levitt LJ, O'Donnell M, et al: Improved results of treatment of adult acute lymphoblastic leukemia. *Blood* 1987; 69:1242.
9. Amadori S, Montuoro A, Meloni G, et al: Combination chemotherapy for acute lymphocytic leukemia in adults: Results of a retrospective study in 82 patients. *Am J Hematol* 1980; 8:175.

10. Willemze R, Drenthe-Schonk AM, van Rossum J, Haanen C: Treatment of acute lymphoblastic leukemia in adolescents and adults. Comparison of two schedules for CNS leukaemia prophylaxis. *Scand J Haematol* 1980; 24:421.
11. Hussein KK, Dahlberg S, Head D, et al: Treatment of acute lymphoblastic leukemia in adults with intensive induction, consolidation, and maintenance chemotherapy. *Blood* 1989; 73:57–63.
12. Bloomfield CD, Goldman AI, Alimena G, et al: Chromosomal abnormalities identify high-risk and low-risk patients with acute lymphoblastic leukemia. *Blood* 1986; 67:415–420.
13. Rodriguez V, Hart JS, Freireich EJ, et al: POMP combination chemotherapy of adult leukemia. *Cancer* 1973; 32:69–75.
14. Bollum FJ: Terminal deoxynucleotidyl transferase as a hematopoietic cell marker. *Blood* 1979; 54:1203.
15. Greaves MF, Janossy G, Peto J, Kay H: Immunologically defined subclasses of acute lymphoblastic leukaemia in children: Their relationship to presentation features and prognosis. *Br J Haematol* 1981; 48:179–197.
16. Greaves MF, Lister TA: Prognostic importance of immunologic markers in adult acute lymphoblastic leukemia. *N Engl J Med* 1981; 304:119–120.
17. Sen L, Borella L: Clinical importance of lymphoblasts with T markers in childhood acute leukemia. *N Engl J Med* 1975; 292:828–832.
18. Sobol RE, Mick R, Royston I, et al: Clinical importance of myeloid antiger expression in adult acute lymphoblastic leukemia. *N Engl J Med* 1987; 316:1111.
19. Sobol RE, Royston 1, LeBien TW, et al: Adult acute lymphoblastic leukemia phenotypes defined by monoclonal antibodies. *Blood* 1985; 65:730–735.
20. Korsmeyer SJ, Arnold A, Bakhshi A, et al: Immunoglobulin gene rearrangement and cell surface antigen expression in acute lymphocytic leukemias of T cell and B cell precursor origins. *J. Clin Invest* 1983; 71:301–313.
21. Tawa A, Hozumi N, Minden M, et al: Rearrangement of the T cell receptor B chain gene in non-T, non-B acute lymphoblastic leukemia of childhood. *N Engl J Med* 1985; 313:1033.
22. Chen Z, Le Paslier D, Dausset J, et al: Human T-cell rearranging genes gamma are very frequently rearranged in B-lineage acute lymphoblastic leukemias but not in chronic B-cell proliferations. *J. Exp Med* 1987; 165–1000.
23. Smith LJ, Curtis JE, Messner HA, et al: Lineage infidelity in acute leukemia. *Blood* 1983; 61:1138–1145.
24. Greaves MF, Chan LC, Furley AJW, et al: Lineage promiscuity in hematopoietic differentiation and leukemia. *Blood* 1986; 67:1–11.
25. Mertelsmann R, Koziner B, Ralph P, et al: Evidence for distinct lymphocytic and monocytic populations in a patient with terminal transferase positive acute leukemia. *Blood* 1978; 51:1051–1056.
26. Bradstock KF, Hoffbrand AV, Ganeshaguru K, et al: Terminal deoxynucleotidyl transferase expression in acute nonlymphoic leukemia. An analysis by immunofluorescence. *Br J Haematol* 1981; 47:133.
27. Mirro J, Kitchingman G, Williams D, et al: Clinical and laboratory characteristics of acute leukemia with the 4; 11 translocations. *Blood* 1986; 67:689.
28. Nagasaka M, Maeda S, Maeda H, et al: Four cases of t(4;11) acute leukemia and its myelomonocytic nature in infants. *Blood* 1983; 61:1174–1181.

29. Hooberman AL, Westbrook CA, Davey F, et al: Molecular detection of the Philadelphia chromosome (Ph^1) in adult acute lymphoblastic leukemia (ALL): Clinical, cytogenetic and immunophenotypic correlations in a CALGB study. *Blood* 1989; 74(suppl):52a.
30. Jain K, Arlin Z, Mertelsmann R, et al: Philadelphia chromosome and terminal transferase-positive acute leukemia: Similarity of terminal phase of chronic myelogenous leukemia and denovo acute presentation. *J Clin Oncol 1983;* 1:669–676.
31. Heisterkamp N, Jenkins R, Thibodeau S, et al: The *bcr* gene in Philadelphia chromosome positive acute lymphoblastic leukemia. *Blood* 1989; 73:1307–1311.
32. Groffen J, Stephenson JR, Heisterkamp N, et al: Philadelphia chromosomal breakpoints are clustered within a limited region, *bcr,* on chromosome 22. *Cell* 1985; 36:93.
33. Schaefer-Rego K, Arlin ZA, Shapiro L, et al: Molecular heterogeneity of adult Philadelphia chromosome positive ALL. *Cancer Res* (in press).
34. Forman SJ, O'Donnell MR, Nademanee AP, et al: Bone marrow transplantation for patients with Philadelphia chromosome positive acute lymphoblastic leukemia. *Blood* 1987; 70:587.
35. Gaynor J, Chapman D, Little C, et al: A cause-specific hazard rate analysis of prognostic factors among 199 adults with acute lymphocytic leukemia: The Memorial Hospital experience since 1969. *J. Clin Oncol* 1988; 6:1014.
36. Hoelzer D, Thiel E, Loffler H, et al: Prognostic factors in a multicenter study for treatment of acute lymphoblastic leukemia in adults. *Blood* 1988; 71:123.
37. Pinkel D: Five year follow-up of "total therapy" of childhood lymphocytic leukemia. *JAMA* 1971; 215:648.
38. Rivera G, Dahl GV, Bowman WP, et al: VM-26 and cytosine arabinoside combination chemotherapy for initial induction failures in childhood lymphocytic leukemia. *Cancer* 1980; 46:1727.
39. Dahl GV, Rivera GK, Look AT, et al: Teniposide plus cytarabine improves outcome in childhood acute lymphoblastic leukemia presenting with a leukocyte count $>100 \times 10^9/1$. *J Clin Oncol* 1987; 5:1015.
40. Hryniuk W, Bush H: The importance of dose intensity in chemotherapy of metastatic breast cancer. *J Clin Oncol* 1984; 3:1281–1288.
41. De Vita VT: Dose–response is alive and well. *J Clin Oncol* 1986; 4:1157–1159.
42. Arlin ZA, Gee TS, Mertelsmann R, et al: Treatment of acute lymphoblastic leukemia (ALL) in adults: Comparability of results using extended and brief consolidation therapy. *Proc Am Assoc Cancer Res* 1983; 24:119.
43. Stryckmans P, Marie JP, Debusscher L, et al: Chemotherapy of adult acute lymphoblastic leukemia (ALL). Protocol 58791. A randomized study [abstr]. *Blood* 1985; 66 (suppl 1): 209.
44. Kantarjian HM, Walters RS, Smith TL, et al: Identification of risk groups for development of central nervous system leukemia in adults with acute lymphocytic leukemia. *Blood* 1988; 72:1784–1789.
45. Ommaya A: Subcutaneous reservoir and pump for sterile access to ventricular cerebrospinal fluid. *Lancet* 1963; 2:983–984.
46. Shapiro WR, Young DF, Mehta BM: Methotrexate: Distribution in cerebrospinal

fluid after intravenous, ventricular and lumbar injections. *N Engl J Med* 1975, 293:161–166.
47. Morra E, Lazzarino M, Inverardi D, et al: Systemic high-dose ara-C for the treatment of meningeal leukemia in adult acute lymphoblastic leukemia and non-Hodgkin's lymphoma. *J Clin Oncol* 1986; 4:1207–1211.
48. Thomas ED, Storb R, Clift, RA, et al: Bone marrow transplantation. *N Engl J Med* 1975; 292:832–843.
49. Thomas ED, Sanders JE, Fluorney N, et al; Marrow transplantation for patients with acute lymphoblastic leukemia: A long-term follow-up. *Blood* 1983; 62:1139–1141.
50. Dinsmore R, Kirkpatrick D, Flomenberg N, et al: Allogeneic bone marrow transplantation for patients with acute lymphoblastic leukemia. *Blood* 1983; 62:381–388.
51. Barrett AJ, Horowitz MM, Gale RP, et al: Marrow transplantation for acute lymphoblastic leukemia: Factors affecting relapse and survival. *Blood* 1989, 74:862–871.
52. Vernant JP, Marit G, Maraninchi D, et al: Allogeneic bone marrow transplantation in adults with acute lymphoblastic leukemia in first complete remission. *J Clin Oncol* 1988; 6:227–231.
53. Woods WG, Nesbit ME, Ramsa NKD, et al: Intensive therapy followed by bone marrow transplantation for patients with acute lymphocytic leukemia in second or subsequent remission: Determination of prognostic factors (A report from the University of Minnesota Bone Marrow Transplantation Team). *Blood* 1983; 61:1182–1189.
54. Goldman JM, Apperly JF, Jones L, et al: Bone marrow transplantation for patients with chronic myelogenous leukemia. *N Engl J Med* 1986; 314:202–207.
55. Arlin ZA, Hagonbeek A, Feldman E, Andreeff M: Implications of "cell kill" for the treatment of acute myelogenous leukemia: Can the cure rate be increased? *Acta Haematol* 1989; 82:175–178.
56. Arlin ZA, Hiddemann W, Feldman E, et al: Further thoughts on "cell kill" in acute leukemia. (submitted) 1990.
57. Lotzova E, Savary CA, Herberman RB: Induction of NK cell activity against fresh human leukemia in culture with interleukin 2. *J Immunol* 1987; 138:2718.
58. Roy DC, Soiffer RJ, Anderson KC, et al: Autologous bone marrow transplantation with CD9/CD10 depleted marrow for adult patients with relapsed ALL. *Blood* 1989; 74; (suppl 1):196.
59. Ritz J, Sallan SE, Bast RC, et al: Autologous bone marrow transplantation in CALLA positive acute lymphoblastic leukemia after in vitro treatment with J5 monoclonal antibody and complement. *Lancet* 1982; 2:60.
60. Yeager AM, Kaizer H, Santos GW, et al: Autologous bone marrow transplantation in patients with acute nonlymphocytic leukemia, using ex vivo marrow treatment with 4-hydroperoxycyclophosphamide. *N Engl J. Med* 1986; 315:141–147.
61. Yeager AM, Kaizer H, Braine HG, et al: Autologous bone marrow transplantation (ABMT) in acute leukemia: Phase I and II studies of ex-vivo marrow treatment with 4-hydroxyperoxycyclophosphamide (4HC). *Int J Cell Cloning* 1985; 3:237–238.
62. Ramsay N, LeBien TW, Nesbit M, et al: Autologous bone marrow transplantation for patients with acute lymphoblastic leukemia in second or subsequent remission:

Results of bone marrow treated with monoclonal antibodies BA-1, BA-2, BA-2 plus complement. *Blood* 1985; 66:508.
63. Hagenbeek A, Lowenberg B (eds): *Minimal Residual Disease in Acute Leukemia*. Dordrecht, Netherlands, Martinus Nijhoff, 1986.
64. Arlin ZA, Feldman E: Can we increase the cure rate of adults with acute lymphoblastic leukemia? *Leukemia* 1989; 3:318–320.
65. Arlin ZA, Ahmed T, Mittelman A, et al: A new regimen of amsacrine with high dose cytarabine is safe and effective therapy for acute leukemia. *J Clin Oncol* 1987; 5:371–375.
66. Arlin ZA, Feldman E, Kempin S, et al: Amsacrine with high dose cytarabine is highly effective therapy for refractory and relapsed acute lymphoblastic leukemia in adults. *Blood* 1988; 72:433–435.
67. Hiddemann W, Buchner TH, Heil G, et al: Treatment of refractory acute lymphoblastic and acute undifferentiated leukemia in adults with high dose cytosine arabinoside and mitoxantrone (HAM). *Leukemia* (in press).
68. Kantarjian HM, Walters RL, Keating MJ, et al: Mitoxantrone and high-dose cytosine arabinoside for the treatament of refractory acute lymphocytic leukemia. *Cancer* 1990; 65:5–8.
69. Arlin ZA, Feldman EJ, Ahmed T, et al: Philadelphia chromsome positive (Ph^1) lymphoblastic leukemia (ALL) is resistant to effective therapy for Ph^{-1} ALL. *Acta Haematol* 1989; 81:217–218.

4

Treatment of Chronic Myelogenous Leukemia

Hagop Kantarjian* and Moshe Talpaz

University of Texas
M. D. Anderson Cancer Center
Houston, Texas

Chronic myelogenous leukemia (CML) is a clonal myeloproliferative disorder of the hematopoietic pluripotent stem cell (1–5). It accounts for 15–25% of leukemias. The clonal nature of the disease has been documented by chromosomal analysis, by glucose-6-phosphodehydrogenase (G6PD) isoenzyme studies, and by molecular probes (6–8). The disease involves the myeloid, erythroid, megakaryocytic, monocytic, eosinophilic, basophilic, B-cell lymphoid, and sometimes T-cell lymphoid series (9–12). The marrow stromal cells are not clonal (13–15). They may be affected through the hematopoietic–stromal interaction, resulting in secondary myelofibrosis, and they may be important for evolution into the CML advanced stages (16–19).

The Philadelphia chromosome (Ph) is present in the leukemic cells of 95% of patients with CML. This was originally described as a shortened long arm of chromosome 22 (20), which was later identified as a balanced reciprocal translocation of genetic material between the long arms of chromosomes 9 and 22 [t(9;22)(q34;q11)] (21). This easily recognized marker expedites the diagnosis of CML, and helps in the evaluation of novel treatments, through their capacity to suppress the Ph-positive leukemic cells.

Chronic myelogenous leukemia progresses from an indolent chronic phase, into accelerated and blastic phases. This multistep evolution suggests that differ-

---

*Dr. Kantarjian is a Scholar of the Leukemia Society of America

Table 1 Presenting Clinical and Laboratory Features by Year of Diagnosis in Patients with Ph-Positive CML

Characteristic	Percentage with characteristic: Before 1976 (N = 162)	1976–1982 (N = 153)	After 1982 (N = 155)	P value
Clinical				
Age ≥ 60 yr	23	13	11	<0.01
Weight loss ≥ 15 lb	25	14	11	<0.01
Hepatomegaly	48	46	20	<0.01
Splenomegaly	80	72	57	<0.01
Symptoms at diagnosis	86	86	55	<0.01
Peripheral Blood				
Hemoglobin <12g/dL	64	55	49	0.02
WBC count ≥ 100 × $10^3/\mu L$	76	63	53	<0.01
Platelet count ≥ 700 × $10^3/\mu L$	27	30	22	NS
Blasts >0%	71	56	44	<0.01
Basophils ≥7%	20	14	16	NS
Marrow				
Blasts ≥5%	17	14	10	NS
Basophils ≥3%	40	41	42	NS
Cytogenetic clonal evolution	9	12	14	NS

NS, not significant.

ent mechanisms might operate in the various phases of CML (22) and provides different targets for therapy.

The *chronic phase* of CML lasts for a median of 3–4 years when patients are treated with conventional therapy. In the past, most patients presented with signs and symptoms related to leukocytosis, splenomegaly, or thrombocytosis. In recent years, the percentage of asymptomatic patients diagnosed on routine physical examination or blood counts has increased from 15 to 45% (Table 1). Patients are also presenting with smaller degrees of tumor burden, as measured by the degree of anemia, leukocytosis, hepatosplenomegaly, and weight loss (see Table 1). Fewer than 10% of patients are first seen in the accelerated or blastic phase.

Accelerated phase CML is manifested by increased resistance to therapy, accentuated proliferation, and maturation arrest. Its criteria are variable and are often based on (1) either subjective features (e.g., short WBC doubling time, increased drug requirement), or (2) features still consistent with prolonged survival (e.g., blasts greater than 5–10%; basophils greater than 10%). A definition based on the appearance of characteristics associated with a subsequent survival of less than 1.5 years has been proposed (23) (Table 2). Its

Table 2 Criteria of Accelerated Phase CML

A. Univariate analysis of patient survival after development of presumed accelerated phase characteristic

Characteristic	*Median survival (mo)*
Peripheral blasts ≥15%	8.6
Marrow blasts ≥15%	10.9
Peripheral blasts + promyelocytes ≥30%	4.7
Marrow blasts + promyelocytes ≥30%	17.4
Peripheral platelets < 100 × $10^3/\mu L$	14.9
> 2 × $10^6/\mu L$	27.2
Hemoglobin <7g/dL	16.0
Nucleated red cells ≥15%	23.0
Cytogenetic clonal evolution	7.0
Extramedullary disease	10.0

B. Proposed multivariate analysis-selected criteria for accelerated phase CML
- Cytogenetic clonal evolution
- Peripheral blasts 15% or more
- Peripheral blasts and promyelocytes 30% or more
- Peripheral basophils 20% or more
- Platelets less than 100 × $10^3/\mu L$ unrelated to chemotherapy

C. Other criteria used for entry on studies
- Triad of WBC greater than 50 × $10^3/\mu L$, hematocrit less than 25, and platelets lower than 100 × $10^3/\mu L$ not controlled by therapy
- Progressive splenomegaly or adenopathy
- Marrow or peripheral blasts 10% or greater
- Marrow or peripheral basophils ± eosinophils 10% or greater
- Persistent unexplained fever or bone pains

uniform use will facilitate the analysis of trials in accelerated phase CML. Sixty to seventy percent of patients develop accelerated phase CML before death or blastic transformation: 20–30% die in accelerated phase or of myelofibrosis-associated complications; the others evolve into a blastic phase (24–26). *Blastic phase* is defined by the presence of 30% or more blasts in the peripheral blood or bone marrow, or extramedullary disease (24). The development of blastic phase without any antecedent accelerated phase occurs in 20–30% of patients. However, most of them manifest evidence of clinical and hematological resistance to therapy. In our experience, the sudden onset of blastic phase without resistance to therapy, and without accelerated disease features, occurs in fewer than 5% of patients.

The past 10 years have witnessed a revolution in the fields of the biological and therapeutic research in CML. Molecular studies have aided an understanding of the mechanisms associated with the chronic and transformed phases of CML (27–35). The insertion of the abnormal molecular messages associated with CML into normal fibroblasts or hemopoietic cells have resulted in their malignant transformation (36–40) and the development of CML animal models (41,42). These models will be useful in studying the development and progression of CML and should provide better preclinical conditions for testing therapeutic regimens. The relentless progression of CML from the chronic to the fatal accelerated and blastic phases with conventional therapy led to the investigation of new approaches in the chronic phase of CML. Two of them, allogeneic bone marrow transplantation (BMT) and interferon alpha (IFN-α) are promising.

In this review we will discuss the results of conventional and investigational therapies in CML, as well as the potential molecular-targeted approaches. To understand the rationale and the results of such treatments, we will review (1) the biology and pathophysiology of CML, (2) the concepts underlying some of the investigational programs, and (3) the prognostic factors that define the disease aggressiveness and individual patient outcome.

BIOLOGY AND PATHOPHYSIOLOGY

The easy access to blood and marrow sampling has established CML as a prime model to study the multistep evolution of a tumor. Although similar processes may cause other tumors, studying their mechanism of evolution from localized to metastatic stages is difficult owing to sampling problems. Chronic myelogenous leukemia is hypothesized to progress through many phases: (1) an early phase of proliferation of Ph-negative clonal cells; (2) a phase of proliferation of Ph-positive clonal cells, known also as Ph-positive chronic phase CML; and (3) a phase of transformation from chronic to accelerated and blastic phases, within which several abnormal processes may interact. The early phase of Ph-negative clonal proliferation has been proposed based on (1) the documentation of Ph-negative CML patients, who were later shown to develop Ph-positive CML (43–45), an observation possibly explained by inaccurate cytogenetic studies; and (2) in vitro studies isolating Ph-negative clonal cells from patients with CML (22,46), an important finding that requires confirmation.

Different mechanisms control the various CML phases. To understand them, we will review the molecular, cellular, and cytogenetic studies pertinent to the CML pathophysiology.

Molecular and Cytogenetic Observations

Studies of the molecular events in CML have been facilitated by the existence of the cytogenetic fingerprint, the Ph chromosome. The breaks in chromosome 22 associated with the Ph abnormality are localized within a narrow segment measuring 5.8 kilobases (kb), referred to as the breakpoint cluster region *(bcr)*

(27,28). The reciprocal genetic translocation t(9;22)(q34;q11) transposes the normal cellular Abelson (c-*abl*) gene sequence from chromosome 9 and attaches it to the 5' *bcr* region on chromosome 22 (29). This creates a new fusion gene with transforming properties, the *bcr/abl* hybrid oncogene (30). In turn, the *bcr/abl* DNA sequence is translated into abnormal messages at the RNA and protein levels, the 8.5-kb mRNA (31) and the 210-kd (P210) protein. The latter shows increased tyrosine kinase activity (33,34), an important mediator of oncogenesis (47) (Fig. 1).

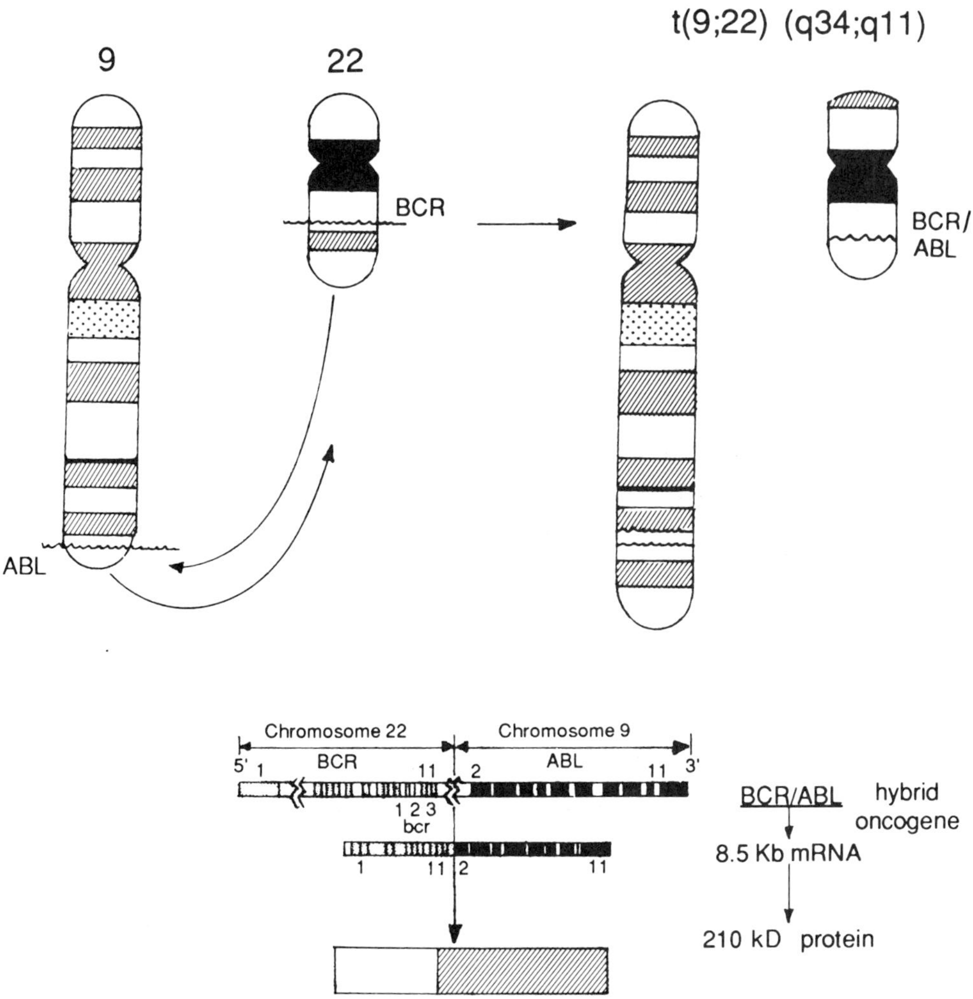

Figure 1 Cytogenetic and molecular abnormalities in CML.

A causal association between the *bcr/abl*-related signals and the pathophysiology of CML has been confirmed by several experiments. A sine qua non for causality would be established through cellular transformation following transfection of the abnormal messages and, conversely, through normalization of the transformed cells by blocking of the abnormal messages (e.g., antisense blockage). Transfection of NIH/3T3 fibroblasts with the P210 *bcr/abl* gene product resulted in the isolation of few transformants that express high levels of P210 kinase activity. Morphological transformation of the fibroblasts required the addition of NH_2-terminal viral *gag* sequences (P220 *gag/bcr/abl*) that contain the myristyl fatty acid moiety needed to anchor the cytoplasmic *bcr/abl* message to the cellular membrane, a necessary step for transformation (36). Similar results were obtained through *bcr/abl* transfection of hematopoietic cells (37). Recently, Daley and associates introduced cDNA encoding P210 *bcr/abl* into mouse marrow cells with a retroviral vector, and reinfused them into lethally irradiated mice (41). Three to eight weeks later, 15% of the mice developed one of three forms of myeloproliferation: (1) a CML picture with leukocytosis, thrombocytosis, and splenomegaly (50% of mice); (2) severe monocytosis or macrophage tumors with organ involvement (25%); and (3) an acute lymphoid leukemic picture (25%). The leukemic cells contained the *bcr/abl* provirus and had a stable expression of P210. Thus the introduction of the P210 *bcr/abl* into mice hematopoietic cells recapitulated the pathogenesis of human CML. This provided strong support that the *bcr/abl* abnormality is tightly linked to the development of chronic phase CML and contributed, perhaps with other intermediate messages, to the evolution into other CML stages (e.g., lymphoid blastic phase, extramedullary disease). Experiments in transgenic mice and other tumors models have produced similar supportive evidence (35,42).

In vitro studies show that introduction of the *bcr/abl* message into growth factor-dependent cell lines may reduce their growth factor requirements (39,48,49). The *bcr/abl* may emancipate CML clones from the requirement of growth factors for proliferation, which would still be needed for normal stem cell growth.

Although the *bcr/abl* abnormality is associated with a CML picture, there are two important questions: (1) Can a chronic phase CML syndrome develop independent of the *bcr/abl* message? (2) Does the *bcr/abl* abnormality contribute to disease transformation?

Available clinical and laboratory observations may partly answer the first question. In Ph-negative CML, a subset of patients without *bcr* rearrangement have a clinical picture and prognosis similar to Ph-positive disease, but have a low frequency of blastic transformation (50,51). This suggests that alternative events (e.g., excessive growth factor production, increased cellular sensitivity to growth factors) may induce a picture that mimics CML, without the presence of the *bcr/abl* abnormality. Supportive evidence is derived from animal models (52) and from the association of juvenile CML and chronic myelomonocytic leukemia (CMML) with growth factor production (53,54). In juvenile CML, excessive production of granulocyte–macrophage colony-stimulating factor (GM-CSF), increased growth of CML colonies with GM-CSF incubation, and suppression of colony growth with anti-GM-CSF antibodies have been observed (53). Interleukin-6 (IL-6) and GM-CSF may act as autocrine growth factors in CMML (54).

The role of the *bcr/abl* abnormality in disease transformation is uncertain. Against such a role are (1) the development of blastic phase CML in patients who have lost the Ph or related *bcr/abl* abnormality (55,56), and (2) the presence of nonrandom chromosomal abnormalities (double Ph, trisomy 8, isochromosome 17) in 50–60% of patients with CML transformation (24,45,57). In favor of such a role are (1) the low incidence of blastic transformation in the subset of patients with typical CML who are Ph-negative without *bcr* rearrangement (50,51), and (2) the development of different morphological pictures, including lymphoid transformation, in mice infused with hemopoietic cells containing the *bcr/abl* abnormality (41).

From the existing information, it is suggested that (1) the *bcr/abl* abnormalities are the initiating event for chronic phase CML in most (Ph-positive CML), but not all cases of CML, (2) the *bcr/abl* abnormalities play a facilitory role in disease transformation, and (3) other mechanisms contribute to CML transformation into the terminal phases.

Identification of the mechanisms of disease transformation other than the *bcr/abl* abnormalities will provide targets for oncogene-directed programs. Suppression of these mechanisms for long periods may induce differentiation and burnout of the chronic phase CML clones, or maintain a durable chronic phase CML picture (analogous to the indolent courses of polycythemia vera or essential thrombocytosis). Molecular abnormalities of CML transformation are under investigation. Amplification of the *bcr/abl* oncogene, possibly by the double Ph chromosome, has been observed in the K562 CML line and, occasionally, in CML blastic phase (58–60). Amplification of the *myc* oncogene may occur with trisomy 8 and could be suppressed by therapeutic intervention (61, 62). Isochromosome 17 represents either a duplication of the messages present on the long arms or a disappearance of antioncogene messages present on the short arm. The *G-CSF* gene localized to 17q11 may participate in disease transformation (63). *p53,* localized on the short arm of chromosome 17, has been reported to be a suppressor gene under certain circumstances (64,65). Its inactivation (deletion or alteration) through the isochromosome 17 abnormality may facilitate CML transformation. Rearrangements or deletions of *p53* are rare in chronic phase CML, but vary in prevalence from 5 to 20% in CML accelerated and blastic phases (66–68). Wetzler et al. reported that interleukin-1β, released by the leukemic clones, may also stimulate the bone marrow stroma to secrete growth factors that promote disease transformation in a paracrine fashion (19). Thus, disease progression from chronic to transformed phases may proceed through different pathways, by the production or deletion messages associated with the cytogenetic abnormalities. The *bcr/abl* abnormality, as discussed, also contributes to disease transformation. In fact, patients evolving from a Ph-positive chronic phase CML to a Ph-negative blastic phase had an unusually indolent progression, suggesting a modulating role of the *bcr/abl* abnormality (55,56). Finally, *ras* oncogene mutations may be involved in the monocytic transformation of CML (69–75). Although rare in Ph-positive CML (70,71), *ras* mutations occur in 40–50% of patients with chronic myelomonocytic leukemia (72, 73), and in acute myelocytic leukemia with monocytic expression (74,75).

Cellular Studies in Chronic Myelogenous Leukemia

The reasons for the growth advantage of Ph-positive clones over the normal stem cells in CML are unknown. The proliferation of CML cells is higher than normal cells in semisolid agar or methycellulose cultures (76,77). In contrast, liquid (Dexter) cultures favor the growth of normal over CML cells (78–82). This suggests that the mechanisms enhancing CML growth in vivo may persist in semisolid cultures, but are abolished in liquid culture. The latter, while attempting to mimic the hemopoietic microenvironment, lacks several of its components.

Recognized differences between CML and normal cells are summarized in Table 3. Discordant maturation has been suggested as the primary defect in CML. A rapid cytoplasmic maturation induces the cells to enter the later maturational compartment, whereas a retarded nuclear maturation allows these more mature leukemic progenitors to undergo more divisions and have a longer life-span than comparable normal mature progenitors (83,84). The CML progenitor cells have a reduced capacity to adhere to the marrow stroma (85). The expression of Ia antigen is decreased or absent on granulocyte–macrophage

Table 3 Observations of Abnormal Cellular Events in Patients with CML

Discordant nuclear (delayed) and cytoplasmic (accelerated) maturation (83,84)
Decreased adhesiveness of CML cells to the marrow matrix (85)
Decreased expression of Ia antigen (86,87)
Decreased natural killer (NK) function (88,89)
Decreased adherent lymphocyte activated killer (A-LAK) cell activity with disease progression (91)
Decreased expression of LFA-3 cytoadhesion molecules (92)
Decreased autologous proliferative T lymphocyte response (93)

colony-forming unit (GM-CFU) colonies in patients with CML, compared with normal bone marrow (86,87). The Ia antigenic determinants are expressed in myeloid progenitor cells early in differentiation and diminish with progressive maturation, indicating their possible role as cell surface signals for differentiation (86,87). Despite possessing normal or increased numbers of circulating natural killer (NK) cells, patients with CML exhibit a profound functional deficiency in NK-cell activity (88). This NK-deficient activity may be mediated through a defective production of interleukin-2 (IL-2) by T-helper or NK cells (89). Verfaillie et al. identified a population of interleukin-2-activated peripheral blood NK cells, referred to as adherent lymphokine-activated killer cells (A-LAK) (90). These cells were benign (not derived from the CML clone), highly cytotoxic, and their activity was diminished with longer disease duration and with transformation into the accelerated and blastic phases (91). The CML progenitor cells are also deficient in cell surface cytoadhesion molecules, such as LFA-3 (92). The LFA-3 antigen is the target by which the CD2 receptor, present on T cells, binds T cells to target cells. The binding of T cells to normal late progenitor cells through the CD2–LFA-3 interaction may negatively regulate hematopoisis. With LFA-3 deficiency this normal regulatory control may be lost (93).

Hypothesis for the Development of Chronic Myelogenous Leukemia

From the previous discussion, we postulate the following model for the development of CML (Fig. 2). The proliferative advantage of CML cells over normal cells results from the *bcr/abl* changes, inducing the emancipation of CML from the requirements for growth factors, which are still needed by normal cells, thereby releasing CML cells from the negative feedback mechanisms (still persistent in normal cells) through changes in the cell surface cytoadhesion or other molecules. These cell surface changes (e.g., poorly formed cytoadhesion molecules) decrease adhesion to marrow stroma and recognition by peripheral suppression or differentiation signals (T cells, NK cells, A-LAK cells). By earlier detachment from the marrow stroma, the disrupted matrix—hematopoietic interaction produces poor maturation of other surface antigens (e.g., la antigens). Thus, CML progenitor cells temporarily escape recognition by differentiation signals, and spend a longer period in the proliferative phase. Interleukin-2 production by NK cells or T-helper cells, A-LAK cells, or other accessory inhibitory cells may contribute to suppressing or differentiating CML cells. Chronic myelogenous leukemia is not completely autonomous, and many patients exhibit regulation-induced oscillations of their white blood cell and platelet counts (94). Once established, the large CML clonal pool may exert a leukemic inhibitory activity that suppresses the normal stem cells (95).

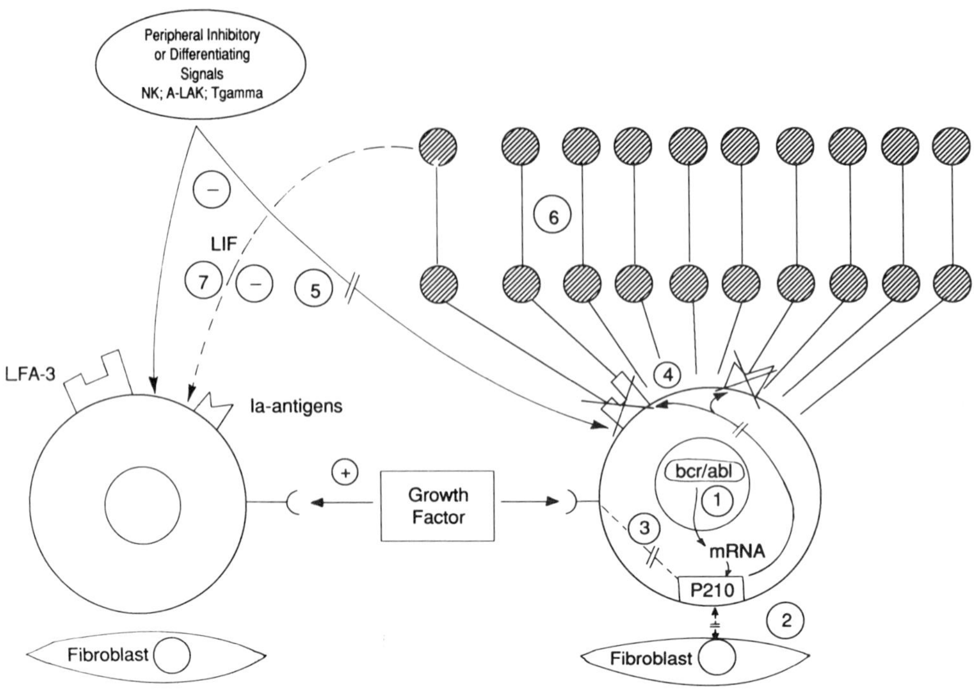

Figure 2 CML versus normal cell proliferation model: Unlike normal cells, the *bcr/abl* abnormality in CML (1) delays nuclear maturation, (2) loosens the matrix–hemopoietic interaction, (3) emancipates cells from normal growth factor requirement, (4) reduces Ia-antigen and LFA-3 expression, thereby (5) preventing the occurrence of negative-feedback mechanism on CML cells, while this persists in normal cells. CML cells proliferate in the late progenitor stage and produce a large CML pool (6), which in turn, suppresses normal stem cell proliferation through the leukemia inhibitory activity (LIA) (7).

CONCEPTS UNDERLYING THE THERAPY IN CHRONIC MYELOGENOUS LEUKEMIA

The Normal Residual Stem Cell Pool

The existence of a normal suppressed stem cell pool in patients with CML has been proved by in vitro and in vivo observations. In vitro growth of CML marrow in a semisolid medium results in the development of pure Ph-positive and Ph-negative colonies (96,97). Liquid (Dexter) cultures of CML marrow cells induces a selective growth advantage for Ph-negative nonclonal hemopoietic cells in the adherent hemopoietic niches and in the nonadherent cell fraction

(78–82). This occurs over a period of 3–8 weeks, with simultaneous gradual disappearance of Ph-positive clones. Treatment with intensive chemotherapy (98–103), high-dose hydroxyurea (104), interferons (105–110), or, occasionally, busulfan overdosage (111,112), results in the appearance of diploid nonclonal cells and in suppression of the Ph-positive clones. Although this phenomenon is transient with modalities such as intensive chemotherapy and high-dose hydroxyurea, it is sustained in 15–25% of patients treated with interferon alpha.

In acute leukemia, long-term suppression of the leukemic cells has been associated with a cure fraction. Treatment strategies since 1973 have attempted to reproduce this phenomenon in CML (i.e., induce long-term suppression of the Ph-positive cells and expansion of the normal stem cell pool). Evidence suggests that an enrichment of the ratio of Ph-negative/Ph-positive cells occurs with diminished CML tumor burden, and that this ratio is higher in the adherent hemopoietic niches, compared with the nonadherent hemopoietic cells (Fig. 3). This resulted in several strategies aimed at reversing the growth advantage to favor normal stem cell proliferation. If this reversal is durable, it will imply long-term suppression of the *bcr/abl* abnormalities that drive CML and, consequently, a favorable change in its natural course, with potential long-term survival as in acute leukemia.

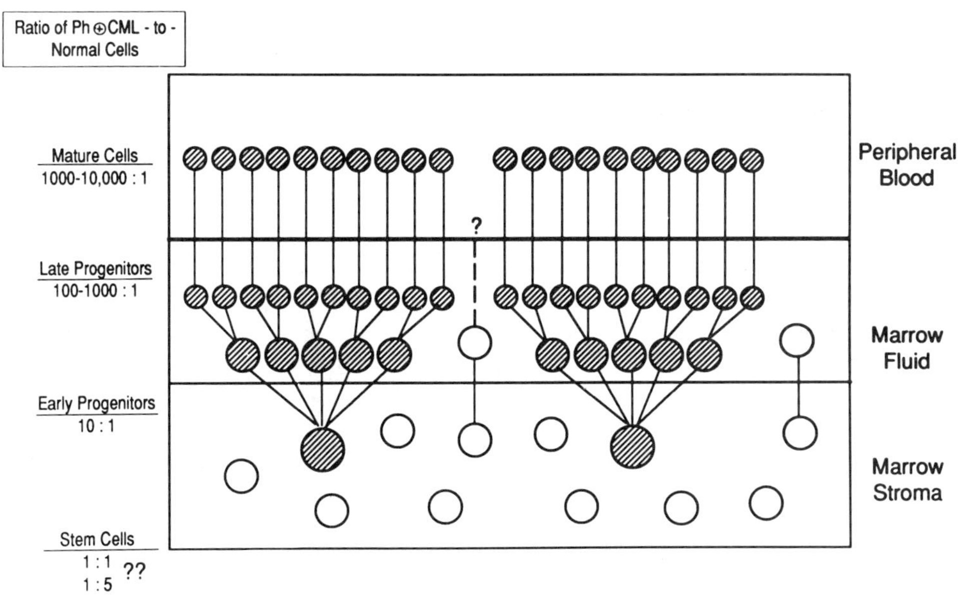

Figure 3 Distribution and ratio of CML and normal cells in marrow and peripheral blood.

Depletion of the normal stem cell pool and acquisition of additional mechanisms of disease resistance and aggressiveness occur with longer duration of CML. This is suggested by the experience with IFN-α and allogeneic BMT in different CML phases (early chronic, late chronic, accelerated blastic). Hence, programs designed to replace the CML clones with normal stem cells are better introduced in the earlier phases of CML.

Mechanisms of Action of Various Modalities in Chronic Myelogenous Leukemia

The rationales behind the treatments in CML are different. One strategy is to eliminate both the CML and normal cells in the bone marrow and replace them with "purged" or "unpurged" host cells (autologous BMT) or normal donor cells (allogeneic or syngeneic BMT). A second possibility is to reduce the CML tumor burden to a minimum, preferable through selective chemotherapy, to improve the normal/CML cell ratio. This is the mechanism associated with intensive chemotherapy, high-dose hydroxyurea, and busulfan overdosage. A third possibility is to reprogram CML cells to behave like normal cells. This may be one of the mechanisms of action of IFN-α in CML, and possibly the mechanism of future differentiation agents. A final possibility is to target the abnormal molecular events in CML, to destroy them selectively in vitro or in vivo (93). Oncogene-targeted programs provide selective therapy, without host toxicity.

PROGNOSTIC FACTORS AND RISK CATEGORIES

The clinical course of CML is variable. Several pretreatment characteristics have been associated with a worse prognosis by univariate analysis (Table 4) (113–128). Many of these prognostic factors have interactions. Multivariate analysis studies accounting for such interrelations have identified variables with independent prognostic impact. This resulted in multivariate analysis-derived prognostic models that categorize patients into low-, intermediate-, and high-risk groups, with median survivals of 4.5, 3, and 2 years, respectively (113–117). At least three of these models, or staging systems have now been validated in independent populations (121,122). We have recently proposed a synthesis staging system that (1) incorporates the reproducible prognostic factors across different CML populations (i.e., not population-specific), (2) assigns the patient stage based on simple enumeration of poor prognosis features, and (3) accounts for accelerated phase features at diagnosis, which are generally not incorporated into multivariate analysis-derived models because of their infrequent occurrence (122) (Table 5). The proposed staging system was superior to existing prognostic models when tested in a population of 406 patients with CML: it identified

Table 4 Characteristics Associated with Poor Prognosis in Ph-Positive CML

Clinical
Older age
Symptoms at diagnosis
Significant weight loss
Hepatomegaly
Splenomegaly
Poor performance
Black race
Peripheral blood
Anemia
Thrombocytosis; thrombocytopenia
Increased blasts, or blasts + promyelocytes
Increased basophils
? Increased peripheral nucleated red cells or eosinophils
Bone Marrow
Increased blasts, or blast + promyelocytes
Increased basophils
Megakaryocytopenia
Collagen fibrosis; reticulin fibrosis grade 3–4
Cytogenetic clonal evolution
? Absence of cells with normal karyotype at diagnosis
Treatment-associated
Longer time to achieve hematological remission with busulfan chemotherapy
Short remission duration
Total dose of busulfan or hydroxyurea therapy required in the first year to control the disease
Lack of significant suppression of Ph-positive metaphases with intensive chemotherapy
Poor initial response to interferon alpha therapy
Lack of significant suppression of Ph-positive metaphases with interferon alpha therapy

Source: Data extracted from Refs. 113–128.

additional risk groups within most of the stages of other systems, whereas the latter did not produce risk subsets within the stages of synthesis system (122).

Staging systems and patient prognosis are relevant to the choice of therapy. This is particularly important, since one form of treatment, allogeneic BMT, can potentially result in 40–70% long-term disease-free survival, but is associated with a first-year mortality of 20–40%, depending on patient age, CML phase, and other factors. For this purpose, Sokal et al. have developed a staging system for younger patients (117). This model was used to assess the patient hazard ratio per unit time, compared with expected outcome with allogeneic BMT, and

Table 5 Proposed Synthesis Staging System for CML

Stage	Number of poor-prognosis characteristics	
		Poor-prognosis characteristic
1	0 or 1	Age $\geq$60 yr
2	2	Spleen $\geq$10 cm below costal margin
		Blasts $\geq$3% in blood or $\geq$3% in marrow
		Basophils $\geq$7% in blood or $\geq$3% in marrow
3	$\geq$3	Platelets $\geq$ 700 $\times$ $10^3/\mu L$
		Accelerated phase characteristics
4	Any accelerated phase characteristic	Cytogenetic clonal evolution
		Blasts $\geq$15% in blood
		Blasts + promyelocytes $\geq$30% in blood
		Basophils $\geq$20% in blood
		Platelets < 100 $\times$ $10^3/\mu L$

resulted in computer-generated models that set upper and lower time limits for initiation of allogeneic BMT in individual CML patients (123,124).

Treatment-associated prognostic factors have not been incorporated into staging systems. In fact, they may be the most sensitive indices of patient prognosis, since they measure the individual in vivo disease aggressiveness. This is analogous to the situation in other tumors, such as acute leukemia, for which achievement of complete remission (CR) is the most important determinant of long-term disease-free survival. Treatment-associated prognostic factors in CML include the time of achievement of a remission and its duration, the total drug dose requirement in the first year of treatment (119,120,125,126), initial response to IFN-α therapy (1,107), and the induction of a cytogenetic response (Ph suppression) with intensive chemotherapy (98,100,127) or with IFN-α (1,107).

THERAPY OF CHRONIC PHASE CHRONIC MYELOGENOUS LEUKEMIA

Historical Perspective

Irradiation was introduced as a treatment modality in 1902, and was the mainstay of CML therapy for the next half century (129–131). Irradiation was given to the whole body, spleen, bones, tumor masses, or in the form of radioactive phosphorus. Splenic irradiation often resulted in an "abscopal" diminution of the peripheral white cell counts. This was possibly due to irradiation of cells in transit through the splenic bed, irradiation of the splenic CML-forming colonies, or suppression of spleen-produced regulatory factors (131). Irradiation resulted in symptomatic relief and improved quality of life. However, most patients in chronic phase still died of related complications (leukostasis, organ failure).

Effective anti-CML chemotherapy unmasked the natural course of CML: with control of the chronic phase, few patients (fewer than 5%) now die of its complications, whereas the majority transform into, and die of complications of accelerated (20–30%) or blastic phase CML (60–70%). Busulfan and hydroxyurea, introduced in 1952 and 1962, respectively, into the management of CML, provide disease control in chronic phase, and survival prolongation, at the cost of minimal toxicity and discomfort. Unfortunately, they do not alter the relentless progression into the accelerated and blastic phases, perhaps because they do not suppress the mechanisms of CML transformation. Their discovery was a mixed blessing, since it delayed the application of new investigations to the chronic phase of CML. In the 1980s, the favorable results with allogeneic BMT and IFN-α encouraged investigation of other new agents or modalities that we will discuss.

Busulfan

Busulfan (1,4-diamethanesulfonyloxybutane), a sulfonic acid alkylating agent, became the first available oral agent with anti-CML activity (132–134). Among comparable populations and in controlled trials, busulfan provided better disease control and longer survival, compared with irradiation. The median survival ranged from 30 to 42 months with busulfan, compared with 6–32 months with irradiation (135–138). Busulfan was also superior to other single agents, including cyclophosphamide, mercaptopurine, chlorambucil, melphalan, and mitobronitol (dibromomannitol) (139–142). In studies comparing busulfan with hydroxyurea, the median survivals of treated patients were similar (Table 6). Busulfan affects early progenitor cells, and hydroxyurea late progenitor cells. This explains the delayed initial effect of busulfan on leukocytosis, but the later prolonged disease control. In contrast, hydroxyurea has an immediate anti-leukocytosis effect which is of shorter duration.

Busulfan is generally given as 2–10 mg orally daily for 7–10 days, or in a tapered daily dosage until the WBC count reaches about $20 \times 10^3/\mu L$. Treatment should then be discontinued because the delayed action of busulfan can result in protracted myelosuppression. The use of busulfan in a long-term schedule of a daily dose to keep the WBC count at a lower range of 5×10^3 to $10 \times 10^3/\mu L$ is difficult and, in fact, dangerous, because of the drug's properties. The serious side effects of busulfan include life-threatening, often fatal, myelosuppression (5–10% of patients); skin hyperpigmentation, and an addisonian-like wasting syndrome; and organ fibrosis affecting the lungs, liver, endomyocardium, and bone marrow (143). Because of the latter problems, and the emergence of autologous and allogeneic BMT as important treatment modalities, the use of

Table 6 Philadelphia Chromosome Suppression and Survival with Different Treatments in Chronic Phase CML

Therapy	Median survival (mo)	Patients (%) with suppression of Ph-positive metaphases to fewer than 35%
No treatment	19	0
Irradiation	6–32	0
Busulfan	30–42	Rare (fewer than 5%)
Hydroxyurea		
Conventional-dose	30–45	Rare (fewer than 5%)
High-dose	?	30
Mitobronitol (dibromomannitol)	36–43	?
Melphalan	29	0
Other single agents	30–35	0
Single agents and splenectomy	36–45	0
Intensive chemotherapy		
L5 and L15	50–58	33–47
Ara-C + 6TG ± other	?	20–50
COAP	55–65	Not done
ROAP, DOAP	55–60	53–68

Abbreviations: ara-C, cytarabine; OAP, vincristine, ara-C, and prednisone; COAP, cyclophosphamide + OAP; ROAP, zorobicin (Rubidazone) + OAP; DOAP, daunorubicin + OAP.

busulfan has decreased considerably. The low cost and durability of responses with busulfan make it a favored anti-CML agent in many countries where the cost of medical care is vital. However, when socioeconomic aspects are less important, busulfan should be replaced by hydroxyurea in most patients. One possible exception is in elderly patients who are not candidates for BMT, and in whom infrequent follow-ups are desired for social and financial considerations.

Hydroxyurea

Hydroxyurea is a ribonucleotidase inhibitor of DNA synthesis, and is cell cycle-specific. It induces rapid disease control and is, together with cytarabine (cytosine arabinoside) and leukapheresis, an excellent choice to control initial severe leukocytosis. The duration of disease control with hydroxyurea is shorter than with busulfan, requiring more frequent monitoring and drug administration (144–150). Serious toxic effects are less frequent and include drug allergies such as fever and skin rashes, or mucositis. The conventional dose schedule of hydroxyurea is 1–5 g orally daily (e.g., 4–5 g for leukocytosis values greater than 100 $\times$ $10^3/\mu L$, and 1–3 g for lower values). The dose is halved with each halving of the WBC count until it reaches 10–20 $\times$ $10^3/\mu L$. Courses can be repeated when leukocytosis reappears.

Other schedules of hydroxyurea have been proposed. A tighter control of the disease process, keeping the tumor burden in the lowest safe range, may decrease the probability of clonal transformation, may prolong chronic phase duration and survival, and may decrease the leukemic-inhibitory effect of CML clones over normal stem cells. Several trials are presently using hydroxyurea in an adjustable daily dosage that keeps the WBC count between 2 $\times$ 10^3 and 4 $\times$ $10^3/\mu L$ and that measure the effect of the "low-dose chronic-exposure" schedule on Ph suppression, duration of chronic phase, and survival.

An alternative schedule is to use hydroxyurea in an intensive regimen (104). Kolitz et al. treated 12 patients with 2 g/m^2 daily, the dose was increased by 1 g every 2 weeks until the granulocyte count was fewer than $10^3/\mu L$. Nine patients showed evidence of Ph suppression. The regimen toxicity was acceptable. This schedule could be used to debulk tumor before BMT, interferon therapy, or other modalities. Other high-dose schedules of busulfan and hydroxyurea have been attempted, without improvement in the results over conventional schedules (151–153).

Other Single Agents

Agents investigated for their efficacy against CML have included mercaptopurine (139), chlorambucil (140,154), melphalan (155,156), mitobronitol (dibromomannitol) (142, 157, 158), and cyclophosphamide (141). These drugs are inferior to busulfan for remission induction or survival (139–142). They are useful when busulfan or hydroxyurea cannot be given because of unacceptable side effects. When significant thrombocytopenia is part of the disease process, cyclophosphamide is preferred for its selective effect against granulopoiesis.

Thrombocytosis in CML may become resistant to busulfan or hydroxyurea. In such instances, thrombocytapheresis is of transient benefit. Three modalities may be useful: thiotepa, IFN-α, and anagrelide. In our experience, thiotepa, given as 75–100 mg/m^2 intravenously every 2–3 weeks, reduces thrombocytosis within 3–6 weeks (two to three doses). Pulmonary toxicity may occur. Interferon-α controls thrombocytosis in 50–75% of patients with essential thrombocytosis (159–163), and in 50–60% of those with thrombocytosis associated with Ph-positive CML (164). A decrease in the marrow megakocytosis is also observed (163). The effect on the clonal nature of the disease is under investigation. Anagrelide reduces thrombocytosis in more than 90% of patients with essential thrombocytosis with minimal toxicity. Like IFN-α, its effect is rapid (within 1 week) but disappears quickly with discontinuation of therapy (165, 166). Marrow megakaryocytosis persists with anagrelide therapy, suggesting that its effect is an arrest in the maturation of megakaryocytes or in their release.

The effect of anagrelide in CML-associated thrombocytosis needs evaluation. A combination of agents (e.g., hydroxyurea plus thiotepa, IFN-α, or anagrelide) may be ideal to control various components of CML myelopoiesis.

Leukapheresis

Leukapheresis was proposed to control CML without (1) exposing the leukemic cells to the selective pressure of antineoplastic agents that could induce cellular resistance and transformation, or (2) exposing the host to drug teratogenicity. Intensive leukapheresis can control CML, but is cumbersome, expensive, and does not alter the disease course (167–169). Leukapheresis is still indicated as an initial approach to prevent severe leukostasis-associated complications (pulmonary failure, cerebrovascular accidents) and in pregnant patients with CML to avoid the teratogenic effects of drugs on the fetus (170). In the latter group, repeated leukapheresis as needed for WBC counts above 80×10^3 to $100 \times 10^3/\mu L$ is successful. Leukapheresis is also used in investigational CML programs to collect peripheral stem cells for autologous transplantation.

Spleen-Oriented Therapies

Splenectomy in CML was based on morphological, kinetic, and cytogenetic observations demonstrating that evolved CML clones can originate in splenic tissues (171–174). Removal of the splenic niche of CML transformation may delay the onset of blastic phase in some patients and prolong survival. Splenectomy occasionally resulted in disappearance of clonal evolution from the peripheral blood. Controlled studies have failed to demonstrate a beneficial effect from splenectomy performed during the chronic phase on duration of chronic phase or survival in the total CML population (175–177). It could be argued that splenectomy is useful only in the small subset of patients (perhaps 10–20%) in whom the spleen is the first site of disease transformation. Since it is difficult to identify such patients, controlled studies in this subset are not feasible. Splenectomy may provide prognostic information. Hester et al. observed a worse prognosis in patients showing CML involvement in the perisplenic lymph nodes at the time of splenectomy (99).

Other proposed benefits from splenectomy include an easier management of blastic phase and better prognosis in that phase, and an earlier marrow recovery and improved prognosis following BMT. In our experience, splenectomy performed in chronic phase did not improve the prognosis in blastic phase, as measured by remission rate and survival (24). Its impact on quality of life and supportive care requirements was not evaluated. Splenectomy before autologous or allogeneic BMT may be associated with earlier hematopoietic recovery, but not an improved prognosis (178–182). Splenectomy is now reserved for symptomatic or painful splenomegaly, unresponsive to therapy, or for significant anemia or thrombocytopenia associated with hypersplenism. The approach to massive splenomegaly (e.g., 10 cm or more below the costal margin) prior to allogeneic or autologous BMT is uncertain.

Intra-arterial splenic perfusion with cytarabine (ara-C) in conventional doses was reported by Canellos et al. to induce transient responses (183). To intensify this regional approach, we treated ten patients with CML and refractory splenomegaly with high-dose ara-C, 1.0–1.5 g/m^2 by continuous intra-arterial splenic infusion over 24 hours daily for 3 days, and cisplatin intrasplenic short infusions of 20–25 mg/m^2 daily for 3 days. One partial response (10%) was observed, although several patients showed transient reductions of splenomegaly. Toxicity was considerable owing to locoregional problems and myelosuppression.

Intensive Chemotherapy

Mechanism of Action

Intensive chemotherapy eliminates a large pool of CML clones. Presumably, this removes the leukemic-inhibitory activity of CML cells and allows the regeneration of the CML and normal stem cells at similar proliferative rates. Subsequently, the expanded CML clones reestablish the mechanisms that favor their proliferative growth, leading to resuppression of the normal stem cells, and explaining the transient nature of cytogenetic response with intensive chemotherapy.

Treatment Results

Intensive chemotherapy refers to regimens that induce marrow hypoplasia and peripheral pancytopenia. These have generally included ara-C for its selective inhibition of CML cells over normal progenitor cells (184–186). The L5 and L15 regimens of Memorial Sloan–Kettering Cancer Center have used ara-C with thioguanine and asparaginase for three cycles, together with splenectomy and splenic irradiation. Significant suppression of the Ph-positive metaphases, to fewer than 35%, was observed in a third of the patients. The median survivals were 58 months for the L5 and 50 months for the L15 study (98,103,127). A similar incidence of Ph suppression was reported in other studies (187–189).

Two studies from our institution used intensive chemotherapy containing vincristine, ara-C, prednisone, and cyclophosphamide (COAP) or anthracyclines [zorubicin (Rubidazone)—ROAP; daunorubicin—DOAP] (99,100). Combination chemotherapy was given for three induction cycles, followed by maintenance with hydroxyurea. Suppression of Ph to fewer than 35% Ph-positive metaphases was observed in 53% of patients treated with ROAP or DOAP (100). Intensive chemotherapy was associated with median survivals of 50–65 months, compared with 30–45 months with conventional therapy (99,100,113). This survival advantage may be due to more favorable patient selection. However, when patients were analyzed within different prognostic categories, survival prolongation with intensive chemotherapy was associated with intermediate-risk (median survival 58 versus 34 months; $p < 0.01$) and high-risk disease (median survival 33 versus 15 months, $p = 0.02$), whereas low-risk patients had a similar survival with intensive or conventional chemotherapy (median survival 55 versus 58 months) (113).

In these studies, increasing the treatment intensity induced a greater suppression of Ph-positive metaphases (see Table 6). The Ph suppression was transient, lasting for a median of 4–8 months.

Clinical Use

Intensive chemotherapy has significant myelosuppression-associated morbidity and requires careful monitoring. In conventional practice, cycles of intensive chemotherapy may be used (1) in patients with poor-prognosis CML, (2) to overcome emerging disease resistance to one form of therapy (e.g., hydroxyurea, interferons), or (3) to suppress signs of disease acceleration or clonal evolution. In the investigational setting, they could be used for in vivo purging, to collect stem cells for later autologous transplantation.

Interferons

Interferons (IFNs) are small, naturally occurring proteins produced in response to various stimuli. They are classified by their physicochemical and antigenic properties into three groups: alpha, beta, and gamma. The IFNs have a wide range of biological activities, including antiviral, antiproliferative, immunomodulatory, differentiating, and oncogene regulatory properties (190,191). They bind to specific cell surface membrane receptors, inducing intracellular messages such as activation of a 2',5'-oligoadenylate synthetase enzyme and an endonuclease that cleaves single-stranded RNA. Interferon alpha and IFN-β are similar in structure and biological activity and bind to the same cell surface receptors. Interferon gamma has different structural and biological properties and binds to different receptors (192–194).

Mechanisms of Action in Chronic Myelogenous Leukemia

The mechanisms of action of IFNs may vary with different malignant conditions. In CML, antiproliferation may suppress CML clones (194–196), perhaps through a selective action on the late progenitor cells (197). Both IFN-α and IFN-γ suppress the growth and differentiation of normal and CML myeloid progenitor cells in vitro (198) and induce granulocytopenia in vivo (199). In vitro incubation of CML cells with IFN-γ results in the growth of colonies with a normal karyotype (200).

Other immunomodulatory mechanisms may be important. IFN-α establishes readherence of the CML cells to the stroma (201); normalizes expression of cytoadhesive molecules such as LFA-3 (92,93), through which the suppressive activity of the effector T-gamma cells on CML clones is reestablished; enhances Ia antigen expression on CML cells, perhaps allowing their recognition and their differentiation or suppression by the peripheral hemopoietic signals (202); and increases NK cell activity (203,204). A decreased production of IFN-α, but not IFN-γ, was reported in patients with CML, suggesting that the beneficial effect of IFN-α was from replacing a deficient regulatory substance (205).

Interferon Alpha

The original studies in CML used a partially pure form of IFN-α (Cantell interferon). The recombinant DNA technology enabled large-scale production of pure IFN-α (interferon alpha) and its rapid evaluation in different stages of CML.

The unique treatment observations with the first study of human IFN-α in CML required the development of standardized criteria for hematological and cytogenetic responses (105–107,164,206). A complete hematological response (CHR) was defined as normalization of the peripheral counts with the WBC count fewer than $10 \times 10^3/\mu L$, absence of immature peripheral cells (blasts, promyelocytes, myelocytes), and disappearance of signs and symptoms of CML disease, including palpable splenomegaly. Patients with CHR were subdivided by the degree of Ph suppression into (1) minor cytogenetic response (Ph suppression between 35% and 90%, (2) partial cytogenetic response (Ph suppression between 1% and 34%), and (3) complete cytogenetic response (Ph suppression to 0%). Among 51 patients treated with human IFN-α, $3–9 \times 10^6$ units/m^2 intramuscularly daily to maintain the WBC count between 2×10^3 and $10 \times 10^3/\mu L$, 36 achieved CHR (71%). Forty-one percent of patients had suppression of Ph-positive metaphases, which was durable in 7 patients (33%; 14% of total) for more than 39–62 months. Disappearance of *bcr* rearrangement was documented by molecular studies in all patients with a complete cytogenetic remission. Hematological responses required a median of 14 weeks of IFN-α treatment, and cytogenetic responses developed after a median of 9 months of therapy. One-quarter of patients achieving CHR showed cyclic oscillations of the WBC counts. The cyclic phenomenon needs to be recognized to avoid confusion with resistance to therapy, and indicates that, in some patients with CML, the disease remains under partial control feedback signals.

These results have been confirmed using recombinant IFN-α in several studies (Table 7). Among 418 patients, 254 achieved CHR (61%) and 170 (41%) had a cytogenetic response. Response to IFN-α was associated with several host and disease characteristics including the population mix, extent of prior therapy, duration of chronic phase CML, and IFN-α dose schedule (Table 8). Patients in early chronic phase CML (diagnosis for fewer than 12 months) had significantly higher hematological and cytogenetic response rates, compared with patients with late chronic phase CML (107). Responses were also better in patients with low-risk, compared with intermediate- or high-risk disease (105,107,108). The

Table 7 Summary of the Experience with IFN-α Therapy in Chronic Phase CML

Study (Ref.)	No. treated	No. (%) CHR	No. (%) Ph suppression
Talpaz et al. (105)	51	36 (71)	21 (41)
Talpaz et al. (106,107)	57	35 (61)	25 (44)
M. D. Anderson Cancer Center (unpublished)	71	62 (87)	51 (58)
Alimena et al. (108)	63	29 (46)	27 (43)
Niederle et al. (109)	41	23 (56)	14 (34)
Ozer et al. (110)	107	59 (55)	32 (30)
Freund et al. (207)	28	10 (36)	
	418	254 (61)	170 (41)

dosage schedule of IFN-α is critical for achieving hematological and cytogenetic responses. The CHR rate was 25% among patients receiving a low-dosage schedule of IFN-α, 2×10^6 units/m^2 three times weekly, compared with 48% for those receiving a higher dosage schedule of 5×10^6 units/m^2, three times weekly (108). One-third of patients not responding to the low dosage achieved CHR with the higher dosage (108). Two studies using lower dosages of IFN-α, between 6×10^5 and 2×10^6 units/m^2, three times a week, had very low CHR rates (10–20%), and no evidence of Ph suppression (207,208). In our studies, IFN-α is used a 5×10^6 units/m^2 daily when tolerated, and as long as the WBC count is above $2 \times 10^3/\mu$L and the platelet count above $60–80 \times 10^3/\mu$L. This may explain the higher incidence of major (partial and complete) cytogenetic responses seen in our studies, compared with other trials (20–30% versus 5–10%). Thus, studies, the objective of which is to induce major cytogenetic responses, should consider a schedule of IFN-α at a dosage of 5×10^6 units/m^2 daily or, if intolerable, the maximally tolerated individual dose.

The projected median survival of patients with early chronic phase CML was 62 months, which compares favorably with previous experience using conventional therapy [hydroxyurea (Hydrea), busulfan] or intensive combination chemotherapy (Fig. 4). The initial response to IFN-α was a treatment-associated prognostic parameter. Patients achieving CHR had a 4-year survival rate of 82%, compared with 32% for patients who had PHR or resistant disease. This indicates the value of interferon response in further decisions on individual therapy.

Table 8 Variables Affecting Response to IFN-α in Ph-Positive CML

		Suppression (%)		
Constant	Variable	CHR	Ph Suppression	Suppression to <35% Ph-positive metaphases
IFN-α dose 5×10^6 units/m^2	CML phase			
	Early chronic	60–80	40–50	20–30
	Late chronic	50–60	10–20	<10
	Accelerated	30–40	<10	0
	Blastic	20–30	<10	0
Early chronic phase	Risk category			
	Low	80–90	60	40
	Intermediate	50–60	40	20–30
	High	20–60	10–20	5–10
Early chronic phase CML	IFN-α dose			
	5×10^6 units/m^2 daily	80	50–60	40
	5×10^6 units/m^2 TIW[a]	70	40	20
	2×10^6 units/m^2 TIW	30–40	20	5–10
	$<2 \times 10^6$ units/m^2 TIW	20–30	<10	0

[a]TIW, three times per week.

Recombinant Interferon Gamma

Interferon gamma has shown a definite, but lower activity, compared with IFN-α in patients with CML. In three studies, hematological response rates ranged from 27% to 64%, and cytogenetic response rates from zero to 27% (209–211). As with in vitro studies, there was a partial lack of cross-resistance between IFN-α and IFN-γ (209–211). This, and the in vitro synergism of IFN-α and IFN-γ, encouraged combined trials.

Interferon Alpha plus Interferon Gamma Combinations

Combinations of IFN-α and IFN-γ have been used in different dosage schedules. At Phase II dosages of each individual drug, the combination of IFN-α and

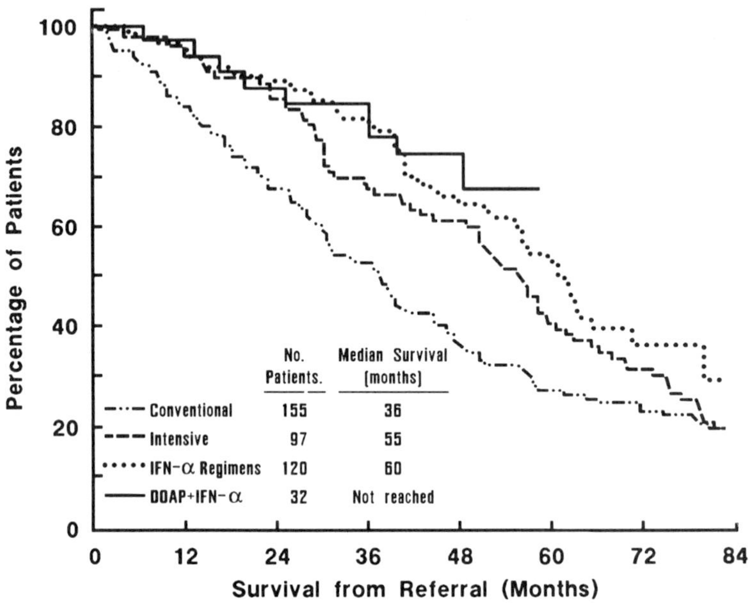

Figure 4 Survival in CML by different treatments.

IFN-γ is toxic. Interferon-α, 5×10^6 units/m^2 daily, with a dose of IFN-γ 0.025 mg/m^2 daily, patterned after the in vitro synergistic experience, does not show better hematological or cytogenetic response rates, compared with IFN-α alone (212,213). Other studies using alternate-day or alternate-week therapy with IFN-α and IFN-γ are maturing.

Toxicities of Interferons

Interferon therapy is associated with early and late side effects. Early side effects include fever, chills, flulike symptoms, headache, nausea, vomiting, diarrhea, anorexia, and a postnasal drip. These are mild to moderate and rarely dose-limiting. Tachyphylaxis develops rapidly to the early side effects. Interferon-α therapy is usually started at half-dose for the first 3–7 days to improve patient tolerance. Serious late side effects are dose-limiting in 10% or fewer of patients. These include severe anorexia and weight loss; neurotoxicity with frontal lobe signs (depression, poor concentration, apathy) and parkinsonian-like syndrome; immune-mediated events (thrombocytopenia, hemolysis, hypothyroidism, nephrotic syndrome), and other toxicities.

A peculiar syndrome of severe musculoskeletal pains occurs with development of interferon resistance. This is associated with increased blastic activity by bone scan, which reverts upon discontinuation of IFN-α. The etiology of this syndrome is unknown. A recent study has shown increased leukotriene-C_4 levels in CML cells, compared with normal cells (214). Interferon alpha may release leukotriene-C_4 from CML granulocytes in patients with increasing counts and IFN-α resistance, resulting in severe inflammation. This syndrome should be recognized early, since continuation of IFN-α may lead to catastrophic pleuropericardial complications (effusions, cardiovascular compromise). The appropriate management includes discontinuation of IFN-α, narcotic analgesia for pains, and hydroxyurea to reduce the WBC count. In severe cases, steroid therapy (prednisone 100 mg daily for 5 days) will rapidly alleviate the pains.

Immune-mediated events are infrequent with interferon therapy. These include immune-mediated thrombocytopenia, hemolytic syndrome and anemia, hypothyroidism, and cardiac and renal failure. Interferon therapy is known to worsen an existing rheumatological condition, and occasional patients developed rheumatoid arthritis or systemic lupus erythematosus. Severe marrow hypoplasia has been reported with interferon therapy. Its etiology is undetermined, but could be due to depletion of the CML clones in a bone marrow devoid of normal stem cells, immune-mediated hypoplasia, or damage to marrow stroma, with a dysfunction in the stromal-hemopoietic interaction.

A triad of depression, fatigue, and insomnia is observed frequently in patients with CML on interferon therapy. This could be related to disruption of the normal circadian rhythm. A small dose of an antidepressant (amitriptyline, 25–50 mg at bedtime) can significantly improve these side effects.

Interferon gamma is associated with a higher frequency of systemic symptoms, including fever, fatigue, and weight loss, whereas the musculoskeletal syndrome occurs frequently with IFN-α. Neurotoxicity, as well as other side effects, are more frequent in elderly patients. A dose of IFN-α of 5×10^6 units/m^2 daily is tolerated by young patients, but not by older patients (e.g., multiple myeloma, hairy cell leukemia) whose tolerance to doses higher than 3×10^6 units/m^2 three times weekly is poor.

Durability and Significance of Major Cytogenetic Responses with Interferon-α Therapy

Once patients achieve a major (complete or partial) cytogenetic response, documented on at least two occasions at 3- to 6-month intervals, these responses are durable, in most patients, as long as IFN-α therapy is continued. Tables 9 and 10 summarize the incidence of cytogenetic responses achieved with IFN-α regimens in early chronic phase CML. Twenty-eight percent of patients achieve a major cytogenetic response, and 23% have a durable cytogenetic response. Cytogenetic response is durable in 25 of 33 patients with major cytogenetic response (76%), compared with only 3 of 16 patients with minor cytogenetic response (12%) (see Table 10). Cytogenetic responses are durable for 12–84

Table 9 Major Cytogenetic Responses with IFN-α Therapy in Early Chronic Phase CML

		No. (%)				
		Ph suppression	Durable Ph suppression			
Regimen	No. Treated		Total	Minor	Major	Duration (mo)
Human IFN-α	51	21	7	1	6	40–82+
Recombinant IFN-α	35	21	12	1	11	26–54+
IFN-α + IFN-γ	34	17	9	1	8	12–30+
Total	120	59(49)	28(23)	3	25	12–82+

Table 10 Patterns of Ph Suppression with IFN-α Regimens in Early Chronic Phase CML

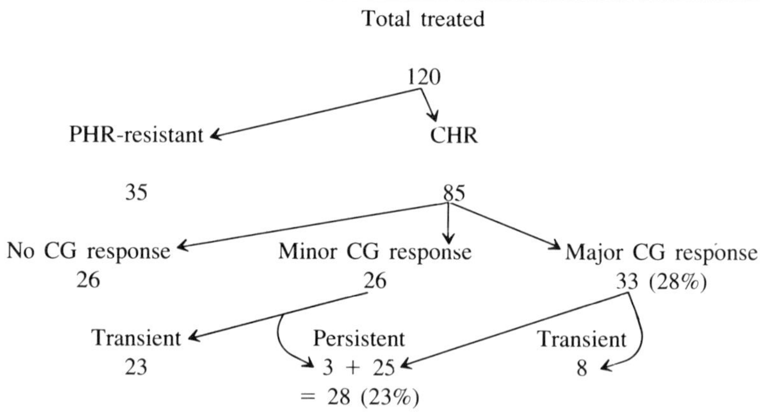

months or more in 20% of patients with Ph-positive early chronic phase CML, or 50% of those who have any cytogenetic response within 6 months of IFN-α therapy (Fig. 5).

Patients achieving a complete or partial cytogenetic response have a significantly better survival than those obtaining CHR with minimal or no Ph suppression, or those with partial hematological response or resistant disease (Fig. 6). The foregoing findings on the durability of major cytogenetic responses and the

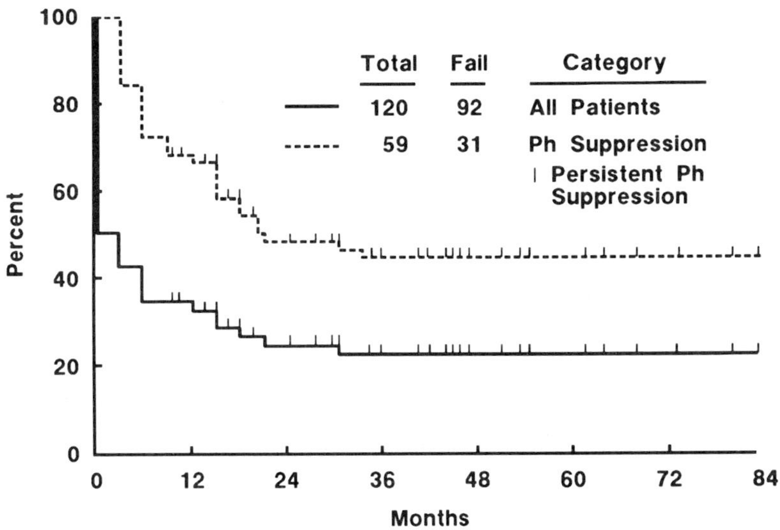

Figure 5 CG response duration with IFN-α.

association with prolonged survival, support trials designed to obtain a major cytogenetic response.

Most patients who develop durable major cytogenetic responses show some Ph suppression after 6 months of IFN-α therapy at 5×10^6 units/m^2 daily, and Ph suppression to fewer than 50% Ph-positive metaphases after 12 months of treatment. These guidelines allow the selection of patients for continued IFN-α-containing therapies versus changing to alternative treatments.

Combined-Modality Treatments

Combined-modality approaches are based on the in vitro synergism of IFN-α and chemotherapeutic agents, such as ara-C, anthracyclines, and others (214,215). These agents are individually effective in patients with CML. Interferon alpha was investigated in combination with intensive chemotherapy, hydroxyurea or busulfan, and low-dose ara-C.

Interferon Alpha plus Intensive Chemotherapy

The study was based on the divergent therapeutic effects of each modality in relation to prognostic categories and Ph suppression. Intensive chemotherapy improved survival in intermediate- and high-risk patients and produced dramatic but short-lasting cytogenetic responses (100,113). On the other hand, IFN-α induced moderate but durable cytogenetic responses.

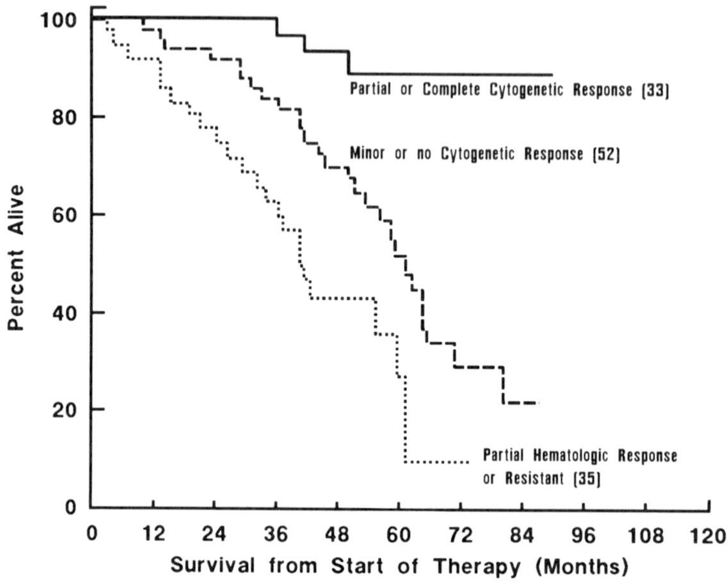

Figure 6 Survival by CG response to IFN-α.

Intensive chemotherapy consisted of three cycles of daunorubicin, vincristine, ara-C, and prednisone (DOAP) followed by maintenance with IFN-α at 3–9 $\times$ 10^6 units/m^2 daily to maintain the WBC count between 2 $\times$ 10^3 and 8 $\times$ $10^3/\mu L$ (217). With induction chemotherapy, 28 (86%) of 32 patients achieved a cytogenetic response and, 21 (66%) a major cytogenetic response. The cytogenetic response persisted in 8 patients (25%) for a median of 30 or more months (range 12–60 or more months), a percentage not different from that with IFN-α alone. After a median follow-up of 40 months, 20 patients are alive in chronic phase, 16 of them on IFN-α therapy. The projected 4-year survival rate is 75%, which is encouraging compared with previous experience.

Interferon Alpha plus Busulfan

A similar strategy using initial therapy with busulfan followed by IFN-α maintenance was reported by Bergsagel et al. (218). The WBC doubling time, measured following busulfan induction alone versus busulfan induction and IFN-α maintenance, showed a significant prolongation with IFN-α maintenance. This suggests that IFN-α suppresses the CML clones and may delay the onset of blastic phase.

Interferon Alpha plus Hydroxyurea

The use of IFN-α and hydroxyurea is prompted by several observations: (1) Hydroxyurea exerts an excellent antiproliferative effect against CML clones in both chronic and advanced phases; (2) some of the IFN-α toxicities (fever, chills, musculoskeletal pains) may be alleviated by rapid control of leukocytosis; (3) IFN-α and hydroxyurea are synergistic in vitro; and (4) studies with high doses of hydroxyruea have resulted in cytogenetic responses (104). Thus, the combination of IFN-α and hydroxyurea may improve the incidence of hematological and cytogenetic response rates and reduce the toxicity of IFN-α.

In a pilot study at our institution, 15 patients with hematological resistance to IFN-α alone were treated with IFN-α, 5×10^6 units/m^2 daily, and hydroxyurea 0.5–3 g daily, to keep the WBC count between 2×10^3 and 8×10^3 μL. Twelve of the 15 patients achieved CHR, and 1 (6%) showed Ph suppression to 55% Ph-positive metaphases. The median dose of hydroxyurea with the combination was 50% of that needed when hydroxyurea had been given alone. None of the 4 patients who experienced musculoskeletal pains with hematologic resistance to IFN-α alone had recurrence of the toxicity with the combination. Guilhot et al. treated 24 patients with IFN-α and hydroxyurea, with or without later ara-C. A CHR was obtained in 18 (75%) and a cytogenetic response in 13 (54%), including 9 (37%) with a complete cytogenetic response. A cytogenetic response was noted in 7 of 12 previously treated patients (58%) (217). This combination has also been investigated by other groups (220,221). So far, the results suggest that the combination is associated with faster remissions, a higher CHR rate, lower requirement of drug dosages, and a lower frequency of leukocytosis-mediated IFN-α toxicities. Whether the incidence of cytogenetic responses is higher warrants further evaluation.

Interferon Alpha plus Cytarabine

In vitro studies have shown a preferential inhibitory effect of ara-C against CML, compared with normal colonies (184). Sokal et al. induced Ph suppression in two of four patients in chronic phase CML treated with low-dose ara-C (222). This led to a trial of IFN-α and low-dose ara-C in advanced stages of CML. The CHR rates were improved with the combination, compared with IFN-α therapy alone, in both late chronic and accelerated phases. The Ph suppression rates were similar (223). Among 16 patients with accelerated phase and cytogenetic clonal evolution, 5 (31%) showed variable degrees of suppression of the evolved clones, indicating the potential value of ara-C for controlling the more aggressive phase of CML.

Interferons Alpha Following Bone Marrow Transplantation

Clinical or cytogenetic leukemic relapse occurs in 20–30% of patients with Ph-positive CML undergoing allogeneic BMT in chronic phase and 50–90% of patients in the accelerated or blastic phases. Interferon alpha maintenance after allogeneic BMT in acute lymphocytic leukemia reduces the incidence of relapse (224). In CML, Arcese et al. administered IFN-α in 16 patients with CML relapse following allogeneic BMT, and obtained a complete cytogenetic response in 3 (19%) (226). Similar results were reported by others (226–228). Maintenance IFN-α post-allogeneic BMT in remission may reduce the incidence of hematological and cytogenetic relapse, particularly among high-risk patients. This approach requires careful investigation, since IFN-α can potentially increase the frequency of graft failure and GVHD, and it may be poorly tolerated following allogeneic BMT. Maintenance IFN-α following autologous BMT may also prolong the duration of Ph suppression.

Differentiating Agents

Differentiating agents used in chronic phase CML may accelerate the maturation of late progenitor cells. This may reduce the CML pool, decrease the leukemic-inhibitory activity of the CML clones on normal cells, "burnout" CML clones, and decrease the probability of clonal evolution. The use of bacille Calmette-Guerin (BCG) as a differentiating agent for chronic phase CML maintenance was not associated with prolongation of remission duration or survival (229). Retinoic acid reduces the number of CML GM-CFU after 14 days of culture (230). However, the use of *cis*-retinoic acid with chemotherapy in CML was not beneficial (231). Whether α-*trans*-retinoic acid would be a better differentiating agent will be of interest.

Bone Marrow Transplantation

Bone marrow transplantation involves delivery of supralethal doses of chemotherapy or irradiation to eradicate the CML cells, and repopulation of the bone marrow with normal hematopoietic stem cells. The source of hematopoietic stem cells may be a related histocompatibility antigen (HLA)-matched donor (*allogeneic* BMT), an identical twin (*syngeneic* BMT), or the patient himself (autologous peripheral stem cell transplantation, *autologous* BMT). Only 35% of patients will have an HLA-matched sibling. To circumvent this limitation, BMT has been extended successfully to include related HLA-mismatched donors, unrelated HLA-matched donors, and unrelated donors with minor HLA-mismatching. The initial studies of BMT involved the use of allogeneic BMT in the advanced phases of CML (232,233). As the safety and efficacy of the procedure were established, allogeneic BMT was applied in the chronic phase of CML. Exciting results have recently been reported with autologous stem cell transplantation (peripheral or marrow). We will summarize these results in chronic phase CML.

Syngeneic Bone Marrow Transplantation

This form of transplantation lacks host–donor histoincompatibility and permits evaluation of the antileukemic effect and toxicity of the chemoirradiation preparative regimen without the contribution of the immunological graft-versus-leukemia (GVL) effect. The long-term follow-up demonstrates a significantly higher incidence of leukemic relapse compared with allogeneic BMT (234,235). This is particularly striking in chronic phase CML, for which the cumulative incidence of relapse was 50–60%, compared with 5–35% for allogeneic BMT. This suggests a value of minor histocompatibility mismatching in inducing GVL and reducing the risk of leukemic relapse.

Allogeneic Bone Marrow Transplantation

Allogeneic BMT in chronic phase CML was prompted by the poor results in accelerated and blastic phases, mainly owing to leukemic relapse, and the encouraging data with syngeneic BMT in chronic phase CML, and with allogeneic BMT in acute myelogenous leukemia (AML) in first remission (similar to chronic phase CML) compared with AML relapse (similar to CML accelerated or blastic phase). Disease-free survival can now be achieved in 40–80% of patients in chronic phase (235–241). Unlike the situation in the accelerated and blastic phases, the mortality in chronic phase CML is mostly due to GVHD, interstitial pneumonitis (cytomegalovirus, idiopathic), and venoocclusive disease (235–241).

The most important determinant of patient outcome following allogeneic BMT is the CML phase during which BMT was performed (Table 11). However, in chronic phase, prognosis is associated with several variables, including the patient's age, the manipulation of the donor marrow, the development of chronic GVHD following allogeneic BMT, and possibly the time from diagnosis to BMT.

Patients younger than 20 years old have a long-term survival rate of 70%, compared with 40% for older patients, mostly because of a higher mortality rate in the latter group and some increase in leukemic relapse among those who are 40 years or older (see Table 11) (237–239). T-cell depletion of the donor marrow, in an attempt to decrease GVHD mortality, has been associated with a relapse rate of 50% or more compared with 5–30% with unmanipulated bone marrows (242–244). Regardless of the transplant T-cell status, patients who develop chronic GVHD are less likely to relapse, compared with those who do not (risk of relapse 5–10% versus 20–30%; relative risk about 3). Survival rates, however, were similar, indicating that the decreased mortality from smaller degrees of GVHD was counterbalanced by leukemic relapse-associated deaths (233,234,245).

The association of chronic phase duration with prognosis postallogeneic BMT is perhaps the most important and controversial issue. It creates the dilemma of an earlier choice of a high-risk procedure associated with a 1-year mortality of 20–50%, but potential cure, versus delaying the procedure for a period at the risk of decreasing the success rate from BMT. The initial reports from Seattle have indicated that allogeneic BMT performed within 12–18 months was associated with significantly better long-term survival rates, compared with later transplantation (70% versus 55%) (see Table 11). This was not corroborated by the data from the International Bone Marrow Transplantation Registry (IBMTR), which showed similar survival rates with early or late BMT in chronic phase CML. This may be related to the population characteristics (e.g., patient age, definition of chronic and accelerated phase) or the type and extent of prior therapy (e.g., busulfan versus other modalities). In fact, Thomas et al. (236) showed a strong correlation between transplantation in early chronic phase and a younger patient age. The simplest explanation is that when CML is diagnosed in a very young patient in the community, he or she is referred directly for allogeneic BMT because of the known better results in this age group. Older patients are usually treated for a longer period with other modalities and are referred in late chronic phase CML. Thus, the better prognosis could be age related rather than owing to the chronic phase duration. In the same study (236), previous exposure to busulfan therapy was correlated with a higher transplantation mortality (51% versus 13%), and with an increased mortality from interstitial pneumonitis (19% versus 0%). This is possibly due to busulfan-induced fibrosis, with marrow and pulmonary damage.

Although splenomegaly has been shown, in some studies, to indicate worse prognosis (235), splenectomy or splenic irradiation before BMT has not improved overall survival (237,238). A positive cytomegalovirus (CMV) titer in the patient prior to BMT has been associated with lower survival, also because of increased mortality.

Strategies to Improve the Results of Allogeneic Bone Marrow Transplantation in Chronic Myelogenous Leukemia

Such strategies include (1) improvement in the preparative regimens, (2) better GVHD prophylaxis and therapy, (3) better CMV prophylaxis and therapy, and (4) maintenance therapy post-BMT.

Whereas the combination of high-dose cyclophosphamide (CTX) and total body irradiation (TBI) is the standard preparative regimen in allogeneic BMT, investigators have sought to improve on the marrow eradicative properties of these regimens, to decrease leukemia relapse, without worsening toxicity. Studies have investigated higher doses of TBI, TBI fractionation, replacement of CTX by etoposide, the addition of etoposide or cytarabine to the standard CTX–TBI regimen, or replacement of TBI by busulfan (246–248). Although these preliminary trials are encouraging, longer follow-ups are required before an optimal regimen could be recommended for CML allogeneic BMT.

Table 11 Results of Syngeneic and Allogeneic BMT in Different CML Phases

Characteristic	Study	No. patients	Survival (%) (at X yr)	Relapse (%)
CML phase	Seattle			
Syngeneic				
Chronic	23	78 (10)	57	
Accelerated	10	20 (10)	65	
Blastic	9	22 (10)	80	
Allogeneic				
Chronic	Seattle	164	55 (6)	25
	IBMTR	956	53 (5)	12
Accelerated	Seattle	75	22 (6)	50
	IBMTR	392	29 (5)	54
Blastic	Seattle	69	15 (6)	75
	IBMTR	188	16 (5)	45
Second chronic	IBMTR	50	25 (5)	40–50
Other characteristics				
Patient age(yr)	IBMTR			
0–10		22	90 (4)	11
11–20		100	65 (4)	9
21–30		282	53 (4)	29
31–40		362	48 (4)	10
More than 40		180	48 (4)	41
	Seattle			
30 or less		70	65 (6)	17
31–40		68	55 (6)	32
More than 40		30	42 (6)	28
T-cell depletion	IBMTR			
Yes		187	62 (3)	52
No		586	62 (3)	9
Duration of chronicity (mo)	Seattle			
<12		79	70 (5)	
12–36		61	50 (5)	
>36		35	28 (5)	
	IBMTR			
<18		202	57 (3)	18
18 or more		202	54 (3)	13

Source: Data summarized from Refs. 235, 240, 245.

Graft-versus-host disease remains a leading cause of morbidity and mortality in allogeneic BMT. The GVHD-associated problems can be reduced by better therapy of acute and chronic GVHD or by prevention of their occurrence. Despite optimal immunosuppressive therapy with cyclosporine, methotrexate or steroids, moderate to severe acute GVHD occurs in 20–45% of patients receiving HLA-matched related allogeneic BMT, and in 60% or more of those treated with HLA-mismatched related or HLA-matched unrelated allogeneic BMT. Chronic GVHD also complicates 20–40% of cases (249–252). The pathophysiology of GVHD is complex, but appears to be mediated by donor immunocompetent T cells attacking recipient tissues. From animal models, T-cell depletion appeared to be an effective method for GVHD prevention (253–257). T-cell depletion in human allogeneic BMT is obtainable by various methods, including single or multiple monoclonal anti-T-cell antibodies alone, or with complement, ricin, or other toxin-conjugated antibodies, antibodies conjugated to iron beads that are later removed physically by magnetic beads, soybean lectin agglutination, E-rosette formation, and elutriation (258–265). In general, studies of T-cell-depletion allogeneic BMT have reduced the incidence and severity of acute GVHD from 20 to 50% down to less than 20%, but increased the incidence of graft failure (from less than 3% to as much as 8–50%) (266–269), and of leukemic relapse (from 5 to 30% up to more than 50%) (242,244,249). Graft failure can be reduced by more intensive preparative regimens or by posttransplantation immunosuppression (249,269,270). Leukemic relapse after T-cell-depleted allogeneic BMT is perhaps due to nonselective removal of T cells which include subsets determining GVHD and others determining GVL. The T cells that induce GVHD versus GVL are possibly separate, as shown in animal models and with clinical experience. For instance, T-cell-depleted allogeneic BMT is associated with a higher incidence of leukemic relapse than with unmanipulated marrow transplant, even after correction for the GVHD effect. Relapse is also higher with syngeneic BMT, compared with allogenic BMT without GVHD, implying a GVL effect. Recent studies performing selective T-cell depletions are encouraging. These have included using anti-CD5, anti-T12, and anti-CD8 monoclonal antibodies (271–274).

Therapy of established GVHD can also be improved through discovering agents with suppressive activity against GVHD-producing mechanisms. Two such promising agents are Xomazyme, an anti-CD5 monoclonal antibody conjugated to a ricin A chain, and thalidomide (275–278).

Improvements in supportive care and therapy of infections will undoubtedly make allogeneic BMT a safer procedure. These include (1) the use of laminar air flow rooms that may potentially reduce GVHD complications and infections, particularly aspergillus infections; (2) the availability of newer antifungal agents such as fluconazole and itroconazole, and (3) measures to prevent or treat CMV. The latter encompass the use of CMV-negative blood products in CMV-negative patients, and high-dose gama globulin or ganciclovir for therapy and prophylaxis (280–283).

The use of postallogeneic BMT maintenance therapy to decrease the incidence of CML relapse is an interesting concept. Potential agents are IFN-α (224–229), interleukin-2 (284), or conventional drugs (hydroxyurea or ara-C).

Unrelated-Matched and Related-Mismatched Allogeneic Bone Marrow Transplantation

Only 35–40% of patients have genotypically HLA-matched siblings for allogeneic BMT. Ten percent will additionally have a family member with one HLA haplotype genotypically identical to one haplotype of the patient, and the other haplotype phenotypically compatible for at least one of the three major HLA loci. Allogeneic BMT conducted from such donors shows a higher frequency of graft failure and moderate to severe GVHD with increasing degrees of histoincompatibility. Comparing the groups phenotypically matched or mismatched at one, two, or three loci, the incidence of moderate to severe GVHD was 40%, 65%, 75%, and 95%, respectively. Compared with a genotypically identical transplant, for which graft failure was observed in 2%, this incidence increased to 7% for phenotypically HLA-matched donors, 9% for one-locus mismatch, and 21% for two-loci mismatch (285, 286). These problems may be overcome through more intensive preparative regimens, posttransplantation immunosuppression, and improved GVHD prophylaxis and therapy. Presently, family donors with phenotypic HLA-matching or one-locus mismatch may be considered for allogeneic BMT.

Another source of marrow donors are unrelated persons who match for HLA-A, B, C, and DR loci with the patient. This is particularly useful in CML, in which the nature of the disease allows enough time for a donor search. An expanded donor bank of 10^5–10^6 volunteers may increase the probability of finding an unrelated donor to 25–50% (287). Preliminary studies are encouraging, but show, as expected, a significantly higher incidence of graft failure, moderate to severe acute GVHD, and chronic GVHD. These studies have targeted very young patients, the median age being 20–25 years (288–290). Among 102 patients treated for CML, the incidence of graft failure was 10%, and that of moderate to severe acute GVHD was 50–70% (289). The 1.5–2 years survival rate is about 30–40% and may be expected to worsen with longer follow-up in view of the use of T-cell-depleted marrows and expected high incidence of CML relapse. However, this potentially curative procedure could be offered to a subset of younger patients with CML, particularly with better management of problems related to graft failure and GVHD.

Autologous Stem Cell Transplantation

Autologous stem cell transplantation in chronic phase CML was prompted by the promising results in the transformed phases (discussed later) despite the resistant nature of the leukemia, the consistently better results with CML modalities (IFN-α, allogeneic BMT) in chronic versus transformed phases, and the appearance of Ph-negative cells in patients infused with 100% Ph-positive autologous cells following marrow ablative therapy. In chronic phase CML, restoration of diploid hematopoiesis following autologous stem cell transplantation was noted in 40–80% of patients. In the study of Hughes et al. (290), 10 of 13 patients (77%) exhibited 5–30% Ph-negative cells in the marrow after hematopoietic recovery. Meloni et al. treated 34 patients with autologous stem cell transplantation, using busulfan and melphalan for myeloablation: 15 of them (44%) showed Ph suppression at 2 months following BMT, including 4 (12%) with a complete cytogenetic response (291). Others have reported similar findings (292, 293). Diploid hematopoiesis is transient in most instances, although occasional long-term persistence of Ph-negativity has been observed (290, 293). The reason for the proliferative advantage of Ph-negative cells after autologous stem cell transplantation is unclear, but, in part, may be due to removal of the negative regulation exerted by the vast excess of Ph-positive myeloid cells on the growth of normal progenitors.

The degree of Ph-negative hematopoiesis could be further enhanced through the use of autologous stem cells that have been enriched in diploid cells by in vitro or in vivo purging (294–300). McGlave et al. treated ten patients with high-dose cyclophosphamide and TBI followed by reinfusion of autologous marrow stem cells that had been incubated in vitro with IFN-γ for 24 hours: three patients recovered with 100% diploid hematopoiesis (297). The contribution of IFN-γ to the degree of Ph-negativity needs further evaluation. A second in vitro purging approach relies on the proliferative advantage provided by the liquid culture system to Ph-negative cells. Barnett et al. demonstrated Ph-negative hematopoietic recovery following marrow ablative therapy and reinfusion of marrows grown in liquid culture for 7–10 days (298). A third possibility is an in vitro positive selection of hematopoietic normal stem cells, using antibodies directed against early progenitor cells, or based on the differential stromal adhesiveness of Ph-negative and Ph-positive progenitors (93, 299–301). Finally, the use of in vitro purging of CML cells with chemotherapy may be considered (295, 296). In vivo purging of CML marrows may be achieved following therapy with interferons or intensive chemotherapy, with or without growth factors.

In summary, the experience with autologous stem cell transplantation in chronic phase CML is encouraging and provides different treatment avenues in patients who do not benefit from established modalities. This could be further developed by using tandem autologous stem cell transplantation, infusion of stem cells enriched in vitro or in vivo with normal stem cells, and the use of posttransplantation maintenance therapy (chemotherapy, interferon, interleukin-2).

Choice of Therapy in Chronic Phase Chronic Myelogenous Leukemia

The choice of therapy in CML is difficult and may be clarified in the future with longer follow-up of the results of various treatments. The dilemma arises from (1) the relatively indolent nature of chronic phase CML, which provides a long survival with minimally toxic conventional therapy; (2) the availability of allogeneic BMT, a procedure with proved curative potential, but a high 1-year mortality rate; (3) the availability of IFN-α, a modality with a 20–25% long-term complete (10–15%) or near complete (5–10%) disappearance of disease with continued therapy in early chronic phase CML; (4) the high success rate of either modality in the earliest stages of the disease; and (5) the reputed unpredictable course of chronic phase CML with the possible sudden onset of disease transformation that would jeopardize the benefit from allogeneic BMT.

In an attempt to investigate the latter question, we reviewed the outcome of the last 260 patients referred to our institution with early chronic phase CML: 10 of them (4%) developed blastic phase in the first year and 9 (3%) in the second year. The onset of blastic phase was predictable (i.e., preceded by resistance to IFN-α therapy in chronic phase) in 16 patients, whereas 4 (2%) has a sudden onset of blastic phase (3 of them with lymphoid morphology). Thus, with careful follow-up, the development of unpredictable disease transformation was low in the first 2 years from diagnosis.

The choice of initial therapy is influenced by the experience of various investigators. Syngeneic BMT is considered as soon as possible in all patients who have such donors because of the high success rate and lack of GVHD complications. Some centers recommend allogeneic BMT in early chronic phase CML for all patients up to aged 50–55 years. At our institution, allogeneic BMT is offered as a frontline approach to all patients younger than 20 years because of the very low risk of GVHD. In older patients, an initial trial with IFN-α-based therapy is recommended. Patients who achieve any Ph suppression after 6 months of therapy, or Ph suppression to fewer than 50% Ph-positive metaphases after 12 months, continue the treatment as long as the cytogenetic response persists. Otherwise, they are offered allogeneic BMT or other investigational modalities with high-risk but curative potential (unrelated matched or related mismatched BMT) or with a capacity to induce a major cytogenetic response (intensive chemotherapy or autologous BMT with or without in vivo/in vitro purging).

Although conventional therapy is still widely applied in the medical community, we believe it should be used for restricted conditions. Busulfan therapy is indicated only for elderly patients for whom BMT cannot be performed and in whom frequent follow-ups are difficult. Hydroxyurea is preferably used in conjunction with other modalities such as IFN-α, in the context of investigational trials, in patients being considered for BMT, or in those who have failed to respond to newer regimens and who do not wish to consider investigational treatments. The indications for specific treatment modalities (cyclophosphamide, mercaptopurine, leukapheresis) have already been discussed.

Future treatment recommendations will depend on the improvement of allogeneic (conditioning regimens, GVHD prophylaxis and therapy, CMV prophylaxis and therapy, post-BMT maintenance) and autologous BMT (conditioning regimens, purging methods, post-BMT maintenance), versus the long-term follow-up results of IFN-α combinations and the discovery of new agents with anti-CML activity.

THERAPY OF ACCELERATED AND BLASTIC PHASE CHRONIC MYELOGENOUS LEUKEMIA

Earlier studies have been carried out in blastic phase CML because of the poor definition of the accelerated phase. The better results observed with allogeneic bone marrow transplantation and biological response modifiers in the accelerated phase, compared with the blastic phase, have encouraged investigations in a rigorously defined accelerated phase of CML.

Although morphologically resembling de novo acute leukemia, the blastic phase of CML is more resistant to therapy. Factors associated with better prognosis include a lymphoid blast cell morphology and the absence of thrombocytopenia or cytogenetic clonal evolution (24–26).

The treatments in blastic phase CML have followed the successful leads in acute leukemia, including intensive chemotherapy to induce marrow hypoplasia and normal stem cell regeneration, differentiating agents to induce maturation of blast cells and a return to chronic phase, and marrow ablative regimens with allogeneic and autologous BMT.

Intensive Chemotherapy

Intensive chemotherapy combinations include cytarabine (ara-C), anthracyclines, amsacrine, etoposide, azacitidine, cyclophosphamide, mercaptopurine, hydroxyurea, and other agents. With remission criteria of acute leukemia, complete remission rates of 10–20% have been reported (Table 12) (302–311). Our recent programs show higher remission rates (32% versus 15%; $p=0.01$) and significant, but modest, survival prolongations (24 versus 15 weeks; $p=0.03$) compared with older treatments (24).

Patients with lymphoid blastic phase CML have different clinical characteristics and a more favorable prognosis (313–317). They tend to develop a sudden onset of blastic phase, and have a higher percentage of marrow blasts and lower platelet counts (317). A high response rate is seen with vincristine and steroid-containing programs and with other antilymphoid regimens such as methotrexate

Table 12 Intensive Chemotherapy in Blastic Phase CML

Study (Ref.)	Regimen[a]	Patients	% CR	Median survival (wk)
Canellos et al. (302)	VP	30	13	20
Hayes et al. (303)	ara-C + carmustine + VP	86	4	6
Spiers et al. (304)	TRAMPCOL	19	42	—
Coleman et al. (305)	Hydroxyurea, VP, mercaptopurine	202	13	12
Schiffers et al. (306, 307)	Etoposide + azacitidine	62	4	5–23
Winton et al. (308)	DATA	30	0	5
Dutcher et al. (309)	Mitoxantrone + azacitidine	21	10	—
		12 (accelerated)	25	—
M. D. Anderson Cancer Center (24, 310, 317)	ADOAP, ROAP, COAP, AMSA-OAP	48	27	—

[a]VP, vincristine and prednisone; ara-C, cytosine arabinoside; TRAMPCOL, thioguanine, daunorubicin, ara-C, methotrexate, prednisone, cyclophosphamide, yincristine, L-asparaginase; DATA, daunorubicin, azacitidine, thioguanine, ara-C; OAP, vincristine, ara-C, prednisone; ADOAP, ROAP, DOAP, COAP, AMSA-OAP, OAP + doxorubicin (Adriamycin), zorubicin (Rubidazone), daunorubicin, cyclophosphamide, or amsacrine.

plus asparaginase (317). Complete response rates of 40–70% are obtained with combinations including vincristine, anthracyclines, and steroids, especially among patients whose blasts express the common acute lymphocytic leukemia antigen (CALLA-positive) (313).

Few studies have extended blastic phase intensive regimens into the accelerated phase. Dutcher et al. (309) recently treated 12 patients with accelerated phase CML using mitoxantrone and azacitidine. The complete response rate was 25%, compared with 10% for those treated in blastic phase. This supports the trend for earlier intervention in the transformed phases.

Differentiating Agents

Agents that induce in vitro leukemic cell differentiation include low doses of ara-C, thioguanine, homoharringtonine, azacitidine, hydroxyurea, plicamycin (mithramycin), retinoids, and interferons (318, 319). Although anecdotal reports showed some activity for low-dose ara-C in CML blastic phase, the response rate in larger series was disappointing. DiRaimondo et al. reported only one response among seven patients with blastic phase CML receiving low-dose ara-C (320). Retinoids have been investigated in myelodysplastic syndrome and acute leukemia with variable results. All *trans*-retinoic acid has recently shown dramatic results in two studies in patients with acute promyelocytic leukemia (321, 322) and may be useful in the accelerated and blastic phases of CML. The combination of several differentiating agents, including low-dose ara-C, *cis*-retinoic acid, vitamin D, and IFN-α produced two partial responses among three patients with CML blastic phase (323).

Plicamycin, an inhibitor of RNA synthesis, induces in vitro differentiation of blast cells and reduction of *abl* and *myc* oncogenic expression (62). Koller and Miller treated nine patients with CML blastic phase with low doses of plicamycin, 1 mg/m^2 intravenously two to three times weekly and hydroxyurea, and observed six responses, all with a myeloid blast cell morphology (Table 13) (324). A follow-up study resulted in two partial remissions among six patients with myeloid blastic phase (33%), but no responses among 15 patients with undifferentiated blastic phase (325). In two other studies, 1 complete response was obtained among 16 patients (6%) with CML blastic phase (326, 327). Antimi et al. suggested a possible value of plicamycin and hydroxyurea in the accelerated phase, with all four treated patients reverting to a second chronic phase (327).

Tiazofurin is a nucleoside analogue that is metabolized to thiazole-4-carboxamide adenine dinucleotide (TAD). TAD acts as a false cofactor to produce potent inhibition of inosine monophosphate dehyrogenase (IMPD) activity, to decrease production of guanine triphosphate (GTP) pools, and to inhibit cellular proliferation (328). As the active metabolite of tiazofurin, TAD is concentrated 20-fold higher in leukemic cells, compared with normal cells, resulting in a selective leukemic cell kill (329). Tricot et al. (330), using a pharmacologically directed approach, treated patients with tiazofurin, 2200–7700 mg/m^2 daily for 15 days, the dose adjusted to achieve inhibition of GTP pools to less than 20% in blast cells, and of IMPD activity to less than 10%. They observed partial responses in all five patients with CML blastic phase, the response defined as a decrease in peripheral blast count by 90% or more, and of marrow blasts by 75% or more. Responses were characterized by lack of marrow hypoplasia, suggesting differentiation to be the primary antileukemic effect. Tiazofurin has substantial side effects and requires administration under careful supervision.

Table 13 Therapy of Blastic Phase CML with Differentiating Agents and Interferons

Study (Ref.)	Therapy	No. patients	No. responses (%)
DiRaimondo (320)	Low-dose ara-C	7	1 (14)
Koller and Miller (324)	Plicamycin[a] + hydroxyurea		
	Myeloid	6	6 (100)
	Other	3	1 (33)
Koller et al. (325)	Plicamycin + hydroxyurea		
	Myeloid	6	2 (33)
	Undifferentiated	15	0 (0)
Trumper et al. (326)	Plicamycin + hydroxyurea	9	1 (11)
Antimi et al. (327)	Plicamycin + hydroxyurea	7	0 (0)
Tricot et al. (328)	Tiazofurin	5	5 (100)
M. D. Anderson Cancer Center (107)	Interferon alpha ± interferon gamma	24	5 (21)
Alimena et al. (108)	Interferon alpha	9	1 (11)

[a]Plicamycin is the current generic name for the older designation of "mithramycin."

The important leads of differentiating agents in CML blastic phase need to be confirmed (tiazofurin) or explored (all-*trans*-retinoic acid), and their potential role in the accelerated phase of CML evaluated.

Biological Agents

Anecdotal reports had shown the capacity of IFN-α to suppress cytogenetic clonal evolution and to control disease transformation (331). Extensive investigation of IFN-α and IFN-γ showed their limited role in producing remissions (107, 108) (see Table 13). The overall remission rate was 10–30% with IFN-α regimens, mostly in the accelerated phase; the overall response rate in the blastic phase was 10% or fewer (107, 108).

With use of low-dose ara-C at 15 mg/m^2 daily for 3 weeks and IFN-α at 5×10^6 units daily in patients with CML, 10 of 20 (50%) patients with accelerated phase CML achieved CHR, 3 of them (15%) showing additional minimal Ph suppression. Interferon-alpha hydroxyurea (Hydrea) are under evaluation for remission induction and maintenance in these stages.

Colony-stimulating factors (CSF) have produced exciting results in several tumor categories. Following intensive chemotherapy or autologous bone marrow transplantation, CSFs have been associated with shortening of the duration of myelosuppression and a decreased incidence of infections (332, 333). In vitro leukemic growth enhancement by CSFs dictated a cautious approach in trials of CSFs in myeloid tumors (334, 335). Granulocyte–macrophage CSF (GM-CSF) in myelodysplastic syndrome resulted in improvement in the granulocyte counts (336). In acute myelogenous leukemia, intensive chemotherapy followed by GM-CSF resulted in regrowth of the normal stem cells. These trials suggest that GM-CSF after intensive chemotherapy may revert CML blasts into mature chronic phase granulocytes, or may induce normal stem cell growth.

Autologous Stem Cell Transplantation

The underlying hypothesis for autologous stem cell transplantation (marrow or peripheral blood) in the accelerated and blastic phases of CML is that the stem cells collected in chronic phase, and reinfused after eradication of the accelerated or blastic phase clones with chemoirradiation, will reestablish a second chronic phase of equal duration to the first from the time of stem cell collection. The stem cells were often harvested in chronic phase with preponderance of Ph-positive clones, except for few patients who had stem cell storage after chemotherapy-induced Ph suppression (338). Studies of autologous stem cell transplantation have had limited success. Whereas 50–60% of patients achieved a second chronic phase, it was generally short-lasting. The median survival time from transplantation was 6 months, with fewer than 25% of patients surviving 1 year (Table 14) (337–341). Cytogenetic studies often showed recurrence of the original blastic phase clone.

To enhance leukemic cell eradication, Reiffers et al. performed double autologous stem cell transplantation with peripheral stem cells collected at diagnosis in 17 patients with CML transformation (341). All patients engrafted promptly. Six of 15 patients evaluated (40%) showed transient Ph suppression to a range of 10–84%. At the time of analysis 8 patients had relapsed after a median of 11 months, whereas 8 were still in a second chronic phase for a median of 11 plus months, 2 of them have a second chronic phase longer than the first one.

Allogeneic Bone Marrow Transplantation

The results of syngeneic or allogeneic bone marrow transplantation in the accelerated and blastic phases of CML are less favorable than in the chronic phase. The programs resulted in a high leukemic recurrence rate, ranging from

Table 14 Autologous Bone Marrow Transplantation in the Blastic Phase of CML

Study	No. treated	Achieving a second chronic phase (%)	Median survival from transplantation (mo)
Haines et al. (337)	51	94	6
Reiffers et al. (341)	45	76	4.5
Preisler et al. (339)	17	29	4
Dantas et al. (340)	11	55	7
Vellekoop et al. (338)	10	60	5

30% to 60% in the accelerated phase and from 40% to 90% in the blastic phase of CML. Cure, however, is still possible in 10–15% of patients with blastic phase and in 15–30% of those with accelerated phase (see Table 11). Thus, patients with available donors must be considered for syngeneic or allogeneic bone marrow transplantation, despite the risks and expenses involved. Transplantation in second chronic phase has consistently yielded higher cure fractions. This could be due to the decreased tumor burden at the time of the transplantation, or to the selection of patients with intrinsically more sensitive disease or with better tolerance to therapy. Although no definite recommendation can be made for the timing of transplantation (blastic phase or after induction of a second chronic phase), induction of a second chronic phase prior to BMT may be a valuable therapy-associated selection procedure when risk and cost analyses are important.

SPECIAL CONSIDERATIONS

Philadelphia Chromosome-Negative Chronic Myelogeneous Leukemia and Chronic Myelomonocytic Leukemia

About 90% of patients with a morphological and clinical diagnosis of CML demonstrate the Ph chromosome by cytogenetic studies. The remaining 10% of patients with Ph-negative CML form a spectrum of heterogeneous diseases.

One-third to one-half of them show *bcr* rearrangement by molecular analysis (380–385). These patients have the same molecular pathophysiology as Ph-positive CML, similar clinical and laboratory features, respond to interferon therapy, and have a favorable prognosis, with a median survival of 3–5 years. They should be treated as Ph-positive CML.

About 10–25% of patients have Ph-negative CML without *bcr* rearrangement and without monocytosis. In them, the disease may be driven by molecular events unrelated to the *bcr/abl* abnormalities, but mimicking them (e.g., excessive growth factor production or increase sensitivity to growth factor stimulation). They respond poorly to IFN-α, but may still have prolonged survival (345). Interestingly, unlike Ph-positive CML, their rate of blastic transformation is low, indicating the possible role of the *bcr/abl* events in disease transformation. Most patients die of complications related to marrow failure and fibrosis or with accelerated disease features (48, 49).

Finally 25–50% of patients have CMML. These patients have a "hybrid" disease with myeloid proliferation, erythroid and megakaryocytic dysplasia, and monocytic expression. The incidence of *ras* oncogene mutation is high (40–50%) and may be linked to monocytosis and to prognosis in general (71, 72). They present with high WBC counts together with monocytosis, anemia, and thrombocytopenia. These patients tend to be older and have higher percentages of marrow and peripheral blasts (345, 347). They respond poorly to IFN-α and have a poor prognosis, with a median survival of 12–18 months. Survival is associated with the degree of anemia, thrombocytopenia, peripheral and marrow blasts, and patient age (347).

Treatment of patients with CMML and those with Ph-negative CML and no *bcr* rearrangement is unsatisfactory. Hydroxyurea, busulfan, low-dose ara-C alone or with anthracyclines, plicamycin, oral etoposide (VP16), and interferons (alpha and gamma), all have been associated with a low incidence of remissions, ranging between 10% and 20% (71).

Indication for Molecular Studies in Chronic Myelogenous Leukemia

The molecular abnormalities in CML at the DNA, RNA, and protein levels opened new possibilities for their value in diagnosis, prognosis, and for follow-up of patients on therapy.

Molecular studies of *bcr* rearrangement in patients with a morphological diagnosis of CML are probably more expensive than routine cytogenetic studies to detect the Ph abnormality, particularly if more than one enzymatic analysis is required to detect *bcr* rearrangement. In patients with Ph-negative CML, studies for *bcr* rearrangement are useful to define the subset of patients with Ph-negative CML and *bcr* rearrangement who have a favorable prognosis and who respond to therapies similar to those for Ph-positive CML.

In Ph-positive CML, the relation of the site of the breakpoint on chromosome 22 to prognosis is controversial (348–351). Initial studies have reported that a 3' breakpoint is more frequent in blastic, compared with chronic phase, and that in chronic phase it was associated with a shorter remission duration and survival

(348–350). Other studies on large populations have not confirmed the prognostic impact of the *bcr* breakpoint. The two RNA messages (L6 versus K28) resulting from alternate splicing may be better correlated with response to therapy and with prognosis (353).

Patients with Ph-positive acute leukemia or with de novo Ph-positive CML blastic phase have similar presentations. Two different molecular abnormalities have been recognized in Ph-positive acute leukemia: the P210-related abnormalities and the P190-related abnormalities (354, 355). The clinical and prognostic correlations of these two molecular events are being investigated.

Molecular studies for detection of *bcr* rearrangement have been used in lieu of karyotypic analysis to follow up the effect of therapy (interferon, BMT) on Ph suppression. The sensitivity of the method is in the range of 1–5%. Molecular analysis for *bcr* rearrangement is equivalent, but not superior to cytogenetic studies in detecting residual Ph-positive disease. Ongoing efforts to quantitate the *bcr* rearrangement signal (by densitomeric analysis), and correlate it with the cytogenetic results, will enable expedient assessment of the degree of Ph suppression by therapy.

The polymerase chain reaction (PCR), a highly sensitive technique to detect minimal residual disease in $1{:}10^5$ to $1{:}10^6$ cells (356) has been adapted to the analysis of the *bcr/abl* RNA message in CML (357, 358). This permitted the examination of minimal residual disease after various treatments. Our studies show residual disease by PCR analysis in all patients rendered Ph-negative by IFN-α therapy (358). The results postallogeneic BMT are variable, with detection of residual disease by PCR ranging from 0% to 96% (358–362). In one instance, all seven patients studied in complete remission 5–7 years after allogeneic BMT had no evidence of residual disease, whereas an additional five patients receiving T-cell-depleted allogeneic BMT had residual disease 2.5–5 years in remission (361, 363). On the other hand, Pignon et al. observed residual disease by PCR in 16 of 17 patients (96%) studied in CR after allogeneic BMT (359). The technique has several limitations, including a high incidence of false-positive and false-negative results and the lack of knowledge of the cell lineage giving the positive result (lymphoid, myeloid). Detection of the *bcr/abl* event in fewer than 10^4 cells may not be relevant for predicting subsequent relapse (363). Several investigators are now evaluating the significance of minimal residual disease by PCR analysis and its relation with long-term prognosis.

Oncogene and Cellular-Directed Approaches in Chronic Myelogenous Leukemia

The molecular aberrations in CML present new opportunities for oncogene or cellular-directed therapies. If successful, they will provide leukemic cell elimination, without toxicity to the host cells.

Specific antibodies or antisense oligonucleotides can be developed against the P210 protein abnormality (364). A blocking of the abnormal message can, as with other tumors, normalize the malignant cellular behavior (365, 366). Since the location of the P210 protein is intracellular, the development of vehicles to internalize the blocking agents is needed. These could be used alone or after conjugation with toxins that enhance cellular destruction once internalized with the blocking agent. Analogous strategies have been used successfully against cells expressing the interleukin-2 receptors and CD5 (367, 368). These strategies could be applied to in vitro purging of bone marrow or, it is hoped, as in vivo therapy in humans to selectively kill or normalize the behavior of Ph-positive cells.

Another approach is to recognize and exploit the cellular differences between normal and CML cells. For example, if CML cells are confirmed to be CD34-positive but LFA-3-negative, a positive selection of the CD34-positive and LFA-3-positive normal stem cells could be carried out that would effectively purge marrows of the CML cells (93). Thus, combinations of these multiple approaches (monoclonal antibodies, antisense oligonucleotides, conjugated toxins, positive selection) could result in nontoxic, selective antileukemic programs that improve prognosis in CML.

Is the Prognosis of Patients with Chronic Myelogenous Leukemia Improving?

The survival of all patients treated at our institution by CML phase is shown in Figure 7. In chronic phase, allogeneic BMT offers long-term disease-free survival in 40–70% of patients, demonstrating the unequivocal improvement in prognosis with this modality. Bone marrow transplantation is applicable to the minority of patients with CML. The analysis of the beneficial effect of new modalities, such as IFN-α, is complicated by a suggested improved survival in CML owing to earlier diagnosis. In fact, as shown in Table 1, CML is diagnosed in a higher percentage of patients in an asymptomatic stage and with lower tumor burden. To address the question, we investigated the outcome of all patients referred with Ph-positive early chronic phase CML since 1971. We excluded patients referred before that time to avoid bias from improvement in supportive care. Patients referred between 1971 and 1981 received conventional or intensive chemotherapy, whereas those referred since 1981 were treated with IFN-α-containing regimens. The survival of the latter group was significantly better. This difference persisted even among patients referred in asymptomatic disease (see Fig. 7). It is interesting that the median survival of asymptomatic patients has not yet been reached (median follow-up of 5 years) with a projected 5-year survival of 65%.

The best proof of improved prognosis with IFN-α therapy is the achievement of a disease-free survival plateau in treated patients. This is, we hope, expected

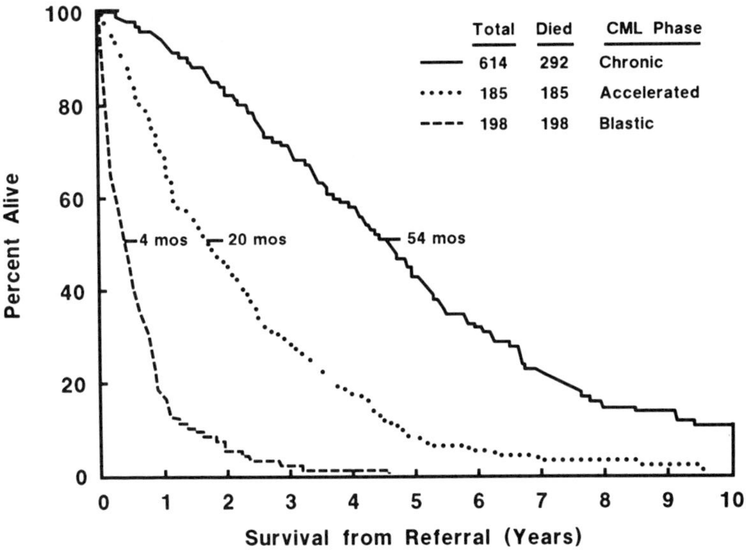

Figure 7 Survival by CML phase.

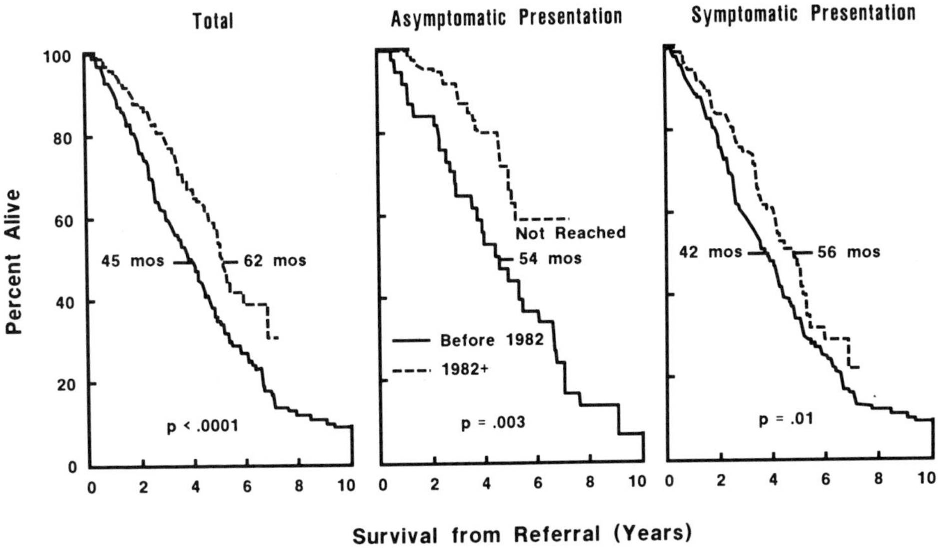

Figure 8 Survival in early chronic phase Ph-positive CML by year of referral; and within groups referred with asymptomatic or symptomatic disease.

in 20% of patients, based on the results shown in Figure 5. With conventional regimens, about 20–25% are alive *with* disease at 5 years. Thus, a follow-up of 6 years or longer, showing a plateau of survival *without* disease on IFN-α therapy will demonstrate its unequivocal therapeutic value. Discovery of additional modalities that are equally as effective as IFN-α may raise the disease-free survival plateau with the combination, making such approaches of even greater value in CML therapy.

REFERENCES

1. Kantarjian HM, Talpaz M, Gutterman JU: Chronic myelogenous leukemia—Past, present, and future. *Hematol Pathol* 1988; 2:91–120.
2. Canellos GP: Chronic granulocytic leukemia. *Med Clin North Am* 1976; 60:1001–1018.
3. Golde DW, Champlin RE: Chronic myelogenous leukemia: Recent advances. *Blood* 1985; 65:1039–1047.
4. Goldman JM, Lu Dao-Pei: New approaches in chronic granulocytic leukemia—origin, prognosis, and treatment. *Semin Hematol* 1982; 19:241–256.
5. Koeffler HP, Golde DW: Chronic myelogenous leukemia–new concepts. *N Engl J Med* 1981; 304:1201–1209.
6. Fialkow PJ, Jacobson RJ, Papayannopoulou T: Chronic myelocytic leukemia. Clonal origin in a stem cell common to the granulocyte, erythrocyte, platelet and monocyte/macrophage. *Am J Med* 1977; 63:125–130.
7. Barr RD, Fialkow PJ: Clonal origin of chronic myelocytic leukemia. *N Engl J Med* 1973; 289:307–312.
8. Yoffe G, Chinault A, Talpaz M, et al: Philadelphia chromosome positive and negative chronic myelogenous leukemia by DNA by hybridization analyses. *J Exp Hematol* 1987; 15:725–728.
9. Martin PJ, Najfeld V, Hansen HA, et al. Involvement of the B-lymphoid system in chronic myelogenous leukemia. *Nature* 1980; 287:49–50.
10. Golde DW, Burgaleta C, Sparkes RS, Cline MJ: The Philadelphia chromosome in human macrophages. *Blood* 1977; 49:367–371.
11. Koeffler HP, Levine AM, Sparkes M, Sparkes RS: Chronic myelocytic leukemia: Eosinophils involved in the malignant clone. *Blood* 1980; 55:1063–1068.
12. Denegri JF, Naiman SC, Gillen J, Thomas JW: In vitro growth of basophils containing the Philadelphia chromosome in the acute phase of chronic myelogenous leukaemia. *Br J Haematol* 1978; 40:351–355.
13. Greenberg BR, Wilson FD, Woo L, Jenks HM; Cytogenetic of fibroblastic colonies in Ph^1-positive chronic myelogenous leukemia. *Blood* 1978; 51:1039–1044.
14. Maniatis AK, Amsel S, Mitus WJ, Coleman N: Chromosome pattern of bone marrow fibroblasts in patients with chronic granulocytic leukemia. *Nature* 1969; 222:1273–1279.
15. O'Brien S, Kantarjian H, Shtalrid M, et al: Lack of breakpoint cluster region rearrangement in marrow fibroblasts of patients with Philadelphia chromosome-positive chronic myelogenous leukemia. *Hematol Pathol* 1988; 2:25–29.

16. Yonekura S, Nagao T, Arimori S: Increased growth and collagen synthesis of bone marrow fibroblasts from patients with chronic myelocytic leukaemia. *Br J Haematol* 1985; 61:93–99.
17. Francis GE, Michalevicz R, Wickremasinghe RG: Chronic myeloid leukaemia and the Philadelphia translocation: Do the c-*sis* oncogene and platelet-derived growth factor provide the link? *Leuk Res* 1983; 7:817–820.
18. Michallet M, Leger J, Chabannon C, et al: Long term bone marrow cultures in patients with chronic granulocytic leukemia before and after bone marrow transplantation: Persistence of an altered bone marrow environment after BMT [abstr]. *Blood* 1987; 70(suppl 1):311a.
19. Wetzler M, Kurzrock R, Lowe D, et al: Alteration in bone marrow stromal growth factor expression—a possible mechanism of disease progression in chronic myelogenous leukemia. *Proc Am Assoc Cancer Res* 1990; 31:30(abstr 179).
20. Nowell PC, Hungerford DA: A minute chromosome in human chronic granulocytic leukemia. *Science* 1960; 132:1497–1502.
21. Rowley JD: A new consistent chromosomal abnormality in chronic myelogenous leukemia identified by quinacrine fluorescence and Giemsa staining. *Nature* 1973; 243:290–294.
22. Fialkow PJ, Martin PJ, Najfeld V, et al: Evidence for a multi-step pathogenesis of chronic granulocytic leukemia. *Blood* 1981; 58:158–163.
23. Kantarjian HM, Dixon D, Keating MJ, et al: Characteristics of accelerated disease in chronic myelogenous leukemia. *Cancer* 1988; 61:1441–1446.
24. Kantarjian HM, Keating MJ, Talpaz M, et al: Chronic myelogenous leukemia in blast crisis: An analysis of 242 patients. *Am J Med* 1987; 83:445–454.
25. Allen SL, Coleman M: Terminal-phase chronic myelogenous leukemia: Approaches to treatment. *Cancer Invest* 1985; 3:491–503.
26. Rosenthal S, Canellos GP, DeVita VT Jr, Gralnick HR: Characteristics of blast crisis in chronic granulocytic leukemia. *Blood* 1977; 49:705–714.
27. Groffen J, Stephenson JR, Heisterkamp N, et al: Philadelphia chromosomal breakpoints are clustered within a limited region, *bcr*, on chromosome 22. *Cell* 1984; 36:93–99.
28. Heisterkamp N, Stam K, Groffen J, et al: Structural organization of the *bcr* gene and its role in the Ph^1 translocation. *Nature* 1985; 315:758–761.
29. Heisterkamp N, Stephenson JR, Groffen J, et al: Localization of the c-*abl* oncogene adjacent to a translocation break point in chronic myelocytic leukaemia *Nature* 1983; 306:239–242.
30. Shtivelman B, Lipshitz B, Gale RP, Canaani E: Fused transcript of *abl* and *bcr* genes in chronic myelogenous leukaemia. *Nature* 1985; 315:550–554.
31. Stam K, Heisterkamp N, Grosveld G, et al: Evidence of a new chimeric *bcr*/c-*abl* mRNA in patients with chronic myleocytic leukemia and the Philadelphia chromosome. *N Engl J Med* 1985; 313:1429–1433.
32. Konopka JB, Watanabe SM, Witte ON: An alteration of the human c-*abl* protein in K562 leukemia cells unmasks associated tyrosine kinase activity. *Cell* 1984; 37:1035–1042.
33. Koeltzer W, Kurzrock R, Smith L, et al: The human cellular *abl* gene product in

the chronic myelogenous leukemia cell line K562 has an associated tyrosine protein kinase activity. *Virology* 1985; 140:230–238.

34. Kurzrock R, Gutterman J, Talpaz M: The molecular genetics of Philadelphia chromosome positive leukemias. *N Engl J Med* 1988; 319:990.
35. Goldman JM, Grosveld G, Baltimore D, Gale RP: Chronic myelogenous leukemia—the unfolding saga. *Leukemia* 1990; 4:163–167.
36. Daley GO, McLaughlin J, Witte ON, Baltimore D: The CML-specific P210 *bcr/abl* protein, unlike v-*abl,* does not transform NIH/3T3 fibroblasts. *Science* 1987; 237:532.
37. McLaughlin J, Chianese E, Witte O: In vitro transformation of immature hematopoietic cells by the P210 *bcr/abl* oncogene product of the Philadelphia chromosome. *Proc Natl Acad Sci USA* 1987; 84:6558–6562.
38. Chung SW, Wong PMC, Shen-Ong G, et al: Production of granulocyte–macrophage colony-stimulating factor by Abelson virus-induced tumorigenic mast cell lines. *Blood* 1986; 68:1074–1081.
39. Chung SW, Ruscetti S, Wong P: Formation of factor independent hemopoietic multilineage colonies after Abelson virus infection. *Blood* 1988; 71:973–977.
40. Young JC, Witte ON: Selective transformation of primitive lymphoid cells by the *bcr/abl* oncogene expressed in long-term lymphoid or myeloid cultures. *Mol Cell Biol* 1988; 8:4079–4087.
41. Daley GQ, Van Etten RA, Baltimore D: Induction of chronic myelogenous leukemia by the P210 *bcr/abl* gene of the Philadelphia chromosome. *Science* 1990; 247:824–829.
42. Hariharan IK, Harris AW, Crawford M, et al: A *bcr*–v-*abl* oncogene induces lymphomas in transgenic mice. *Mol Cell Biol* 1989; 9:2798–2805.
43. Lisker R, Caras L, Mutchinick O, et al: Late appearing Philadelphia chromosome in two patients with chronic myelogenous leukemia. *Blood* 1980; 56:812–814.
44. Sandberg AA: Cytogenetic staging of chronic myeloid leukemia. *Boll 1st Sieroter Milan* 1989; 57:247–256.
45. Rowley JD: Ph^1-positive leukaemia, including chronic myelogenous leukaemia. *Clin Haematol* 1980; 9:55–81.
46. Gupta CM, Dalousek DK, Eaves CJ, Eaves AC: Cytogenetic studies of early myeloid progenitor compartments in Ph^1 positive chronic myeloid leukemia. I. Persistence of Ph^1 negative committed progenitors that are suppressed from differentiating in vivo. *Br J Haematol* 1984; 56:633–644.
47. Hunter T, Cooper JA: Protein-tyrosine kinases. *Annu Rev Biochem* 1985; 54:897–930.
48. Daley GQ, Baltimore D: Transformation of an interleukin 3-dependent hematopoietic cell line by the chronic myelogenous leukemia-specific $P210^{bcr/abl}$ protein. *Proc Natl Acad Sci USA* 1988; 85:9312–9316.
49. Laneuville P, Tellier R, Fauser A: Introduction of $p210^{bcr/abl}$ into a human factor dependent myeloid cell line by retroviral mediated gene transfer reduces growth factor dependence. *Blood* 1989; 74(suppl 1):199a (abstr 744).
50. Kantarjian H, Kurzrock R, Talpaz M: Philadelphia chromosome-negative chronic

myelogenous leukemia and chronic myelomonocytic leukemia. *Hematol Oncol Clin North Am* 1990; 4:405–430.

51. Kurzrock R, Kantarjian H, Shtalrid M, et al: Philadelphia chromosome-negative chronic myelogenous leukemia without breakpoint cluster region rearrangement—a chronic myeloid leukemia with a distinct clinical course. *Blood* 1990; 74:445–452.
52. Chang J, Metcalf D, Lang R, et al: Non-neoplastic hematopoietic myeloproliferative syndrome induced by dysregulated multi-CSF (IL-3) expression. *Blood* 1989; 73:1487–1497.
53. Gualtieri R, Emanuel P, Zuckerman D, et al: Granulocyte-macrophage colony stimulating factor is an endogenous regulator of cell proliferation in juvenile chronic myelogenous leukemia. *Blood* 1989; 74:2360–2367.
54. Everson M, Brown C, Lilly M: Interleukin-6 and granulocyte–macrophage colony stimulating factor are candidate growth factors for chronic myelomonocytic leukemia cells. *Blood* 1989; 74:1472–1476.
55. Hagemeijer A, Smit EME, Lowenberg B, Abels J: Chronic myeloid leukemia with permanent disappearance of the Ph^1 chromosome and development of new clonal subpopulations. *Blood* 1979; 53:1–14.
56. Bartram CR, Janssen JWG, Becher R, et al: Persistence of chronic myelocytic leukemia despite deletion of rearranged *bcr*/c-*abl* sequences in blast crisis. *J Exp Med* 1986; 164:1389–1396.
57. Lawler SD: The cytogenetics of chronic granulocyte leukemia. *Clin Haematol* 1977; 6:55–75.
58. Collins SJ, Groudine MY: Rearrangement and amplication of c-*abl* sequence in the human chronic myelogenous leukemia cell line K562. *Proc Natl Acad Sci USA* 1983; 80:4313–4817.
59. Collins SJ: Breakpoints on chromosomes 9 and 22 in Philadelphia chromosome-positive chronic myelogenous leukemia (CML). Amplification of rearranged c-*abl* oncogenes in CML blast crisis. *J Clin Invest* 1986; 78:1392–1396.
60. Andrews DF III, Collins SJ: Heterogeneity in expression of *bcr–abl* fusion transcript in CML blast crisis. *Leukemia* 1987; 1:713–724.
61. Jonak, GJ, Knight E Jr: Selective reduction of c-*myc* mRNA in Daudi cells by human β interferon. *Proc Natl Acad Sci USA* 1984; 81:1747–1750.
62. Koller C, Campbell V, Polansky D: In vivo differentiation of blast-phase chronic granulocytic leukemia—expression of c-*myc* and c-*abl* protooncogenes. *J Clin Invest* 1985; 76:365–369.
63. Le Beau M, Lemons R, Carrino J, et al: Chromosomal localization of the human *G-CSF* gene to 17q11 proximal to the breakpoint of the t(15;17) in acute promyelocytic leukemia. *Leukemia* 1987; 1:795–799.
64. Finlay CA, Hinds PW, Levin MJ: The *p53* protooncogene can act as a suppressor of transformation. *Cell* 1989; 57:1083–1093.
65. Hershkowitz I: Functional inactivation of genes by dominant negative mutations. *Nature* 1987; 329:219–222.
66. Kelman Z, Prokocimer M, Peller S, et al: Rearrangements in the *p53* gene in Philadelphia chromosome positive chronic myelogenous leukemia. *Blood* 1989; 74:2318.

67. Ahuja H, Bar-Eli M, Advani SH, et al: Alterations in the *p53* gene and the clonal evolution of the blast crisis of chronic myelocytic leukemia. *Proc Natl Acad Sci USA* 1989; 86:6783.
68. Mashal R, Shtalrid M, Talpaz M, et al: Rearrangement and expression of *p53* in the chronic phase and base crisis of chronic myelogenous leukemia. *Blood* 1990; 75:180.
69. Bos JL: *ras* Oncogenes in hematopoietic malignancies. *Hematol Pathol* 1988; 2:55–63.
70. Collins SJ, Howard M, Andrews DF, et al: Rare occurrence of N-*ras* point mutatins in Philadelphia chromosome positive chronic myeloid leukemia. *Blood* 1989; 73:1028–1032.
71. LeMaistre A, Lee M-S, Talpaz M, et al: *ras* Oncogene mutations are rare late stage events in chronic myelogenous leukemia. *Blood* 1989; 73:889–891.
72. Padua RA, Carter G, Hughes D, et al: *ras* Mutations in myelodysplasia detected in amplification, oligonucleotide hybridization, and transformation. *Leukemia* 1988; 2:503–510.
73. LeMaistre, A, Hirsch-Ginsberg C, Kantarjian H, et al: *ras* Mutations are rare events in Philadelphia-negative/*bcr*-negative chronic myelogenous leukemia (Ph^1-*bcr*-CML) but prevalent in chronic myelomonocytic leukemia (CMML). *Blood* 1990; (in press)
74. Farr CJ, Saiki RK, Erlich HA, et al: Analysis of *ras* gene mutations in acute myeloid leukemia by polymerase chain reaction and oligonucleotide probes. *Proc Natl Acad Sci USA* 1988; 85:1629–1633.
75. Janssen JWG, Steenvoorden ACM, Lyons J, et al: *ras* Gene mutations in acute and chronic myelocytic leukemias, chronic myeloproliferative disorders, and myelodysplastic syndromes. *Proc Natl Acad Sci USA* 1987; 84:9228.
76. Moore MAS, Williams N, Metcalf D: In vitro colony formation by normal and leukemic human hematopoietic cells. Characterization of the colony-forming cells. *JNCI* 1973; 50:603–610.
77. Spiers ASD, Bain BJ, Turner JE: The peripheral blood in chronic granulocytic leukaemia: Study of 50 untreated Philadelphia-positive cases. *Scand J Haematol* 1977; 18:25–38.
78. Coulombel L, Kalousek DK, Eaves CJ, et al: Long-term marrow culture reveals chromosomally normal hematopoietic progenitor cells in patients with Philadelphia chromosome-positive chronic myelogenous leukemia. *N Engl J Med* 1983; 308:1493–1498.
79. Dube ID, Kalousek DK, Coulombel L, et al: Cytogenetic studies of early myeloid progenitor compartments in Ph^1-positive chronic myeloid leukemia. Long-term culture reveals the persistence of Ph^1-negative progenitors in treated as well as newly diagnosed patients. *Blood* 1984; 63:1171–1177.
80. Dube ID, Arlin ZA, Kalousek DK, et al: Nonclonal hemopoietic progenitor cells detected in long-term marrow cultures from a Turner syndrome mosaic with chronic myeloid leukemia. *Blood* 1984; 64:1284–1287.
81. Hogge DE, Coulombel L, Kalousek DK, et al: Nonclonal hemopoietic progenitors in a G6PD heterozygote with chronic myelogenous leukemia revealed after long-term marrow cultures. *Am J Hematol* 1987; 24:389–394.

82. O'Brien S, Kantarjian H, Talpaz M, et al: The effect of long-term marrow culture on the nonadherent Philadelphia chromosome-positive clones in chronic myelogenous leukemia—preliminary observations. *Hematol Pathol* 1987; 1:167–172.
83. Strife A, Clarkson B: Biology of chronic myelogenous leukemia—is discordant maturation the primary defect? *Semin Hematol* 1988; 25:1–19.
84. Strife A, Lambek C, Wisniewski D, et al: Discordant maturation as the primary biological defect in chronic myelogenous leukemia. *Cancer Res* 1988; 48:1035–1041.
85. Gordon MY, Dowding CR, Riley GP, et al: Altered adhesive interactions with marrow stroma of haematopoietic progenitor cells in chronic myeloid leukemia. *Nature* 1987; 328:342–344.
86. Moore MAS, Broxmeyer HE, Sheridan APC, et al: Continuous human bone marrow culture: Ia antigen characterization of probable pluripotential stem cells. *Blood* 1980; 55:682.
87. Schlossman F, Chess L, Humphreys RE, Strominger JL: Distribution of Ia-like molecules on the surface of normal and leukemic human cells. *Proc Natl Acad Sci USA* 1976; 73:1288.
88. Fujimiya Y, Bakke A, Chang WC, et al: Natural killer-cell immunodeficiency in patients with chronic myelogenous leukemia. I. Analysis of the defect using the monoclonal antibodies HNK-1 (LEU-7) and B73.1. *Int J Cancer* 1986; 37:639–649.
89. Chang W-C, Fujimiya Y, Casteel N, Pattengale P: Natural killer cell immunodeficiency in patients with chronic myelogenous leukemia. III. Defective interleukin-2 production by T-helper and natural killer cells. *Int J Cancer* 1989; 43:591–597.
90. Verfaillie C, Miller W, Kay N, McGlave P: Adherent lymphokine-activated killer cells in chronic myelogenous leukemia—a benign cell population with potent cytotoxic activity. *Blood* 1989; 74:793–797.
91. Verfaillie C, Kay N, Miller W, McGlave P: Diminished A-LAK cytotoxicity and proliferation accompanying disease progression in chronic myelogenous leukemia. *Blood* 1990; 76:401–408.
92. Upadhyaya G, Deisseroth A, Emerson S: CML progenitor cells are deficient in cell surface LFA-3; modulation by alpha-interferon in vitro and in vivo. *Blood* 1988; 72(suppl 1):231a (abstr 836).
93. Deisseroth A, Herst V, Wedrychowski A, et al: Future directions in molecular and genetic therapy for leukemias and solid tumors. *Cancer Bull* 1990; 43:173–180.
94. Vodopick H, Rupp EM, Edwards CI, et al: Spontaneous cyclic leukocytosis and thombocytosis in chronic myelogenous leukemia. *N Engl J Med* 1972; 286:284–289.
95. Olofsson T, Olsson I: Suppression of normal granulopoiesis in vitro by a leukemia-associated inhibitor (LAI) of acute and chronic leukemia. *Blood* 1980; 55:975–982.
96. Chervenick PA, Ellis LD, Pan SF, Lawson AL: Human leukemic cells: In vitro growth of colonies containing the Philadelphia (Ph^1) chromosome. *Science* 1971; 174:1134–1136.

97. Shadduck RK, Nankin HR: Cellular origin of granulocyte colonies in chronic myeloid leukaemia. *Lancet* 1971; 2:1097–1098.
98. Cunningham I, Gee T, Dowling M, et al: Results of treatment of Ph^1+ chronic myelogenous leukemia with an intensive treatment regimen (L-5 protocol). *Blood* 1979; 53:375–396.
99. Hester JP, Waddell CC, Coltman CA Jr, et al: Response of chronic myelogenous leukemia patients to COAP–splenectomy. *Cancer* 1984; 54:1977–1982.
100. Kantarjian HM, Vellekoop L, McCredie KB, et al: Intensive combination chemotherapy (ROAP) and splenectomy in the management of chronic myelogenous leukemia. *J Clin Oncol* 1985; 3:192–200.
101. Singer JW, Arlin ZA, Najfeld V, et al: Restoration of nonclonal hematopoiesis in chronic myelogenous leukemia (CML) following a chemotherapy-induced loss of the Ph^1+ chromosome. *Blood* 1980; 56:356–360.
102. Singer JW, Adamson JW, Arlin AZ, et al: Chronic myelogenous leukemia: In vitro studies of hematopoietic regulation in a patient undergoing intensive chemotherapy. *J Clin Invest* 1981; 67:1593–1598.
103. Goto T, Nishikori M, Arlin Z: Growth characteristics of leukemia and normal hematopoietic cells in Ph^1+ chronic myelogenous leukemia and effects of intensive treatment. *Blood* 1982; 59:793–803.
104. Kolitz J, Kempin S, Schluger A, et al: Phase II trial of high dose hydroxyurea in chronic myelogenous leukemia. *Blood* 1989; 74(suppl 1):155a (abstr 577).
105. Talpaz M, Kantarjian HM, McCredie KB, et al: Clinical investigation of human alpha interferon in chronic myelogenous leukemia. *Blood* 1987; 69:1280–1288.
106. Talpaz M, Kantarjian HM, McCredie K, et al: Hematologic remission and cytogenetic improvement induced by recombinant human interferon alpha A in chronic myelogenous leukemia. *N Engl J Med* 1986; 314:1065–1069.
107. Kantarjian HM, Talpaz M, Gutterman J: Biologic therapy of chronic myelogenous leukemia. *Oncology* 1987; 1:35–40.
108. Alimena G, Morra E, Lazzarino M, et al: Interferon alpha-2b as therapy for Ph^1-positive chronic myelogenous leukemia. A study of 82 patients treated with intermittent or daily administration. *Blood* 1988; 72:642–647.
109. Niederle N, Kloke O, Osieka KR, et al: Interferon alpha-2b in the treatment of chronic myelogenous leukemia. *Semin Oncol* 1987; 16:29–35.
110. Ozer H, Dear K, Testa J, et al: Prolonged administration of subcutaneous α-interferon induces major clinical and complete cytogenetic remissions in untreated Philadelphia chromosome positive chronic myelogenous leukemia. *Proc Am Soc Clin Oncol* 1990; 9:203 (abstr 783).
111. Djaldetti M, Padeh B, Pinkhas J, Deries A: Prolonged remission in chronic myeloid leukemia after one course of busulfan. *Blood* 1966; 27:103.
112. Finney R, McDonald GA, Baikie AG, Douglas AS: Chronic granulocytic leukaemia with Ph^1 negative cells in bone marrow and a ten year remission after busulphan hypoplasia. *Br J Haematol* 1972; 28:283.
113. Kantarjian HM, Smith TL, McCredie KB, et al: Chronic myelogenous leukemia: A multivariate analysis of the associations of patient characteristics and therapy with survival. *Blood* 1985; 66:1326–1335.

114. Tura S, Baccarani M, Corbelli G, et al: Staging of chronic myeloid leukaemia. *Br J Haematol* 1981; 47:105–119.
115. Cervantes F, Rozman C: A multivariate analysis of prognostic factors in chronic myeloid leukemia. *Blood* 1982; 60:1298–1304.
116. Sokal JE, Cox EB, Baccarani M, et al: Prognostic discrimination "good-risk" chronic granulocytic leukemia. *Blood* 1984; 63:789–799.
117. Sokal JE, Baccarani M, Tura S, et al: Prognostic discrimination among younger patients with chronic granulocytic leukemia. Relevance to bone marrow transplantation. *Blood* 1985; 66:1352–1357.
118. Sokal J, Gomez G, Baccarani M, et al: Prognostic significance of additional cytogenetic abnormalities at diagnosis of Philadelphia chromosome-positive chronic granulocytic leukemia. *Blood* 1988; 72:294–298.
119. Wareham NJ, Johnson SA, Goldman JM: Relationship of the duration of the chronic phase in chronic granulocytic leukemia to the need for treatment during the first year after diagnosis. *Cancer Chemother Pharmacol* 1982; 8:205–210.
120. Prabhu M, Kochupillai V, Sharma S, et al: Prognostic assessment of various parameters in chronic myeloid leukemia. *Cancer* 1986; 58:1357–1360.
121. Tura S: Italian Cooperative Study Group on Chronic Myeloid Leukemia: Prospective confirmation of a prognostic classification for Ph+ chronic myeloid leukemia. *Br J Haematol* 1988; 69:463–466.
122. Kantarjian H, Keating M, Smith T, et al: Proposal for a simple synthesis prognostic staging system in chronic myelogenous leukemia. *Am J Med* 1990; 88:1–8.
123. Segal GB, Simon W, Lichtman MA: Variables influencing the timing of marrow transplantation in patients with chronic myelogenous leukaemia. *Blood* 1986; 68:1055–1064.
124. Simon W, Segel GB, Lichtman MA: Upper and lower time limits of marrow transplantation for patients with chronic myelogenous leukaemia. *Br J Haematol* 1988; 70:31–36.
125. Bergsagel DE: The chronic leukemias: A review of disease manifestations and the aims of therapy. *Can Med Assoc J* 1967; 96:1616–1620.
126. Inball A, Modan M, Mary A: A retrospective study of patients with chronic myeloid leukemia diagnosed and treated at the Chaim Sheba Medical Center during the years 1966–76. *Isr J Med Sci* 1978; 14:1259–1264.
127. Clarkson B: Chronic myelogenous leukemia: Is aggressive treatment indicated? *J Clin Oncol* 1985; 3:135.
128. Dekmezian R, Kantarjian HM, Keating MJ, et al: The relevance of reticulin stain—measured fibrosis at diagnosis in chronic myelogenous leukemia. *Cancer* 1987; 59:1739–1743.
129. Minot GR, Buckman TE, Isaacs R: Chronic myelogenous leukemia: Age, incidence, duration and benefit derived from irradiation. *JAMA* 1924; 82:1489–1494.
130. Reinhard EH, Neely L, Samples DM: Radioactive phosphorus in the treatment of chronic leukemias: Long-term results over a period of 15 years. *Ann Intern Med* 1959; 50:942.
131. Barrett AJ, Longhurst P, Humble JG, Newton KA: Effect of splenic irradiation on

circulating colony-forming cells in chronic granulocytic leukaemia. *Br Med J* 1977; 14:1259.

132. Haddow A, Timmis GM: Myleran in chronic myeloid leukaemia. Chemical constitution and biological action. *Lancet* 1953; 1:207.
133. Galton DAG: Myleran in chronic myeloid leukaemia. *Lancet* 1953; 1:208.
134. Haut, A, Abbott WS, Wintrobe MM, Cartwright GE: Busulfan in the treatment of chronic myelocytic leukemia: The effect of long term intermittent therapy. *Blood* 1961; 17:1.
135. Conrad FG: Survival in chronic granulocytic leukemia. Splenic irradiation vs busulfan. *Arch Intern Med* 1973; 131:684–685.
136. Gollerkeri MP, Shah GB: Management of chronic myeloid leukemia: A five-year survey with a comparison of oral busulfan and splenic irradiation. *Cancer* 1971; 21:596.
137. The Working Party for Therapeutic Trials in Leukemia. Chronic granulocytic leukemia—a comparison of radiotherapy and busulfan. *Br Med J* 1968; 1:203–208.
138. Sokal JE: Evaluation of survival data from chronic myelocytic leukemia. *Am J Hematol* 1979; 1:493–500.
139. Southeastern Cancer Chemotherapy Cooperative Study Group: Comparison of 6-mercaptopurine and busulfan in chronic granulocytic leukemia. *Blood* 1963; 21:89.
140. Rundles RW, Grizzle J, Bell WN: Comparison of chlorambucil and Myleran in chronic lymphocytic and granulocytic leukemia. *Am J Med* 1959; 27:424–432.
141. Kuang DT, Close HP, Whittington RM, Patno ME: Comparison of busulfan and cyclophosphamide in the treatment of chronic myelocytic leukemia. *Cancer* 1971; 27:603–612.
142. Silver RT, Mick R, Cooper R, et al: A comparative study of dibromomannitol and busulfan in the treatment of chronic myeloid leukemia—a study of Cancer and Leukemia Group B. *Cancer* 1987; 60:1442–1448.
143. Feingold ML, Koss LG: Effects of long-term administration of busulfan. *Arch Intern Med* 1975; 124:66.
144. Fishbein WN, Carbone PP, Freireich EJ: Clinical trials of hydroxyurea in patients with cancer and leukemia. *Clin Pharmacol Ther* 1964; 5:574.
145. Kennedy BJ, Yarbro JW: Metabolic and therapeutic effects of hydroxyurea in chronic myeloid leukemia. *JAMA* 1966; 195:1038
146. Kennedy BJ: Hydroxyurea therapy in chronic myelogenous leukemia. *Cancer* 1972; 29:1052.
147. Tanzer J, Briere J, Aucleic A, et al: Long term results for 47 patients with Ph^1+ chronic myelogenous leukemia given hydroxyurea as major treatment. *Blood* 1979; 54:212a.
148. Schwartz, JH, Canellos GP: Hydroxyurea in the management of hematologic complications of chronic granulocytic leukemia. *Blood* 1975; 46:11.
149. Bolin RW, Robinson WA, Sutherland J, Hamman R: Busulfan vs hydroxyurea in long-term therapy of chronic myelogenous leukemia. *Cancer* 1982; 50:1683–1686.

150. Rushing D, Goldman A, Gibbs G, et al: Hydroxyurea versus busulfan in the treatment of chronic granulocytic leukemia. *Am J Clin Oncol* 1982; 5:307.
151. Sullivan JR, Hurley TH, Bolton JH: Treatment of chronic myeloid leukemia with repeated single doses of busulfan. *Cancer Treat Rep* 1977; 51:43.
152. Vicariot M, Goldman JM, Catovsky D, Galton DAG: Treatment of chronic granulocytic leukaemia with repeated single doses of busulphan. *Eur J Cancer* 1979; 15:559–563.
153. Schwarzenberg L, Mathe G, Pouillart P, et al: Hydroxyurea, leucopheresis, and splenectomy in chronic myeloid leukaemia at the possible phase. *Br Med J* 1973; 1:700.
154. Krakoff IH, Karnofsky DA, Burchenal JH: Remissions induced by chlorambucil in chronic granulocytic leukemia. *JAMA* 1958; 166:629.
155. Hauch T, Logue G, Laszlo J, et al: Treatment of chronic granulocytic leukemia with melphalan. *Blood* 1978; 51:571.
156. Seeler RA, Hahn KO: Chronic granulocytic leukemia responding to melphalan. *Cancer* 1971; 27:284.
157. Dibromannitol Cooperative Study Group: Survival of chronic myeloid leukaemia patients treated by dibromomannitol. *Eur J Cancer* 1973; 9:583.
158. Canellos GP, Young RC, Nieman PE, DeVita VT Jr: Dibromomannitol in the treatment of chronic granulocytic leukemia: A prospective randomized comparison with busulfan. *Blood* 1975; 45:197.
159. Talpaz M, Kurzrock R, Kantarjian H, et al: Recombinant interferon-alpha therapy of Philadelphia chromosome-negative myeloproliferative disorders with thrombocytosis. *Am J Med* 1989; 86:554–558.
160. Gisslinger H, et al: Long-term interferon therapy for thrombocytosis in myeloproliferative disorders. *Lancet* 1989; 1:634–637.
161. Giles F, et al: Alpha-interferon therapy for essential thrombocytopenia. *Lancet* 1988; 1:70–72.
162. Lazzarino M, et al: Interferon alpha-2b as treatment for Philadelphia-negative chronic myeloproliferative disorders with excessive thrombocytosis. *Br J Haematol* 1989; 72:173–177.
163. Gugliotta L, et al: In vivo and in vitro inhibitory effect of alpha-interferon on megakaryocyte colony growth in essential thrombocythaemia. *Br J Haematol* 1989; 71:177–181.
164. Talpaz M, Mavligit G, Keating M, et al: Human leukocyte interferon to control thrombocytosis in chronic myelogenous leukemia. *Ann Intern Med* 1983; 99:789–792.
165. Silverstein M, Petitt R: The use of anagrelide in thrombocythemic states. *Blood* 1989; 74(suppl 1):200a (abstr 746).
166. Silverstein M, Petitt R, Solberg, et al: Anagrelide—a new drug for treating thrombocytosis. *N Engl J Med* 1988; 318:1292–1294.
167. Vallejos CS, McCredie KB, Brittin GM, Freireich EJ: Biological effects of repeated leukapheresis of patients with chronic myelogenous leukemia. *Blood* 1973; 42:925–933.
168. Goldman JM, Lowenthal RM, Buskard NA, et al: Chronic granulocytic leukemia-

selective removal of immature granulocytic cells by leukapheresis. *Semin Hematol* 1975; 8:28–40.
169. Lowenthal RM, Buskard NA, Goldman JM, et al: Intensive leukapheresis as initial therapy for chronic granulocytic leukemia. *Blood* 1975; 46:835–844.
170. Fitzgerald D, Rowe JM, Heal J: Leukapheresis for control of chronic myelogenous leukemia during pregnancy. *Am J. Hematol* 1986; 22:213–218.
171. Neiman F, Brandt L, Nilsson PG: Cytogenetic evidence for splenic origin of blastic transformation in chronic myelogenous leukemia. *Scand J. Haematol* 1974; 13:87–90.
172. Spiers ASD, Ermidou-Sazeidis C, Richards HGH: Chronic granulocytic leukaemia: Clinical course, blood and bone marrow changes after chemotherapy and splenectomy. *Haematologica* 1979; 64:616.
173. Baccarani M, Zaccaria A, Santucci AM, et al: A simultaneous study of bone marrow, spleen, and liver in chronic myeloid leukaemia: Evidence for differences in cell composition and karyotypes. *Ser Haematol* 1975; 8:81–112.
174. Mitelman F: Comparative cytogenic studies of bone marrow and extra-medullary tissues in chronic myeloid leukaemia. *Ser Haematol* 1975; 8:113.
175. Ihde DC, Canellos GP, Schwartz JH, DeVita VT: Splenectomy in the chronic phase of chronic granulocytic leukemia. Effects in 32 patients. *Ann Intern Med* 1976; 84:17–21.
176. Medical Research Council's Working Party for Therapeutic Trials in Leukemia: Randomized trial of splenectomy in Ph^1 positive chronic granulocytic leukaemia, including an analysis of prognostic factors. *Br J Haematol* 1983; 54:415.
177. The Italian Cooperative Study Group on Chronic Myeloid Leukemia: Results of a prospective randomized trial of early splenectomy in chronic myeloid leukemia. *Cancer* 1984; 54:333–338.
178. Goldman JM, Johnson SA, Islam A, et al: Haematological reconstitution after autografting for chronic granulocytic leukemia in transformation: The influence of previous splenectomy. *Br J Haematol* 1980; 45:223–231.
179. Gratwohl A, Goldman J, Gluckman E, Zwaan F: Effect of splenectomy before bone marrow transplantation on survival in chronic granulocytic leukaemia. *Lancet* 1985; 2:1290–1291.
180. Gluckman E, Devergie A, Bernheim A, et al: Splenectomy and bone marrow transplantation in chronic granulocytic leukemia. *Lancet* 1983; 1:1392–1393.
181. Martin PJ, Clift RA, Fisher LD, et al: HLA-identical marrow transplantation during accelerated-phase chronic myelogenous leukemia: Analysis of survival and remission duration. *Blood* 1988; 72:1978–1984.
182. McGlave P, Arthur D, Haake R, et al: Therapy of chronic myelogenous leukemia with allogeneic bone marrow transplantation. *J Clin Oncol* 1987; 5:10033.
183. Canellow GP, Sutliffe SB, DeVita VT, Lister TA: Treatment of refractory splenomegaly in myeloproliferative disease by splenic artery infusion. *Blood* 1979; 53:1014.
184. Sokal JE, Leong SS, Gomez GA: Preferential inhibition by cytarabine of CFU-GM from patients with chronic granulocytic leukemia. *Cancer* 1987; 59:197–202.
185. Kirshner J, Preisler HD: In vitro drug sensitivity studies of colony-forming units in

culture in chronic myelocytic leukemia: Lack of specificity between chronic-phase patients and normal donors. *Cancer Res* 1983; 43:6094–6095.
186. Spiro TE, Mattelaer M-A, Efira A, Stryckmans P: Sensitivity of myeloid progenitor cells in healthy subjects and patients with chronic myeloid leukemia to chemotherapeutic agents. *JNCI* 1981; 66:1053–1059.
187. Brodsky L, Fuscaldo KE, Kahn SB, et al: Chronic myelogenous leukemia: A clinical and experimental evaluation of splenectomy and intensive chemotherapy. *Ser Haematol* 1975; 8:143.
188. Sharp JC, Joyner MV, Wayne AW, et al: Karyotypic conversion in Ph^1-positive chronic myeloid leukaemia with combination chemotherapy. *Lancet* 1979; 1: 1370–1372.
189. Smalley RV, Vogel J, Huguley CM, et al: Chronic granulocytic leukemia: Cytogenetic conversion of the bone marrow with cycle-specific chemotherapy. *Blood* 1977; 50:107.
190. Goldstein D, Laszlo J: Interferon therapy in cancer: From imagination to interferon. *Cancer Res* 1986; 46:4315.
191. Clark JW, Longo DL: Interferons in cancer therapy. In DeVita VT Jr, Hellman S, Rosenberg LSA (eds): *Cancer: Principles and Practice of Oncology,* 4th ed. Philadelphia, JB Lippincott, 1987.
192. Branca A, Baglioni C: Evidence that types I and II interferons have different receptors. *Nature* 1981; 294:768.
193. Rubin BY, Gupta SL: Differential efficacies of human type I and type II interferons as antiviral and antiproliferative agents. *Proc Natl Acad Sci USA* 1980; 77:5928–5932.
194. Denz H, Lechleitner M, Marth CH, et al: Effect of human recombinant alpha-2 and gamma-interferon on the growth of human cell lines from solid tumors and hematologic malignancies. *J Interferon Res* 1985; 5:147–157.
195. Oladipupo Williams CK, Svet-Moldavskaya I, Vicek J, et al: Inhibitory effects of human leukocyte and fibroblast interferons on normal and chronic myelogenous leukemic granulocytic progenitor cells. *Oncology* 1981; 38:356–360.
196. Talpaz M, Spitzer G, Hittelman WN, et al: Changes in granulocyte–monocyte colony-forming cells among leukocyte-interferon-treated chronic myelogenous leukemia patients. *Exp Hematol* 1986; 14:668–671.
197. Galvani D, Cawley J: Mechanisms of action of α-interferon in chronic granulocytic leukemia—evidence for preferential inhibition of late progenitor cells. *Br J Haematol* 1989; 73:475–479.
198. Broxmeyer HE, Lu L, Platzer E, et al: Comparative analysis of the influences of human gamma, alpha and beta interferons on human multipotential (CFU-GEMM), erythroid (BFRL-E) and granulocyte-macrophage (CFU-GM) progenitor cells. *J Immunol* 1983; 131:1301–1305.
199. Ernstoff MS, Kirkwood JM: Changes in the bone marrow of cancer patients treated with recombinant interferon alpha-2. *Am J Med* 1984; 76:593.
200. McGlave P, Mamus S, Vilen B, Dewald G: Effect of recombinant gamma interferon on chronic myelogenous leukemia bone marrow progenitors. *Exp Hematol* 1987; 15:331.

201. Osterholz J, Dowding C, Goldman J: Interferon-alpha enhances the binding of CFU-GM from the marrow of patients with chronic myeloid leukemia (CML) to preformed stroma in long-term bone marrow culture. *Blood* 1989; 74(suppl 1):320a (abstr 1208).
202. Lyding J, Li WJ, Arlinghaus RB, Deisseroth A: Alpha interferon activates class 1 histocompatibility gene expression in chronic myelogenous leukemia cells [abstr]. *Blood* 1987; 70(suppl 1):263a.
203. Pattengale P, Sundstrom C, Yu A, Levine A: Lysis of fresh leukemic blasts by interferon-activated human natural killer cells. *Nat Immunol Cell Growth Regul* 1984; 3:165–180.
204. Riccardi C, Giampietri A, Migliorati G, et al: Generation of mouse natural killer (NK) cell activity: Effect of interleukin-2 (IL-2) and interferon (IFN) on the in vivo development of natural killer cells from bone marrow (BM) progenitor cells. *Int J Cancer* 1986; 38:553–562.
205. Stryckmans P, Dorval C, Clauss I, et al: Decreased production of alpha interferon by peripheral blood cells in patients with chronic myeloid leukemia. *Blood* 1989; 74(suppl 1):76a (abstr 276).
206. Talpaz M, McCredie K, Mavligit GM, Gutterman JU: Leukocyte interferon-induced myeloid cytoreduction in chronic myelogenous leukemia. *Blood* 1983; 62:689–692.
207. Freund M, Von Wussow P, Diedrich H, et al: Recombinant human interferon (IFN) alpha-2b in chronic myelogenous leukemia—dose dependency of response and frequency of neutralizing anti-interferon antibodies. *Br J Haematol* 1989; 72:350–356.
208. Gastl G, Aulitzky Q, Tilg H, et al: Dose related effectiveness of alpha interferon in chronic myelogenous leukemia. *Blut* 1987; 54:251–252.
209. Kurzrock R, Talpaz M, Kantarjian H, et al: Therapy of chronic myelogenous leukemia with recombinant interferon-gamma. *Blood* 1987; 70:943–947.
210. Silver RT, Reich SD, Coleman M, et al: Gamma interferon (IFN) has activity in treating chronic myeloid leukemia (CML) (abstr). *Blood* 1986; 68(suppl 1):232a.
211. Russo D, Fanin R, Zuffa E: Treatment of Ph + chronic myeloid leukemia by gamma interferon. *Blut* 1989; 59:15–20.
212. Talpaz M, Kurzrock R, Kantarjian H, et al: Therapy of Philadelphia positive chronic myelogenous leukemia with recombinant alpha-2 interferon and recombinant gamma interferon. *Blood* 1988; 72(suppl 1):229a.
213. Kloke O, Wandl U, Opalka B: A randomized trial of interferon (IFN) alpha or IFN alpha plus IFN gamma for the treatment of Philadelphia chromosome (Ph) positive chronic myelogenous leukemia (CML). *Blood* 1989; 74:277a (abstr 1046).
214. Stenke L, Samuelson J, Palmblad J, et al: Elevated white blood cell synthesis of leukotriene C_4 in chronic myelogenous leukemia but not in polycythemia vera. *Br J Haematol* 1990; 74:257–263.
215. Imanishi J, Tanaka A: Experimental research for clinical application of interferon. *Jpn J Cancer Chemother* 1984; 11:53–59.
216. Welander CE, Morgan TM, Homesley HD, et al: Combined recombinant human interferon alpha2 and cytotoxic agents studied in a clonogenic assay. *Int J Cancer* 1985; 35:721.

217. Kantarjian H, Talpaz M, Keating M: Combined modality therapy with intensive chemotherapy (DOAP) followed by alpha interferon maintenance in chronic myelogenous leukemai. *Am Assoc Cancer Res* 1988; 29:210 (Abstr 836).
218. Bergsagel DE, Haas RH, Messner HA: Interferon alfa-2b in the treatment of chronic granulocytic leukemia. *Semin Oncol* 1986; 13:29–35.
219. Guilhot F, Dreyfus B, Brizard A, Huret JL: Cytogenetic remissions in chronic myelocytic leukemia using interferon alpha-2a and hydroxyurea with or without low-dose cytosine arabinoside. *Leuk Lymphoma* 1990; (in press).
220. Shtalrid M, Lugassy G, Berrebi A: High response rate to recombinant interferon alpha in chronic myeloid leukemia after intensive cytoreductive chemotherapy. *Blood* 1989; 74(suppl 1):370a (abstr 1411).
221. Anger B, Porzsolt F, Leichtle R, et al: A Phase I/II study of recombinant interferon alpha 2a and hydroxyurea for chronic myelocytic leukemia. *Blut* 1989; 58:275–278.
222. Sokal J, Bigner S: Low-dose cytosine arabinoside in early and advanced chronic granulocytic leukemia. *Blood* 1986; 66(suppl 1):233a, (abstr 810).
223. Kantarjian H, Keating M, McCredie K, et al: Treatment of advanced stages of Philadelphia chromosome-positive chronic myelogenous leukemia with alpha interferon and low-dose cytosine arabinoside. *Blood* 1989; 74(suppl 1):235a (abstr 878).
224. Meyers J, Flournoy N, Sanders J: Prophylactic use of human leukocyte interferon after allogeneic marrow transplantation. *Ann Intern Med* 1987; 107:809–816.
225. Arcese W, Alimena G, Maura F, et al: Recombinant alpha 2 interferon for Ph + chronic myeloid leukemia relapse after T-cell depleted BMT. *Bone Marrow Transplantation* 1988; 3(suppl 1):185.
226. Higano C, Raskind W, Durnam D, Singer J: Alpha interferon induces cytogenetic remissions in patients who relapse with CML after allogeneic bone marrow transplantation. *Blood* 1989; 74:83a (abstr 307).
227. Newland AC, Jones L, Mlr N, Slocombe GW: Alpha 2 interferon in chronic myeloid leukemia following relapse post-allogeneic transplant. *Br J Haematol* 1987; 66:147–148.
228. Borgies, Ferrant A, Delannoy A, et al: Interferon alpha induced and maintained complete remission in chronic granulocytic leukemia in relapse after bone marrow transplantation. *Bone Marrow Transplantation* 1989; 4:127–128.
229. Sokal J, Aungst C, Grace J: Immunotherapy in well controlled chronic myeloid leukemia. *NY State J Med* 1973; 73:1180.
230. Aglietta M, Piacibello W, Stacchinia, et al: In-vitro effect of retinoic acid on normal and chronic myeloid leukemia granulopoiesis. *Leuk Res* 1985; 9:879–883.
231. Arlinz, Mertelsmann R, Berman E, et al: 13-*cis*-Retinoic acid does not increase the true remission rate and the duration of true remission (induced by cytotoxic chemotherapy) in patients with chronic phase chronic myelogenous leukemia. *J Clin Oncol* 1985; 3:473–476.
232. Doney K, Buckner CD, Thomas ED, et al: Allogeneic bone marrow transplantation for chronic granulocytic leukemia. *Exp Hematol* 1981; 9:966–971.
233. McGlave PB, Miller WJ, Hurd DD, et al: Cytogenetic conversion following

allogeneic bone marrow transplantation for advanced chronic myelogenous leukemia. *Blood* 1981; 58:1150–1152.
234. Fefer A, Cheever M, Thomas ED, et al: Disappearance of Ph-positive cells in four patients with chronic granulocytic leukemia after chemotherapy, irradiation and bone marrow transplantation from an identical twin. *N Engl J Med* 1979; 300:333–337.
235. Fefer A, Thomas ED: Bone marrow transplantation for the treatment of chronic myelogenous leukemia. In, DeVita V, Hellman S, Rosenberg S (eds.): *Important Advances in Oncology*. JB Lippincott, Philadelphia, 1990, pp 143–158.
236. Thomas ED, Clift RA, Fefer A, et al: Marrow transplantation for the treatment of chronic myelogenous leukemia. *Ann Intern Med* 1986; 104:155.
237. Goldman JM, Apperley JF, Jones L, et al: Bone marrow transplantation for patients with chronic myeloid leukemia. *N Engl J Med* 1986; 314:202–207.
238. McGlave P, Arthur D, Haake R, et al: Therapy of chronic myelogenous leukemia with allogeneic bone marrow transplantation. *J Clin Oncol* 1987; 5:1033.
239. Goldman JM, Gale RP, Horowitz MM, et al: Bone marrow transplantation for chronic myelogenous leukemia in chronic phase: Increased risk for relapse associated with T cell depletion. *Ann Intern Med* 1988; 108:806–814.
240. Snyder DS, McGlave PB: Treatment of chronic myelogenous leukemia with bone marrow transplantation. *Bone Marrow Transplant* 1990; 4:535–557.
241. Delage R, Ritz J, Anderson KC: The evolving role of bone marrow transplantation in the treatment of chronic myelogenous leukemia. *Chronic Leuk* 1990; 4:369–388.
242. Apperley JF, Jones L, Hale G, et al: Bone marrow transplantation for patients with chronic myeloid leukaemia: T-cell depletion with Campath-1 reduces the incidence of graft-versus-host disease but may increase the risk of leukaemic relapse. *Bone Marrow Transplantation* 1986; 1:53–66.
243. Arthur CK, Apperly JF, Guo AP, et al: Cytogenetic events after bone marrow transplantation for chronic myeloid leukemia in chronic phase. *Blood* 1988; 71:1179–1186.
244. Butturini A, Gale RP: The role of T-cells in preventing relapse in chronic myelogenous leukemia. *Bone Marrow Transplant* 1987; 2:351–354.
245. Advisory Committee of the International Bone Marrow Transplant Registry: Report from the International Bone Marrow Transplant Registry. *Bone Marrow Transplantation* 1989; 4:221.
246. Tutschka PJ, Copeland EA, Klein JP: Bone marrow transplantation for leukemia following a new busulfan and cyclophosphamide regimen. *Blood* 1987; 70:1382–1388.
247. Santos GW, Tutschka PJ, Brookmeyer R, et al: Marrow transplantation for acute nonlymphocytic leukemia after treatment with busulfan and cyclophosphamide. *N Engl J Med* 1983; 309:1347.
248. Blume KG, Beutler E, Bross KJ, et al: Bone marrow ablation and allogeneic marrow transplantation in acute leukemia. *N Engl J Med* 1980; 302:1041.
249. Champlin R: T-cell depletion of bone marrow transplantation—effect on graft rejection, graft-versus-host disease, graft-versus leukemia, and survival. In,

McGuire WL, Champlin R (eds): *Bone Marrow Transplantation*. Boston, Kluwer Academic Publishers, 1990, pp 99–111.

250. Sullivan K: Chronic graft-versus-host disease. In, McGuire WL, and Champlin R (eds): *Bone Marrow Transplantation*. Boston, Kluuwer Academic Publishers, 1990, pp 79–98.
251. Forman SJ, Blume KG, Krance RA, et al: A prospective randomized study of acute graft-v-host disease in 107 patients with leukemia: Methotrexate/prednisone v cyclosporine A/prednisone. *Transplantation Proc* 1987; 19:2605.
252. Storb R, Deeg HJ, Whitehead J, et al: Methotrexate and cyclosporine compared with cyclosporine alone for prophylaxis of acute graft-versus-host disease after marrow transplantation for leukemia. *N Engl J Med* 1986; 314:729–735.
253. Dicke KA, Van Hooft J, Van Bekkum DW: The selection elimination of immunologically competent cells from bone marrow and lymphomatic cell mixtures. *Transplantation* 1968; 6:562–570.
254. Wagemaker G, Vriesendorp HM, Van Bekkum DW: Successful bone marrow transplantation against major histocompatibility barrier in rhesus monkeys. *Transplantation Proc* 1981; 13:875–880.
255. Korngold R, Sprent J: Lethal graft-versus-host disease after bone marrow transplantation across minor histocompatibility barriers in mice. Prevention by removing mature T cells from marrow. *J Exp Med* 1978; 148:1687–1698.
256. Hamilton BC, Bevan MJ, Parkman R: Antirecipient cytotoxic T-lymphocyte precursors are present in the spleens of mice with acute graft-versus-host disease due to minor histocompatibility antigens. *J Immunol* 1981; 126:621.
257. Sakamoto K, Sachs DH, Shimada S, et al: Bone marrow transplantation in miniature swine III. Graft-versus-host disease and the effect of T cell depletion of marrow. *Transplantation* 1988; 45:869–875.
258. Waldmann H, Hale G, Cividalli G, et al: Elimination of graft-versus-host disease by in vitro depletion of alloreactive lymphocytes with monoclonal rat anti-human lymphocytic antibody (CAMPATH-1). *Lancet* 1984; 2:483–486.
259. Filipovich AH, McGlave PB, Ramsay NKC, et al: Pretreatment of donor bone marrow with monoclonal antibody OKT3 for prevention of acute graft-versus-host disease in allogeneic histocompatible bone marrow transplantation. *Lancet* 1982; 1:1266–1270.
260. Prentice H, Janossy G, Trejdosiewicz L, et al: Depletion of T lymphocytic in donor marrow prevents significant graft-versus-host disease in matched allogeneic leukemia marrow transplant recipients. *Lancet* 1984; 1:472–476.
261. Mitsuyasu R, Champlin RE, Gale RP, et al: Depletion of T lymphocytes from donor bone marrow for the prevention of graft-versus-host disease following bone marrow transplantation. *Ann Intern Med* 1986; 105:20–26.
263. Maraninchi D, Gluckman E, Blaise D, et al: Impact of T-cell depletion on outcome of allogeneic bone marrow transplantation for standard-risk leukemias. *Lancet* 1987; 2:175–178.
264. Filipovich A II, Vallera DA, Youle RJ, et al: Ex-vivo treatment of donor bone marrow with anti-T-cell immunotoxins for prevention of graft vs. host disease. *Lancet* 1984; 1:469–472.

265. Treleaven JG, Gibson FM, Ugelstad J, et al: Removal of neuroblastoma cells from bone marrow with monoclonal antibodies conjugated to magnetic microspheres. *Lancet* 1984; 1:70–83.
266. Patterson J, Prentice HG, Brenner MK, et al: Graft rejection HLA-matched T lymphocyte depleted bone marrow transplantation. *Br J Haematol* 1986; 63:221–230.
267. Kernan NA, Flomengerg N, Dupont B, et al: Graft rejection in recipients of T-cell-depleted HLA-non-identical marrow transplants for leukemia. *Transplantation* 1987; 43:842–847.
268. O'Reilly RJ, Collins NH, Kernan N, et al: Transplantation of marrow-depleted T cells by soybean lectin agglutination and E-rosette depletion: Major histocompatibility complex-related graft resistance in leukemic transplant recipients. *Transplantation Proc* 1985; 17:455–459.
269. Martin PJ, Hansen JA, Buckner C: Effects of in vitro depletion of T cells in HLA-identical allogeneic marrow grafts. *Blood* 1985; 66:664–672.
270. Bozdech MJ, Sondel PM, Trigg ME, et al: Transplantation of HLA haploidentical T cell depleted marrow for leukemia: Addition of cytosine arabinoside to the transplant conditioning prevents graft rejection. *Exp Hematol* 1985; 13:1201–1210.
271. Smith BR, Rappeport JM, Lipton JM, et al: Marrow T cell depletion with anti-Leu-1 monoclonal antibody (Mab) and complement in matched and mismatched bone marrow transplantation (BMT). *Blood* 1984; 64(suppl 1):221a.
272. Korngold R, Sprent J: Variable Capacity of L3T4+ T cells to cause lethal graft-versus-host disease across minor histocompatibility barriers in mice. *J Exp Med* 1987; 165:52–64.
273. Maraninchi D, Mawas C, Guyotat D, et al: Selective depletion of marrow-T cytotoxic lymphocytes (CD5) in the prevention of graft-versus-host disease after allogeneic bone marrow transplantation. *Transplant* 1988; 1:91–94.
274. Champlin RE, Winston H, Gajewski J, et al: Selective depletion of CD8 positive T lymphocytes for prevention of graft-versus-host disease after allogeneic bone marrow transplantation. *Blood* 1990; 76:418–423.
275. Kernan NA, Byers V, Brochstein J, et al: Anti-T cell ricin-A-chain immunotoxin for treatment of steroid resistant acute graft-versus-host disease. *Blood* 1986; 68(suppl 1):1011.
276. Byers V, Henslee P, Kernan N, et al: Therapeutic response to a pan-T lymphocyte monoclonal antibody–ricin A chain immunotoxin in steroid refractory graft versus host disease. *Blood* 1987; 70(suppl 1):1071.
277. Vogelsang GB, Hess AD, Gordon G, Santos GW: Treatment and prevention of acute graft-versus-host disease with thalidomide in a rat model. *Transplantation* 1986; 41:644–647.
278. Vogelsang GB, Taylor S, Gordon G, Hess A: Thalidomide, a potent agent for the treatment of graft-versus-host disease. *Transplant Proc* 1986; 18:904–906.
279. Vogelsang G: Acute graft-versus-host disease. In, Champlin R (ed): *Bone Marrow Transplantation*. Boston, Kluwer Academic Publishers, 1990, pp 55–78.

280. Shepp DH, Dandliker PS, DeMiranda P, et al: Activity of 9-[2-hydroxy-1-(hydroxymethyl)ethoxymethyl]+guanine in the treatment of cytomegalovirus pneumonia. *Ann Intern Med* 1985; 103:368–373.
281. Emanuel D, Cunningham I, Jules-Elysee K, et al: Cytomegalovirus pneumonia after bone marrow transplantation successfully treated with the combination of ganciclovir and high-dose intravenous immune globulin. *Ann Inter Med* 1988; 109:777–782.
282. Reed EC, Bowden RA, Dandliker PS, et al: Treatment of cytomegalovirus pneumonia with ganciclovir and intravenous cytomegalovirus immunoglobulin in patients with bone marrow transplants. *Ann Intern Med* 1988; 109:783–788.
283. Schmidt GM, Kovacs A, Zaia JA, et al: Ganciclovir/immunoglobulin combination therapy for the treatment of human cytomegalovirus-associated interstitial pneumonia in bone marrow allograft recipients. *Transplantation* 1988; 46:905–907.
284. Hauch M, Gazzola M, Small T, et al: Anti-leukemia potential of IL-2 activated NK cells after bone marrow transplantation for chronic myelogenous leukemia. *Blood* 1990; 75:2250–2262.
285. Beatty PG, Clift RA, Mickelson EM, et al: Marrow transplantation from related donors other than HLA-identical siblings. *N Engl J Med* 1985; 313:765–771.
286. Anasetti C, Amos D, Beatty PG, et al: Effect of HLA compatibility of engraftment of bone marrow transplants in patients with leukemia or lymphoma. *N Engl J Med* 1989; 320:197–204.
287. Beatty PG, Dahlberg S, Mickelson EM, et al: Probability of finding HLA-matched unrelated marrow donors. *Transplantation* 1988; 45:714–718.
288. McGlave P, Scott E, Ramsay N, et al: Unrelated donor bone marrow transplantation therapy for chronic myelogenous leukemia. *Blood* 1987; 70:877–881.
289. Beatty P, Ash R, Hows JM, McGlave PB: The use of unrelated bone marrow donors in the treatment of patients with chronic myelogenous leukemia: Experience of four marrow transplant centers. *Bone Marrow Transplant* 1989; 4:253.
290. Hughes T, Brito-Babapulle F, Marcus RE: Transient Ph-negativity after autografting with blood-derived stem cells for patients with chronic myeloid leukemia in chronic phase. *Bone Marrow Transplant* 1989; 4(suppl 1):51.
291. Meloni G, DeFabritiis P, Alimena G, et al: Autologous bone marrow or peripheral blood stem cell transplantation for patients with chronic myelogenous leukemia in chronic phase. *Bone Marrow Transplant* 1989; 4(suppl 4):92–95.
292. Butturini A, Keating A, Goldman J, Gale P: Autotransplants in CML-strategies and results. *Lancet* 1990; 1: 335:1255–1258.
293. Kantarjian HM, Talpaz M, Spinolo J, et al: High-dose of cyclophosphamide, BCNU and etoposide (CBV) induce cytogenetic responses in most patients with advanced stages of Philadelphia chromosome-positive chronic myelogenous leukemia. *Blood* 1989; 74(suppl 1):273a.
294. Degliantoni G, Mangoni L, Rizzole V: In vitro restoration of polyclonal hematopoiesis in a chronic myelogenous leukemia after in vitro treatment with 4-hydroperoxycyclophosphamide. *Blood* 1985; 65:753–757.

295. Ball E: In vitro purging of bone marrow for autologous marrow transplantation in acute myelogenous leukemia using myeloid-specific monoclonal antibodies. *Bone Marrow Transplant* 1988; 3:387–392.
296. Chang J, Moregenstern G, Coutinho L, et al: The use of bone marrow cells grown in long-term culture for autologous bone marrow transplantation in acute myeloblastic leukemia—an update. *Bone Marrow Transplant* 1989; 4:5–9.
297. McGlave P, Miller W, Arthur D, et al: Ph^1 mosaicism after autologous transplantation for CML with gamma interferon treated bone marrow. *Blood* 1989; 74(suppl 1):281a (abstr 1061). 1989.
298. Barnett M, Eaves C, Phillips G, et al: Rapid reconstitution of Philadelphia chromosome-negative hematopoiesis in patients with chronic myeloid leukemia transplanted with cultured autologous bone marrow to support intensive therapy. *Bone Marrow Transplantation* 1989; 4:345.
299. Andrews RG, Singer JW, Bernstein ID: Precursors of colony forming cells in human can be distinguished from colony forming cells by expression of the CD33 and CD34 antigens and light scatter properties. *J Exp Med* 1989; 169:1721–1731.
300. Bensinger WI, Berenson RJ, Andrews RG, et al: The use of purified hematopoietic progenitors for autologous marrow transplantation. *Bone Marrow Transplant* 1989; 4(suppl 2):86.
301. Berenson RJ, Andrews RG, Bensinger WI, et al: Antigen CD43+ marrow cells engraft lethally irradiated baboons. *J Clin Invest* 1988; 81:951–955.
302. Canellos GP, DeVita VT, Whang-Peng J, Carbone PP: Hematologic and cytogenetic remission of blastic transformation in chronic granulocytic leukemia. *Blood* 1971; 38:671–679.
303. Hayes DM, Ellison RR, Glidewell O, et al: Chemotherapy for the terminal phase of chronic myelocytic leukemia. *Cancer Chemother Rep* 1974; 58:233–247.
304. Spiers AS, Goldman JM, Catovsky D, et al: Multiple-drug chemotherapy for acute leukemia. The TRAMPCOL regimen: Results in 86 patients. *Cancer* 1977; 40:20–29.
305. Coleman M, Silver R, Pajak T: Combination chemotherapy for terminal phase chronic granulocytic leukemia—Cancer and Leukemia Group B studies. *Blood* 1980; 29:55.
306. Schiffer CA, DeBellis R, Kasdorf H, Wiernik P: Treatment of the blast crisis of chronic myelogenous leukemia with 5-azacytidine and VP-16-213. *Cancer Treat Rep* 1982; 66:267–271.
307. Schiffer CA, Anderson K, Colman M, Cuttner J: Therapy for chronic myelogenous leukemia in blast crisis with etoposide and 5-azacytidine administered by continuous infusion: A Cancer and Leukemia Group B study. *Cancer Treat Rep* 1985; 69:1027–1028.
308. Winton EF, Miller D, Vagler WR: Intensive chemotherapy and daunorubicin, 5-azacytidine, 6-thioguanine and cytarabine (DATA) for the blastic transformation of chronic granulocytic leukemia. *Cancer Treat Rep* 1981; 64:389.
309. Dutcher J, Arlin Z, Paietta E, et al: Phase II study of mitoxantrone and 5-azacytidine in patients with accelerated or blastic crisis chronic myelogenous leukemia. Twenty-Second Congress of ISH, Milan, Italy: 172(OP-TU-6-7), 1988.

310. Iacoboni SJ, Plunkett WK, Kantarjian H, et al: High dose cytosine arabinoside: Treatment and cellular pharmacology of chronic myelogenous leukemia blast crisis. *J Clin Oncol* 1986; 4:1079–1088.
311. Kantarjian H, Walters R, Keating M, et al: Treatment of the blastic phase of chronic myelogenous leukemia with mitoxantrone and high-dose cytosine arabinoside. *Cancer* 1988; 62:672–676.
312. Herzig RH, Phillips GL, Lazarus HM, et al: High-dose cytarabine for the treatment of blastic phase chronic myelogenous leukemia. *Cancer Treat Rep* 1985; 69:881–883.
313. Walters RS, Kantarjian HM, Keating MJ, et al: Therapy of lymphoid and undifferentiated chronic myelogenous leukemia in blast crisis with continuous vincristine and Adriamycin infusion plus high-dose Decadron (VAD). *Cancer* 1987; 60:1708–1712.
314. Rosenthal S, Canellos GP, Whang-Peng J, Gralnick HR: Blast crisis of chronic granulocytic leukemia. Morphologic variants and therapeutic implications. *Am J Med* 1977; 63:542–547.
315. Janossy G, Woodruff RK, Pippard MJ, et al: Relation of "lymphoid" phenotype and response to chemotherapy incorporating vincristine–prednisone in the acute phase of Ph^1 positive leukemia. *Cancer* 1979; 43:426–431.
316. Marks SM, Baltimore D, McCaffrey R: Terminal transferase as a predictor of initial responsiveness to vincristine and prednisone in blastic chronic myelogenous leukemia. *N Engl J Med* 1978; 293:812.
317. Kantarjian H, Keating M, Talpaz M, et al: Characteristics and outcome of patients with chronic myelogenous leukemia in lymphoid blastic crisis. *Am Soc Clin Oncol* 1988; 7:193 (abstr 748.)
318. Koeffler HP: Induction of differentiation of human acute myelogenous leukemia cells: Therapeutic implications. *Blood* 1983; 62:709–721.
319. Bloch A: Induced cell differentiation in cancer therapy. *Cancer Treat Rep* 1984; 68:199–205.
320. Di-Raimondo F, Milone G, Guglielmo P, et al: Treatment of CML blast crisis with low dose ara-C. Br J Haematol 1985; 60:773–774.
321. Yu-Chen Y, Shu-rong C, Jin-ren C: Use of all-*trans* retinoic acid in the treatment of acute promyelocytic leukemia. *Blood* 1988; 72:567–572.
322. Dego SL, Chomienne P, Ballerini P, et al: All-*trans* retinoic acid—a novel differentiation therapy for acute promyelocytic leukemia. *Proc Am Soc Clin Oncol* 1990; 9:207(abstr 802).
323. Robert K-H, Hellstrom E, Einhorn S, Gahrton G: Acute myelogenous leukemia of unfavourable prognosis treated with retinoic acid, vitamin D^3, alpha-interferon and low doses of cytosine arabinoside. *Scand J Haematol Suppl* 1986; 34:61–77.
324. Koller CA, Miller DM: Preliminary observations on the therapy of the myeloid blast phase of chronic granulocytic leukemia with plicamycin and hydroxyurea. *N Engl M Med* 1986; 315:1433–1438.
325. Koller C, Keating M, Walters R, et al: Mithramycin and hydroxyurea in chronic myelogenous leukemia and other hematologic malignancies. *Blood* 1988; 72(suppl 1):209a (abstr 747).
326. Trumper L, Lie JVD, Goudsmit R, et al: Therapy of the myeloid blast phase of

chronic granulocytic leukemia with plicamycin and hydroxyurea: A retrospective analysis. 22nd Congress of ISH, Milan, Italy SYM-TU-6-6, 1988.
327. Antimi M, Poeta GD, Cianciulli P, et al: Plicamycin and hydroxyurea in the treatment of blast phase and accelerated phase of the Ph[1] chronic myelogenous leukemia. 22nd Congress of ISH, Milan, Italy OP-TU-6-6, 1988.
328. Weber G: Biochemical strategy of cancer cells and the design of chemotherapy: GHA Clowes Memorial Lecture. *Cancer Res* 1983; 43:3466–3492.
329. Jayaram HN, Pillwein K, NIchols CR, et al: Selective sensitivity to tiazofurin of human leukemic cells. *Biochem Pharmacol* 1986; 35:2920–2032.
330. Tricot G, Jayaram H, Weber G, Hoffman R: Tiazofurin is a potent antiproliferative agent and induces differentiation in patients with leukemia. *Am Assoc Cancer Res* 1988; 29:210 (abstr 835).
331. Talpaz M, Trujillo JM, Hittelman WN, et al: Suppression of clonal evolution in two chronic myelogenous leukaemia patients treatment with leukocyte interferon. *Br J Haematol* 1985; 60:619.
332. Gabrilove JL, Jakubowski A, Scher H, et al: Effect of granulocyte colony-stimulating factor on neutropenia and associated morbidity due to chemotherapy for transitional-cell carcinoma of the urothelium. *N Engl J Med* 1988; 318:1414–1422.
333. Brandt SJ, Peters WP, Atwater SK, et al: Effect of recombinant human granulocyte–macrophase colony-stimulating factor on hematopoietic reconstitution after high-dose chemotherapy and autologous bone marrow transplantation. *N Engl J Med* 1988; 318:869–876.
334. Vellenga E, Delwel HR, Touw IP, Lowenberg B: Patterns of acute myeloid leukemia colony growth in response to recombinant granulocyte–macrophase colony-stimulating factor (rGM-CSF). *Exp Hematol* 1987; 15:652–656.
335. Elias L: The basis for treatment of myelodysplastic syndrome and acute nonlymphoblastic leukemia with biologic agents. *Leukemia* 1988; 2:400–402.
336. Vadhan-Raj S, Keating M, LeMaistre A, et al: Effects of recombinant human granulocyte–macrophase colony-stimulating factor in patients with myelodysplastic syndromes. *N Engl J Med* 1987; 17:1545–1552.
337. Haines LE, Goldman JM, Worsley AM, et al: Chemotherapy and autografting for chronic granulocytic leukaemia in transformation: Probably prolongation of survival for some patients. *Br J Haematol* 1984; 58:711–721.
338. Vellekoop L, Zander AR, Kantarjain HM, et al: Piperazinedione, total body irradiation, and autologous bone marrow transplantation in chronic myelogenous leukemia. *J Clin Oncol* 1986; 4:906–911.
339. Preisler HD, Raza A, Higby D, et al: Treatment of myeloid blastic crisis of chronic myelogenous leukemia. *Cancer Treat Rep* 1984; 11:1351–1355.
340. Dantas ME, Robinson WA, Thomas MR: Autologous marrow infusion in blastic crisis of chronic myeloid leukemia. *Blood* 1981; 58:1721.
341. Reiffers J, Gorin N, Michallet M, et al: Autografting for chronic granulocytic leukemia in transformation. *Bone Marrow Transplant* 1989; 4 (suppl 1):52.
342. Bartram CR: Rearrangement of the c-*abl* and *bcr* genes in Ph-negative CML and Ph-positive acute leukemias. *Leukemia* 1988; 2:63–64.

343. Dreazen O, Klisak I, Rassool F, et al: Do oncogenes determine the clinical features in chronic myeloid leukaemia? *Lancet* 1987; 1:1402–1405.
344. Ganesan TS, Rassool LF, Guo AP, et al: Rearrangement of the *bcr* gene in Philadelphia chromosome-negative chronic myeloid leukemia. *Blood* 1986; 68:957–960.
345. Kantarjian HM, Shtalrid M, Kurzrock R, et al: Significance and correlations of molecular analysis results in patients with Philadelphia chromosome-negative chronic myelogenous leukemia and chronic myelomonocytic leukemia. *Am J Med* 1988; 85:639–644.
346. Shtalrid M, Talpaz M, Blick M, et al: Philadelphia-negative chronic myelogneous leukemia with *bcr* rearrangement: Molecular analysis and clinical characteristics. *J Clin Oncol* 1988; 6:1569–1575.
347. Kantarjian HM, Keating MJ, Walters RS, et al: Clinical and prognostic features of Philadelphia chromosome-negative chronic myelogenous leukemia. *Cancer* 1986; 58:2023–2030.
348. Eisenberg A, Silver R, Soper L, et al: The location of breakpoints within the breakpoint cluster region *(bcr)* of chromosome 22 in chronic myeloid leukemia. *Leukemia* 1988; 2:642.
349. Schaefer-Rego K, Dudek H, Popenoe D, et al: CML patients in blast crisis have breakpoints localized to a specific region of the *BCR*. *Blood* 1987; 70:448–455.
350. Mills KI, MacKenzie ED, Birnie GD: The site of the breakpoint within the *bcr* is a prognostic factor in Philadelphia-positive CML patients. *Blood* 1988; 72:1237–1241.
351. Shtalrid M, Talpaz M, Kurzrock R, et al: Analysis of breakpoints within the *bcr* gene and their correlation with the clinical course of Philadelphia-positive chronic myelogenous leukemia. *Blood* 1988; 72:485.
352. Jaubert J, Martiat P, Dowding C, et al: The position of the M-*BCR* breakpoint does not predict the duration of chronic phase or survival in chronic myelogenous leukemia. *Br J Haematol* 1990; 74:30–35.
353. Lee M, Kantarjian H, Deisseroth A, et al: Clinical usage of polymerase chain reaction (PCR) to analyze the *bcr/abl* splicing patterns and minimal residual disease in Philadelphia chromosome-positive chronic myelogenous leukemia [abstr]. *Blood* 1989; 74(suppl 1):199a.
354. Kurzrock R, Shtalrid M, Romero R, et al: A novel c-*abl* protein in Philadelphia-positive acute lymphoblastic leukemia. *Nature* 1987; 325:631.
355. Clark SS, McLaughlin J, Crist WM, et al: Unique forms of the *abl* tyrosine kinase distinguish Ph^1-positive CML from Ph^1-positive ALL. *Science* 1987; 237:85–86.
356. Eisenstein B: The polymerase chain reaction—a new method of using molecular genetics for medical diagnosis. *N Engl J Med* 1990; 322:173–183.
357. Lee M, LeMaistre A, Kantarjian H, et al: Detection of two alternative *bcr/abl* mRNA junctions and minimal residual disease in Philadelphia chromosome-positive chronic myelogenous leukemia by polyamerase chain reaction. *Blood* 1989; 73:2165–2170.
358. Lee MS, Chang KS, Freireich EJ, et al: Detection of minimal residual *bcr/abl* transcripts by a modified polymerase chain reaction. *Blood* 1988; 72:893–897.

359. Pignon J, Hermnni T, Vernant J, et al: Detection of specific *bcr/abl* mRNA using the polymerase chain reaction (PCR) in CML after bone marrow transplantation. *Bone Marrow Transplant* 1989; 4(suppl 1):23.
360. Lange W, Synder DS, Castro R, et al: Detection by enzymatic amplification of *bcr/abl* mRNA in peripheral blood and bone marrow cells of patients with chronic myelogenous leukemia. *Blood* 1989; 73:1735–1741.
361. Morgan GJ, Hughes T, Janssen JW, et al: Polymerase chain reaction for detection of residual leukaemia. *Lancet* 1989; 1:928–929.
362. Roth M, Antin J, Bingham E, Ginsberg D: Detection of Philadelphia chromosome-positive cells by the polymerase chain reaction following bone marrow transplant for chronic myelogenous leukemia. *Blood* 1989; 74:882–885.
363. Hughes TP, Goldman JM: Biological importance of residual leukemic cell relapse after BMT for CML: Does the polymerase chain reaction help? *Bone Marrow Transplant* 1990; 5:3–6.
364. von Deneren J, Hermans A, Meeuwsen T, et al: Antibody recognition of the tumor specific *bcr–abl* forming region in chronic myeloid leukemia. *J Exp Med* 1989; 169:87–98.
365. Wickstrom E, Bacon T, Gonzalez A, et al: Human promyelocytic leukemia HL-60 cell proliferation and c-*myc* protein expression are inhibited by antisense pentadecadeoxynucleotide target against c-*myc* mRNA. *Proc Natl Acad Sci USA* 1988; 85:1028–1032.
366. Zamecnik PC, Goodchild J, Taguchi Y, Sarin P: Inhibition of replication and expression of human T-cell lymphotropic virus type 3 in cultured cells by exogenous synthetic oligonucleotides complementary to viral RNA. *Proc Natl Acad Sci USA* 1986; 83:4143–4146.

5

Treatment of Chronic Lymphocytic Leukemia

Michael J. Keating

University of Texas
M. D. Anderson Cancer Center
Houston, Texas

Chronic lymphocytic leukemia (CLL) is a disease characterized by an accumulation of lymphocytes that morphologically appear to be mature. In almost all cases (>95%) the cells are of the B-lymphocyte lineage, as demonstrated by the presence of surface membrane immunoglobulin (SmIg) and evidence of immunoglobulin gene rearrangement (1–3). Monoclonality is demonstrated by the presence of only κ or λ light chains on the surface of the cell. A few cases are of T-lymphocyte lineage, as demonstrated by expression on the surface of the cells of antigens recognized by monoclonal antibodies against the sheep erythrocyte rosette receptor (CD2) (4). The cells of most patients with T-cell CLL have a mature T-helper cell phenotype and express CD4 surface antigen. Some cases express CD8 surface antigen, rather than CD4, and most of these are considered to be cases of T-γ-lymphoproliferative disorder and express a variety of surface antigen characteristics of natural killer (NK) cells (4).

Chronic lymphocytic leukemia was first described in 1845 (5). Subsequently, more precise definitions of CLL have been developed, and related disorders such as Waldenstrom's macroglobulinemia, hairy cell leukemia, and prolymphocytic leukemia have been well-defined. Chronic lymphocytic leukemia has been separated from diffuse well-differentiated lymphocytic lymphoma (DWDLL) by the presence of >30% lymphocytes in the bone marrow and >4000 monoclonal lymphocytes per microliter in the peripheral blood. Other investigators require the lymphocyte count to be >15,000/μL in the peripheral blood before CLL is diagnosed (6,7). Other variants such as follicular small-cleaved cell lymphoma in a leukemic phase and villous lymphoma have also been separated from typical CLL (4).

Although typical CLL is a B-cell leukemia, it was discovered that, surprisingly, nearly all cases express a surface antigen (CD5) that was formerly thought to be present only on the surface of T lymphocytes (8). CD5 is a 67-kd protein originally defined on normal mature T lymphocytes, but not normal B lymphocytes. A few normal lymphocytes that share the phenotype of B-cell CLL (CD5+ and B-cell antigen+) are present in normal lymph nodes, especially at the periphery of the general center (9). These are also present in the blood of patients with rheumatoid arthritis and after allogeneic bone marrow transplantation (10,11). Controversy still exists over whether these cells are the cells of origin of B CLL or whether the presence of the CD5 antigen is an aberrant expression of genes associated with the malignant clone.

The most common B-cell antigens used to diagnose CLL are CD19 and CD20, which are present on the surface of almost all cases of B-cell CLL (12). The CLL cells are almost always positive for the Ia antigen, the C3 complement receptor (CD3dR+, but not C3bR+), the Epstein–Barr virus receptor, and for the mouse red blood cell (MRBC) rosette receptor (17). Several cases (approximately 25%) have now been reported who express interleukin-2 (IL-2) receptor (CD25) (14). Thus, most cases of B-cell CLL have SmIg (of weak intensity), are κ- or λ-positive, MRBC rosette positive, Ia+, and are CD5+, CD19+, and CD20+. The SmIg is usually IgM alone or IgM and IgD.

CLINICAL PRESENTATIONS

Most cases of CLL are diagnosed because of the discovery of enlarged lymph nodes or, coincidentally, while a patient is being examined on a routine physical examination or for another illness. Ninety-five percent of cases are over 50 years of age, with a 2:1 male preponderance. External lymphadenopathy is present in the majority of patients (60–70%), and hepatomegaly (20–25%) and splenomegaly (40–50%) are less commonly found. Most patients have a markedly elevated white blood cell (WBC) count, although some, who resemble cases of diffuse well-differentiated lymphocytic lymphoma, have a modest increase in the lymphocyte count (4000–15,000/μL) (15). Patients who predominantly have splenomegaly, with minimal or no lymph node enlargement and marked lymphocytosis, are often cases of the prolymphocytic variant of CLL. Most patients with CLL have a normal hemoglobin level and platelet count at diagnosis, but 10–25% of patients will have a hemoglobin level less than 11 g/dL or a platelet count of fewer than 100,000/μL. Careful examination of the morphology of the lymphocytes in the peripheral blood and bone marrow smear, combined with immunological markers, will readily allow differentiation of B-cell CLL from PLL, hairy cell leukemia and its variants, splenic lymphoma with villous lymphocytes, and follicular lymphoma and T-cell CLL (4).

STAGING

The outcome of B CLL is heterogeneous. Patients who present with extensive tumor burden or marrow compromise (anemia, neutropenia, or thrombocytopenia) are at risk of dying within 2 years, whereas others who present with lymphocytosis; normal red cell, neutrophil, and platelet counts; and minimal tumor burden, can live for more than 20 years without requiring treatment (15–17).

These prognostic features were first noted by Galton, in 1966, who paid particular attention to the extent of tumor burden as measured by lymphadenopathy, enlargement of liver or spleen, and the degree of increase in the white blood cell count (19). He also noted that some patients, if observed when receiving no treatment, had a steady increase in the white cell count and were called type I (progressive disease). Type II patients had indolent disease with no increase in white cell count over long periods. Others noted similar associations. On the basis of these studies, Rai and co-workers proposed a five-category staging system that has remained as a clinically useful system until the present time (Table 1) (15). It is remarkable that a system developed from a mixture of patients, with or without previous treatment, could lead to such a consistently reproducible system. Although the Rai system has been repeatedly validated in independent studies, it has been suggested that there are probably three, rather than five stages, with the outcome of stage II resembling stage I more than being intermediate between stages I and III. Stages III and IV have a fairly similar poor prognosis. However, applying the Rai system to patients treated at the M. D. Anderson Cancer Center from 1970 to 1985, shows a clear difference between stages I and II (Fig. 1).

Table 1 Rai Staging System in CLL

Rai stage	Lymphocytosis	Lymphoadenopathy	Hepato- or splenomegaly	Hemoglobin (g%)	Platelets ($\times 10^3/\mu L$)
0	+	—	—	≥11	≥100
I	+	+	—	≥11	≥100
II	+	±	+	≥11	≥100
III	+	±	±	<11	≥100
IV	+	±	±	Any	<100

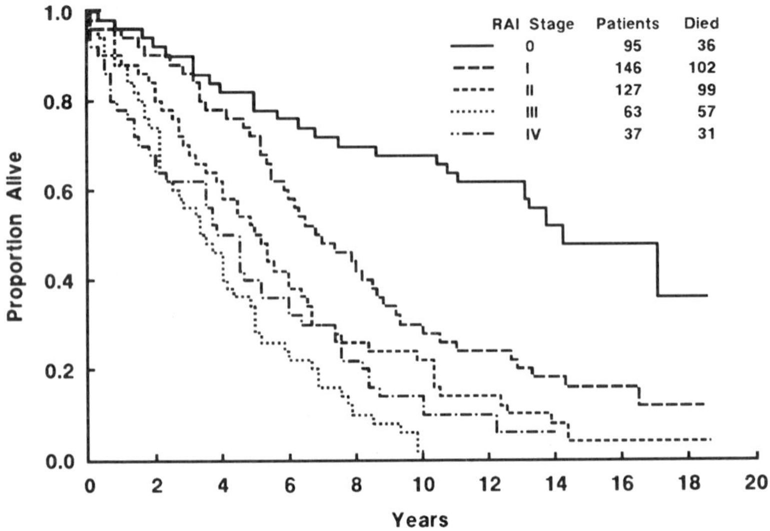

Figure 1 Application of Rai staging system to M. D. Anderson patients 1970–1984.

Binet et al. sought to simplify the Rai system and have proposed a three-stage system (Table 2) (18). Stage C patients resemble Rai stage III and IV, having evidence of marrow failure with a hemoglobin level lower than 10 g/dL (versus lower than 11 g/dL for Rai stage III) or a platelet count below 100,000/μL, or both. The Binet system has also been prospectively validated in several studies, including the M. D. Anderson data (Fig. 2).

The International Workshop on CLL (IWCLL) has adopted a hybrid Rai–Binet system in which the Binet stages are subdivided according to Rai stage within the Binet stage (1). The Rai system is indicated in parentheses [e.g., A(0), A(I), B (I), B(II), and so on]. Despite this proposal, most investigators use either the Rai or Binet systems. Other staging systems, such as those of Jaksic (17) and Lee (20) have not been widely applied. Lee et al., noted that elevated levels of serum lactic dehydrogenase (LDH), uric acid, or alkaline phosphatase were adverse factors, as were advanced age and external lymphadenopathy (20).

PROGNOSTIC FACTORS

The significance of other prognostic factors, such as sex, lymphocyte count, lymphocyte morphology, granulocyte count, bone marrow biopsy pattern, γ-globulin level, lymphocyte doubling time, and karyotype have been reviewed by

Table 2 Binet Staging System in CLL

Binet stage	Lymphocytosis	Lymphoadenopathy	Hepato- or splenomegaly	Hemoglobin (g%)	Platelets ($\times 10^3/\mu L$)
A	+	±	±	≥10	≥100
		(<3 Lymphatic groups[a] positive)			
B	+	±	±	≥10	≥100
		(≥3 Lymphatic groups[a] positive)			
C	+	±	±	<10	or <100

[a]Cervical, axillary, inguinal nodes; liver; spleen; are each considered one group whether unilateral or bilateral.

Montserrat (21). Most studies suggest that males have a slightly inferior survival, compared with females, and several studies suggest that a white cell count higher than 50,000/μL is an independent prognostic factor (22). No consistent association between lymphocyte size, morphology, and presence of nuclear clefts has been noted. A large study of immunophenotype and prognosis in 500 patients has not demonstrated an association of antigen expression with survival (23). With one exception, which showed that low IgG and IgA levels were associated with

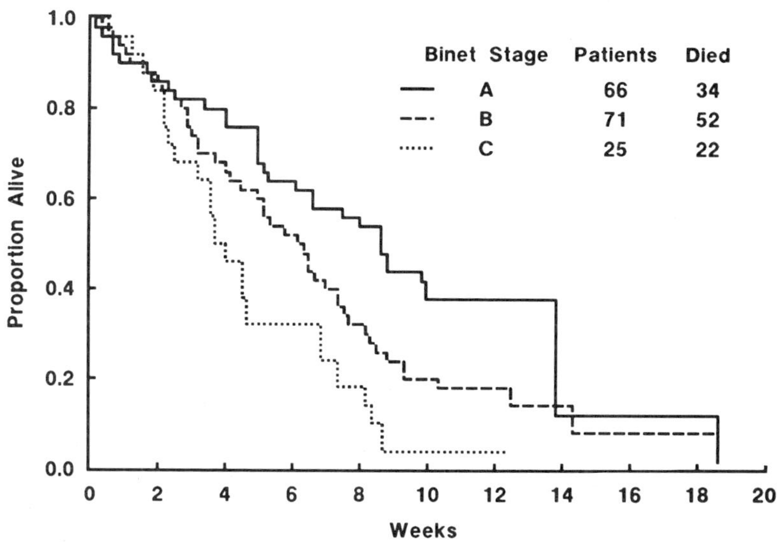

Figure 2 Application of Binet staging system to a subset of M. D. Anderson patients 1970–1984.

more advanced stages and short survival, no association of immunoglobulin level with survival has been noted (24). The karyotype of patients appears to be correlated with survival (25,26). Although complex abnormalities are associated with a poor prognosis, whether this finding is more common in advanced-stage disease, as an independent factor, is uncertain. The effect on prognosis of common changes, such as trisomy of chromosome 12 or presence of 14q+ abnormalities, is still being studied (25,26).

Not surprisingly, a doubling time for peripheral blood lymphocytes of fewer than 12 months correlates with a tendency to progressive disease and a high presenting white cell count. A short doubling time is associated with a poor prognosis and can separate Binet stage A and B patients into good- and poor-risk groups (27). This observation is in keeping with a short survival of patients with a high degree of tritiated thymidine incorporation (28).

BONE MARROW BIOPSY

Several investigators have demonstrated the presence of different patterns of lymphocytic infiltration in the bone marrow (29). Rozman and his co-workers have proposed the most-used classification for bone marrow histology, namely, a four-pattern system: (1) *nodular*—large, nonparatrabecular collections of mature lymphocytes; (2) *interstitial*—replacement of hemopoietic tissue by lymphocytes; (3) *mixed*—mixture of (1) and (2); and (4) *diffuse*—extensive nonnodular replacement of hemopoietic cells. As the disease progresses in stage, a greater proportion of patients have a diffuse pattern in the bone marrow (30). The approximate incidence of diffuse histologies in the three Binet stages is A (10–15%), B (40%), and C (80%). Although the prognostic significance of the four-pattern system is not clearly defined, most investigators believe that a diffuse pattern is a poor prognostic factor, and the Spanish group found it to be more significant than tumor burden, marrow compromise, and white cell count (31). Pangalis et al. (32) support this finding and found a diffuse pattern to be a good predictor for probability of disease progression (33).

TREATMENT

When to Treat Chronic Lymphocytic Leukemia

Most disseminated malignancies are treated at the time of diagnosis, as they are usually associated with a short survival without effective treatment. Additionally, most treatments for neoplasia are more effective when the tumor burden is small, possibly because fewer clones resistant to available regimens have evolved. Analysis of prognostic factors and the development of staging systems in CLL have caused this conventional wisdom to be questioned. The prognosis for CLL varies from a median survival of 10–15 years for newly diagnosed patients with Rai stage 0, to 18–36 months for Rai stage III to IV patients. Twenty-five years ago Galton first raised the question of whether the indolent (type II) patients required treatment (19).

Because of the poor prognosis of Rai stages III and IV or Binet C patients (1,16,18), most physicians will initiate treatment immediately in an attempt to change the natural history of the disease. One question remaining in this group is whether a different approach should be taken for patients whose anemia or thrombocytopenia is due to immune destruction, rather than failure of marrow production (34). Some studies suggest that such patients have a better prognosis than other advanced-stage patients (35,36), although this has not been a consistent finding (37). Most patients respond to treatment with corticosteroids, with an improvement in the hemoglobin level or platelet count. If patients achieve a remission after treatment of an immune lytic syndrome, they should probably be treated according to the postcorticosteroid therapy stage.

At the other extreme, a group of patients has been defined who have "smoldering" CLL (38). Such patients have fewer than three involved lymphoid sites, a nondiffuse marrow histology, a hemoglobin level higher than 13 g/dL, a lymphocyte count below 30,000/μL, and a lymphocyte doubling time of more than 12 months. These findings are based on an analysis of the time to progression of Binet stage A patients. More rapid progression was noted for patients with more lymphoid enlargement, more rapid doubling time, and a higher lymphocyte count. Smoldering CLL patients have a survival similar to an age- and sex-matched population without the disease. Few physicians would recommend treatment of such patients. The indication for treatment of patients who fall between these two extremes is still not well-defined. Most studies initiate treatment for patients with CLL when they have become Binet stage C or Rai stage III to IV, have evidence of progressive disease, or have active disease. Features of active disease include unexplained weight loss (>10% in less than 6 months), fever of more than 100°F (37.8°C) for more than 2 weeks, night sweats, or extreme fatigue (7). Disease outside the liver and spleen nodes or marrow, or progressive or painful enlargement of lymph nodes, massive hepatomegaly, splenomegaly, or lymphadenopathy are other common indications for treatment. These indications have been recommended in the set of guidelines for clinical studies published by the National Cancer Institute (NCI)-sponsored working group on CLL (7). These guidelines were published to obtain a reasonable degree of homogeneity for patients entering clinical trials.

Immediate Versus Delayed Treatment of Binet Stage A Patients with Chronic Lymphocytic Leukemia

The French Cooperative Group on CLL, in protocol CLL80, initiated a study in which patients were randomly allocated to receive immediate treatment with continuous daily chlorambucil (0.1 mg/kg daily by mouth) or no treatment until progressive disease developed (39). A total of 309 patients were allocated to no treatment and 303 to initial chlorambucil. Although no significant difference was noted between the two groups, a slightly superior survival was noted for the no-treatment group. Adjustment for prognostic factors (a dubious technique in randomized clinical trials) led to this difference being significant ($p = 0.03$). Chlorambucil was significantly superior than no treatment in delaying progression to stages B or C, but was somewhat inferior from a survival viewpoint. An increase in epithelial neoplasms (11 in the chlorambucil group versus 3 in the no-treatment group) was noted. The conclusion was that the Binet stage A patients should not be treated until progression to a more advanced stage was noted. Longer follow-up of this study, together with presentation of data on the proportion of patients in the no-treatment arm treated each year after entry into the study should help clarify the treatment issues for the early-stage disease. The duration of treatment of stage A patients and therapeutic goals have still not been clearly defined.

No current study has addressed the timing of intervention in Binet stage B patients. Other studies of patients with Rai stages I and II disease with randomized assignment to no treatment or chlorambucil have been conducted. Similar results to the French study were noted, with delay of progressive disease with chlorambucil treatment, but no influence on survival (40).

Questions that still remain are whether physicians should attempt to achieve complete remission using the criteria of normal blood, bone marrow, and x-ray findings, or whether the goal should be more complete eradication of the disease, using immunophenotypic and molecular biology probes to identify residual disease. On the other hand, is "control" of the disease adequate, based on the contention that there is no curative strategy for such patients?

Chlorambucil and Steroids: A Weak Gold Standard?

The two major drugs used as initial treatment for CLL are chlorambucil (CLB) and prednisone. These agents are often given concurrently, although many physicians use CLB as a single agent, with prednisone being added if control of the disease is not satisfactory. Although chlorambucil has been used to treat CLL for more than 30 years, data on its effectiveness is limited to a relatively few patients. Knospe, in 1974, reported the results of CLB administration at a dose of 0.4 mg/kg once each 2 weeks, with escalating doses, in 62 patients with CLL (41). The response rate was 31/53 (58%) in patients not previously refractory to alkylating agents, with 5 (9%) of the evaluable patients achieving a CR (defined as normal peripheral blood indexes, normal clinical examination, and fewer than 30% lymphocytes in the differential cell count on the bone marrow aspirate). Earlier studies that used clinical bone marrow criteria describe complete response (CR) rates of 2/62 (3%) and 2/32 (6%) (42,43).

Han, in 1973, reported a CR rate of 1/11 (9%) in patients treated with CLB as a single agent at a dose of 2–4 mg/day continuously (44). This group of patients was part of a randomized, double-blind, placebo-controlled study comparing CLB plus placebo with CLB plus prednisone. Three (20%) of 15 patients treated with CLB plus prednisone achieved a CR, although only 1 was shown to have fewer than 30% lymphocytes on the differential count of a bone marrow aspirate. Overall, excellent to good responses occurred in 5/11 CLB patients, compared with 13/15 patients treated with CLB plus prednisone ($p = 0.02$). A fall in the hematocrit, the platelet count, or both, was more noticeable in the CLB-alone arm. Although survival was slightly superior for the CLB plus prednisone group, no significant difference was noted.

Sawitsky et al., in 1977, reported on the results of a three-arm randomized study in patients with Rai stage III and IV disease (45). Prednisone alone was compared with daily CLB plus prednisone and monthly CLB plus prednisone. The response rates were 11, 37, and 47%, respectively. No differences in survival among the three arms of the study was found. Thus, the evidence that CLB plus prednisone is superior to either drug alone is based on two small studies, neither of which shows a significant increase in survival.

A major difficulty in evaluating the effectiveness of CLB as a single agent is the difference in the doses and schedules used in various studies. In addition, as most of the early studies were conducted before the development of the conventional endpoints presently used for clinical studies, comparability of results is difficult (46,47). Little information is provided on the duration of treatment, time to treatment failure, and subsequent treatment. These weaknesses are coupled with the natural history of CLL, a disease with comparatively long median survival. More recent studies of CLB plus prednisone have also been conducted without a standard dose or schedule having been developed (Table 3).

A study by Jaksic is illuminating for the CLB versus CLB plus prednisone question (48). Chlorambucil was administered as a single high dose (75 mg every 4 weeks), combined with prednisone (30 mg/day for 7 days every 4 weeks), after a more intensive prednisone regimen for the first 6 weeks of treatment. This combination (CLB + prednisone) was compared with a high dose of CLB (15 mg) given daily to complete remission or dose-limiting toxicity (48). The preliminary results of this study are striking. The response rate is 90% for the 129 patients in CLB-alone arm, compared with 50% in 52 patients in the CLB plus prednisone arm of the study. The dose of CLB, given as a single agent, was five to six times greater than that given in the combination arm. This study demonstrated a highly significant survival advantage for the high-dose single-agent arm of the study. Some remaining questions posed by this study include: (1) What is the optimal dose and schedule for CLB as a single agent? (2) Does prednisone significantly add to the clinical response and survival of CLB when the latter is given in full dosage?

Table 3 Variations in Dose, Schedule, and Response Rate for Chlorambucil and Prednisone in CLL

Author	Ref.	CLB dose + schedule	Total 4-wk CLB dose	Prednisone (mg) dose + schedule	Total 4-wk prednisone dose	Response (%)
Keller	61	30 mg/m² q2w	60 mg/m²	80 mg/day q2w	≈400 mg	74%
Sawitsky	45	0.4–0.8/kg q4w	16–32 mg/m²	0.8 mg/kg ×7 q4w	216 mg	47%
		0.08/kg/day continuous	90 mg/m²	0.8 mg/kg ×7 q4w	216 mg	38%
Montserrat	59	0.4 mg/kg q2w	32 mg/m²	60 mg/m² ×5 q2w	600 mg	59%[a]
Idestrom	62	10 mg/day continuous	≈150 mg/m²	30 mg/m² contin.	≈220 mg	61%
Jaksic	48	75 mg q4w	≈ 40 mg/m²	30 mg/m² ×7 q4w	≈220 mg	60%
FCGCLL (N)	55	0.3 mg/kg ×5 q4w	60 mg/m²	40 mg/m² ×5 q4w	200 mg	53%[b]
Montserrat	60	0.4 mg/kg ×2 days q2w	64 mg/m²	60 mg/m² ×4 q2w	480 mg	75%[c]
Hansen	58	10 mg/m² ×5 q4w	50 mg/m²	40 mg/m² ×5 q4w	200 mg	71%[c]

[a]Stage C.
[b]Stage B.
[c]Stages B and C.

Combinations Other Than Chlorambucil Plus Prednisone

Alkylating agents, other than CLB, have been studied to a limited degree in CLL. Although busulfan and triethylenemelamine have been studied in CLL, the only other alkylating agent studied to a reasonable degree is cyclophosphamide (CYT). Single-agent CYT data is sparse. The only study comparing its efficacy with CLB showed roughly equal results (49). The efficacy of the combination of cyclophosphamide, vincristine (VCR), and prednisone (CVP) in indolent lymphoma led to studies of CVP in CLL. Liepman et al., in 1978, reported on the results of CVP in 36 patients (23 previously untreated) who received CVP (50). The dosage of CYT was 2 g/m^2 every 4 weeks. The response rate was excellent with 16/36 (44%) patients achieving a CR and 10 (28%) a PR, for an overall response rate of 72%. Complete response rates were higher in the previously untreated patients, 12/23 (52%) compared with 4/13 (31%). The CRs in this study were not always documented by bone marrow biopsy, and morphologically several patients had poorly differentiated lymphocytic lymphoma.

Oken has studied CVP at lower doses of CYT. Both oral and intravenous (IV) schedules were studied (51). Eight (44%) of 28 patients who had received previous treatment with chlorambucil responded to CVP, compared with 8/13 (61%) in the Leipman study. Montserrat et al. studied 18 previously treated stage C patients with CVP with 5 (28%) responding (52). The response rate for the 27 untreated stage C patients was 9/27 (33%). In this study, the patients were compared with CLB plus prednisone. Although the response rate was higher with the CLB plus prednisone arm of the study, the survival curves were identical. The doses for these two studies were remarkably lower than those in the Leipman study (800 mg/m^2, Oken; 600 mg/m^2, Montserrat; 2000 mg/m^2, Leipman), again raising the question of the dose–response characteristics of alkylating agents in CLL, as was previously discussed for chlorambucil.

The use of multiple alkylating agents together with the use of VCR plus prednisone has been studied in the M-2 protocol, by Kempin et al. (53). The M-2 used vincristine 0.03 mg/kg (1.2 mg/m^2) IV, carmustine (BCNU) 0.05 mg/kg (2 mg/m^2) IV, and cyclophosphamide 10 mg/kg (400 mg/m^2) IV on day 1, together with melphalan 0.25 mg/kg (10 mg/m^2) PO daily for 4 days, and prednisone 1 mg/kg (14 mg/m^2) PO daily for 7 days, then a reduced dosage for a further 7–28 days, as necessary. Courses were repeated at 5-week intervals. Criteria for response were clearly defined, and the bone marrow biopsy had to be normal for a CR to be achieved. Eleven (17%) of 63 evaluable patients obtained a CR and 28 (44%) a PR, for an overall response rate of 61%. Seven of the CR patients had no evidence of disease when bone marrow lymphocyte subsets were analyzed by immunophenotyping. The CR rate for previously untreated patients was 11/37 (30%) versus 0/26 for the previously treated patients. The overall response rate for untreated patients was 30/37 (81%), compared with 9/26 (35%) in the previously treated group. The median survival was dated from the time of diagnosis and, therefore, is difficult to compare with other studies.

Surprisingly, doxorubicin has not been reported to be active as a single agent in CLL. However, several combination studies have now been reported suggesting that anthracycline-containing regimens have a significant role in CLL. The French Cooperative Group on CLL conducted a randomized comparison of COP (CVP) versus COP plus doxorubicin (CHOP) in previously untreated Binet stage C patients (39,54). Fifty-nine patients were initially reported, 29 receiving COP (cyclophosphamide, 300 mg/m^2 daily PO and prednisone, 40 mg/m^2 daily PO, each for 5 days each month, and vincristine, 1 mg/m^2 on day 1). Thirty patients received CHOP, with doxorubicin, 25 mg/m^2 IV, given on day 1, together with cyclophosphamide, vincristine, and prednisone as in the COP regimen. Eighteen (60%) of the CHOP patients improved to Binet state A, and 6 (20%) to stage B. Only 5 (17%) of the COP patients improved to stage A, 6 (21%) to stage B, and 15 (52%) remained stage C. The median survival of the COP patients was approximately 21 months, and 77% of the CHOP patients were still alive at 2 years. The survival of the CHOP stage C patients was significantly superior to the COP patients and approached the historical experience of the French group's stage B patients.

An updated analysis shows a persistent survival advantage for the CHOP patients (median 56 months), compared with 26 months for the COP patients (39). No suggestion of a plateau has appeared for the CHOP patients, suggesting that no patients are being cured. The reported survival is impressive for a population of stage C patients.

More recently, the same CHOP regimen has been compared with CLB 0.3 mg/kg (12 mg/m^2) PO, and prednisone 40 mg/m^2 daily for 5 days each month, for 3 years (55). This study is being conducted in stage B patients in the CLL-85 protocol of the French Cooperative Group on CLL. The CHOP courses were given each month for 6 months, then each 3 months for another ten courses. Eighty-one patients have been evaluated after at least 6 months on the CHOP regime and 72 after 6 months of CLB–prednisone. Twenty-two (27%) of the patients given CHOP have obtained a CR, and 40 (50%) have improved to stage A. The comparable figures for the CLB plus prednisone arm of this study are 11/72 (15%) and 27/72 (38%). Thus 77% of the CHOP-treated patients have had an excellent response, compared with 53% of the CLB–prednisone group. No survival data is yet available.

The M. D. Anderson group has conducted a study of cyclophosphamide, doxorubicin (Adriamycin), and prednisone (CAP) in patients with previously untreated chronic lymphocytic leukemia (56). The CAP regimen was given to complete clinical remission, followed by 18 months of cyclophosphamide–prednisone maintenance. Forty-seven patients with previously untreated CLL received CAP. The dose of cyclophosphamide was 750 mg/m^2 IV on day 1, doxorubicin 50 mg/m^2, and prednisone 100 mg/day on days 1 through 5. Courses were repeated at 3-week intervals. A maximum cumulative dose of 450 mg/m^2 of doxorubicin (nine courses of CAP) was given. Twenty-three (48%) of 47 patients obtained a CR, and 11 (23%) obtained a PR. Twelve of the 20 CRs occurred on the CAP phase of the study, and the additional 8 occurred during the cyclophosphamide–prednisone maintenance phase of the study. Marrow biopsy criteria were used to define response, in addition to clinical and peripheral blood findings. All patients in that study have been followed for 10 years, and the median survival was 60 months. No patient remains free of disease. Surprisingly, no impact of response on survival was noted. This appears to be related to a high incidence of death due to second malignancies, cardiovascular and cerebrovascular events in the responding patients. The doxorubicin regimen was well-tolerated. The CAP–CP regimen has resulted in the highest complete remission rate that has been reported in chronic lymphocytic leukemia. A surprising feature of this study was a very high CR rate in Binet stage C patients. Fourteen of 17 patients responded with 9/17 patients achieving a CR. The median survival of the Binet stage C patients was 80 months, comparable with the survival figures being reported by the French Cooperative Group on CLL for Binet C patients treated with their version of CHOP, which has a dosage of doxorubicin of 25 mg/m^2/daily.

Subsequent to the CAP study the M. D. Anderson group initiated a POACH protocol with doxorubicin 15 mg/m^2 IV on days 1, 8, and 15; cyclophosphamide 500 mg/m^2 IV on day 1; vincristine 2 mg IV on day 1; cytarabine (ara-C) 25 mg/m^2 q12h, subcutaneously, on days 1 through 5; and prednisone 100 mg PO daily on days 1 through 7 (57). Thirty-four patients received POACH as initial treatment, and 7 (21%) obtained a CR and 12 (45%) a PR. Four of the PR patients had residual foci in the bone marrow as the only evidence of disease and had fewer than 30% lymphocytes in the bone marrow aspirate and would be considered as CRs by response parameters quoted in several other studies. The authors describe these patients as having "nodular" partial remissions. The median survival was 60 months. The response rates were 5/10 (50%) for stage A, 11/15 (73%) for stage B, and 3/9 (33%) for stage C. The response rate was significantly inferior for previously treated patients, with only 2 (6%) obtaining a CR and 6 (19%) a PR. The median survival of the previously treated patients was 15 months.

A Danish study has compared CHOP (71 patients) with CLB plus prednisone (73 patients) as initial treatment for CLL (58). The CHOP regimen used cyclophosphamide 750 mg/m^2 IV on day 1; doxorubicin 50 mg/m^2 IV on day 1; and vincristine 1 mg/m^2 IV on day 1, with prednisone 40 mg/m^2 PO on days 1 through 5. Courses were repeated each 4 weeks. The chlorambucil dose for the control arm was 10 mg/m^2 daily for 5 days, and the prednisone dose was 40 mg/m^2 PO for 5 days. The study was restricted to patients in stages B and C. The

CR rate (clinical—no bone marrow criteria) was 63% for the CHOP arm and 29% for the CLB plus prednisone arm. No significant survival advantage was noted for either arm.

COMPARATIVE CLINICAL TRIALS IN CHRONIC LYMPHOCYTIC LEUKEMIA

In recent years, several groups have conducted clinical trials in CLL. The majority of these studies have compared a new regimen with CLB plus prednisone. As mentioned earlier, great variability exists in the doses and schedules for CLB and prednisone (see Table 3). Montserrat et al. compared CLB plus prednisone with CVP in 96 patients with stage C CLL (59). The response rate was higher for the CLB—prednisone arm [30/51 (59%)] than for the CVP arm [14/45 (31%)]. Only 8% and 2% achieved a CR in respective arms of the study. The response rates were higher for the untreated patients in the CLB–prednisone arm, 24/34 (71%) versus 9/27 (33%), ($p < 0.05$), but not for the previously treated patients [CLB–prednisone, 6/17 (35%) versus CVP 5/18 (28%)]. Although no survival difference was noted for the two arms of the study, responders had a superior survival, compared with nonresponders ($p < 0.001$), and the previously untreated patients had a better survival.

A Danish study has compared CHOP with CLB–prednisone in 550 previously untreated stage B and C patients (58). A significantly higher clinical CR rate was noted for the CHOP arm of the study, compared with CLB–prednisone (63% versus 29%). Again, no survival advantage was noted for either arm of the study, although complete responders faired better than partial responders or resistant patients. The CHOP regimen was very well-tolerated, despite the age of the population.

Montserrat has compared CLB–prednisone with cyclophosphamide, melphalan, and prednisone (CMP) in stage B and C patients (60). Forty-eight patients have been assigned to each arm of the study. The response rate was 75% for CLB–prednisone and 54% for CMP arm. Again, no survival difference was noted between the two arms, but responding patients had a survival advantage. The response rate was higher for stage B patients than for stage C in both of these studies. Keller et al. (61) treated patients with CLB and prednisone initially. Of 178 evaluable patients, 22% obtained a CR and 52% a PR. Responders then randomly received consolidation treatment with ara-C 25 mg/m^2 q12h for eight doses and cyclophosphamide 25 mg/m^2 q12h orally for eight doses for four cycles or additional CLB and prednisone. No difference in time to progression in survival was noted for the two postremission arms of the study. Idestrom compared CLB–prednisone with continuous low-dose or intermittent prednimustine (a chlorambucil ester of prednisone) (62). The response rates were

61, 55, and 57%, respectively. No difference in survival was noted for the three arms of the study.

The results of the French Cooperative Group on CLL protocol CLL-80 for stage A (intermediate versus delayed in CLB) and stage C (CHOP versus COP) have already been mentioned (39,54). The same group has compared CLB (150 patients) with COP (139 patients) in stage B patients (55). The survival data was identical in the two arms of the study. No difference in the response rate, judged by change in stage, was noted. Catovsky et al. have conducted two MRC trials for the United Kingdom Study Group on CLL (CLL-1 and CLL-2) (40). In CLL-1, stable Rai stages I–II patients were assigned to CLB immediately versus no treatment until progression. Progressive stage I patients were randomized to CLB versus COP and progressive stage II and all stage III and IV patients were randomized to CLB versus COP versus splenic irradiation. No significant survival advantage was noted, although CLL deaths were less frequent for the splenic irradiation arm than for the CLB arm in the last stratification. In CLL-2, stage A patients were again assigned to immediate or delayed CLB; stages B and C, with a spleen larger than 5 cm, were assigned to CLB or CLB–prednisone; and stages B and C with splenomegaly ≥5 cm to CLB or CLB–prednisone or splenic irradiation. In this ongoing trial no survival or response differences have been noted.

As mentioned earlier, Jaksic et al. have conducted a trial for the International Society for Chemo and Immunotherapy (IGLI) CLL study group, comparing continuing high-dose CLB with intermittent CLB–prednisone (48). The CLB had a significantly higher response rate and significantly prolonged survival, compared with CLB–prednisone. This is the only study that has demonstrated a survival advantage for any regimen, when compared with CLB–prednisone. Although the variability in doses and schedules for CLB–prednisone does not allow comparability of regimens, it appears that there is no convincing evidence that the addition of prednisone to CLB given in adequate doses significantly affects response or survival. Jaksic's study suggests that CLB can be delivered safely at higher doses than are usually recommended and that the high doses may be associated with a higher response rate and better survival.

My conclusions from these studies are that, despite chlorambucil being available for many years, the optimal dose and schedule has not yet been defined. In addition, the role of prednisone in the management of CLL again has not been defined, as there is little evidence that the addition of prednisone to CLB significantly improves response rate or survival. Recent studies with CHOP regimens or the CAP regimen suggest that a high response rate can be achieved in Binet stage C patients with anthracycline regimens (54,56,58). Early results suggest a similar finding in Binet stage B patients. It appears that we have underestimated the ability of elderly patients to tolerate anthracycline-containing regimens, as all studies of cyclophosphamide–anthracycline combination programs have been well-tolerated. Although a higher response rate has been noted for the CHOP studies, it is disturbing that the largest study reported by the Danish group has not led to a survival advantage, compared with CLB–prednisone, although longer follow-up of that study may lead to a survival advantage.

Currently, it appears that Binet stage A patients do not benefit from immediate treatment with regimens that have so far been administered. New approaches to the management of stages B and C patients certainly are warranted, with further investigation of higher doses of alkylating agents being recommended. Liepman's study (50) of high-dose CVP giving better results than had been reported with lower-dose schedules also supports the concept of dose–intensity relationships in alkylating agent therapy in CLL.

Eligibility and Response Criteria

Gradually, well-defined criteria for response have evolved in CLL (6,7). A review of the response criteria used historically in the studies quoted in the foregoing will illustrate a shift from terminology such as "good" or "excellent" response to formal criteria for CR and PR. These have now been codified by both the International Working Group on CLL (6) and the NCI-Workshop on CLL (7). The criteria for CR for these two sets of recommendations are remarkably similar. The major difference that exists is in the criteria for PR, which in the IWGCLL recommendation, is based on the shift in Binet stage, whereas in the NCI criteria, more emphasis is placed on numerical changes in disease parameters. Until the relative usefulness of each of these two sytems is established prospectively, it is hoped that investigators will report their studies by using both sets of criteria to allow comparability. This approach will be more meaningful if the recommended guidelines for eligibility for studies are followed or precisely stipulated in reports of studies. Both of the recommended response criteria allow for persistence of residual lymphoid nodules in the bone marrow, on the basis that these may be residual normal lymphoid cells.

Significance of Complete Remission

Complete remissions in CLL were initially reported to be rare. In recent studies several reports have quoted CR rates of 20–43% (53,56,57,61,62). Some of these reports have been clinical CRs, rather than requiring bone marrow criteria to be fulfilled. Most recent reports have required fewer than 30% lymphocytes to be present in the bone marrow before a patient can be considered to have had a CR. As noted earlier, IWGCLL and NCI-Workshop on CLL have allowed residual foci on nodules of lymphocytes to present in the bone marrow biopsy of CR patients (6,7). One difficulty is to determine whether nodules are monoclonal (suggesting residual disease) or polyclonal (suggesting normal lymphoid tissue). One variable that could be evaluated for prognostic significance will be whether these nodules are occasional or multiple and what sized nodules are present. Most studies report a distinct survival advantage for patients who achieve a CR over that for the PR patients (53,57,61,62), although this is not always true (56). One conflicting factor is that earlier-stage patients tend to have higher response rates than advanced-stage patients. The question that arises is whether the overall advantage is due to the biology of the patients or their disease, or is consequent upon the response. Technology is now available using flow cytometry to identify cells that coexpress CD5 in B-cell markers (e.g., CD19 and CD20). These cells appear to be malignant CLL phenotypes. The percentage of these cells among the mononuclear cells in blood and bone marrow can now be documented precisely permitting an immunophenotypic CR to be defined.

NEW AGENTS IN CHRONIC LYMPHOCYTIC LEUKEMIA

In the last 5 years, clinical trials have demonstrated three clinically useful purine analogues in CLL. These agents, fludarabine monophosphate, pentostatin (2-deoxycoformycin; DCF), and 2-chlorodeoxyadenosine (CDA) have structural similarities. The chemical structures are shown in Figure 3. Deoxycoformycin predominantly acts as an inhibitor of adenosine deaminase (63), whereas fludarabine monophosphate (64) and 2-chlorodeoxyadenosine (65), analogues of adenosine, are relatively refractory to deamination by adenosine deaminase.

Fludarabine phosphate (9-*β*-*d*-arabinofuranosyl-2-fluoroadenine-5'-phosphate) is an adenine nucleoside related to vidarabine (adenine arabinoside;

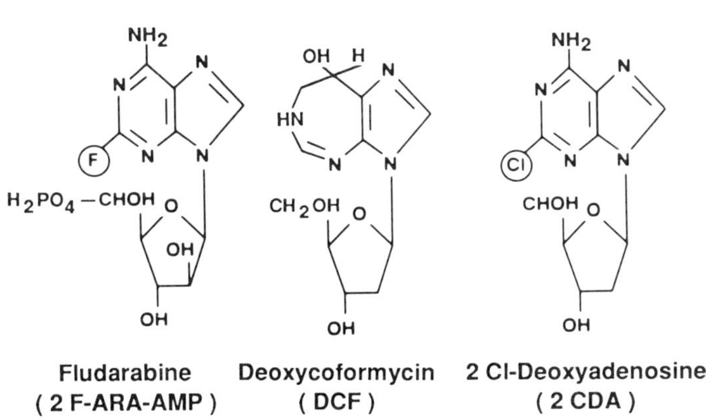

Figure 3 Chemical structures of fludarabine, pentostatin, and 2-clorodeoxyadenosine.

ara-A). Vidarabine was limited in efficacy as an antitumor agent because of rapid inactivation by adenosine deaminase and poor solubility (66,67). The addition of a fluorine atom to the adenine moiety conferred relative resistance to deamination and the addition of the monophosphate to the sugar moiety markedly enhanced solubility. After injection into humans, fludarabine phosphate is rapidly dephosphorylated in vivo to 2-F-araA. The 2-F-araA is taken up into cells and phosphorylated to 2-F-araATP which is thought to be the form of the drug necessary for its cytotoxic effect. The rate-limiting enzyme in phosphorylation is deoxycytidine kinase (68).

Grever and colleagues were the first group of investigators to conduct a Phase II study of fludarabine monophosphate in CLL (60). The response rate was 9/26 (35%). Subsequently, investigators at the M. D. Anderson have conducted a number of studies with fludarabine monophosphate. In the initial Phase I–II protocol, fludarabine was administered initially at a dose of 25–30 mg/m^2 daily for 5 days every 4 weeks (70). Sixty-eight patients with CLL were entered into the study. Sixty-three patients had received prior cytotoxic therapy for CLL, and the remaining 5 patients had previously been treated for diffuse well-differentiated lymphocytic lymphoma that had progressed into a leukemic phase. Eighty-seven percent of the patients had received prior alkylating agents. Thirty-nine (57%) of the 68 patients achieved either a CR or PR. Nine (13%) achieved a CR, 11 a nodular CR (residual foci in the bone marrow being the only evidence of disease), and 19 (28%) a PR. Nineteen patients failed to respond because of refractory disease. The median survival of the 68 patients in this study was 16 months. The survival of the CR and nodular CR patients was identical. Patients who achieved PR had a significantly inferior survival than that of CR and nodular CR patients. Improvement in Rai stage occurred in 5/13 patients with Rai stage I, 5/10 patients with Rai stage II, 9/19 with Rai stage III, and 10/24 with Rai stage IV disease. The drug was well tolerated with minimal nausea, vomiting, alopecia, or diarrhea. The major toxicity was an incidence of febrile episodes, with pneumonias and fevers of unknown origin occurring in 15% and 16% of courses, respectively. Other minor infections occurred in 11% of courses. The 57% CR plus PR rate is the highest response rate that has been reported in refractory patients with CLL. Regimens, such as CLB and prednisone, CVP, and the M-2 regimen, obtained partial response rates of 25–35% in previously treated patients (52,53,59). The POACH regimen resulted in a response rate of 26% in 31 patients, using the same entry and response criteria as used in the fludarabine study (57).

Because of the activity of fludarabine as a single agent in previously treated patients with CLL and the reported additive action of prednisone when combined with other cytotoxic agents, such as CLB, in the treatment of CLL, a new protocol was designed to combine fludarabine and prednisone (71). The dose of fludarabine was maintained at 30 mg/m^2 daily for 5 days IV, and prednisone was added at a dose of 30 mg/m^2 orally for 5 days. Courses were repeated every 4 weeks. One hundred and one patients have been entered on the protocol. The CR rate was 12/101 (12%), nodular PR 24%, PR 19%, and resistant disease 33%. The response rate and survival characteristics were almost identical with those noted with fludarabine as a single agent, with no current evidence that the addition of prednisone improved tolerance, response rate, or survival. Response was strongly correlated with Rai and Binet stage and pretreatment white blood cell count. The serum albumin level was strongly predictive for response and survival, a level lower than 3.5 g/dL being predictive for probability of dying within the first three courses of treatment.

As fludarabine was highly effective in previously treated patients, it was introduced into the management of patients with previously untreated disease who were Rai stages III–IV (64). After initial success in this subset of patients, patients with previously untreated Rai stages 0–II CLL who demonstrated clear evidence of progressive disease were treated with fludarabine as their initial treatment regimen (72). Thirty-three patients received fludarabine, at a dose of 30 mg/m^2 daily for 5 days every 4 weeks, as a single agent. Twenty-six (79%) of the 33 patients have obtained a CR or PR. Eleven patients (33%) achieved a CR, 13 patients (39%) a nodular PR, and 2 (6%) a PR. Of the 7 patients who failed to respond, 3 died of infection during the first three cycles of treatment. The CR rate was 42% for 19 patients with Rai stage 0–II disease compared with 3/14 (21%) for Rai stages III–IV.

Pentostatin (2-deoxycoformycin; DCF) is an adenosine deaminase inhibitor with activity in CLL. Grever et al. treated 25 patients with refractory CLL. The dose was 4 mg/m^2 each 2 weeks (73). One CR and 4 PRs were noted, for a response rate of 20%. The results of another study of 29 patients treated with 5 mg daily for 3 days every 3 weeks were reported in a review (74). Seven of 29 responded, with 1 CR and 6 PRs. Dillman reported on 39 patients who had received 4 mg weekly for 3 weeks, then every 2 weeks (75). Nine patients achieved a PR, and 1 a CR; 11 patients have a clinical improvement. Riddell has used a similar regimen in 16 patients, and 7 had an improvement in peripheral blood findings, but no criteria for objective response were reported (76). The toxicities of the drug, particularly at the lower-dose schedules, have been minor. Myelosuppression, nausea, vomiting, stomatitis, conjunctivitis, and elevations in renal function tests occurred, as well as an increased incidence of infection with herpesviruses, *Candida* species, and *Pneumocystis carinii* (14).

2-Chlorodeoxyadenosine has been studied by Piro and co-workers (65). Eighteen patients with relapsed or refractory CLL, all except 1 being Binet stage C, received treatment with 2-CDA as a 7-day continuous infusion. The dose varied from 2 to 4 mg/m^2 per day. Four patients achieved a partial remission, and 6 patients a clinical improvement.

As pentostatin and 2-CDA, have been studied in relatively few patients, their exact roles in the management of CLL is poorly defined. Fludarabine, on the other hand, appears to be a major new drug in the management of chronic lymphocytic leukemia which will be administered in comparative trials in the United States and other countries.

Biological Response Modifiers

The most widely studied biological response modifier in CLL is recombinant interferon alpha (rIFN-α). Early studies conducted in previously treated patients demonstrated a low response rate (responses being less than a PR in most studies) (77–80). Eight PRs occurred in 45 patients treated in these studies. Two-thirds of the patients had previously been treated with chemotherapy. Foon et al. reported acceleration of CLL in 5/19 patients treated in his study (77). Most recent reports have evaluated the activity of rIFN-α in untreated early-stage patients. Pangalis et al. have reported a decrease in lymphocyte count by more than 50% in 5/10 patients in one study, and 10/26 in a second study (81,83). In the latter study, 3/26 had a decrease in the size of their spleen and lymph nodes, but no change in marrow infiltrate. Others have reported a >50% decrease in lymphocyte count in 6/10 (59%) patients (82,84). In the first of these studies, an increase in the absolute granulocyte count was noted in 8/10 patients (82). In the second, a decrease in an elevated pretreatment T-lymphocyte count was noted in 6/7 patients and, of interest, the serum immunoglobulin G level increased by more than 0.3 g/L in 3/7 patients studied (84). There are no reported clinical trials of interferon beta or gamma in CLL.

Recombinant interleukin-2 (rIL-2) has been administered to 12 refractory patients with CLL (85). The basis of this study was the observation that natural killer (NK) cell activity was decreased in CLL and IL-2 is able to increase NK cell number and function. The lymphocyte count decreased in 7/10 patients with B-cell CLL and three patients had a decrease in node size and 2 in spleen size. The authors suggested that in 3 of 5 patients treated with therapy to which they were previously refractory, chemosensitivity was restored.

Future studies of biological response modifiers will almost certainly be as adjuncts to chemotherapy to prolong the disease-free intervals, as reported in multiple myeloma, to enhance response in patients with minimal residual disease after chemotherapy, to restore normal immune function, or together with chemotherapy to enhance response rates.

Monoclonal Antibodies

As the majority of the B-CLL cells express T101 (CD5), clinical trials have been conducted with anti-T101 antibodies. The clinical results have been disappointing, with transient reductions in circulating lymphocyte count, but not significant change in tumor burden, as measured in liver, spleen, or node size, or bone marrow infiltration (86,87). The idiotype of the immunoglobulin expressed on the surface of CLL cells is specific for the malignant cells. Anti-idiotype antibodies have been developed and used to treat CLL, again with disappointing results. Many problems exist for the therapy of CLL with antibodies. Modulation of the antigen on the surface of the CLL cells (loss of expression), presence of circulating antigen (including idiotypic immunoglobulin), biclonality or polyclonality of tumor cells, somatic mutations of the immunoglobulin, and development of human anti-mouse antibody (HAMA) responses are challenges to be overcome before successful application of this treatment is more common. Recent reports of more satisfactory responses for a blocked whole ricin conjugated with anti-B-4 (anti-CD19) in B-cell lymphoma suggests that continued exploration in this area will be productive (88).

Consolidation Therapy

Only one study has addressed the role of postinduction chemotherapy in patients with CLL. Keller et al. administered six additional courses of CLB–prednisone or four courses of cyclophosphamide and Ara-C to patients who had responded with a complete or partial remission to CLB–prednisone (61). Of 102 patients 82 completed consolidation courses. Further improvement of PR patients to CR occurred equally in both arms of the study, and survival was equivalent. Both regimens were well tolerated. The continued response to CR with further treatment of CLL in patients who have achieved a PR after 6 to 9 months of treatment, suggests the need for further studies of the duration of treatment in this disease.

AUTOIMMUNE COMPLICATIONS OF CHRONIC LYMPHOCYTIC LEUKEMIA

Anitbodies to hematopoietic cells are common in B-cell CLL and autoimmune hemolytic anemia (AIHA) is reported to occur in 10–25% of patients sometime during the course of their disease (89). Antibodies are not produced by the malignant B cells, and the mechanism of antibody production is uncertain. The prevailing opinion is the high prevalence of autoantibody production is due to an imbalance of the CD4 and CD8 T lymphocyte subsets in CLL. One feature that needs further explanation is the reason for the antibody production to be directed against the hematopoietic cells, as there is no increase in other autoantibodies in CLL (90).

Two recent studies have evaluated the incidence of autoantibodies in CLL and found 12/100 (12%) and 12/195 (8%) to be positive (90,91). In the latter study, the incidence in nonprogressive Binet stage A patients was 3/105 versus 12/94 progressive stage A or stages B and C patients ($p < 0.02$) (90). Autoimmune thrombocytopenia and neutropenia, and pure red cell aplasia occur, but are less common (1–2%) (90). Despite the low incidence of autoimmune thrombocytopenia, a high incidence (74%) of autoantibodies against platelets has been reported using the Dixon direct and indirect tests (91). Despite the positive antibody tests, hemoglobin levels and platelet counts are often normal. The hemoglobin or platelet counts, per se, appear to be an important prognostic factor, regardless of the presence or absence of autoantibodies.

The vast majority of the antibodies are warm IgG antibodies, directed at the Rh system, most commonly against the C antigen. As in other AIHA cases, the recommended treatment initially is to use prednisone at a dose of 60–100 mg/day until evidence for hemolysis is absent. At that time (usually 2–4 weeks), the prednisone dose can be tapered by 20–25% of the dose per week and can eventually be discontinued. Three of four patients will have a good response, but several patients will relapse. In patients whose AIHA is refractory to steroids or recurrent, a splenectomy is usually effective. A similar approach, without as much supporting data, is recommended for thrombocytopenia in CLL when immune destruction is postulated as the cause. Again, splenectomy is often effective, at least initially. The use of intravenous immunoglobulin, which is rapidly effective in many cases of idiotypic thrombocytopenic purpura (ITP), has not been investigated adequately in AIHA, neutropenia, and thrombocytopenia which are associated with CLL.

Cyclosporine has been reported to be effective in sporadic cases of anemia, neutropenia, and thrombocytopenia caused by impaired marrow production. Tura et al. recently reported on the use of cyclosporine in three cases of pure red cell aplasia (RCA) at a dose of 6–9 mg/kg daily (92). All three patients had a marked sustained response, beginning within a week of the start of therapy. T-cell-mediated suppression of erythropoiesis is thought to be the mechanism of RCA. It is proposed that cyclosporine helps by decreasing IL-2 production, and may decrease the inhibiting T-cell effect.

SPLENECTOMY IN CHRONIC LYMPHOCYTIC LEUKEMIA

As mentioned earlier, splenectomy is indicated in CLL patients with refractory or recurrent autoimmune hemolytic anemia or thrombocytopenia. Several other justifications for a splenectomy exist in CLL.

An enlarged spleen that sequesters both red cells and platelets may destroy cells without the demonstrated presence of antibodies and may remain as a site of a significant tumor burden in many patients. Rapid expansion of the spleen may be painful in later stages of the disease. Splenectomy has been recommended for early stages of CLL when splenomegaly is the predominant site of the CLL, but the pure splenic type of typical B-type CLL (not the prolymphocytic variant) has a good prognosis. Most investigators recommend a splenectomy only for those thought to have a reasonable marrow reserve (93,94). Ferrant performed splenectomies in 20 patients in whom ferrokinetic studies suggested that adequate erythropoietic function still existed in the marrow (93). They also measured the splenic red cell volume to predict the probable increase in hematocrit after splenectomy. Most of the patients had an improvement in well-being and a markedly reduced transfusion requirement. Seven of 9 patients with a preoperative hematocrit level of less than 30% increased to more than 35% and in 9/10 patients with a platelet count of fewer than 100,000/μL the count increased to more than 150,000/μL. No survival advantage was demonstrated. The outcome of splenectomy in unselected patients without ferrokinetic parameters is uncertain. Pegourri et al. performed a splenectomy in 43 patients with resistance to initial or subsequent courses of chlorambucil (94). Twenty-four of 33 Rai stage IV patients improved to Rai stage 0–II. The median survival after splenectomy was 48 months.

The results with recombinant erythropoietin in anemia of renal disease promise that this drug will play a major role in improving the red cell production level in CLL and may decrease the need for splenectomy. Similar roles for improvement of neutrophil count with colony-stimulating factors (GCSF and GM-CSF) and platelet count with agents such as IL-3 are predicted for the future.

LEUKAPHERESIS

The indolent nature of CLL suggests that removal of a substantial number of cells will require a relatively long period for these cells to be replaced. This, together with a limited repertoire of agents active in this disease, led to the use of intensive leukapheresis in patients with CLL, especially in those with progressive disease and marrow compromised when further chemotherapy was considered dangerous. In one study, an average of 2.9×10^{11} cells could be removed in each attempt with alternate-day pheresis (95). Thirteen of 20 patients responded with a significant elevation of hemoglobin and platelet levels and a fall in lymphocyte count. In most of the responders, a decrease in the size of lymph nodes and spleen also occurred. Many of the patients had sustained control of their disease for more than 12 months. Other studies have not been as positive. However, pheresis may be useful to prepare patients for splenectomy and depletion of the white cell count in the uncommon CLL patients in whom extreme leukocytosis (>400,000/μL) leads to symptoms of leukostasis (dyspnea, hypoxemia, pulmonary infiltrates, or neurological symptoms).

HYPOGAMMAGLOBULINEMIA

At diagnosis, 20% of patients with CLL have a γ-globulin level of less than 800 mg/dL. The incidence is 29% for patients with stage C disease and 17–18% for stages A and B. Low levels of IgA and IgM are more common than low IgG levels (30 versus 10%) (96). The pathogenesis of the hypogammaglobulinemia is not known and may be due to impaired B-cell function or abnormal T–B-cell interaction. Several substances can induce IgG production in vitro. Eventually, over 50% of patients will have developed hypogammaglobulinemia as their disease progresses and more chemotherapy is given (97). The pattern of infection that occurs in CLL in the early phase is what would be expected in hypogammaglobulinemia, namely a high frequency of bacterial sinopulmonary infections. Low levels of IgG antibodies to *Escherichia coli,* lipopolysaccharides, and *Streptococcus pneumoniae* have been found in CLL (98). Response to vaccination with diphtheria, typhoid, influenza, and mumps is poor (99). Hypogammaglobulinemia is not the only mechanism of infection in CLL, as cell-mediated immunity is also impaired, and later in the disease, neutropenia is not uncommon.

Although treatment of CLL is effective in several patients in eradicating the disease, the γ-globulin level seldom returns to normal. The incidence of infection in CLL has been related to the IgG level. There are several anecdotal reports of decreased infection in patients with CLL and hypogammaglobulinemia who received intramuscular immunoglobulin (98,99). Recent preparations of monomeric IgG for intravenous use have become available. This permits delivery of high doses of IgG intravenously. Levels of immunoglobulin can be maintained by intravenous infusions at 3 to 4-week intervals. In a recent cooperative group clinical trial of intravenous immunoglobulin for prevention of infections in CLL, 41 patients received IV immunoglobulin and 40 patients placebo (100). Patients were well matched for prognostic factors, but more of the placebo patients had a severe decrease in IgG below the level of 350 mg/dL (16/40 placebo versus 11/41 of IV immunoglobulin). A significant decrease in moderate and trivial bacterial infections were noted in the IV immunoglobulin group, compared with placebo (15 episodes versus 31), but not for major infections (8 versus 11). No influence on viral or fungal infections were noted. A major question remains about whether the cost of the treatment warrants the decrease in moderate to trivial bacterial infections.

CONCLUSIONS

Improved knowledge of the biology of lymphoid neoplasms and the development of new cytoreductive agents promise to lead to improved responses in CLL. New biological agents should allow protection from the cytopenia in CLL and encourage attempts to restore normal immune function, especially in patients with minimal residual disease.

REFERENCES

1. Binet JL, Catovsky D, Chandra P, et al: Chronic lymphocytic leukaemia: Proposals for a revised prognostic staging system. *Br J Haematol* 1981; 48:365–367.
2. Melo JV, Catovsky D, Bodger M: Reactivity of the monoclonal antibody RFB1 in chronic B-cell leukaemias. *Scand J Haematol* 1984; 32:417–422.
3. Croce CM, Nowell PC: Molecular basis of human B cell neoplasia, *Blood* 1985; 65:1–7.
4. Bennett JM, Catovsky D, Daniel M-T, et al: Proposals for the classification of chronic (mature) B and T lymphoid leukaemias. The French–American–British (FAB) Cooperative Group. *J Clin Pathol* 1989; 42:567–584.
5. Craigie D: *Edin Med Surg J* 1845; 64:400.
6. International Workshop on Chronic Lymphocytic Leukemia: Chronic lymphocytic leukemia: Recommendations for diagnosis, staging, and response criteria. *Ann Intern Med* 1989; 110:236–238.
7. Cheson BD, Bennett JM, Rai KR, et al: Guidelines for clinical protocols for chronic lymphocytic leukemia: Recommendations of the National Cancer Institute-sponsored working group. *Am J Hematol* 1988; 29:152–163.
8. Royston I, Majda J, Baird S, et al: Human T cell antigens of chronic lymphocytic leukemia cells bearing surface immunoglobulin. *J Immunol* 1980; 125:725–731.
9. Caligaris-Cappio F, Gobbi M, Bofill M, Janossy G: Infrequent normal B lymphocytes express features of B chronic lymphocytic leukemia. *J Exp Med* 1982; 155:623–628.
10. Ault KA, Antin JH, Ginsburg D, et al: Phenotype of recovering lymphoid cell populations after marrow transplantation. *J Exp Med* 1985; 161:1483–1502.
11. Plater-Zyberk C, Maini RN, Lam K, et al: A rheumatoid arthritis B cell subset expresses a phenotype similar to that in chronic lymphocytic leukemia. *Arthritis Rheum* 1985; 28:971–976.
12. Freedman AS, Boyd AW, Bieber FR, et al: Normal cellular counterparts of B cell chronic lymphocytic leukemia. *Blood* 1987; 70:418–427.
13. Freedman AS, Nadler LM: Chronic lymphocytic leukemia: Cell surface phenotype and normal cellular counterparts. In, Polliack A, Catovsky D (eds): *Chronic Lymphocytic Leukemia*. Chur, Switzerland, Harwood Academic Publishers, 1988, pp 47–66.
14. Foa R, Giovarelli M, Jemma C, et al: Interleukin 2 (IL 2) and interferon-(gamma) production by T lymphocytes from patients with B-chronic lymphocytic leukemia: Evidence that normally released IL 2 is absorbed by the neoplastic B cell population. *Blood* 1985; 66:614–619.
15. Galton DAG: B-chronic lymphocytic leukemia: Some diagnostic and clinical aspects. In, Polliack A, Catovsky D (eds): *Chronic Lymphocytic Leukemia*. Chur, Switzerland, Harwood Academic Publishers, 1988, pp 33–45.
16. Rai KR, Sawitsky A, Cronkit EP, et al: Clinical staging of chronic lymphocytic leukemia. *Blood* 1975; 46:219–234.
17. Jasksic B, Vitale B: Total tumor mass score (TTM): A new parameter in chronic lymphocytic leukemia. *Br J Haematol* 1981; 49:405–413.

18. Binet J-L, Auguier A, Dighiero G, et al: A new prognostic class of chronic lymphocytic leukemia derived from a multivariate survival analysis. *Cancer* 1981; 48:198–206.
19. Galton DAG: *Can Med Assoc* 1966; 94:1105–1010.
20. Lee JS, Dixon DO, Kantarjian HM, et al: Prognosis of chronic lymphocytic leukemia: A multivariate regression analysis of 325 untreated patients. *Blood* 1987; 69:929–936.
21. Montserrat E, Rozman C: Prognostic factors in chronic lymphocytic leukemia. In, Polliack A, Catovsky D (eds): *Chronic Lymphocytic Leukemia*. Chur, Switzerland, Harwood Academic Publishers, 1988, pp. 111–122.
22. Rozman C, Montserrat E, Feliu E, et al: Prognosis of chronic lymphocytic leukemia: A multivariate survival analysis of 150 cases. *Blood* 1982; 59:1001–1005.
23. Geisler C, Larsen JK, Andersen E, et al: The CLL2 study: Preliminary results of flow cytometry immunophenotyping in the first 500 patients. *Nouv Rev Fr Hematol* 1986; 30:335–337.
24. Rozman C, Montserrat E, Viñolas N: Serum immunoglobulins in B-chronic lymphocytic leukemia. Natural history and prognostic significance. *Cancer* 1988; 61:279–283.
25. Gahrton G, Juliusson G, Karl-Henrik R: Chromosomal aberrations in chronic lymphocytic leukemia. In, Polliack A, Catovsky D (eds): *Chronic Lymphocytic Leukemia*. Chur, Switzerland, Harwood Academic Publishers, 1988, pp 289–304.
26. Han T, Sadamori N, Block AMW, et al: Cytogenetic studies in chronic lymphocytic leukemia, prolymphocytic leukemia and hairy cell leukemia: A progress report. *Nouv Rev Fr Hematol* 1988; 30:393–395.
27. Viñolas N, Urbano Ispizua A, Reverter JC, et al: Lymphocyte doubling time in chronic lymphocytic leukemia: An update of its prognostic significance. *Blood Cells* 1987; 12:457–70.
28. Juliusson G, Robert KH, Nilsson B, Gahrton G: Prognostic value of B-cell mitogen-induced and spontaneous thymidine uptake in vitro in chronic B-lymphocytic leukaemia cells. *Br J Haematol* 1985; 60:429–36.
29. Rozman C, Montserrat E: Bone marrow biopsy in chronic lymphocytic leukemia. In, Polliack A, Catovsky D (eds): *Chronic Lymphocytic Leukemia*. Chur, Switzerland, Harwood Academic Publishers, 1988, pp 184–191.
30. Montserrat E, Rozman C: Bone marrow biopsy in chronic lymphocytic leukaemia: A study of 208 cases. *Haematologia* 1983; 16:73–79.
31. Rozman C, Montserrat E, Rodriguez-Fernandez JM, et al: Bone marrow histologic pattern—the best single prognostic parameter in chronic lymphocytic leukemia: A multivariate survival analysis of 329 cases. *Blood* 1984; 64:642–648.
32. Pangalis GA, Roussou PA, Kittas C, et al: Patterns of bone marrow involvement in chronic lymphocytic leukemia and small lymphocytic (well differentiated) non-Hodgkin's lymphoma: Its clinical significance in relation to their differential diagnosis and prognosis. *Cancer* 1984; 54:702–708.
33. Pangalis GA, Boussiotis VA, Kittas C: B-chronic lymphocytic leukemia. Disease progression of 150 untreated stage A and B patients as predicted by bone marrow pattern. *Nouv Rev Fr Hematol* 1988; 30:373–375.

34. Rubinstein DB, Longo DL: Peripheral destruction of platelets in chronic lymphocytic leukemia: Recognition, prognosis and therapeutic implications. *Am J Med* 1981; 71:729–732.
35. Geisler C, Hansen MM: Chronic lymphocytic leukaemia: A test of a proposed new clinical staging system. *Scand J Haematol* 1981; 27:279–286.
36. Manoharan A, Phadke KP, Pitney WR: Prognostic factors in chronic lymphocytic leukaemia [letter]. *Lancet* 1980; 1:592.
37. Bernadou A, Bernard J, Bilski-Pasquier G, Bousser J: Prognosis in chronic lymphatic leukemia. *Ann Med Interne (Paris)* 1973; 124:549–560.
38. Montserrat E, Viñolas N, Reverter JC, Rozman C: Natural history of chronic lymphocytic leukemia: On the progression and prognosis of early clinical stages. *Nouv Rev Fr Hematol* 1988; 30:359–361.
39. French Cooperative Group on Chronic Lymphocytic Leukemia: Therapy of chronic lymphocytic leukemia patients—results from the French cooperative trials. *Semin Hematol* 1987; 24:275–290.
40. Catovsky D, Fooks J, Richards S: Prognostic factors in chronic lymphocytic leukaemia: The importance of age, sex and response to treatment survival. The UK Medical Research Council CLL trials 1 and 2. *Br J Haematol* 1989; 72:141–149.
41. Knospe WH, Loeb V Jr, Huguley CM Jr: Bi-weekly chlorambucil treatment of chronic lymphocytic leukemia. *Cancer* 1974; 33:555–562.
42. Han T, Ezdinli EZ, Sokal JE: Complete remission in chronic lymphocytic leukemia and leukolymphosarcoma. *Cancer* 1967; 20:243–252.
43. Kaung DT, Whittington RM, Spencer HH, Patno ME: Comparison of chlorambucil and streptonigrin (NSC-45383) in the treatment of chronic lymphocytic leukemia. *Cancer* 1969; 23:597–600.
44. Han T, Ezdinli EZ, Shimaoka K, Desai DV: Chlorambucil vs combined chlorambucil corticosteroid therapy in chronic lymphocytic leukemia. *Cancer* 1973; 31:502–508.
45. Sawitsky A, Rai KB, Glidewell C, Silver RT: Comparison of daily versus intermittent chlorambucil and prednisone therapy in the treatment of patients with chronic lymphocytic leukemia. *Blood* 1977; 50:1049–1059.
46. Ezdinli EZ, Stutzman L: Chlorambucil therapy for lymphomas and chronic lymphocytic leukemia. *JAMA* 1965; 191:444–450.
47. Galton DAG, Wiltshaw F, Szur L, Dacie JV: The use of chlorambucil and steroids in the treatment of chronic lymphocytic leukemia. *Br J Haematol* 1961; 7:73–97.
48. Jaksic B, Brugiatelli B: High dose continuous chlorambucil vs intermittent chlorambucil plus prednisone for treatment of B-CLL—IGCI CLL-01 trial. *Nouv Rev Fr Hematol* 1988; 30:437–442.
49. Huguley CM Jr: Treatment of chronic lymphocytic leukemia with triethylene melamine (TEM) and chlorambucil (CB-1348). *Cancer Chemother Rep* 1963; 30:27–43.
50. Liepman M, Votaw ML: The treatment of chronic lymphocytic leukemia with COP chemotherapy. *Cancer* 1978; 41:1664–1669.
51. Oken MM, Kaplan ME: Combination chemotherapy with cyclophosphamide, vincristine, and prednisone in the treatment of refractory chronic lymphocytic leukemia. *Cancer Treat Rep* 1979; 63:441–447.

52. Montserrat E, Rozman C: Combination chemotherapy in chronic lymphocytic leukemia: A brief review. *Nouv Rev Fr Hematol* 1984; 26:87–93.
53. Kempin S, Lee BH III, Thaler HT, et al: Combination chemotherapy of advanced chronic lymphocytic leukemia: The M-2 protocol (vincristine, BCNU, cyclophosphamide, melphalan and prednisone). *Blood* 1982; 60:1110–1121.
54. French Cooperative Group on Chronic Lymphocytic Leukemia: Effectiveness of "CHOP" regimen in advanced untreated chronic lymphocytic leukaemia. *Lancet* 1986; 2:1346–1349.
55. French Cooperative Group on Chronic Lymphocytic Leukemia: CHOP regimen versus intermittent chlorambucil–prednisone in stage B chronic lymphocytic leukemia—short term results from a randomized clinical trial. *Nouv Rev Fr Hematol* 1988; 30:449–452.
56. Keating MJ, Hester JP, McCredie KB, et al: Long-term results of CAP therapy in chronic lymphocytic leukemia. *Leuk Lymphoma* 1990; 2:391–397.
57. Keating MJ, Scouros M, Murphy S, et al: Multiple agent chemotherapy (POACH) in previously treated and untreated patients with chronic lymphocytic leukemia. *Leukemia* 1988; 2:157–164.
58. Hansen MM, Anderson E, Christensen BE, et al: CHOP versus prednisone + chlorambucil in chronic lymphocytic leukemia (CLL): Preliminary results of a randomized trial. *Nouv Rev Fr Hematol* 1988; 30:433–436.
59. Montserrat E, Alcala A, Parody R, et al: Treatment of chronic lymphocytic leukemia in advanced stages. A randomized trial comparing chlorambucil plus prednosone versus cyclophosphamide, vincristine, and prednisone. *Cancer* 1985; 56:2369–2375.
60. Montserrat E, Alcala A, Alonso C, et al: A randomized trial comparing chlorambucil plus prednisone vs cyclophosphamide, melphalan, and prednisone in the treatment of chronic lymphocytic leukemia stages B and C. *Nouv Rev Fr Hematol* 1988; 30:429–432.
61. Keller JW, Knospe WH, Raney M, et al: Treatment of chronic lymphocytic leukemia using chlorambucil and prednisone with or without cycle-active consolidation chemotherapy. *Cancer* 1986; 58:1185–1192.
62. Idestrom K, Kimby E, Bjorkholm M, et al: Treatment of chronic lymphocytic leukaemia and well-differentiated lymphocytic lymphoma with continuous low- or intermittent high-dose prednimustine versus chlorambucil/prednisolone. *Eur J Cancer* 1986; 18:1117–1123.
63. Grever MR, Siaw MFE, Jacob WF: The biochemical and clinical consequences of 2'-deoxycoformycin in refractory lymphoproliferative malignancy. *Blood* 1981; 57:406–417.
64. Keating MJ, Kantarjian H, Talpaz M, et al: Fludarabine therapy in chronic lymphocytic leukemia (CLL). *Nouv Rev Fr Hematol* 1988; 30:461–466.
65. Piro LD, Carrera CJ, Beutler E, Carson DA: 2-Chlorodeoxyadenosine: An effective new agent for the treatment of chronic lymphocytic leukemia. *Blood* 1988; 72:1069–1073.
66. LePage GA, Khaliq A, Gottlieb JA: Studies of 9-β-D-arabinofuranosyladenine in man. *Drug Metab Dispos* 1973; 1:756–759.
67. Brockman RW, Schabel FM Jr, Montgomery JA: Biologic activity of 9-β-D-

arabinofuranosyl-2-fluoroadenine. A metabolically stable analog of 9-β-D-arabinofuranosyladenine. *Biochem Pharmacol* 1977; 26:2193–2196.
68. Plunkett W, Chubb S, Alexander L, Montgomery JA: Comparison of the toxicity and metabolism of 9-β-D-arabinofuranosyl-2-fluoroadenine and 9-β-D-arabinofuranosyladenine in human lymphoblastoid cells. *Cancer Res* 1980; 40:2349–2355.
69. Grever MR, Kopecky KJ, Coltman CA, et al: Fludarabine monophosphate: A potentially useful agent in chronic lymphocytic leukemia. *Nouv Rev Fr Hematol* 1988; 30:457–459.
70. Keating MJ, Kantarjian H, Talpaz M, et al: Fludarabine: A new agent with major activity against chronic lymphocytic leukemia. *Blood* 1989; 74:19–25.
71. Keating MJ, Kantarjian H, O'Brien S, et al: Fludarabine (FLU)–prednisone (PRED): A safe effective combination in refractory chronic lymphocytic leukemia (CLL) [abstr]. *Proc Am Soc Clin Oncol* 1989; 8:201.
72. Keating MJ, Kantarjian H, O'Brien S, et al: Fludarabine: A new agent with marked cytoreductive activity in untreated chronic lymphocytic leukemia. *J Clin Oncol* 1991; 9:44–49.
73. Grever MR, Leiby JM, Kraut EH, et al: Low-dose deoxycoformycin in lymphoid malignancy. *J Clin Oncol* 1985; 3:1196–1201.
74. O'Dwyer PJ, Wagner B, Leyland-Jones B, et al: 2-Deoxycoformycin (pentostatin) for lymphoid malignancies. *Ann Intern Med* 1988; 108:733–743.
75. Dillman RO, Mick R, McIntyre OR: Pentostatin in chronic lymphocytic leukemia: A Phase II trial of Cancer and Leukemia Group B. *J Clin Oncol* 1989; 7:433–438.
76. Riddell S, Johnston JB, Bowman D, et al: 2-Deoxycoformycin (DCF) in chronic lymphatic leukemia (CLL) and Waldenstrom's macroglobulinemia (WM). *Proc Am Soc Clin Oncol* 1985; 4:651.
77. Foon KA, Bottino GC, Fer MF, et al: Phase II trial of recombinant leukocyte A interferon in patients with advanced chronic lymphocytic leukemia. *Am J Med* 1985; 78:216–220.
78. Shulof RS, Lloyd MJ, Stallings JJ, et al: Recombinant leukocyte A interferon in B-cell chronic lymphocytic leukemia: In vivo effects on autologous antitumor immunity. *J Biol Resp Mod* 1985; 4:310–323.
79. Talpaz M, Rosenblum M, Kurzrock R, et al: Clinical and laboratory changes induced by alpha interferon in chronic lymphocytic leukemia—A pilot study. *Am J Hematol* 1987; 24:341–350.
80. O'Connell MJ, Colgan JP, Oken MM, et al: Clinical trial of recombinant leukocyte A interferon as initial therapy for favorably histology non-Hodgkin's lymphomas and chronic lymphocytic leukemia. An Eastern Cooperative Oncology Group pilot study. *J Clin Oncol* 1986; 4:128–136.
81. Pangalis GA, Griva E: Recombinant alfa-2b-interferon therapy in untreated, stages A and B chronic lymphocytic leukemia. *Cancer* 1988; 61:869–872.
82. Rozman C, Montserrat E, Vinolas N, et al: Recombinant alpha2-interferon in the treatment of B chronic lymphocytic leukemia in early stages. *Blood* 1988; 71:1295–1298.
83. Boussiotis VA, Pangalis GA: Randomized clinical trial with alpha2b-interferon

stage A untreated B-chronic lymphocytic leukemia patients. *Nouv Rev Fr Hematol* 1988; 30:471–474.

84. Ziegler-Heitbrock HWL, Schlag R, Flieger D, Thiel E: Favorable response of early stage B CLL patients to treatment with IFN-alpha$_2$. *Blood* 1989; 73:1426–1430.
85. Kay NE, Oken MM, Maaza JJ, Bradley EC: Evidence for tumor reduction in refractory or relapsed B-CLL patients with infusional interleukin-2. *Nouv Rev Fr Hematol* 1988; 30:475–478.
86. Foon KA, Schroff RW, Bunn PA, et al: Effects of monoclonal antibody therapy in patients with chronic lymphocytic leukemia. *Blood* 1984; 64:1085–1093.
87. Hertler AA, Schlossman DM, Borowitz MJ, et al: A Phase I study of T101-ricin A chain immunotoxin in refractory chronic lymphocytic leukemia. *J Biol Resp Mod* 1988; 7:97–113.
88. Nadler L, Breitmeyer J, Coral F, et al: Anti-B4 blocked immunotherapy for patients with B cell malignancies: Phase I trial of bolus infusions [abstr]. Proceedings of the 31st Annual Meeting of the American Society of Hematology. *Blood* 1989; 74:121a.
89. Bergsagel DE: The chronic leukemias: A review of disease manifestations and the aims of therapy. *Can Med Assoc J* 1967; 96:1615–1620.
90. Hamblin TJ, Oscier DG, Young BJ: Autoimmunity in chronic lymphocytic leukemia. *J Clin Pathol* 1986; 39:713–716.
91. DeRossi G, Granati L, Gandolfo G, et al: Incidence and prognostic significance of autoantibodies against erythrocytes and platelets in chronic lymphocytic leukemia (CLL). *Nouv Rev Fr Hematol* 1988; 30:403–406.
92. Tura S, Finelli C, Bandini G, et al: Cyclosporin A in the treatment of CLL associated PRCA and bone marrow hypoplasia. *Nouv Rev Fr Hematol* 1988; 30:479–481.
93. Ferrant A, Michaux J-L, Sokal G: Splenectomy in advanced chronic lymphocytic leukemia. *Cancer,* 1986; 58:2130–2135.
94. Pegourie B, Sotto J-J, Hollard D, et al: Splenectomy during chronic lymphocytic leukemia. *Cancer* 1987; 59:1626–1630.
95. Cooper IA, Ding JC, Adams PB, et al: Intensive leukapheresis in the management of cytopenias in patients with chronic lymphocytic leukemia (CLL) and lymphocytic lymphoma. *Am J Hematol* 1979; 6:387–398.
96. Rozman C, Montserrat E, Vinolas N: Serum immunoglobulins in B-chronic lymphocytic leukemia. Natural history and prognostic significance. *Cancer* 1988; 61:279–283.
97. Fairley GH, Scott RB: Hypogammaglobulinaemia in chronic lymphatic leukaemia. *Br Med J* 1961; 2:920–924.
98. Chapel H: Infectious complications in chronic lymphocytic leukemia. In, Polliack A, Catovsky D (eds): *Chronic Lymphocytic Leukemia*. Chur, Switzerland, Harwood Academic Publishers, 1988; pp 249–262.
99. Shaw RK, Szwed C, Boggs DR, et al: Infection and immunity in chronic lymphocytic leukemia. *Arch Intern Med* 1966; 106:467–478.
100. Cooperative Group for the Study of Immunoglobulin in Chronic Lymphocytic Leukemia: Intravenous immunoglobulin for the prevention of infection in chronic lymphocytic leukemia. *N Engl J Med* 1988; 319:902–907.

6

Therapy for Multiple Myeloma and Related Diseases

Bart Barlogie*

University of Texas
M. D. Anderson Cancer Center
Houston, Texas

This chapter will attempt to bring into perspective available treatment options for patients with solitary or multiple myeloma and with Waldenstrom's macroglobulinemia. The practicing hematologist and oncologist may be provided, thereby, with a guide to differential therapy, with the overall goal of achieving the longest possible survival and assuring a high quality of life.

Multiple myeloma and Waldenstrom's macroglobulinemia belong to a group of hematological malignancies that have not yet benefited from progress in cytotoxic and biological therapy. Thus, about 25 years after the introduction of melphalan and chlorambucil, complete remissions with disappearance of monoclonal gammopathy remain rare and, despite recognition of a multitude of prognostic factors, especially in myeloma, survival curves are characterized by a constant death rate, even for patients with the lowest risk. Over the last 5 years, however, insight into the disease's biology has deepened (reviewed in Ref. 1); and promising new regimens (2), novel modes of therapy (3), and new treatment concepts have been developed (4,5). These include the recognition of interferon alpha (IFN-α) as an active agent in early and low-tumor-bulk myeloma (3,6,7); the identification of a steep dose–response effect for glucocorticoid hormones (2,8) and alkylating agents, especially melphalan (11,12); and the demonstration

*Present Address: University of Arkansas for Medical Sciences, Arkansas Cancer Research Center, Little Rock, Arkansas

of acceptable tolerance, even by older patients, of marrow ablative therapy with hematopoietic stem cell support (5,13,14); all of which are undergoing active investigation. Their appropriate use may well lead to a profound improvement in patient prognosis.

When contemplating treatment for patients with myeloma, several important questions concerning age and tumor staging must be posed. Although half of the patients will be older than 65, referral centers must address the needs of younger individuals who deserve special consideration to provide them with today's optimal care and yet preserve organ systems for future curative options. Because of its superior prognosis, with a potential for cure from local treatment, solitary plasmacytoma should be recognized (15). Similarly, benign monoclonal gammopathy represents a laboratory syndrome with clonal and neoplastic tumor cell features, the progression of which to overt myeloma is infrequent and extremely protracted (16,17).

MULTIPLE MYELOMA

The prognosis of patients with multiple myeloma has long been recognized as being associated closely with tumor burden (18). In recent years, determination of a single laboratory test, serum B_2-microglobulin (B2M), has provided better separation of risk groups than had been achieved with the more complex Durie–Salmon staging system (19–21). Most larger studies have, in addition, recognized an independent adverse impact of high tumor cell proliferative activity (22–24), and hypodiploidy as well as low plasma cell RNA content are both reliable indicators of resistance to standard therapy (25).

In an extensive daily practice of myeloma therapy, it has become clear that good-risk patients with more favorable B2M levels (less than 6 mg/L) or Durie–Salmon stages I or II, may deserve entirely different approaches. These will depend on the presence and extent of lytic bone lesions, which lead to the vexing problem of compression fractures and, ultimately, to complete immobilization. Careful radiographic staging with computed tomography (CT) and magnetic resonance imaging (MRI) have led to better definitions of early bone and associated soft-tissue disease, as well as focal marrow involvement, long before bone changes can be appreciated on roentgenograms. To derive a global plan of care aimed at preservation of physical activity, the presence and extent of bone disease should be considered more seriously if the relentless progression with complete immobility because of painful fractures is to be delayed more effectively in the future. Thus, the most effective systemic therapy should be applied promptly whenever multiple lesions involving the weight-bearing skeleton have been uncovered. With a long-term quality of life in mind, the following recommendations have been developed.

New Guidelines for Therapy

Serum B2M levels that are higher than 6 mg/L, hypercalcemia, renal failure, or severe anemia, with a hemoglobin level of less than 10 g/dL, all are sufficient indicators of high bulk disease necessitating initiation of the best available treatment without delay, regardless of extent and severity of bone disease. In the absence of these criteria, diffuse osteoporosis or the presence of more than two vertebral or pelvic lesions, even before visible bone destruction on standard roentgenograms, should prompt the same intensive therapy as already delineated. Patients lacking the aforementioned characteristics of advanced disease and who present with only one or two bone lesions may be offered milder forms of systemic therapy, such as high-dose dexamethasone (DEX) or IFN-α, or a combination thereof, with local radiotherapy as consolidation treatment.

In the absence of bone disease in vertebral bodies and pelvis and with low tumor mass criteria by standard measurements, cytotoxic therapy or high-dose glucocorticoid treatment may be deferred to evaluate such patients' sensitivity to IFN. Given the foregoing general concepts, specific treatment recommendations are put forth utilizing a novel staging system (Tables 1 and 2).

Stage I

Stage I is defined by the presence of normal levels of calcium and creatinine, modest anemia, and mild elevations of B2M and marrow plasmacytosis, but without roentgenographic or CT evidence of osteolytic disease in the spine or pelvis or marked bone marrow abnormalities on MRI scans of the axial skeleton (see Table 1). Such patients may be started on a regimen of recombinant IFN-α at daily doses of 5 MU/m^2. In the event of poor tolerance, frequently seen in patients over aged 65, dose reduction can be implemented by switching to an every-other-day schedule of the same initial dose or to a lower daily dose regiment, but no lower than 2 MU/m^2 three times weekly. Patients should be monitored carefully for changes in their disease indicators, including monoclonal protein in serum and urine, levels of uninvolved immunoglobulin isotypes, marrow plasmacytosis, and MRI examination of focal marrow lesions. In the absence of disease progression, IFN-α should be continued for at least 4 months, or longer, if at least improvement occurs and, certainly, if remission ensues, in which case tolerable doses of IFN-α may be prescribed indefinitely. Improvement would be defined by doubling of previously suppressed normal immunoglobulin levels, halving of myeloma protein in serum or urine, and recovery from anemia. Since IFN-α may aggravate anemia, therapy needs to be discontinued for 1 month at periodic intervals to recognize improvement of disease. An increase in serum B2M level should not be equated with disease progression, since this change also typically accompanies IFN-α therapy in responding patients.

Table 1 Classification of Stages

Stage	Abnormalities present: Laboratory	Abnormalities present: Radiology[b]
I[a]	B2M, but ≤ 6 mg/L Hb, but > 10.5 g/dL Marrow plasmacytosis (PC), but ≤ 30% Plasma cell-labeling index (PC-LI) ≤ 2% Uninvolved Ig suppressed	0
II	Same as in I	≤ 2
III	Same as in II	> 2
IV	B2M > 6 mg/L Hb ≤ 10.5 g/dL Marrow PC > 30% PC-LI > 2% LDH > 2x normal Ca elevated (>10.5 mg/dL) Creatinine elevated (>1.7 mg/dL)	0 or any

[a]Rule out benign monoclonal gammopathy; repeated measurements at monthly intervals recommended before IFN-α to distinguish "indolent myeloma."
[b]Standard bone roentgenograms; CT of spine and pelvis; MRI of spine and pelvis at diagnosis.

Stage II

Such patients have laboratory profiles identical to those with stage I disease, but with the addition of up to two osteolytic or two major bone marrow lesions in spine or pelvis. To achieve prompt disease control, high-dose glucocorticoids in standard fashion as practiced in the vincristine, doxorubicin (Adriamycin), dexamethasone (VAD) program should be evaluated for at least 3 months. In the absence of tumor regression by 75% on CT or MRI studies, similar reduction in myeloma protein and in marrow plasmacytosis, cytotoxic chemotherapy with cyclophosphamide–VAD (C-VAD) or melphalan–prednisone (MP) should be employed, as used for stage III disease. Responding patients should be offered local radiotherapy for response consolidation and IFN-α for remission maintenance at doses and schedules delineated for stage I disease, for at least 2 years, following which a lower-dose schedule should be pursued indefinitely.

Table 2 Proposal for Therapy of Untreated Multiple Myeloma

	Induction	Consolidation	Maintenance
Low risk			
Stage I	IFN 5 MU/m^2	None	IFN-$\alpha \geq 2$ MU/m^2 indefinitely
Stage II	DEX pulsing	XRT to involved bone and marrow	IFN-$\alpha \geq 2$ MU/m^2 indefinitely
High Risk			
Stages III,IV			
< 45 yr	VADiPAM	HDM 200 mg/m^2 or HDM 140 mg/m^2 + TBI 850–1020 cGy auto or allo BMT	CR, none until relapse $<$ CR, IFN-$\alpha \geq 2$ MU/m^2 indefinitely
45–65 yr	VADiPAM	As above	IFN-$\alpha \geq 2$ MU/m^2 indefinitely
		or	
		cyclic reinduction with VADIPAM q 6–8 mo $\times$ 3 yr	IFN-$\alpha \geq 2$ MU/m^2 between reinduction and then indefinitely
> 65 yr Zubrod < 2	VADiPAM or VADiCYCLO	Cyclic reinduction with VAD alternating with cyclophosphamide 3 mo $\times$ 3 yr	IFN-$\alpha \geq 2$ MU/m^2 between reinduction and then indefinitely
Zubrod ≥ 2	Standard VAD alternating with MP	None	Standard MP or IFN-$\alpha \geq 2$ MU/m^2 indefinitely

VAD, DEX, see Table 3.
VADiPAM, standard VAD alternating with IV melphalan 50–70 mg/m^2.
VADiCYCLO, standard VAD alternating with IV cyclophosphamide 1.5–2 g/m^2.

Stages III and IV (High-Risk Myeloma)

The presence of diffuse osteoporosis or of more than two osteolytic lesions in spine or pelvis, without major laboratory abnormalities (stage III); or of markers of advanced systemic disease (high levels of B2M, calcium; renal failure, and severe anemia; stage IV), regardless of bone and bone marrow involvement, should prompt initiation of optimal chemotherapy. Stages III and IV account for

75% of all patients with multiple myeloma, and the following section will review results of published trials and propose regimens likely to have a favorable impact on long-term prognosis.

Which Is the Best Primary Therapy for High-Risk Multiple Myeloma in the 1990s?

The myeloma investigative community seems to be in agreement that the addition of other cytotoxic drugs to standard melphalan and prednisone (MP) has not improved survival markedly (1, 2–29). Promising leads have been reported for the addition of IFN-α to remission-induction therapy, with a M2-like regimen (30) or with IFN-α as maintenance therapy, once response has been accomplished with either standard MP or vincristine, melphalan, cyclophosphamide, prednisone–vincristine, carmustine, doxorubicin, prednisone (VMCP-VBAP) (6).

Several groups have reported pilot trials on the use of high-dose chemotherapy or chemoradiotherapy requiring autologous or allogeneic hemopoietic stem cell support (5,11,13,14). These studies can be summarized by stating that, with allogeneic bone marrow transplantation (BMT), complete remissions can be obtained in about 40% of patients and that their relapse-free and overall survival seems to be more favorable when treatment was administered early, when drug resistance had not yet developed, and tumor burden was less advanced (31). Since multiple myeloma typically affects an elderly patient population and since the mortality from allogeneic transplantation increases sharply with age (mainly from graft-vs-host disease; GVHD), autologous stem cell support with marrow or blood has also been investigated (4,5,11,13,14,32,33). Complete remissions seem to occur at a lower frequency (about 20%) and are less durable than after allogeneic transplantation, even when such approaches have been applied in remission (13,14). Questions on the role of reinfused autologous tumor cells and of a graft-vs-myeloma effect are currently being discussed. Analysis of response kinetics has indicated that high-dose regimens currently in use with autologous stem cell support are not sufficiently cytoreductive. Accordingly, most investigators consider greater cytoreduction, as part of high-dose therapy before transplantation, with maintenance treatment after transplantation, as important strategies to offset the lack of a graft-vs-tumor effect with allogeneic grafts.

An obvious question concerns the management of patients who relapse after marrow ablative therapy. Recent studies from the M. D. Anderson Cancer Center indicate that subsequent survival is longest when the time from marrow ablative to salvage treatment exceeded 6 months, and when tumor burden and tumor grade characteristics such as B2M and LDH, respectively, were low (34).

The current state of therapy development can be summarized by noting that (1) VAD induces marked and fast cytoreduction in about 70% of patients, without prolonging survival, perhaps owing to a preferential effect on differentiated tumor cells (1); (2) high doses of melphalan (HDM) are effective in about 50% of patients with VAD-refractory myeloma and in almost all patients when administered together with TBI; (3) IFN-α is active only when tumor mass is low or cytotoxic drug resistance is not yet established. Thus, there are at least three independently active regimens (VAD, HDM, IFN-α), that can be offered to patients with symptomatic myeloma, and the following general guidelines deserve consideration (see Table 2).

Age Younger Than 45

All younger patients with multiple myeloma should be carefully evaluated for the availability of suitable marrow donors. Depending on the individual's acceptance of a treatment-associated mortality, mainly from GVHD, of 25–30% for the 30–40% chance of durable disease control, such patients may opt for prompt allogeneic BMT applied in remission from standard induction treatment with programs like VAD, with or without cyclophosphamide, or for primary resistant disease. Unlike the situation with acute leukemia and chronic myelogenous leukemia for which a higher relapse-free survival rate of 60–70% can be expected, the inferior prognosis in multiple myeloma probably reflects suboptimal conditioning treatment, justifying deferral of allogeneic BMT, pending further progress to reduce treatment-associated toxicity and improve its efficacy.

The next best option for such patients consists of a program that incorporates maximum cytoreduction with marrow ablation and autologous hemopoietic stem cell support. Fast cytoreduction can be achieved with CVAD, which seems to be insufficient, however, for durable remissions to be achieved with subsequently administered melphalan plus TBI (14). Better cytoreduction can be expected from rotating regimens of VAD and intermediate to high doses of melphalan without marrow support and with added IFN-α as both a cytoreductive and immunorestorative agent. Thus, a program of VADIPAM with initial VAD and alternating cycles of IV melphalan (PAM) at 50–70 mg/M^2 with intervening IFN-α appears ideally suited to achieve maximum cytoreduction before autologous marrow or blood harvest. Marrow-ablative therapy can then be carried out with either high doses of melphalan alone at 200 mg/m^2 (13) or at a lower dose of 140 mg/m^2 with added TBI (5,14), or with standard cyclophosphamide and TBI. With persistence of myeloma protein following marrow ablative therapy, recombinant IFN-α should be given as maintenance treatment indefinitely. In the absence of an allogeneic donor, additional autologous marrow may be harvested when sufficient time has elapsed to permit sufficient hematopoietic recovery with normal marrow cellularity and megakaryopoiesis, as the best indicator of stem cell function. In vitro analysis of hematopoietic precursor growth may aid in the timing of a second marrow harvest to be used for a second high-dose treatment for disease relapse that is no longer responsive to standard therapy. This approach, however, should be considered only if the first high-dose treatment provided a sufficiently long remission of at least 2 years.

There are insufficient data to advocate blood over bone marrow as a source of autologous hematopoietic stem cells. The presence of circulating clonal cells, often with an earlier B-cell phenotype than that of mature plasma cells, calls into question seriously the initial notion that autologous blood stem cell support might be associated with a lower risk of reseeding autologous tumor cells (35,36).

Ages 45 to 65

If patients in this age group have good performance, such that treatment-related mortality is under 10% and their non–tumor-related prognosis is at least 10 years, the foregoing approach, with autologous stem cell support, as delineated for younger patients, can also be pursued. Alternatively, VADIPAM treatment could be offered both for remission induction and for cyclic reinduction every 6–8 months, during which time IFN-α maintenance treatment should be given. Autologous stem cells harvested at the end of the initial induction phase can be used to support marrow ablative treatment when relapse develops during IFN-α maintenance treatment. Thus, cyclic VADIPAM treatment would be discontinued when marked cytoreduction can no longer be maintained during 6–8 months of IFN-α administration.

Aged Older Than 65 with Good Performance

Such individuals may be offered VADIPAM or VAD plus cyclophosphamide (causing, even at high doses, more predictable and shorter duration of myelosuppression than melphalan), with IFN-α maintenance therapy. These patients probably would not benefit from consideration of high-dose therapy, except in unusual circumstances.

Poor Performance Presentation Not Relieved with VAD or VADIPAM

Patients with recurrent pulmonary infections as a result of myelosuppression or with other organ disease related or unrelated to myeloma can be managed with standard MP, alternating with VAD and, subsequent IFN-α maintenance.

Refractory Myeloma

Depending on the history of prior treatment exposure and responsiveness, a variety of regimens with good short-term efficacy and palliation are now available (Table 3). The most crucial variable determining responsiveness to most salvage regimens concerns the presence of primary drug resistance and its duration (1). Thus, except for hypodiploidy or disease with low plasma cell RNA index, VAD effects remissions in 50% of patients if the duration of primary resistance does not exceed 12 months (Fig. 1). In the absence of response to myelosuppressive drug regimens with MP or VMCP-VBAP for over 1 year, VAD is effective in no more than 30% of patients, a result similar to that achieved with dexamethasone (DEX) alone (8). Dexamethasone induces remission both by a direct tumor cytolytic effect and perhaps, indirectly, by suppres-

Table 3 Salvage Regimens for Refractory Myeloma

Regimen	Drug	Dose	Route	Days
DEX	Dexamethasone	40 mg	IV or PO	1–4
				9–12
				17–20
VAD	Vincristine,	0.5 mg	CI[a]	1–4
	doxorubicin,	10 mg/m^2	CI	1–4
	dexamethasone	40 mg	IV or PO	1–4
				9–12
				17–20
HDM	Melphalan	70–140 mg/m^2	IV	1
EDAP	Etoposide,	100–200 mg/m^2	CI	1–4
	Dexamethasone,	40 mg	IV	1–5
	Ara-C,	1 g/m^2	IV	5
	Cisplatin	25 mg/m^2	CI	1–4
HDM	Melphalan,	180 mg/m^2	IV	1–2
	BMT			4
HDM-TBI	Melphalan,	140 mg/m^2	IV	1
	TBI	170 cGy		4–6
		q12hr × 5		
				6 or 7

[a]Continuous infusion.

sion of the recently recognized major myeloma growth factor, interleukin-6 (IL-6), which is produced by many normal tissue accessory cells and by some tumor cells themselves (37–39).

High-dose melphalan (HDM) has been evaluated mainly in VAD-refractory myeloma, and it seems to overcome, but only at doses ≥90 mg/m^2, those conditions of primary drug resistance that are associated with unfavorable nucleic acid features such as hypodiploidy and low RNA content (1,40). Also, in contrast with VAD, HDM ≥ 90 mg/m^2 induced remission rates of over 40%, regardless of the duration of primary drug resistance (see Fig. 1). When autologous hematopoietic stem cells are available, TBI added to melphalan further enhances the incidence and duration of remission (5,14).

A four-drug combination termed EDAP (combining continuous infusions of etoposide and cisplatin, together with dexamethasone pulsing and high-dose cytarabine (cytosine arabinoside), similar to a regimen with great efficacy in aggressive lymphoma) (41) effects remission in 40% of patients, regardless of the foregoing prognostic factors and even after resistance to HDM has been established (42), as well as in high-grade myeloma with high serum levels of LDH (43) (see Fig. 1).

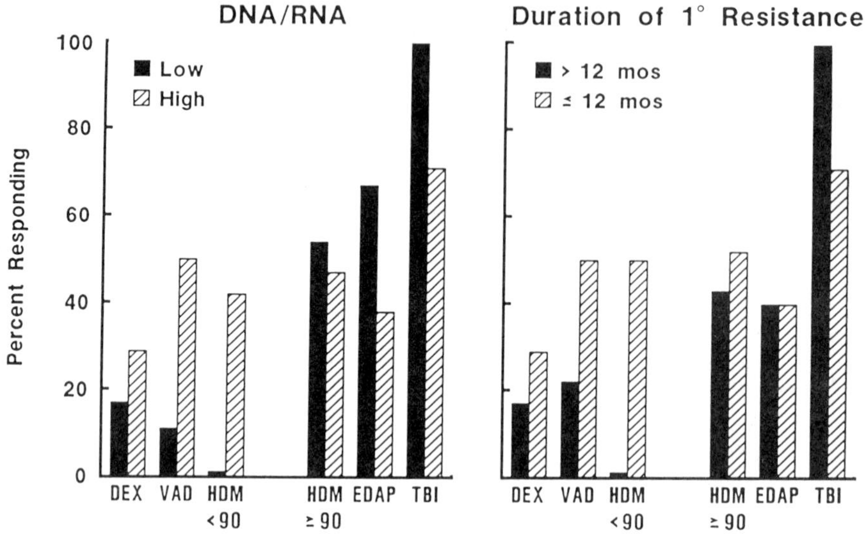

Figure 1 Responses to salvage therapy depended on a variety of pretreatment variables, especially plasma cell DNA–RNA content and long primary drug resistance. The adverse influence of these features was observed mainly after treatment with DEX, VAD, and melphalan at doses of less than 90 mg/m^2, whereas these variables did not affect response to EDAP, higher melphalan doses (>90 mg/m^2), and TBI-containing regimens.

It is conceivable that judicious use of all of the aforementioned salvage programs early during the development of drug resistance might still yield durable disease control. The use of VADIPAM salvage, with consolidation involving melphalan and TBI, would appear logical. Alternatively, EDAP or similar regimens with marked, but short lasting, myelosuppression can be explored in conjunction with hematopoietic growth factors such as granulocyte–macrophage colony-stimulating factor (GM-CSF).

For those patients with refractory myeloma who are younger than 45, suitable allogeneic donors should be identified. Recent notions of successful allotransplantation from HLA-compatible unrelated donors or partially mismatched related donors should all be considered for the young patient seeking more than palliation of typically under 1 year.

Special Conditions

Organ Compromise with Amyloidosis or Light-Chain Deposition Disease

Occasionally, the sequelae of monoclonal plasma cell proliferation lead to the patient's death in the absence of marked tumor progression. For example, amyloidosis and light-chain deposition disease can impair renal and cardiac function irreversibly. Therefore, it is mandatory to recognize the onset of such conditions promptly; for example, in the context of persistent renal failure, despite marked improvement in Bence Jones proteinuria, or when cardiomegaly develops without recognized risk factors including excessive doses of doxorubicin. The only known possibly effective intervention in such circumstances consists of treatment directed at reducing an even relatively small tumor burden so that further apposition of light chains or amyloid, with the attendant risk of irreversible organ damage, can be postponed. If this goal cannot be accomplished with standard-dose regimens, high-dose therapy requiring hematopoietic stem cell support should be seriously considered, especially in younger patients.

Although persistence of renal failure, per se, does not seem to affect survival adversely, independently of tumor burden (44), renal transplantation may reduce morbidity and permit the younger patient to undergo more safely high-dose therapy regimens.

Life-Threatening Metabolic Conditions

Hypercalcemia or renal failure represent oncologic emergencies requiring immediate intervention. Renal failure most often results from hypercalcemia or Bence Jones proteinuria with light chain cast nephropathy (44). Prompt hydration and initiation of active cytoreductive therapy are warranted.

Infections

Recurrent infections may interfere with the effective chemotherapeutic management of patients with high-risk myeloma. Intravenous immunoglobulins, which appear to be promising in chronic lymphocytic leukemia, deserve exploration in multiple myeloma as well (45). In addition, broad-spectrum antibiotics, such as trimethoprim–sulfamethoxazole or ciprofloxacin, can be useful in reducing the incidence and severity of infections in myeloma patients with already depressed immune status, which is often further aggravated by cytotoxic therapy.

Spinal Cord Compression

The clinical suggestion of spinal cord compression should always lead to proper delineation of the underlying problem, especially in those patients for whom the disease is newly diagnosed. When symptoms are vague, primary chemotherapy under close supervision is often successful. Marked resistance to chemotherapy seems to forecast resistance to ionizing radiation, especially in hypodiploid myeloma and disease with low RNA content. For the long-term management, it would appear better to treat early signs of cord compression with chemotherapy to establish treatment efficacy in vivo. There are rare circumstances of discordant genetic markers between marrow and soft tissue disease underlying the cord problem, which can be recognized only by proper tissue analysis, using fine-needle aspiration. In case of a solitary plasmacytoma, partial resection and tissue examination for ploidy would appear crucial to assure best local control. In hypodiploidy, HDM should be applied before or along with ionizing radiation.

Discussion and Perspective

Myeloma covers a broad spectrum of clinical disease syndromes. Symptoms result from marrow replacement with suppression of hematopoiesis, also by humoral factors (see Ref. 1) leading to anemia and, less frequently, to pancytopenia. The mechanisms of immunoparesis are still obscure.

Osteolytic lesions result from tumor cell release of cytokines (interleukin-1-β and tumor necrosis factor-β; TFN-β). Renal failure occurs most frequently in association with hypercalcemia and light chain cast nephropathy. Occasional multiorgan involvement is a consequence of amyloidosis and light chain deposition disease. Although only rarely leading to overt myeloma, benign monoclonal gammopathy may be a typical forerunner of the fully expressed disease syndrome in a high percentage of patients. Absence of all other laboratory and clinical abnormalities, including preserved normal immunoglobulins, supports this diagnosis, which does not require therapy, but does require regular follow-up. Solitary plasmacytoma of soft tissue or bone needs to be recognized with the aid of extensive high-resolution radiographic-imaging techniques and blood and bone marrow examination, so that potentially curative radiotherapy after surgical resection, in case of larger masses, or after high-dose alkylating agent therapy, in case of hypodiploid disease, can be administered.

The management of systemic multiple myeloma requires novel treatment approaches to improve patients' long-term prognosis. The use of non–cross-resistant drugs or drug combinations for patients with high B2M levels (>6mg/L) or with diffuse bone disease holds promise for greater cytoreduction in a larger proportion of patients who, dependent upon their age at disease presentation, would benefit from marrow ablative high-dose therapy as further remission consolidation with either autologous or allogeneic hematopoietic stem cell support. The additional use of IFN-α appears justified in view of promising results in patients with low tumor mass. It is hoped that the inclusion of patients with diffuse bone disease in this aggressive treatment schema will delay or even prevent the clinically vexing problems resulting from compression fractures.

Glucocorticoids and IFN-α with local radiation may suffice initially in patients with earlier disease stage and with limited bone lesions and, thereby, preserve sensitivity to cytotoxic drugs required in later disease phases.

Refractory myeloma provides the opportunity to develop novel and more effective treatment approaches. The key prognostic indicators for remission include the history of prior drug resistance and its duration. Combinations of VAD and HDM with stem cell-supported marrow ablative therapy for consolidation appear promising. With the notion that various interleukins, most notably IL-6, affect myeloma cell proliferation and differentiation, at least in vitro (37), clinical trials can be envisioned with radioisotope-conjugated IL-6 for localization of lethal therapy to IL-6 receptor-bearing tumor cells; alternatively, IL-6 may recruit myeloma cells into active proliferation for better subsequent cell kill by cytotoxic agents, an approach already under investigation in acute myeloid leukemia. Such exciting insights into disease biology and the already established role of IFN-α suggest strongly that more physiologically oriented approaches can be developed for the management of myeloma to correct abnormal expression or transduction of proliferation signals and, thereby, effectively prevent disease progression. If abnormal expression of c-*myc* (46) and H-*ras* oncogenes (47,48) emerge as crucial triggers or mediators of myeloma, molecular approaches of gene suppression can also be envisioned.

WALDENSTROM'S MACROGLOBULINEMIA

Only few systematic clinical trials have been reported for the management of patients with Waldenstrom's disease. Chlorambucil alone, or combined with glucocorticoids, and more recently, the M2 protocol have shown efficacy (49,50). Prognostic factors have not yet been clearly established, but are likely to include indicators of overall tumor burden, such as anemia (as a consequence of marked marrow lymphocytosis or TNF-α), lymphadenopathy and splenomegaly, and perhaps serum B2M levels.

Like other centers, we also have applied treatments that are active in myeloma and in CLL for the management of patients with macroglobulinemia. From experience with about 30 patients, high doses of glucocorticoids induced remissions in 15–20% of patients, VAD was active in a third, and HDM has produced marked remission in half-a-dozen individuals treated. The marked efficacy of fludarabine for refractory and, especially untreated, CLL (51) seems to extend to Waldenstrom's macroglobulinemia, with an estimated response rate of 50%. The EDAP regimen deserves exploration in refractory disease, especially when there is evidence of transformation to a higher histological grade.

It is currently impossible to provide the practicing hematologist–oncologist with treatment guidelines as detailed as for myeloma. A nationwide data base would be a first step to more reliably assess the prognosis of such patients in relationship to potential risk factors and therapeutic management.

ACKNOWLEDGMENT

The author gratefully acknowledges the invaluable help of Ms Kimberly Pruitt in preparing this manuscript. Supported in part by grants CA37161, CA28771 and CA23077 from the National Cancer Institute, National Institutes of Health, Bethesda, Maryland.

REFERENCES

1. Barlogie B, Epstein J, Selvanayagam P, Alexanian R: Plasma cell myeloma—new biological insights and advances in therapy. *Blood* 1989; 73:865–879.
2. Barlogie B, Smith L, Alexanian R: Effective treatment of advanced multiple myeloma refractory to alkylating agents. *N Engl J Med* 1984; 310:1353–1356.
3. Mellstedt H, Ahre A, Bjorkholm M, et al: Interferon therapy in myelomatosis. *Lancet* 1979; 1:245–247.
4. Barlogie B, Hall R, Zander A, et al: High dose melphalan with autologous bone marrow transplantation for multiple myeloma. *Blood* 1986, 67:1298.
5. Barlogie B, Alexanian R, Dicke K, et al: High dose chemoradiotherapy and autologous bone marrow transplantation for resistant multiple myeloma. *Blood* 1987; 70:869–72.
6. Mandelli F, Avvisati G, Amadori S, Boccadoro M, Gernone A, Lauta VM, Marmont F, Petrucci MT, Tribalto M, Vegna ML, Dammacco F., Pileri A: Maintenance treatment with alpha-2b recombinant interferon significantly improves response and survival duration in multiple myeloma patients responding to conventional induction chemotherapy results of an Italian randomized study. *N Engl J Med* 1990; 322(20):1430–1434.
7. Quesada JR, Alexanian R, Hawkins M, et al: Treatment of multiple myeloma with recombinant alpha-interferon. *Blood* 1986; 67:275–278.
8. Alexanian R, Barlogie B, Dixon D: High dose glucocorticoid treatment of resistant myeloma. *Ann Intern Med* 1986; 105:8.
9. McElwain TJ, Powles RL: High-dose intravenous melphalan for plasma-cell leukaemia and myeloma. *Lancet* 1983; 1:822.
10. Selby PF, McElwain TJ, Nandi AC, et al: Multiple myeloma treated with high dose intravenous melphalan. *Br J Haematol* 1987; 66:55.
11. Selby P, Zulian G, Forgeson G, et al: Developments in treatment of myeloma. *Acta Haematol* 1989; (in press).
12. Barlogie B, Alexanian R, Smallwood L, et al: Prognostic factors with high dose melphalan for refractory multiple myeloma. *Blood* 1988; 72:2015.
13. Gore ME, Viner C, Meldrum M, Bell J, Milan S, Zuiable A, Slevin M, Selby PJ, Clark PI, Millar B, Maitland JA, Judson IR, Tillyer C, Malpas JS, McElwain TJ: Intensive treatment of multiple myeloma and criteria for complete remission. *Lancet* 879, October 14, 1989.
14. Jagannath S, Barlogie B, Dicke KA, Alexanian R, Zagars G, Cheson B, LeMaistre

FC, Smallwood L, Pruitt K, Dixon DO: Autologous bone marrow transplantation in multiple myeloma: Identification of prognostic factors. *Blood,* 1990; 76:1860–1866.

15. Knowling MA, Haarwood AR, Bergasagel DE: Comparison of extramedullary plasmacytomas with solitary and multiple plasma cell tumors of the bone. *J Clin Oncol* 1983; 1:255.
16. Alexanian R: Localized and indolent myeloma. *Blood* 1980; 56:521.
17. Kyle RA, Greipp R: Smoldering multiple myeloma. *N Engl J Med* 1980; 302:1347.
18. Durie BGM, Salmon SE: A clinical staging system for multiple myeloma. Correlation of measured myeloma cell mass with presenting clinical features, response to treatment and survival. *Cancer* 1975; 36:842.
19. Child JA, Norfolk DR, Cooper EH: Serum beta-2 microglobulin in myelomatosis: Potential value in stratification and monitoring. *Br J Haematol* 1986; 63:406.
20. Bataille R, Grenier J, Sany J: beta-2 Microglobulin in myeloma: Optimal use for staging, prognosis and treatment—a prospective study of 160 patients. *Blood* 1984; 63:468.
21. Alexanian R, Barlogie B, Fritsche H: beta-2-Microgloblin in multiple myeloma. *Am J Hematol* 1985; 20:345.
22. Durie BGM, Salmon SE, Moon TE: pretreatment tumor mass, cell kinetics and prognosis in multiple myeloma. *Blood* 1980; 55:364.
23. Latreille J, Barlogie B, Dosik G, et al: Ploidy and proliferative characteristics in monoclonal gammopathies. *Blood* 1982; 59:43.
24. Greipp PR, Katzmann JA, O'Fallan WM, Kyle RA: Value of beta-2 microglobulin level and plasma cell labeling indices as prognostic factors in patients with newly diagnosed myeloma. *Blood* 1988; 72:219.
25. Barlogie B, Alexanian R, Smith L, et al: Prognostic implications of tumor cell DNA and RNA content in multiple myeloma. *Blood* 1985; 66:338.
26. Salmon SE, Haut A, Bonnet JD, et al: Alternating combination chemotherapy improves survival in multiple myeloma. A Southwest Oncology Group study. *J Clin Oncol* 1983; 1:453–457.
27. Alexanian R, Dreicer R: Chemotherapy for multiple myeloma. Cancer 1984; 53:583–588.
28. Peest D, Deicher H, Coldeway R, et al: Induction and maintenance therapy in multiple myeloma: A multicenter trial of MP versus VMCP. *Eur J Cancer Clin Oncol* 1988; 24:1061–1067.
29. Boccadoro M, Marmont F, Tribalto M, Avvisati G, et al: Multiple myeloma: VMCP/VBAP Alternating combination chemotherapy is not superior to melphalan and prednisone even in high-risk patients. *J Clin Oncol* 1991; 9(3):444–448.
30. Oken MM, Kyle RA, Greipp PR, et al: Alternating cycles of VBMCP with interferon (rIFN-alpha 2) in the treatment of multiple myeloma. *Proc Am Soc Clin Oncol* 1988; 7:868.
31. Barlogie B, Gahrton G: Bone marrow transplantation in multiple myeloma—a review. *Bone Narrow Trans,* in press, 1991.
32. Fermand J, Levy Y, Gerota J, et al: Treatment of aggressive multiple myeloma by high-dose chemotherapy and total body irradiation followed by blood stem cells autologous graft. *Blood* 1989; 73:20–23.

33. Ventura GJ, Barlogie B, Hester JP, Yau JC, Le Maistre CF, Wallerstein RO, Spinola JA, Dicke KA, Horwitz LH, Alexanian R: High dose cyclophosphamide, BCNU and VP-16 with autologous blood stem cell support for refractory multiple myeloma. *Bone Marrow Trans* 1990; 5:265–268.
34. Jagannath S, Barlogie B: Repeated high-dose therapy in refractory myelomatosis. 5th International Symposium on Autologous Bone Marrow Transplantation, in press, 1991.
35. Barlogie B, Latreille J, Swartzendruber D, et al: Quantitative cytology in myeloma research. In, Salmon SE (ed): *Clinics in Haematology*. London, WB Saunders, 1982, p 19.
36. Berenson J, Wong R, Kim K, et al: Evidence of peripheral blood B lymphocyte but not T lymphocyte involvement. *Blood* 1987; 70:1550.
37. Kawano M, Hirano T, Matsuda T, et al: Autocrine generation and requirement of BSF-2/IL-6 for human multiple myelomas. *Nature* 1988; 332:83.
38. Klein B, Zhang X-G, Jourdan M, et al: Paracrine but not autocrine regulation of myeloma-cell growth and differentiation by interleukin-6. *Blood* 1989; 73:517–526.
39. Kishimoto T: The biology of interleukin-6. *Blood* 1989; 74:1–10.
40. Barlogie B: Management of Multiple Myeloma. *Blut* 60:1–7, 1990
41. Velasquez W, Cabanillas F, Salvador P, et al: Effective salvage therapy for lymphoma with cisplatin in combination with high dose ara-C and dexamethasone (DHAP). *Blood* 1988; 71:117–22.
42. Barlogie B, Alexanian R, and Cabanillas F: Etoposide, dexamethasone, cytarabine and cisplatin in vincristine, doxorubicin, and dexamethasone-refractory myeloma. *JCO,* 7:1514–1517, 1989.
43. Barlogie B, Smallwood L, Smith T, Alexanian R: High serum levels of lactic dehydrogenase identify a high-grade lymphoma-like myeloma. *Ann Intern Med* 1989; 110:521–525.
44. Alexanian R, Barlogie B and Dixon D: Renal Failure in Multiple Myeloma: Pathogenesis and Prognostic Implications. *Arch Intern Med* 150:1693–1695, 1990.
45. Bunch C, Chapel HM, Dicato M, et al: Intravenous immunoglobulins for the prevention of infection in chronic lymphocytic leukemia: A randomized controlled clinical trial. *N Engl J Med* 1988; 319:902–907.
46. Selvanayagam P, Blick M, Narni F, et al: Alteration and abnormal expression of the c-*myc* oncogene in human multiple myeloma. *Blood* 1988; 71:30.
47. Tsuchiya H, Epstein J, Selvanayagam P, et al: Correlated flow cytometric analysis of H-*ras* p21 and nuclear DNA in multiple myeloma. *Blood* 1988; 72:796.
48. Seremetis S, Inghirami G, Ferrero D, et al: Transformation and plasmacytoid differentiation of EBV-infected human B lymphoblasts by *ras* oncogenes. Science 1989; 243:660–663.
49. Cohen R, Bohannon R, Wallerstein R: Waldenstrom's macroglobulinemia. A study of ten cases. *Am J Med* 1966; 41:274.
50. Case DC: Combination chemotherapy (M-2) protocol (BCNU, cyclophosphamide, vincristine, melphalan, and prednisone) for Waldenstrom's macroglobulinemia: Preliminary report. *Blood* 1982; 59:934–937.
51. Kantarjian HM, Alexanian R, Koller CA, Kurzrock R and Keating MJ: Fludarabine Therapy in macroglobulinemic lymphoma. *Blood* 75:1928–1931, 1990.

7

Hairy Cell Leukemia

Jorge R. Quesada

OnCol, Center for I.V. Therapies and Cancer Therapeutics
Houston, Texas

Hairy cell leukemia has been recognized as a distinct entity since 1958 (1). The origin of the malignant cell remained elusive until recently, when monoclonal antibodies and molecular probes to detect immunoglobulin gene rearrangements have clarified the B-cell nature of the great majority of cases (2–4). However, hairy cells can express monocytelike characteristics, phagocytic properties, and express the membrane receptor for interleukin-2, suggesting a unique stage of differentiation (4).

The natural history of hairy cell leukemia (HCL) is variable, with most typical cases progressing over a period of several years (1, 5). Occasionally, however, there are patients who harbor the disease indolently and without evidence of progression. Rarely, spontaneous remissions after an infectious process have been described (6, 7). These observations suggest that HCL is an entity that may be, under certain circumstances, still responsive to cell growth regulatory signals from the host's immune system.

Hairy cell leukemia characteristically infiltrates the bone marrow, spleen, and liver, resulting in pancytopenia and moderate to severe immunological deficits. Autopsy studies, however, have revealed infiltration of multiple other organs at a subclinical level (8). The impaired hematopoiesis and the state of immunodeficiency results in an increased susceptibility both to bacterial and opportunistic infections, the main cause of morbidity and mortality in HCL.

The pathogenetic mechanisms responsible for the pancytopenia in HCL remain unknown. A typical feature in the examination of the bone marrow of these patients is an increased amount of fibrin deposition, which frequently result in dry bone marrow taps (5). It is suspected that the abnormalities of the bone marrow stroma, a direct inhibitory influence from the malignant cells, or displacement of normal hematopoietic cell precursors by the leukemic infiltration may participate in the development of pancytopenia. Furthermore, hematopoiesis is regulated by complex cellular interactions between mononuclear phagocytes, lymphocytes, and bone marrow stromal cells by the production of growth factors or inhibitory signals. It is not known whether the immunological deficits described in HCL may play a significant role in the defective hematopoiesis caused by subnormal or absent production of hematopoietic growth factors.

A variety of abnormal functions of the immune system have been described in patients with HCL (9–11). Monocytopenia and defects of the monocyte function are ubiquitous to these patients. Cellular immunity defects include impaired delayed hypersensitivity to recall antigens, decreased antibody-dependent cellular cytotoxicity, decreased natural killer cell cytotoxicity, absolute deficiencies of B and T cells, inverted T-helper/T-suppressor cell ratio, and decreased lymphocyte responsiveness to mitogens and allogeneic and autologous cells (12). Humoral immunity, conversely, remains largely intact, as manifested by the capacity of these patients to synthesize antibodies. Nonetheless, a severe cellular immune deficit may be associated with a reduced humoral reactivity.

An impaired capacity to produce endogenous interferon has also been reported (14, 15). Patients with active disease and pancytopenia have a profound deficiency in their ability to produce endogenous interferon alpha. Even patients with a normal complement of monocytes and lymphocytes may show a subnormal production of interferon alpha (14).

THE CLINICAL EVALUATION OF HAIRY CELL LEUKEMIA

The diagnosis of HCL continues to be made primarily on the basis of a good clinical index of suspicion and morphological assessment of the bone marrow (1, 5). In any patient who presents with pancytopenia and splenomegaly, particularly in the abscence of peripheral adenopathy, HCL should be a diagnostic consideration. Bone marrow biopsy is mandatory because of the frequent occurrence of dry taps.

It is beyond the scope of this review to expand on the histological diagnosis of HCL. In addition to the typical morphological appearance of the malignant cells, a positive stain with tartrate-resistant acid phosphatase is a helpful histological feature, but it is not pathognomonic (16). Bone marrow trephine biopsy specimens generally demonstrate a homogeneous infiltrate by mononuclear cells in loose spongy arrangement and increased reticulin and collagen fibers. In some cases, electron microscopy may provide valuable assistance in the morphological identification of these cells. The surface phenotype of the malignant cells is a helpful aid in the initial diagnosis, since almost all patients will have evidence of a monoclonal population of cells with B-cell features (2). One important phenotypic characteristic has been the description of a high expression of receptors for interleukin-2 (IL-2) in the surface of the hairy cells (4). Furthermore, soluble receptors in the serum are found in almost all patients, and titers above 10,000 are virtually diagnostic of HCL (17, 18).

Pancytopenia and splenomegaly are the most typical clinical features at diagnosis (1, 5). A rather common presentation is the finding of cytopenias in a patient, complicated with an infection. However, approximately 10–20% of the patients may have leukocytosis at diagnosis (rarely above 50,000 leukocytes per milliliter). Circulating hairy cells in the peripheral blood smears can be easily identified in 20–40% of the patients at diagnosis.

Occasionally, less frequent manifestations of the disease may be the presenting clinical feature. These include retroperitoneal adenopathy (19), cutaneous vasculitis (20), hypergammaglobulinemia and monoclonal proteins, hyperviscosity syndrome, or bone lesions (21). Rarely, HCL may present with polyarteritis nodosa (22), concurrent second malignancies (23, 24), or central nervous system manifestations (25). When clinically warranted, baseline evaluation should include a computerized tomography (CT) scan of the abdomen, serum electrophoresis, and a screening bone scan. We have found subclinical retroperitoneal adenopathy in as many as 25% of patients. Occasionally, this may be extensive enough to suggest lymphoma and, rarely, may be associated with chylous ascites and pleural effusions (19).

Evaluation of the immunological status is not required for diagnostic purposes, but a baseline assessment of some selected laboratory tests may provide the clinician with an estimate of the degree of the immunodeficiency, if present. Serological studies in HCL have revealed increased titers of antibodies to Epstein-Barr virus and to cytomegalovirus in 80% of patients (26). The geometric titers are as high as those found in patients with acquired immunodeficiency syndrome (AIDS). Flow cytometry phenotyping of peripheral blood is now widely available and enables quantitation of T-cell subpopulations.

TREATMENT OF HAIRY CELL LEUKEMIA

Review of Older Therapies

Until recently, splenectomy was the only treatment immediately available for patients with HCL. Splenectomy resulted in improvement of peripheral blood indexes in approximately 75% of the patients and, occasionally, long-term control of the disease was observed (27–30). However, in most patients, the improvement in the hematological indexes was transient. Furthermore, splenectomy was unlikely to benefit those individuals who did not have splenomegaly of moderate or substantial degree (27). Splenectomy did not seem to influence the incidence of infections and, thus, the overall survival did not improve, despite the improvement of hematological values (27, 28).

For those patients who failed to respond to splenectomy, or those relapsing from an initial response, treatment choices were limited and, in general, were unsatisfactory. Traditional antileukemic chemotherapy with single agents or with drugs in combination, was effective in inducing remissions in HCL (31–33). However, because of the poor regenerative capacity of their bone marrow, this modality of treatment was complicated by severe and prolonged myelosuppression, precluding its more widespread application. Low doses of chlorambucil were better tolerated and capable of improving some hematological indexes. However, this treatment modality did not improve granulocytopenia nor did it decrease the risk of infectious complications; accordingly, it failed to improve survival of patients (34). Long-term remission of the disease was reported in one patient treated with radiochemotherapy followed by bone marrow transplantation from an identical twin brother (35). This approach unfortunately, is feasible only in exceptional cases. Consequently, chemotherapy was used in the past only at the expense of toxicity, a high risk of potentially fatal infections, and the need for sophisticated supportive systems. In a large series, traditional antileukemic chemotherapy was found to be detrimental to the outcome of patients with HCL (32).

Androgenic hormones and lithium carbonate were used in an effort to enhance myelopoiesis, but without significantly consistent benefits (36). Leukapheresis was used with success as palliative therapy for the occasional patient who appeared with high peripheral blood counts (37). However, no long-term remissions were obtained, and patients required frequent pheresis to maintain the hematological improvement (38). Quesada et al. (39) used transfusion of allogeneic mononuclear cells and immunostimulation with the methanol extraction residue (MER) of bacille Calmette-Guerin (BCG). The rationale behind this approach was to stimulate the production of growth factors from healthy mononuclear cells to enhance hematopoiesis or to exert a direct antitumor effect. Transfusions of allogeneic mononuclear cells from siblings sharing at least one haplotype improved the hematological indexes in 4 of 11 patients treated and, in 3 of the 4 responsive patients, the benefit was long-lasting (25, 45, and 53 months) (36). Unfortunately, the methodology involving the mononuclear cell transfusions was cumbersome and of limited applicability. Perhaps the most important contribution of that study was to further strengthen the notion that biological therapy coud be of distinct clinical benefit in HCL.

Modern Approaches to the Treatment of Hairy Cell Leukemia

The treatment of hairy cell leukemia has improved significantly in the decade of the 1980s, mainly because of the introduction of recombinant interferon-alfa (IFN-α) and pentostatin (deoxycoformycin; DCF). Currently, the prognosis has improved dramatically, and evidence of improved survival is beginning to emerge. The clinician confronting patients with newly diagnosed disease is presented with choices not available 5 years ago. Yet, because of the peculiar features in the course of the disease and the heterogeneity in clinical presentations, the optimal choice of therapy for the individual patient must be judged carefully, including even the use of older treatment strategies (40, 41).

Observation with No Treatment

A small subset of patients with HCL follow a favorable course with an indolent nonprogressive disease (42). Conceivably, they may represent a group of patients in whom the proliferation of the malignant cells is still under partial control by normal regulatory growth signals. One possible mechanism to explain the behavior of the disease in these patients could be the ability of their circulating mononuclear cells to produce endogenous interferon alpha in response to ubiquitous environmental factors, in contrast with the typical patient in whom there is a deficiency in interferon production.

In general, in newly diagnosed patients with one or two cytopenias (no blood product dependency) and no history of severe or recurrent infections, judicious observation is reasonable. Approximately 2% of patients followed at M.D. Anderson Hospital continue to be observed without any treatment. Similarly, patients in whom splenectomy has been performed, who have adequate peripheral blood count values and have no history of recurrent infections, may continue to be observed without additional treatment for prolonged periods. Approximately 5% of our patients belong to this category. An unusual situation is the patient who may undergo spontaneous remission of HCL following an infection (6, 7), for whom observation may be also indicated.

Bone marrow studies should be performed at regular intervals (every 6–12 months). A bone marrow cellularity below 50% is usually associated with little or moderate disruption of blood cell production and should serve as an additional criteria to determine whether a patient should be recommended for therapeutic intervention. More recently, the finding of soluble IL-2 receptor in patients with HCL, may provide a useful serum marker as a guide for the need of treatment. Preliminary data show a correlation between disease status and level of IL-2 receptors in sera (18). The usefulness of this assay, however, awaits additional studies in all stages of the disease, including indolent course. Finally, evidence of severe immunodeficiency by existing methods of evaluation (flow cytometry phenotyping, delayed skin reactivity, natural killer (NK) activity, or other) may assist the clinician in determining whether therapy is needed, regardless of the status of the hematological indexes.

Splenectomy

Golomb and collaborators (43) have best studied the natural history of patients who have undergone splenectomy as the primary modality of treatment with HCL. In a retrospective study of 267 patients, 194 had splenectomy. Of these,

123 patients (63%) had a recurrence of the disease within a median of 82 weeks. These investigators identified a subgroup of patients in whom relapse occurred shortly after splenectomy, who were characterized by a hypercellular bone marrow and leukemic infiltrates above 70%. In patients with bone marrow cellularity greater than 85%, the median time to relapse was 24 weeks, whereas the median time to relapse in patients with less than 50% cellularity was 123 weeks.

Clearly, there are individual patients who derived major clinical benefit and may attain a well-balanced host–tumor relationship for prolonged periods following splenectomy. For this reason, the role of splenectomy in newly diagnosed patients must continue to be considered. However, the therapeutic impact of IFN-α and DCF in both treated and previously untreated patients, has greatly limited the indications of splenectomy. In patients wth minimally enlarged spleen or those without splenomegaly, splenectomy does not result in satisfactory or durable remissions (27). Also, a hypercellular bone marrow predicts a poor outcome for this surgical procedure. For these subsets of patients and those at high surgical risk, systemic treatment with either IFN-α or DCF is presently preferable to splenectomy.

Indications for splenectomy remain spleen rupture or spleen infarct, which are rare complications of patients with splenomegaly (44). Consideration for splenectomy should still be given to patients with massively enlarged spleens and evidence of severe hypersplenism. In those instances, splenectomy may be the quickest way to obtain a prompt improvement of hematological indexes. In the patient with pancytopenia, moderately enlarged spleen, and bone marrow cellularity of less than 50%, the potential benefit of splenectomy must be weighed against the surgical risk and the small, but lifelong, risk of hazardous bacterial infections associated with the removal of this organ, including the syndrome of overwhelming postsplenectomy infection (45, 46). Interestingly, splenectomy has been shown to decrease the production of colony-stimulating factor(s) (CSFs) and of IFN in some experimental models (47, 48). This effect could be adverse for a patient with HCL undergoing splenectomy, should similar deficits occur in humans.

Alpha Interferons

The efficacy of interferons alpha against hairy cell leukemia has been amply documented. Interferon alpha was the first agent to show consistent improvement in the bone marrow with an attendant recovery of peripheral hematological indexes. Such improvement was associated with reduction in morbidity and mortality.

Our original observations, identifying IFN-α as an effective treatment against HCL, were published in 1984 (49). Of the first seven patients included in that report, three achieved complete remissions (CR) and four achieved partial remissions (PR). The response criteria were not limited to the peripheral blood indexes, but included the disappearance (CR) or more than 50% reduction (PR) of bone marrow leukemic infiltrate and reduction or disappearance of the splenomegaly or retroperitoneal nodes. In contrast with previous existing modalities of treatment at that time, IFN-α resulted in consistent reduction of the HCL infiltration in the bone marrow.

The results of those preliminary studies were subsequently confirmed by multiple investigators with both partially purified interferon and recombinant interferon alpha (50–58). Recently, we have reviewed our experience in 106 patients treated with natural or recombinant interferon alpha-2a (rIFN alpha-2a). In most patients treatment consisted of a daily administration of 3 million units of IFN-α by intramuscular or subcutaneous injection for 6 months, followed by 3 million units three times a week. There were no differences in the result between rIFN alpha-2a and IFN-α

Responses. Ninety-five, 45, and 14 patients completed 12, 24, and more than 24 months of uninterrupted treatment, respectively. Forty-eight patients achieved CR or near CR, 38 had PR, and 17 had a minor response (MR) to therapy. Only 2 patients failed to respond to treatment. The median time to onset of response was 6 months for patients achieving a PR and 14 months for patients achieving a CR.

Patients who achieved CR had, at the beginning of treatment, significantly higher hemoglobin levels, monocyte counts, and a lower bone marrow cellularity value than did patients whose maximal response was PR or MR. The white blood cell (WBC), granulocyte, and platelet counts had no independent predictive value. However, the frequency of CR was lower for patients with pancytopenia. Additionally, patients with a high WBC or with a high leukemic index (product of cellularity times percentage of hairy cells) in the bone marrow before treatment, required prolonged therapy to achieve CR. These profiles may reflect the extent of leukemic systemic involvement. No significant difference in the frequency of CR was found among patients with or without splenectomy, but the onset of CR required significantly longer treatment in splenectomized patients.

Several other investigators have reported similar results (51–58). The paucity of complete remissions in some of these studies is perhaps explained by the selection of patients, treatment doses and schedules, or length of treatment. Many patients continued to obtain benefit from the treatment beyond the first 12 months of therapy (50). Studies designed to terminate therapy early may prove inadequate in achieving PR or CR in HCL. Also, the evaluation of sequential bone marrow specimens involves considerable subjective variability and may explain differences among investigators in the assessment of CR. A histologically normal bone marrow specimen is achieved in approximately 20–25% of the patients. However, we feel that the existence of residual atypical cells, without definite histological characteristics of hairy cells, or the existence of residual fibrosis or other minor histological abnormalities should not rule out a CR, a criterion similarly used in characterizing the response of other leukemic conditions. This and other subjective elements in the definition of a CR may explain the prevalence of CR in the literature, that has varied from zero to 50% of the patients.

Furthermore, it is still unclear whether there may be differences in the prognosis and survival of patients who achieved CR or near-CR compared with those who achieved only a PR. The improvement of the peripheral blood hematological indexes and the reduced morbidity are similar, regardless of the maximal response in the bone marrow.

Duration of Response. The achievement of CR or PR does not equate with cure. Most patients who discontinue treatment will have a relapse of the disease. Criteria of relapse were defined as a drop in the hematological indexes below the response criteria parameters in at least three consecutive blood samples or a doubling of the leukemic index in the bone marrow.

In our series of 106 patients, 64 patients had treatment discontinued after achieving PR or CR. Eighteen of the 30 patients (60%) who had achieved CR at the end of treatment sustained their remission status, without further therapy, for periods ranging from 3 to 36 months (median, 18 months). Thirty-four patients had achieved a PR at the end of treatment and, of these, 6 (18%) have sustained their remission status without further therapy (median, 25 months; range, 12–40 months). In contrast, 40 of the 64 patients (62.5%) who had treatment discontinued after achieving PR or CR had subsequent relapse of the disease, including 12 of the 30 patients who achieved CR (40%) and 28 of the 34 who achieved PR (82%). The median duration of remission without further therapy was 18 months (range, 3–28+ months) for patients in CR and 9 months (range, 3–24+ months) for patients in PR. These data are in agreement with results reported by Ratain and collaborators, who found that the residual leukemic bone marrow infiltration at the completion of treatment was a reliable indicator of relapse (59).

Relapses occurred in patients who discontinued therapy. Only two patients experienced a relapse of the disease after achieving PR while receiving rIFN alpha-2a therapy. In both of these patients, antibodies to rIFN alpha-2a were detected during treatment (see later discussion).

Reinduction. Reinduction of remission is consistently achieved with reinitiation of treatment and, in some patients, a CR is actually achieved during the second or third course of therapy. An increase in the bone marrow leukemic infiltrate should not be considered the sole criterion to reinitiate treatment. Sustenance of normal or adequate peripheral hematological indexes may hold for prolonged periods, despite evidence of bone marrow relapse. The criteria we have used to determine when to reinitiate treatment consisted of a minimum of three consecutive blood counts showing a hemoglobin value less than 12 *g*/dL; a granulocyte count of fewer than $1.5 \times 10^6/mm^3$ or platelet count of fewer than $100,000/mm^3$; or progressive increase in the total WBC to more than 10,000/

mm^3. Of these, progressive decline of the granulocyte count, was found to be the most sensitive indicator of disease relapse and the main indication to restart therapy.

ANTIBODIES. Neutralizing antibodies to rIFN alpha-2a, but not to natural IFN-α were detected in 14 of 78 patients tested. Of these, 9 patients had titers greater than 1200 neutralizing units per milliliter, and 7 experienced loss of an ongoing response to treatment, suggesting that the antibodies blocked the therapeutic activity of the rIFN alpha-2a. Steiss and collaborators had published similar results (60).

The prevalence of antibodies to both rIFN alpha-2a and rIFN alpha-2b have varied in published reports (61, 62). Differences in treatment duration, route of drug administration, blood sampling relative to IFN administration, total cumulative dose at the time of assessment, or assay methodology, all could account for these observations. Also, it remains unresolved whether the molecular structure of the alpha-2a and alpha-2b IFNs, which differ by only one amino acid, may account for the difference in immunogenicity of these proteins. However, loss of response associated with neutralizing antibodies to rIFN alpha-2b has been recently documented in patients with chronic myelogenous leukemia (63). Of note, the antibodies will cross-react with both molecules. Consequently, changing treatment from rIFN alpha-2a to IFN alpha-2b would not result in benefit. However, we have shown that natural IFN-α is capable of reinducing remission in patients with antibodies to rIFN alpha-2a. This is probably best explained by the fact that the natural product contains multiple species of IFN-α, in contrast with the single species in the recombinant preparation (Fig. 1).

Development of antibodies to rIFN alpha-2a occurs infrequently and usually within the first 4 months of therapy. Loss of an ongoing response during this period would most likely be related to the development of antibodies to rIFN alpha-2a. However, failure to achieve PR cannot be equated with this complication, since there are patients who may require several months to reach PR or CR. Similarly, the development of antibodies to rIFN alpha-2a does not necessarily result in relapse. Some patients may sustain remission in the presence of circulating antibodies.

CLINICAL USE. Treatment guidelines are shown in Table 1. The optimal dose of IFN-α has not yet been determined. There is no indication to use doses higher than 3 million units (MU)/day as induction treatment. When we used higher doses, we observed more toxicity, but no evidence of better results, than with the standard dose (50). Induction with 3 MU three times per week is satisfactory (52–58), but we favor an induction course of 4–6 months, with daily doses for a faster achievement of remission. Dosages as low as 0.1–1 MU/day have been reported to have activity and may be indicated in patients with severe pancytopenia to avoid potential complications during the induction phase of treatment (64–65). Indeed, during the first 6–8 weeks of treatment IFN-α may

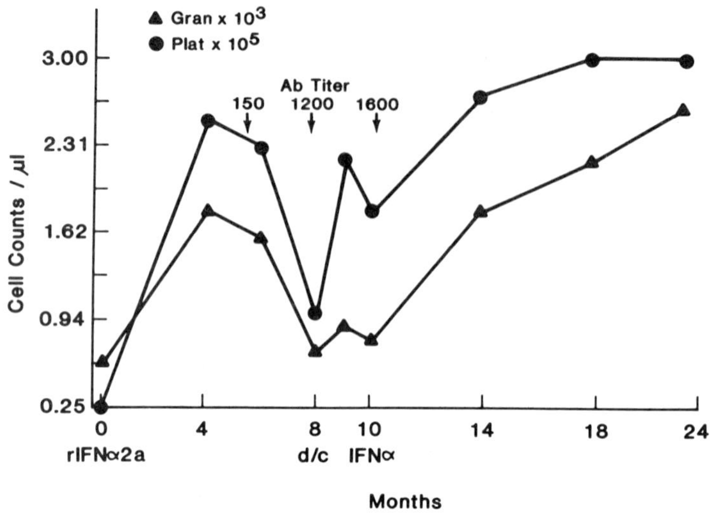

Figure 1 Granulocyte and platelet counts from a patient who developed neutralizing antibodies against rIFN alpha-2a expressed as interferon neutralizing units per microliter (INU-uL), showing initial response to treatment, disease relapse that was coincidental with increasing titers of antibodies, and subsequent response to natural interferon (IFN-α).

produce further decrease in the WBC of leukopenic patients, and moderate to severe infections may complicate the course of approximately 10% of the patients at this stage. Occasionally, profoundly thrombocytopenic patients may experience a drop in the platelet count as well.

It is clear, from clinical observation, that an increased production of blood elements can occur as early as the first week of treatment, and that hematological restoration may precede, by several weeks, any distinct evidence of improvement in the bone marrow. This indirectly suggests that IFN-α may stimulate the production of growth and maturation factors, derived from cells of the immune system, which enhance hematopoiesis. The effects elicited in HCL are in general contrary to the observed hematological effects in other cancer patients in whom anemia, leukopenia, or thrombocytopenia have been observed (66). It is also in contrast with the described in vitro effects of IFN-α in bone marrow colony cell growth. Conceivably, the stimulation of cells capable of producing these signals overrides any inhibitory influence related to the antiproliferative activities of interferon. Recently, Michalevicz and Revel (67) described the existence of a unique hematopoietic stem cell in patients with HCL, which IFN-α promotes to differentiate toward myelomonocytic cell lines. This effect may explain the prompt hematological responses.

Table 1 Alpha Interferons: Treatment Guidelines

Commercial products[a]	Intron-A Roferon-A
Dose and route	1–3 MU daily SC or IM × 4–6 mo then 3 MU tiw
	1–3 MU tiw SC or IM
Length of treatment	Beyond 12 mo (18–36 mo)
Expected response	> 90%
CR	~ 10–25%[b]
PR	~ 50–70%
Median duration of response	~ 12 mo
Indications	Splenectomy relapse
	Newly diagnosed patients with
	Bone marrow cellularity > 50%
	Active infections
	History of infections
	Normal/minimally enlarged spleen
	Blood product dependency
Relative contraindications	Antibodies to alpha interferon

[a]Natural IFN-α available in some states.
[b]Approximately additional 15–25% of patients obtained "near-CR" with residual atypical cells and excess fibrin in the bone marrow.

Typically, the first evidence of response to IFN-α is a rise in the platelet count in patients with thrombocytopenia, which may be documented within the first 2–4 weeks of treatment. In patients with splenomegaly or in those with high WBC counts and circulating hairy cells, prompt reduction in the size of the spleen and rapid drop in the circulating malignant cells may be the first evidence of response.

Improved myelopoiesis in the bone marrow can be documented within the first 4 months of treatment, with attendant increase in the number of granulocytes. Most patients reach more than 1500 granulocytes within 6 months of therapy. In some individuals, administration of IFN-α precludes normalization of the total WBC count. In these patients, interruption of treatment results in brisk increase in the total WBC level, consistent with the effects of IFN-α in nonleukopenic patients. Administration of short courses of steroids shows evidence of a normal hematopoietic activity, similar to that seen in normal individuals. Only a small proportion of patients may have persistent leukopenia, despite improvement of other parameters. This sometimes can be seen in patients with extensive fibrosis of the bone marrow stroma. In other cases, we have seen a persistent lymphocytosis and fluctuating absolute number of granulocytes.

These are morphologically and phenotypically normal lymphocytes and should not be equated with a lack of response.

Profound granulocytopenia is not a contraindication for administration of IFN-α. Treatment was initiated in the presence of active life-threatening infections in 11 patients in our series, all of whom subsequently achieved remission. Anecdotally, some of the best and most durable remissions occurred in patients with concurrent mycobacterial infections.

Restoration of erythropoiesis usually takes the longest to occur. Normalization of hematocrit and hemoglobin levels may require 6–12 months of therapy. This value, however, is usually not affected in the event of relapse. Occasionally, patients may develop polycythemia if continued on IFN-α for a prolonged time. We have discontinued therapy in two patients because of an erythrocyte excess.

Changes in the bone marrow occur gradually. Within 4–6 months there is usually evidence of improvement, consisting of a decrease in overall cellularity, a decrease in leukemic infiltrate, an increase in the number of normal hemopoietic elements, and a normalization of the myeloid/lymphoid cell ratios. Improvement of bone marrow fibrosis and reticulin content does not occur early and may require 12 or more months of treatment to be demonstrable (49, 50, 68, 69). As with other hematological indexes, we have seen continuous improvement in patients receiving 2 or more years of uninterrupted therapy. With prolonged therapy, approximately 25% of our patients normalized the histological and histochemical appearance of their bone marrow. Interferon does not adversely alter the immunohistological phenotype of the normal elements of the bone marrow (70).

Other less frequent manifestations of the disease can also effectively be treated with IFN. Responses have been reported in patients with massive splenomegaly, bulky retroperitoneal adenopathy, hyperviscosity syndrome, and even bone lesions (19, 71–73).

The optimal length of treatment remains unknown. Prolonged therapy beyond 1 year of treatment continues to reduce the leukemic infiltration, resulting in more patients achieving CR. For some individuals, periodic administration (every 6–12 months) may prove satisfactory in the long-term control of the disease. Laboratory or clinical measurements to guide the length of therapy or its reinstitution must be sought and defined. Recently, it has been suggested that the levels of circulating, shedded IL-2 receptors may be associated with the quality of the response and may be predictive of residual disease and leukemic relapse (18, 74). Similarly, the assessment of endogenous IFN-α production may be a useful criterion to determine the length of treatment. An adequate endogenous production of IFN-α by cells of the immune system in patients with HCL may be indicative of restoration of an existing deficit and the ability of regaining autochthonous control of residual disease (75).

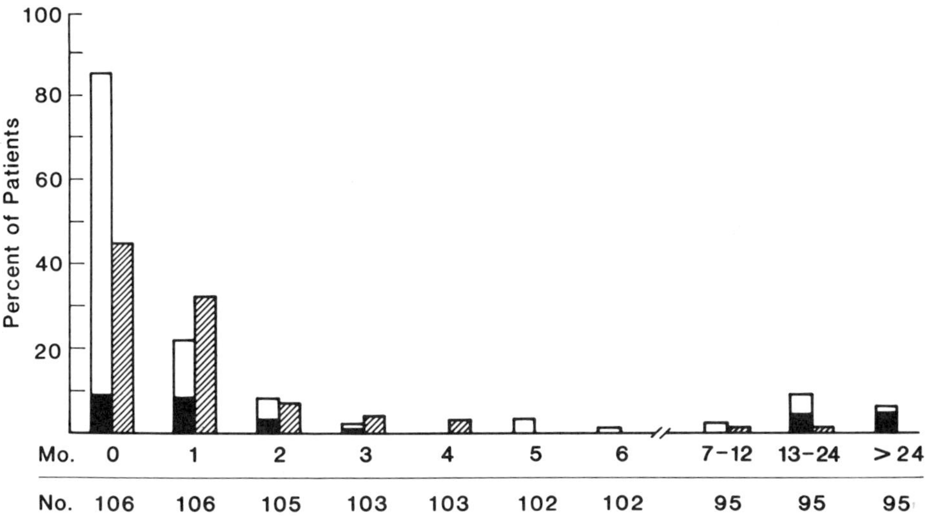

Figure 2 Percentage of patients with history of infections and transfusions of blood products before and after treatment with interferon alpha. Open bars represent suspected or documented bacterial or opportunistic infections; closed bars indicate suspected or documented viral infections or fever of unknown origin. Hatched bars indicate percentage of patients who received transfusions. Bacterial infections after 6 months of treatment were urinary tract infections. Suspected viral infections increased after discontinuation of treatment. Transfusions beyond 4 months were given in connection with elective surgical procedures.

For interferons other than IFN-α, treatment with recombinant interferon gamma was ineffective in eliciting remissions in patients with HCL (76). However, inteferon beta has been used successfully in treating a patient who did not respond to IFN-α (77).

OUTCOME. Over 90% of the patients maintained a normal life-style that included athletic activities. The administration of IFN-α resulted in a significant decrease in the incidence of infections and the need for transfusion of blood products (Fig. 2). No serious infections occurred in any patient beyond 2 months of treatment. Most documented bacterial infections after achievement of a response were those of the urinary tract. Suspected viral infections of the respiratory tract increased after discontinuation of treatment. Transfusions after 4 months were given only in connection with elective surgical procedures. Survival of this group of patients has been superior to that of contemporary and historical controls followed from 1970 to 1985 at M. D. Anderson Hospital (Fig.

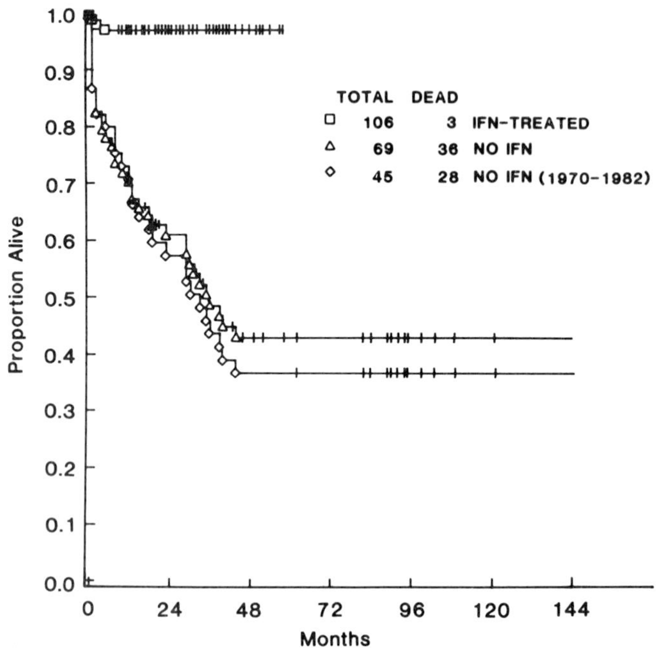

Figure 3 Survival curves (Kaplan–Meier) of 106 patients treated with interferon alpha (squares) and 69 patients who did not receive interferon (triangles). Of these, 45 patients (diamonds) were seen at M. D. Anderson Hospital and Tumor Institute before introduction of interferon alpha (1970–1982).

3). Only three patients in our series died after initiation of treatment with IFN-α: one died of gastric carcinoma, one died of a self-inflicted gunshot, and the other died of pneumonia within the first 2 weeks of treatment.

TOXICITY. The toxicity of low doses of IFN-α is minor, except for unusually sensitive individuals. The most common side effects, such as the influenzalike symptoms experienced on first exposure to IFN-α, are well tolerated and short-lived. As treatment continues and with the improvement of the hematological indexes, most patients will report none or only mild adverse effects. Compliance is excellent, and only rarely persistent constitutional and neurological symptoms are reported. These consist of mental fatigue, mild mental confusion, and poor concentration or mental endurance. Rarely, IFN-α can be associated with persistent low-grade fever. Approximately 10% of the male patients complained of reversible decreased libido (66).

In our series of 106 patients, 24 (22%) had complicating infections or fever of undetermined origin that warranted administration of antibiotics during the initial

8 weeks of treatment. In 4 cases, life-threatening infections necessitated hospitalization. Other rare toxicities observed included a sensorial peripheral neuropathy. Two of these patients received IFN concomitantly with isoniazid, rifampicin, and ethambutol. Occasionally, patients complain of arthralgias with mild inflammation in small joints of the hands. Five other patients developed cutaneous vasculitis during the first 3 months of treatment. All these complications improved with steroids, nonsteroidal anti-inflammatory agents, or temporary discontinuation of treatment.

MECHANISMS OF ACTION. The etiology of HCL remains unknown. Some recent advances in virology and molecular biology may result in the identification of a causative or pathogenetic mechanism in HCL in the near future. Identification of the causative agent should result in a better understanding of the mode of action of IFN in HCL.

Broad antiviral activity defines all IFNs. Inhibition of transforming viruses or viruses that are coadjuvant to the expression of such transforming virus(es) could be a mechanism behind the antitumor activity of IFN in HCL. However, there is no solid evidence that a transforming virus is involved in HCL, with the exception of rare instances of patients who have an HCL variant with predominantly T markers, in whom evidence of infection by the human immunodeficiency virus II (HIV-II) has been demonstrated (78). We and others have shown the absence of HIV-II involvement in the more prevalent B-cell HCL (26, 79).

There is increasing evidence implicating activation of protooncogenes (c-*onc* genes) in B-cell neoplasms. The only indirect evidence of such activity in HCL has been published by Sairenji and collaborators (13), who identified, in transfection experiments, activity of a transforming gene(s) from DNA of hairy cells. Interferon has been shown to suppress the expression of some oncogenes. Thus, if abnormal expression of cellular genes determines the malignant behavior of the hairy cells, inhibition of expression of such genes could explain the action of IFN-α in HCL. Hairy cells are dependent on B-cell growht factor(s) to grow in vitro (80, 81). Furthermore, hairy cells produce B-cell growth factor(s) that could maintain their growth in vitro (82). Inhibition of gene activity responsible for the production of the B-cell growth factor has been postulated as a mechanism of action of IFN-α, but remains to be proved.

The activity of other genes may also participate in the sensitivity or resistance of hairy cells' to IFN-α. In our series, the only two bona fide resistant patients were found to lack the receptor for IL-2 on their cells' surfaces and absence of soluble IL-2 receptors in their plasma. Another resistant case reported in the literature had rearrangement of both immunoglobulin and T-receptor genes (80). These and other patients who do not respond to IFN-α are likely to belong to variants of the typical B-cell HCL.

Interferon, among its multiple biological activities, promotes or induces cellular differentiation in a variety of experimental models (84). Yet, there is no evidence that this might be an actual mechanism of action of IFN-α in HCL (85).

To what extent the immunomodulatory effects of IFN-α participate in its antitumor activity in HCL is still unknown. Extensive literature exists on the multiple activities of IFN-α on both cellular and humoral immunity in vitro and in vivo (86). It is a potent stimulator of cytotoxic effector mechanisms, including NK activity and macrophages. However, studies addressing this possible mechanism of action have failed to demonstrate a direct role of activated immune cells and tumor response in hairy cell leukemia (87–89). Furthermore, hairy cells seem to be poorly sensitive to NK cells in vitro (89, 90).

Finally, the deficiency in production of IFN-α in patients with HCl may play a role in the pathogenesis of the disease and could satisfactorily explain the prompt response to replacement treatment. The origin or nature of this deficiency remains unknown. Conceivably, there could be a genetic deficiency in the IFN system of patients with HCL. Hairy cell leukemia occurs preponderantly in men, and the synthesis of IFN-α has been shown to be influenced by an X-linked locus (91). Alternatively, the defect in IFN-α production could be secondary to suppressive or inhibitory influences derived from the malignant cells, as suggested by some preliminary laboratory work (92). Lastly, an exhaustion of the system, perhaps related to a chronic or recurrent viral infection, could be responsible for the low levels of production (26).

Pentostatin (Deoxycoformicin)

Pentostatin (DCF), a product of *Streptomyces antibioticus,* tightly binds and inhibits the activity of adenosine deaminase (ADA), found predominantly in lymphoid cells. It is lymphocytotoxic and has demonstrated antitumor activity against both T- and B-cell lymphoid neoplasms. In early clinical trials, DCF was associated with prohibitive toxicity. More recently, safer dose schedules have been identified. Low doses of 2–5 mg/m^2, given once a week, or every-other-week, have safely induced remissions in chronic lymphoid neoplasms with low proliferative rates or with high concentrations of ADA, including HCL (93).

Mechanism of Action. The precise mechanism of action of DCF in these disorders remains unclear. Inhibition of ADA is known to result in accumulation of 2'-deoxyadenosine, which is metabolized to dATP. In rapidly dividing cells, accumulation of dATP leads to inhibition of ribonucleotide reductase and impairment of DNA synthesis. However, Ho et al. (94) failed to correlate clinical response of neoplasms with low proliferative rate and DCF-induced suppression of ADA activity, dATP accumulation, ATP depletion, or other typical biochemical effects induced by DCF. In their study, inhibition of *S*-adenosylhomocysteine hydrolase (SAH) best correlate with the clinical response of CLL or HCL to DCF. The inhibition of SAH hydrolase results in accumulation of SAH, which, in turn, inhibits *S*-adenosylmethionine (SAM), a crucial enzyme in methylation reactions that are required in the synthesis and function of DNA and RNA. Interestingly, De Ferra and Baglioni (95) have shown in vitro that IFN-α reduces the SAM/SAH ratio and thus alters ribonucleotide methylation. This could represent a common pathway of antitumor activity for IFN-α and DCF.

RESPONSES. Spiers and collaborators originally described two patients with HCL receiving low doses of DCF who underwent remission of the disease (96). Confirmation of the results in a larger number of patients has been reported by these and other investigators (97–100). Pentostatin has been shown to induce remissions in the various stages of the disease, including patients who have failed to respond to IFN-α (101–103). Pentostatin results in rapid responses, and a higher proportion of patients achieve complete remission with normalization of bone marrow histology.

Over 150 patients with HCL have received therapy with DCF in Phase II clinical trials sponsored by the National Cancer Institute (NCI) (98). The overall response rate exceeds 80%, with 63% CRs and 22% PRs. In contrast with IFNs, which require prolonged administration to achieve maximal response, remissions with DCF are usually obtained after one to eight doses of DCF (2–4 months of treatment). Remissions, as with IFN-α include responses in the bone marrow and the restoration of hematological indexes.

The overall response rate is similar, regardless whether patients had received prior therapy with IFN-α. However, the incidence of CRs is higher for previously untreated patients (99), than for those who had received systemic therapies. Complete remission has been observed more often in patients with newly diagnosed disease, in whom splenectomy has not been performed. No other independent variables that bear on the quality or the duration of the responses have been published.

DURATION OF RESPONSE. Pentostatin-induced remissions are durable and most patients who achieved CR sustain their remission status beyond 12 months after discontinuation of treatment. Since most published series have a median follow-up of fewer than 2 years, the precise duration of remission awaits longer periods of observation and future updates of these data. In random instances, reinduction of remission with DCF has been successfully obtained upon reinitiation of treatment (100). Relapses occurring following DCF treatment have been characterized by reappearance of hairy cells in the bone marrow specimens, but with little or no impact on the peripheral blood indexes.

CLINICAL USE. Treatment guidelines are shown in Table 2. The drug is supplied as a lyophilized powder that is reconstituted with physiologic saline or an equivalent sterile solution. It can be administered as a slow intravenous bolus injection (over 2–5 minutes) or as an infusion over 20–30 minutes. As with IFN-α, the optimal dose or length of treatment have yet to be elucidated. Three main methods of administration have been used consisting of 5 mg/m^2 daily for 2–3 days; 4 mg/m^2 once a week, or 4 mg/m^2 every other week. The latter has

Table 2 Pentostatin (Deoxycoformycin): Treatment Guidelines

Commercial products[a]	Not available
Dose and route	4 mg/m^2 IV once/week or every 14 days
Length of treatment	8–12 doses (4–6 months)
Expected response	> 90%
CR	~ 50–100%
PR	~ 30–40%
Median duration of response	~ >12 mo[b]
Indications	Clinical research studies[c] Interferon alpha failures Antibodies to interferon alpha
Relative contraindications	Active infection, renal dysfunction

[a]Product may be obtained through the Special Exception Mechanism of the NCI.
[b]Median not reached for most studies.
[c]Referral to research studies is encouraged to delineate optimal therapy.

been the preferred dosage in most recent studies and in the community through the Special Exception Mechanism of the NCI (98).

The length of treatment has varied among different studies, but it is infrequent to administer more than 12 doses of DCF. Presently, the NCI recommends two doses beyond the achievement of CR (98). A larger tumor burden or the presence of massive splenomegaly may require twice as many doses as required for the more typical patients to achieve CR (97, 100).

The pattern of response is similar to that observed with IFN-α. Platelets are first to recover, followed by neutrophils, and lastly hemoglobin. Also, splenomegaly and circulating hairy cells responded briskly after the first course of therapy. Neutropenia has been consistently observed following the first course of treatment and may coincide with complicating infections. Because of this adverse effect, investigators seldom initiate therapy with DCF in the presence of active infections.

The response in the bone marrow is significantly faster in patients treated with DCF than in those treated with IFN-α. A histologically normal bone marrow can be seen within 2–4 months of treatment, and sometimes as early as after one course of treatment (70). In contrast, IFN usually requires more than 12 months of therapy to accomplish similar results in approximately 25% of the patients.

TOXICITY. Initial Phase I and II studies with DCF, which average a dose of 25 mg/m^2, were associated with prohibitive toxicity and complicated with severe and fatal infections (104). Low doses are considerably less toxic, but concern with infectious complications remains.

The most frequent toxic effects observed at these doses consist of nausea and vomiting (60–80%), infections (31–50%), and renal or hepatic dysfunction (22%) (96–100). Although severe neurotoxicity, originally reported with high-dose DCF, is avoided, central nervous system effects consisting of lethargy have been reported by some investigators in as many as 62% of patients (99). Other peculiar adverse effects include conjunctivitis (5–20%) and dermatitis that is aggravated or induced by sun exposure (20–35%). Rarely, anaphylactic reactions to DCF have occurred (105).

Hematological toxicity consists of leukopenia (45–60%) and anemia (30–40%), which occur during the initial induction courses. Johnson and collaborators (99), who used three weekly doses at a dose of 4 mg/m^2, have shown that the median day of the nadir with this regimen occurred on day 15, with a median neutrophil count of 230 cells/mL. By the end of the 3-week course the median neutrophil count was over 2000/mL. The hematological toxic effects vary somewhat according to the investigators and the treatment scheme. Hematological toxicity has been reported as minimal with an every-other-week schedule (100).

Acute infections have been the concern of many investigators. These have been caused both by bacterial pathogens and opportunistic organisms. It is still unclear to what degree the lymphotoxic effects of DCF may be contributing to these events, since these types of infections are common in HCL. However, the potent inhibitory effect of DCF on adenosine deaminase may partially simulate the profound immunodeficiency associated with the inborn absence of this enzyme. Recently, evidence of a prolonged immunodeficit in peripheral blood and in the bone marrow of HCL patients in remission who were treated with DCF has been published (70, 106). The clinical effect of such deficit is a matter of controversy. Because of the lymphotoxicity and the myelosuppressive effects, DCF is not recommended for infected patients with HCL in presently approved studies.

Pentostatin remains a controlled experimental agent and, therefore, is available only at some research centers or by request through the Special Exception Mechanism of the NCI.

Other Therapies

RADIOTHERAPY. Radiotherapy has been shown to have a role in the treatment of bone lesions associated to HCL (21). However, IFN-α has also been shown to be effective in certain skeletal complications (72, 73). Radiotherapy should continue to be considered as a strong treatment choice in patients with large single lytic lesions involving the head of the femur or other weight-bearing bones, to produce a quick response and avoid orthopedic complications. In contrast, in patients with more diffuse skeletal involvement in whom radiotherapy may be complicated with myelotoxicity, IFN-α is preferable because of a better therapeutic index. Currently, there are no reports describing responses of bone lesions to DCF.

GROWTH FACTORS. The recent cloning and clinical availability of purified recombinant colony-stimulating factors (CSFs) and erythropoietin makes their use attractive in pancytopenic patients. Quite occasionally there are patients in whom a single blood value may have failed to return to normal, both after IFN as well as after DCF (50, 96). For these patients administration of hematopoietins may contribute to their overall clinical management.

More often, however, clinicians may be confronted with patients who have profound neutropenia in whom both IFN or DCF may be associated with further reduction in the neutrophil count. In this circumstance, the granulocyte colony-stimulating factors (G-CSF or GM-CSF) may be useful adjunctives to other therapies. By producing a sharp and powerful boost in granulocyte production, these patients may undergo subsequent therapy, be it splenectomy, IFN, or DCF in safer clinical conditions. Glaspy and collaborators (107) have shown the feasibility of such an approach. Administration of G-CSF, given subcutaneously in doses of 3–6 mg/kg/daily for 4–6 weeks, increased the neutrophil count of four HCL patients with severe neutropenia. Tolerance to treatment was excellent, except for one patient with existing vasculitis in whom administration of G-CSF resulted in acute neutrophilic dermatosis (Sweet syndrome) (107).

PURINE NUCLEOSIDE ANALOGUE. Chlorodeoxyadenosine (CDA) and fludarabine (FAMP) are purine nucleoside analogues synthetized to overcome the pharmacologic limitations of cytarabine (cytosine arabinoside). Chemical substitutions in the parent molecule have resulted in more stable products resistant to the action of adenosine deaminase. Both CDA and FAMP have been effective in the treatment of advanced chronic lymphoid neoplasms (108, 109). In contrast with DCF, these agents are substrate analogues of adenosine deaminase, rather than enzyme inhibitors. These compounds are converted to their respective triphosphates, which are highly competitive inhibitors of DNA synthesis.

Recently, CDA has been shown to induce prompt remissions in twelve patients with HCL after a single course of the drug, consisting of a 7-day continuous infusion of 0.1 mg/kg daily (110). Eleven patients achieved a complete response, and 1 had a partial response. Treatment was associated with minimal toxicity, and none of the common side effects described for DCF were seen. No infections were observed during the induction course. The median remission duration at the time of last follow-up was 15.5 months (range 7+ to 46+ months), and no patient has yet relapsed. If these results persist with longer follow-up of a larger population, CDA may turn out to be the most active agent against HCL, and may become the first line of therapy for this disease. The use of CDA in HCL and other chronic lymphoid leukemias is being pursued, and

Phase II studies have begun to explore the full range of activity of this compound.

There is very little experience with use of FAMP against HCL. Anecdotally, we treated a patient with HCL who ceased to respond to IFN-α and failed to respond to DCF. He obtained a satisfactory and durable remission after five courses of FAMP. His lack of response to DCF remains unexplained, suggesting different biochemical pathways in their mechanism of action. Because CDA may have an improved therapeutic index over FAMP, it is unlikely that the latter agent will have a major role in the treatment of HCL.

CONCLUSIONS

The outlook for patients with HCL has improved significantly with the introduction of IFN-α and DCF. The U.S. Food and Drug Administration approved rIFNalpha-2a and rIFNalpha-2b in April 1986 as an effective treatment for this disorder, simultaneously with most other countries. Thus, IFN-α is the first therapeutic alternative for the treatment of HCL presently available to clinicians. Therapy with interferon has already resulted in a significant improvement in the quality of life of most of these patients by reducing or eliminating the morbidity factors associated with this disease. When DCF becomes more widely available in the future, the use of these two agents would probably have a significant influence on survival.

The particular indications for each of the presently available therapeutic choices, including conservative observation without treatment or the traditional splenectomy, require further experience with the newly available drugs, as well as identification of prognostic factors or biological indicators that could assist in the clinical decisions. Conceivably a combination of these therapeutic options and adjunctive biological therapy with hematopoietins may provide optimal therapy and a potential cure for HCL. Randomized studies comparing the results of treatment with IFN-α and DCF are presently being conducted to determine the particular benefits and drawbacks of these therapies. Also, controlled studies combining IFN-α and DCF have begun in this country with the objective of utilizing the clinical benefits of both of these agents.

The encouraging results with CDA are being pursued actively through Phase II studies in HCL and other lymphoid neoplasms. Comparison of the results of CDA with IFN-α and DCF will help define the best therapeutic options and sequence in HCL.

Rare variant cases of HCL may show resistance to both IFN-α and DCF. For these HCL variants CDA and FAMP may be of value. These chemotherapeutic agents seem to have a considerably better therapeutic index than other traditional agents. Currently, the use of aggressive drug combinations against HCL cannot be justified (111).

ACKNOWLEDGMENT

Data described was generated during the author's tenure as an Associate Professor of Medicine and Associate Internist at the University of Texas, M. D. Anderson Hospital and Tumor Institute.

REFERENCES

1. Bouroncle BA: Leukemic reticuloendotheliosis (hairy cell leukemia). *Blood* 1979; 53:412–436.
2. Meyers FJ, Cardiff RD, Taylor CR, et al: Hairy cell leukemia has a B cell genotype. *Hematol Oncol* 1984; 2:145–150.
3. Cleary ML, Wood GS, Warnke R, et al: Immunoglobulin gene rearrangements in hairy cell leukemia. *Blood* 1984; 64:99–104.
4. Korsmeyer SJ, Greene WC, Cossman J, et al: Rearrangement and expression of immunoglobulin genes and expression of Tac antigen in hairy cell leukemia. *Proc Natl Acad Sci USA* 1983; 80:4522–4526.
5. Jansen J: Hairy cell leukemia. *Crit Rev Oncol Hematol* 1987; 7:183–217.
6. Hersh EM, Murphy S, Zander A, et al: Host defense deficiency in hairy cell leukemia and its correction by leukocyte transfusion. *Blood* 1980; 56:526–533.
7. Keefer MJ, Weber MJ, Bottomley SS, et al: Peripheral blood remission of hairy cell leukemia after transfusion hepatitis. *Am J Hematol* 1987; 25:277–284.
8. Vardiman JW, Variakojis D, Golomb HM: Hairy cell leukemia: An autopsy study. *Cancer* 1979; 43:1339–1349.
9. Hersh EM, Quesada JR, Keating MJ, et al: Host defence factors and prognosis in hairy cell leukemia. *Leuk Res* 1982; 6:625–637.
10. Seshadri RS, Brown EJ, Zioursky A: Leukemic reticuloendotheliosis. A failure of monocyte production. *N Engl J Med* 1976; 295:181–184.
11. Sabbe LJM, Meijer CJ, Jansen J: T lymphocyte function in hairy cell leukemia. *Clin Exp Immunol* 1980; 42:336.
12. Quesada JR, Reuben J, Scouros MA, Murphy SG: Autologous mixed cell lymphocyte reaction in lymphoid malignancies. Lack of correlation with disease activity or clinical remission. *Cancer Immunol Immunother* 1982; 12:231–239.
13. Sairenji T, Lane MA, Reisert PS, et al: Characterization of Epstein-Barr virus infection on hairy cell leukemia patients. *Semin Oncol* 1984; 11(suppl 2):439–444.
14. Quesada JR, Lepe-Zuniga JL, Gutterman JU: Mid-term observations on the efficacy of alpha-interferon in hairy cell leukemia and status of the interferon system of patients in remission. *Leukemia* 1987; 1:317–319.
15. Porzsolt F, Janik R, Heil G, et al: Deficient IFN alpha production in hairy cell leukemia. *Blut* 1986; 52:185–190.
16. Yam LY, Janckila AJ, Li CY, et al: Cytochemistry of tartrate-resistant acid phosphatase: 15 years' experience. *Leukemia* 1987; 1:285–288.
17. Chilosi M, Semenzato G, Cetto G, et al: Soluble interleukin-2 receptors in the sera of patients with hairy cell leukemia: Relationship with the effect of recombinant alpha-interferon therapy on clinical parameters and natural killer in vitro activity. *Blood* 1987; 70:1530–1535.

18. Steis RG, Marcon L, Clark J, et al: Serum soluble IL 2 receptor as a tumor marker in patients with hairy cell leukemia. *Blood* 1988; 71:1304–1309.
19. Quesada JR, Kantarjian H, Keating M: Massive lymphadenopathy, chylous ascites and pleural effusions in a patient with hairy cell leukemia. Successful treatment with interferon alpha. *Cancer Bull* 1985; 37:88–90.
20. Spann CR, Callen JP, Yam LT, et al: Cutaneous leukocytoclastic vasculitis complicating hairy cell leukemia (leukemic reticuloendotheliosis). *Arch Dermatol* 1986; 122:1057–1059.
21. Quesada JR, Keating MJ, Libshitz HI, Llamas L: Bone involvement in hairy cell leukemia. *Am J Med* 1983; 74:228–231.
22. Thorwarth WT, Jaques PF, Orringer EP: Polyarteritis nodosa in hairy cell leukemia. *J Can Assoc Radiol* 1983; 34:151–152.
23. Downing JR, Grossi CE, Smedberg CT, et al: Diffuse large cell lymphoma in a patient with hairy cell leukemia: Immunoglobulin gene analysis reveals separate clonal origins. *Blood* 1986; 67:739–744.
24. Jacobs RH, Vokes EE, Golomb HM: Second malignancies in hairy cell leukemia. *Cancer* 1985; 56:1462–1467.
25. Knecht H, Budmiger H, Groscurth P, et al: Central nervous system involvement in hairy cell leukemia. *Klin Wochenschr* 1985; 63:423.
26. Quesada JR, Reuben JM, Hopfer RL, et al: Serologic studies in hairy cell leukemia. *Leuk Res* 1986; 10:1169–1174.
27. Jansen J, Hermans J, et al: Splenectomy in hairy cell leukemia: A retrospective multicenter analysis. *Cancer* 1981; 47:2066–2076.
28. Golomb HM, Vardiman JW: Response to splenectomy in 65 patients with hairy cell leukemia: An evaluation of spleen weight and bone marrow involvement. *Blood* 1983; 61:349–352.
29. Magee MJ, McKenzie S, Filippa DA, et al: Hairy cell leukemia. Durability of response to splenectomy in 26 patients and treatment of relapse with androgens in six patients. *Cancer* 1985; 56:2557–2562.
30. Van Norman AS, Nagorney DM, Martin JK, et al: Splenectomy for hairy cell leukemia. A clinical review of 63 patients. *Cancer* 1986; 57:644–648.
31. Joosten P, Hagenbeek A, Lowenberg B, Sizoo W: High dose methotrexate with leucovorin rescue: Effectiveness in relapsed hairy cell leukemia. *Blood* 1985; 66:241–242.
32. Flandrin G, Sigaux F, Sebahoun G, et al: Hairy cell leukemia: Clinical presentation and follow up of 211 patients. *Semin Oncol* 1984; 11(suppl 2):458–471.
34. Golomb HM: Progress report on chlorambucil therapy in postsplenectomy patients with progressive hairy cell leukemia. *Blood* 1981; 57:464–467.
35. Cheever MA, Fefer A, Greenberg PD, et al: Treatment of hairy cell leukemia with chemoradiotherapy and identical bone marrow transplantation. *N Engl J Med* 1982; 307:479–481.
36. Quesada JR, Hersh EM, Gutterman JU: Biologic therapy of hairy cell leukemia. *Semin Oncol* 1984; 11 (suppl 2): 507–510.
37. Yam LT, Klock JC, Mielke CH: Therapeutic leukapheresis in hairy cell leukemia: Review of literature and personal experience. *Semin Oncol* 1984; 11(suppl 2):493–501.

38. Golomb HM, Kraut EH, Oviatt DL, et al: Absence of prolonged benefit of initial leukapheresis therapy for hairy cell leukemia. *Am J Hematol* 1983; 14:49–56.
39. Quesada JR, Hersh EM, Keating M, et al: Hairy cell leukemia: Clinical effects of the methanol extraction residue (MER) of BCG, lithium carbonate and mononuclear cell-enriched leukocyte transfusions. *Leuk Res* 1981; 5:463–476.
40. Quesada JR: Present therapeutic options in the treatment of hairy cell leukemia. In, Brain MC, Carbone PP (eds): *Current Therapy in Hematology-Oncology* 3. New York, Decker Publishers, 1988: pp. 79–82.
41. Catovsky D, Quesada JR, Golomb H: Guidelines for the treatment of hairy cell leukemia. *Leukemia* 1987; 1:405–406.
42. Bouroncle BA: The history of hairy cell leukemia: Characteristics of long-term survivors. *Semin Oncol* 1987, 11(suppl 2):479–485.
43. Golomb HM, Ratain MJ, Vardiman JW: Sequential treatment of hairy cell leukemia: A new role for interferon. In, DeVita VT, Hellman S, Rosenberg SA (eds): *Important Advances in Oncology 1986*. Philadelphia, JB Lippincott, 1986, pp 311–322.
44. Coser P, Prinoth O, Fabris P, et al: Emergency splenectomy in hairy cell leukemia. *Acta Haematol (Basel)* 1985; 52:116–117.
45. Heier HE: Splenectomy and serious infections. *Scand J Hematol* 1980; 24:5–9.
46. Krivit WGS, Giebink GS, Leonard A: Overwhelming postsplenectomy infection. *Surg Clin North Am* 1979; 59:223–229.
47. Fruitstone MJ, Michaels BS, Rudloff DA, et al: Role of the spleen in interferon production in mice. *Proc Soc Exp Biol Med* 1966; 122:1008–1011.
48. Wood PR, Young AM, McKimm-Breschkin JL, et al: Effect of splenectomy on production of interferon and colony-stimulating factor in *Listeria monocytogenes*-infected mice. *Infect Immun* 1984;46:860–861.
49. Quesada JR, Reuben J, Manning JT, et al: Alpha interferon for induction of remission in hairy-cell leukemia. *N Engl J Med* 1984; 310:15–18.
50. Quesada JR, Hersh EM, Manning J, et al: Treatment of hairy cell leukemia with recombinant alpha-interferon. *Blood* 1986; 68:493–497.
51. Aderka D, Michalevicz R, Daniel Y, et al: Recombinant interferon $alpha_c$ for advanced hairy cell leukemia. An Israeli multicenter study. *Cancer* 1988; 61:2207–2213.
52. Damasio EE, Bernasconi C, Castoldi GL, et al: Human lymphoblastoid interferon for hairy cell leukemia: Results from the Italian Cooperative Group. *Leukemia* 1987; 1:331–333.
53. Flandrin G, Castaigne S, Sigaux F, et al: Results of treating 53 hairy cell leukemia patients with alpha-interferon. *Leukemia* 1987; 1:326–328.
54. Golomb HM, Jacobs A, Fefer A, et al: alpha 2 Interferon therapy of hairy cell leukemia: A multicenter study of 64 patients. *J Clin Oncol* 1986; 4:900–905.
55. Machii T, Kitani T, Kimura K, et al: Interferon alpha therapy for hairy cell leukemia and lymphoproliferative disorders simulating hairy cell leukemia (hairy cell leukemia variant): A cooperative group study in Japan. *Rinsho Ketsueki* 1988; 29:2029–2036.
56. Mandelli F, Cafolla-Annino L, Amadori S, et al: The alpha 2 (r) interferon in the treatment of hairy cell leukemia—progressive report of 25 cases. *J Biol Regul Homeostatic Agents* 1987; 1:177–182.

57. Pralle H, Bartel A, Boedewadt-Radzun S, et al: alpha Interferon in the therapy of hairy cell leukemia. Results of 3 prospective multicenter studies in West Germany. *Onkologie* 1988; 11:44–47.
58. Worman CP, Catovsky D, Cawley JC, et al: The UK experience with human lymphoblastoid interferon in HCL: A review of the first 50 cases. *Leukemia* 1987; 1:320–322.
59. Ratain MJ, Golomb HM, Vardiman JW, et al: Relapse after interferon alfa-2b therapy for hairy-cell leukemia: Analysis of prognostic variables. *J Clin Oncol* 1988; 6:1714–1721.
60. Steiss RG, Smith JW, Urba WG, et al: Resistance to recombinant interferon alfa-2a in hairy cell leukemia associated with neutralizing anti-interferon antibodies. *N Engl J Med* 1988; 318:1409.
61. Itri L, Champion M, Dennin RA, et al: Incidence and clinical significance of neutralizing antibodies in patients receiving recombinant interferon alpha-2a by intramuscular injection. *Cancer* 1987; 59:668–674.
62. Spiegel RJ: Clinical overview of alpha interferon. Studies and future directions. *Cancer* 1987; 59:626–631.
63. von-Wussow P, Freund M, Block B, et al: Clinical significance of anti-IFN-alpha antibody titres during interferon therapy. *Lancet* 1987; 2:635–636.
64. von-Wussow P, Freund M, Block B, et al: Low-dose alpha-interferon treatment of hairy cell leukemia. *Klin Wochenschr* 1987; 65:1681–1684.
65. Gastl, G, Werter M, De Pauw B, et al: Comparison of clinical efficacy and toxicity of conventional and optimum biological response modifying doses of interferon alpha 2c in the treatment of hairy cell leukemia. *Leukemia* 1989; 3:453–460.
66. Quesada JR, Talpaz M, Rios A, Gutterman JU: Clinical toxicity of interferon in cancer patients. *J Clin Oncol* 1986; 4:234–243.
67. Michalevicz R, Revel M: Interferons regulate the in vitro differentiation of multilineage lymphomyeloid stem cells in hairy cell leukemia. *Proc Natl Acad Sci USA* 1987; 84:2307–2311.
68. Bardawil RG, Ratain MJ, Ho AD, et al: Pentostatin (2'deoxycoformycin) for the treatment of lymphoid neoplasms. Bone Marrow Transplantation 1989; 4(suppl 1):60–62.
69. Laughlin M, Islam A, Barcos M, et al: Effect of alpha-interferon therapy on bone marrow fibrosis in hairy cell leukemia. *Blood* 1988; 72:936–939.
70. Thaler J, Denz H, Dietze O, et al: Immunohistological assessment of bone marrow biopsies from patients with hairy cell leukemia: Changes following treatment with alpha-2-interferon and deoxycoformycin. *Leuk Res* 1989; 13:377–383.
71. Afeltra A, Caccavo D, Siena MM, et al: Disappearance of huge splenomegaly under alpha interferon treatment of hairy cell leukemia. *Haematologica (Pavia)* 1988; 73:67–70.
72. Grosbois B, Derennes V, Chales G, et al: Multiple bone localizations in hairy cell leukemia. Efficacy of treatment with alpha 2 interferon. *Nouv Rev Fr Hematol* 1986; 28:377–379.
73. Rossi JF, Marcelli C, Dubois A, et al: Regression of excessive bone remodelling by interferon alpha 2a in a patient with hairy cell leukemia. *Eur J Haematol* 1988; 41:191.

74. Reuben JM, Ip S, Quesada JR: Effect of interferon alpha therapy on plasma IL-2 receptors in hairy cell leukemia. *Blood* 1986; 68(suppl 1):32a.
75. Lepe-Zuniga JL, Quesada JR, Baron S, et al: Alpha interferon production in patients with hairy cell leukemia: Correlations with disease activity and remission status. *Hematol Pathol* 1987; 1:157–65.
76. Quesada JR, Alexanian R, Kurzrock R, et al: Clinical studies with recombinant interferon gamma in hairy cell leukemia, multiple myeloma and Waldenstrom's macroglobulinemia. *Am J Hematol* 1988; 29:1–5.
77. Michalevicz R, Aderka D, Frisch B, et al: Interferon beta induced remission in a hairy cell leukemia patient resistant to interferon alpha. *Leuk Res* 1988; 12:845–851.
78. Kalyanaraman VS, Sarngardharan MG, Robert-Guroff M, et al: A new subtype of human T cell leukemia (HTLV II) associated with a variant of hairy cell leukemia. *Science* 1982; 218:571–573.
79. Lion T, Razvi N, Golomb HM, Brownstein RH: B-lymphocytic hairy cells contain no HTLV-II DNA sequences. *Blood* 1988; 72:1428–1430.
80. Paganelli KA, Evans SS, Han T, Ozer H: B cell growth factor-induced proliferation of hairy cell lymphocytes a inhibition by type II interferon in vitro. *Blood* 1986; 67:937–942.
81. Ford RJ, Yoshimura L, Morgan J, et al: Growth factor-mediated tumor cell proliferation in hairy cell leukemia. *J Exp Med* 1985; 162:1–6.
82. Ford RJ, Kwok D, Quesada JR, Sahasrabuddhe CG: Production of B cell growth factor(s) by neoplastic B cells from hairy cell leukemia patients. *Blood* 1986; 67:573–577.
83. Giardina SL, Young HA, Faltynek CR, et al: Rearrangement of both immunoglobulin and T cell receptor genes in a prolymphocytic variant of hairy cell leukemia patient resistant to interferon alpha. *Blood* 1988; 72:1708–1716.
84. Rossi GB: Interferons and cell differentiation. In, Gresser I (ed): *Interferon* 6. London, Academic Press, 1985, pp 31–62.
85. Gressler VH, Weinkauff RE, Franklin WA, et al: Is there a direct differentiation-inducing effect of human recombinant interferon on hairy cell leukemia in vitro? *Cancer* 1989; 64:374–378.
86. De Maeyer-Guignard J, De Maeyer E: Immunomodulation by interferons: Recent developments. In, Gresser I (ed): *Interferon* 6. London, Academic Press, 1985, pp 69–86.
87. Gastl G, Aulitzky W, Leiter E, et al: Alpha-interferon induces remission in hairy cell leukemia without enhancement of natural killing. *Blut* 1986; 52:273–279.
88. Griffiths SD, Cawley JC: The beneficial effects of alpha-interferon in hairy cell leukemia are not attributable to NK cell-mediated cytotoxicity. *Leukemia* 1987; 1:372–376.
89. Lahat N, Aghai E, Kotler A, et al: Discordant effect of interferon on natural killer activity and tumor cell sensitivity to lysis in hairy cell leukemia. *Blood* 1988; 71:1141–1143.
90. Starling GC, Nimmo JC, Hart DN: Hairy cell leukemia cells are relatively NK insensitive targets. *Pathology* 1988; 20:361–365.

91. De Maeyer-Guignard J, Zawatzky R, Dandoy F, et al: An X-linked locus influences early serum IFN levels in mouse. *J Interferon Res* 1983; 3:241–252.
92. Lauria F, Bagnara GP, Guarini A, et al: Reduced bone marrow colony growth in hairy cell leukemia before and after interferon alpha treatment. Possible inhibitory role of a serological factor. *Haematologica (Pavia)* 1988; 73:191–194.
93. Grever MR, Leiby JM, Kraut EH, et al: Low-dose deoxycoformycin in lymphoid neoplasms. *J Clin Oncol* 1985; 3:1196–1201.
94. Ho AD, Kanagasabai G, Knauf WU, et al: Clinical response to deoxycoformycin in lymphoid neoplasms and biochemical changes in circulating malignant cells in vivo. *Blood* 1988; 72:1884–1890.
95. de Ferra F, Baglioni C: Increase in *S*-adenosylhomocysteine concentrations in interferon-treated HeLa cells and inhibition of methylation of vesicular stomatitis virus mRNA. *J Biol Chem* 1983; 258:2118–2123.
96. Spiers AS, Parekh SJ, Bishop MB: Hairy cell leukemia: Induction of complete remission with pentostatin (2'-deoxycoformycin). *J Clin Oncol* 1984; 2:1336–1342.
97. Spiers ASD, Moore D, Cassileth PA, et al: Remissions in hairy cell leukemia with pentostatin (2'-deoxycoformycin). *N Engl J Med* 1987; 316:825–830.
98. Grem JL, King SA, Cheson BD, et al: Pentostatin in hairy cell leukemia: Treatment by the special exception mechanism. *JNCI* 1989; 81:448–453.
99. Johnston JB, Eisenhauer E, Corbett WE, et al: Efficacy of 2'-deoxycoformycin in hairy-cell leukemia: A study of the National Cancer Institute of Canada Clinical Trials Group. *JNCI* 1988; 80:765–769.
100. Kraut EH, Bournoncle BA, Grever MR: Pentostatin in the treatment of advanced hairy cell leukemia. *J Clin Oncol* 1989; 7:168–172.
101. Foon KA, Nakano GM, Koller CA, et al: Response to 2'-deoxycoformycin after failure of interferon-alpha in nonsplenectomized patients with hairy cell leukemia. *Blood* 1986; 68:297–300.
102. Ho AD, Kuse R, Prummer O, et al: 2'-Deoxycoformycin (pentostatin) in hairy cell leukemia: Response in patients refractory to interferon alpha. *Klin Wochenschr* 1987; 65:975–979.
103. Lembersky BC, Ratain MJ, Westbrook C, et al: Rapid response to 2' deoxycoformycin in advanced hairy cell leukemia after failure of interferons alpha and gamma. *Am J Hematol* 1988; 27:60–62.
104. O'Dwyer PJ, Spiers ASD, Marsoni S: Association of severe and fatal infections and treatment with pentostatin. *Cancer Treat Rep* 1986; 70:1117–1120.
105. O'Dwyer PJ, King SA, Eisenhauer E, et al: Hypersensitivity reactions to deoxycoformycin. *Cancer Chemother Pharmacol* 1989; 23:173–175.
106. Urba WJ, Baseler MW, Kopp WC, et al: Deoxycoformycin induced immunosuppression in patients with hairy cell leukemia. *Blood* 1989; 73:38–46.
107. Glaspy JA, Baldwin GC, Robertson PA, et al: Therapy for neutropenia in hairy cell leukemia with recombinant human granulocyte colony-stimulating factor. *Ann Intern Med* 1989; 109:789–795.
108. Piro LD, Carrera CJ, Beutler E, et al: 2-Chlorodeoxyadenosine: An effective new agent for the treatment of chronic lymphocytic leukemia. *Blood* 1988; 72:1069–1073.

109. Keating MJ, Kantarjian H, Talpaz M, et al: Fludarabine: A new agent with major activity against chronic lymphocytic leukemia. *Blood* 1989; 74:19–25.
110. Piro LD, Carrera DA, Carson DA, Beutler E: Lasting remissions in hairy-cell leukemia induced by a single infusion of 2-chlorodeoxyadenosine. *N Engl J Med* 1990; 322:1117–1121.
111. Calvo F, Castaigne S, Sigaux F, et al: Intensive chemotherapy of hairy cell leukemia in patients with aggressive disease. *Blood* 1985; 65:115–119.

8

Controversies in Management of Hodgkin's Disease

Fredrick B. Hagemeister

University of Texas
M. D. Anderson Cancer Center
Houston, Texas

Historically, Hodgkin's disease is one of the best described malignancies in medical literature. It was one of the first tumors to be controlled with radiotherapy, and it is curable with chemotherapy. The disease can be confused with other lymphomas and nonmalignant disorders. The cell of origin remains controversial. Most of the cells in the Hodgkin's disease infiltrate are normal reactive blood constituents. The malignant cell itself represents only 5% or less of the tumor infiltrate. Its cytogenetic, morphological, and chemical properties have been studied in detail, but results are controversial. The cellular and humoral defects associated with the disease have been evaluated extensively, but their etiology has not been clarified. Multiple investigators have studied clinical characteristics of the disease and, for the most part, the clinical course of the disease is predictable, which permits the application of staging techniques predictive of treatment outcome.

Treatment for patients with Hodgkin's disease is often successful and results in durable complete remissions. Investigators have refined treatment techniques in recent years to reduce toxicity and improve quality of life. Issues such as sterility, the incidence of second malignancies, and other complications of radiotherapy and chemotherapy have become more important in initial treatment of the disease. Therapy for patients with relapsing disease with second-line chemotherapy remains a problem. Bone marrow transplantation has been effective in inducing durable remissions in patients with recurrent disease.

In this chapter, we will review new concepts of pathology, with an emphasis on tumor biology and the importance of making distinctions between various subtypes of the disease. We will also discuss treatment options for individual stages of disease, clinically or laparotomy staged, potential complications of treatment, and treatment options that might reduce these complications.

PATHOLOGY

Cell of Origin

In 1832, Thomas Hodgkin first described the disease now named after him (1). Many of the patients described in his original work may not have actually had this malignancy. The cell of origin of the Reed–Sternberg and other abnormal cells in the tumor infiltrate remains unclear. A macrophage origin has been proposed on a morphological basis (2–4). However, there is recent evidence that the disease may be a neoplasm of true lymphocytic origin. The Leu-M1 marker produced by Hsu and Jaffe stains T- and B-lymphoma cells, but also Reed–Sternberg cells (5–7). This marker distinguishes malignant cells from nonmalignant processes, but not one lymphoma subtype from another.

In 1982, Stein and associates produced convincing evidence that the Reed–Sternberg cell is derived from a lymphocytic precursor (8). By using a cell line derived from a tumor from a patient with Hodgkin's disease, they developed a monoclonal antibody, known as Ki-1, which, when coupled with appropriate stains, identified transformed lymphocytes. The Ki-1 antibody does not react with normal unstimulated lymphocytes, but does react with certain fetal cells, mitogen-transformed lymphocytes in vitro, Reed–Sternberg cells and their variants, and certain lymphomas derived from T and B cells, now known as "Ki-1 lymphomas." The Ki-1 antibody does not specifically stain Reed–Sternberg cells or their variants, and cannot be used to distinguish Hodgkin's disease from other lymphomas that appear pathologically similar to Hodgkin's disease.

Morphological Subtypes

At the Rye meeting in 1966, investigators recognized at least six pathologic variants of the disease. These were consolidated into four groups now identified as *nodular sclerosis* (NS), *mixed cellularity* (MC), *lymphocyte-depleted* (LD), and *lymphocyte-predominant* (LP) Hodgkin's disease (9,10). The Reed–Sternberg cells are essential for the diagnosis of Hodgkin's disease, but criteria for denoting the diagnostic cell are controversial (11–13). The diagnostic cellular variants of Hodgkin's disease (lacunar, lymphocyte and histiocytic [L and H], pleomorphic, mononuclear, and pyknotic cells) may suggest the diagnosis of Hodgkin's disease; however, only the Reed–Sternberg (RS) cell, itself, can establish a diagnosis, with the proper histological background. The diagnosis of Hodgkin's disease may be difficult for the pathologist who has difficulty distinguishing between L and H and lacunar cells. Lacunar cells are characteristic of NS, but can occur in some cases of diagnosed MC, which may actually be NS histology without the fibrous bands. The L and H cells, on the other hand, are characteristic of LP, a histologic type that characteristically lacks RS cells. However, an occasional occurrence of LP may be mistakenly diagnosed as MC because diagnostic Reed–Sternberg cells are present. Pleomorphic cells may be found in both LD and NS Hodgkin's disease. Mononuclear variants of the Reed–Sternberg cell suggest Hodgkin's disease and are more common in patients who have early-staged disease, in which there is only focal involvement in the node, with a background of reactive hyperplasia.

Lymphocyte Predominance

Occasionally, Hodgkin's disease is confused pathologically with a variety of other conditions, notably the non-Hodgkin's lymphomas. The two variants of lymphocyte-predominant Hodgkin's disease (nodular, LP-N or diffuse, LP-D) present the greatest problem with misdiagnosis. The LP-N form may be confused with follicular lymphoma if the nodules are construed as being predominant in the pathological interpretation, or as small lymphocytic lymphoma or reactive hyperplasia when the nodules are not well visualized. The LP-D form may be confused with small lymphocytic lymphoma if the characteristic L and H cells cannot be seen because sections are too thick. They may also be confused with the MC subtype if the Reed–Sternberg cell is abundant (13,14).

Investigators have also proposed that there are phenotypic differences between LP-N Hodgkin's disease and the LP-D variant, and that the latter is similar to MC and NS forms of the disease. Pinkus et al. reported important staining differences between the atypical L and H cells from patients with LP-N, and the classic cell seen in the MC and NS subtypes (15). Others have demonstrated J chains in cells of the LP-N variant, suggesting that LP-N may be a different disease from the other subtypes, with characteristics similar to B-cell neoplasms (16–18). Atypical L and H cells are also seen in LP-D, and these stain as B cells, but there are other characteristics suggesting that this variant may be different from LP-N (17,18). The background cells also seem to be of B-cell type, whereas in MC and NS forms, they are of T-cell origin (19).

Regula et al. reported that patients with LP-N Hodgkin's disease had a different natural history from the LP-D, NS, and MC subtypes (20). They concluded that LP-N behaves like a low-grade lymphoma, with a chronic relapsing course and a response to treatment similar to the low-grade B-cell lymphomas. However, Borg-Greck et al. reported that late relapse was infrequent in all pathological subtypes and that, although these diseases may represent separate forms pathologically, there are no clinical differences between these variants (21). Further analysis is needed to determine whether LP-N is a B-cell lymphoma different from LP-D, MC, and NS.

Nodular Sclerosis

The nodular sclerosis subtype is the most easily diagnosed type of Hodgkin's disease because of the visible nodules and fibrous bands. However, RS cells are typically difficult to locate in this subtype, and lacunar cell variants predominate. Accordingly, the diagnosis should be nodular sclerosis, rather than mixed cellularity, if many lacunar cells are present. However, patients with this subtype have a survival similar to patients with MC (22). In some cases, clusters of lacunar cells may resemble large-cell lymphoma cells, especially if the tissue is from an extranodal site. This type is designated the "lacunar cell predominant" variant of NS. Necrosis may be prominent in this variant and is unusual in other subtypes.

Ben-Yehuda-Salz et al. have reported that the syncytial variant of nodular sclerosing Hodgkin's disease is a unique morphologic type (23). Such patients often have clinically advanced disease at diagnosis. It can be confused with other malignancies, especially large-cell lymphoma. Patients with a diagnosis of large-cell lymphoma should be carefully reevaluated to rule out these variants of NS, since treatment outcome may depend on this differentiation (14).

MacLennan and co-workers have devised a grading system for NS Hodgkin's disease (24). A grade II histology, which included specimens with extensive areas of lymphocyte depletion or numerous anaplastic Hodgkin's cells, was associated with a poor response to initial therapy by patients, a higher relapse rate, and lower survival, regardless of stage, compared with patients with grade I histology. Patients with grade II histology also had a high frequency of B symptoms, abnormal erythrocyte sedimentation rates, low hemoglobin levels, thrombocytopenia, and low serum albumin concentration, all considered poor prognostic features. The prognostic value of histologically subdividing nodular sclerosis into two grades has been confirmed in other studies (25,26).

Mixed Cellularity

Mixed cellularity is an intermediate between the nodular and diffuse varieties of LP Hodgkin's disease, and between diffuse fibrosis and reticular LD subtypes. The lymphoma most commonly misdiagnosed as MC Hodgkin's disease is peripheral T-cell lymphoma. This lymphoma represents a wide spectrum of diseases, and the T cells present are truly malignant, whereas the T cells in MC are merely part of a reactive process. Clonality cannot be demonstrated with marker studies for such T-cell lymphomas. However, gene rearrangement studies may distinguish between the two diseases. The diagnosis of peripheral T-cell lymphoma should be considered in patients with MC Hodgkin's disease who present with mediastinal masses or diffuse adenopathy, without extranodal involvement. The distinction is critical, since therapy is different for the two diseases, and peripheral T-cell lymphoma has a worse prognosis than MC.

Lymphocyte Depletion

The lymphocyte depletion form consists of two variants: diffuse fibrosis and reticular types. Both large-cell lymphoma and NS Hodgkin's disease are frequently misinterpreted as LD (27). This diagnosis is rare, and patients with this subtype should have repeat biopsies, and material reevaluated for other diagnostic possibilities.

HODGKIN'S DISEASE: STAGES I AND II

With modern-day chemotherapy and radiation therapy, newer staging techniques, and improvement in pathological analysis, there are now a variety of ways to manage early-staged Hodgkin's disease. Most of the credit for the application of these various treatments can be attributed to the development of improved techniques in multiple fields, and the dedication of pathologists, biologists, and medical and radiotherapeutic oncologists. In this section, we will review concepts of management of the disease, present recent data available on treatment, and discuss current policies for management.

The Importance of Pathology and Staging in Treatment Decisions for Patients with Early-Staged Hodgkin's Disease

Pathology

The Lukes and Butler classification system identified subtypes of Hodgkin's disease that had prognostic relevance to treatment with radiation therapy alone. Patients with mixed cellularity had relapse rates higher than those for patients with other pathological subtypes. However, in later studies, subtype alone was not an important factor (28). Patients with stage II mixed cellularity who were treated with irradiation alone had worse outcomes than those with stage I mixed cellularity disease (29). However, patients with upper torso mixed cellularity disease, staged by lymphangiography, often had involvement of abdominal nodes; therefore, results improved when patients with abdominal disease were excluded from studies (30). For lymphangiogram-staged disease, pathology played little role in the management of patients treated with radiotherapy alone.

Lymphangiography

A lymphangiography study is important for the management of Hodgkin's disease. This radiographic study can detect early changes from Hodgkin's disease within normal-sized nodes that cannot be visualized by computed tomography (CT). If radiotherapy is contemplated as treatment for abdominal disease, visualization of abdominal nodes by lymphangiography is essential (31). When chemotherapy alone is chosen to treat clinically staged II Hodgkin's disease, lymphangiography may not be essential, since chemotherapy alone might control microscopic abdominal disease. However, when the treatment is combined modality therapy or radiotherapy alone, lymphangiography is necessary for staging.

Laparotomy

Staging by laparotomy was first introduced by physicians at Stanford to investigate the possibility of splenic involvement early in the course of the patient's disease (32). In the initial study, all patients, regardless of clinical stage, underwent staging by laparotomy. In this series, the presence of B symptoms was associated with a high likelihood of positive laparotomy findings, the liver was involved only if splenic disease was present, and false-negative results at lymphangiography were frequent.

Subsequently, other investigators have reported their results of findings at laparotomy (33–38). At our institution, male gender, age 40 years or older, and the presence of B symptoms were independent features indicating a higher likelihood of abdominal disease at laparotomy (37). Patients with stage I cervical presentations above the cricoid cartilage, those with LP stage I disease, and females with NS stage IA peripheral node presentations consistently had negative findings for disease at laparotomy. Other investigators have reported similar findings in their studies (38–40). However, all other groups of patients had a risk of positive findings.

Other investigators have tried to develop arithmetic methods that could detect patients who had a very low risk of positive findings for disease at laparotomy. De La Cruz and colleagues studied patients with clinically staged I and II supradiaphragmatic Hodgkin's disease (36). By multivariate analysis, mixed cellularity histologic type, presence of B symptoms, and a higher number of involved upper torso nodal regions were independent predictors for a positive staging laparotomy. By using an index system depending upon these features, they suggested that patients with clinically staged I and II disease have a 4–93% risk of occult abdominal disease, depending on various combinations of features. This system needs confirmation in independent populations to determine its reproducibility.

Studies of findings at laparotomy may be important for determining effectiveness of therapy and the best overall treatment plan. Patients with pathologically staged I and II disease who have features associated with clinically staged III disease may have a higher risk of abdominal relapse, especially when treated with upper torso or extended field irradiation alone. Isolated splenic involvement may be an important feature in selecting therapy for patients with stage III Hodgkin's disease (41). Therefore, exploration of celiac nodes is important, since these are often positive for disease in the patient with splenic involvement (37). The extent of splenic disease may be an important factor for patients treated with irradiation alone (42), but not for those treated with combined modality (43).

Staging Modification: The Cotswolds Conference

Because of the discovery of prognostic factors that influence treatment results, the prognostic importance of stage has changed since the Ann Arbor Conference. A group of experts have recently accepted four new conclusions for staging and response to therapy (42). First, both CT and lymphangiography could be used for evaluation of the chest and infradiaphragmatic lymph nodes, primarily because physicians can easily perform and interpret the CT. Second, criteria for clinical involvement of the spleen and liver were modified to include evidence of focal defects with two imaging techniques; serum abnormalities of liver function were excluded, and criteria for extranodal spread were more completely outlined. Third, the suffix "x" was proposed to designate bulky disease greater than 10 cm in maximum dimension; this included masses that measured more than one-third of the chest at T5–6. Finally, a new category of response to therapy was introduced to accommodate the difficulty of persistent radiological abnormalities of uncertain significance; this was termed *unconfirmed/uncertain* complete remission (CR_u). These recommendations should be incorporated into new studies and included in reports of results.

Conclusions Concerning Staging Methods

Regardless of the technical issues concerning staging methods, staging by lymphangiography and laparotomy still influences therapy for patients with favorable prognoses, especially when radiotherapy will be part of the treatment plan. Computed tomography may not be as accurate as lymphangiography in establishing the presence or extent of minimal abdominal disease. However, in patients with Hodgkin's disease, the CT scan is usually negative for disease when the lymphangiogram is negative. Therefore, it is reasonable to first perform a lymphangiogram when evaluating the patient with an upper torso presentation.

For patients with favorable upper torso presentations and no evidence of abdominal disease by lymphangiography, staging by laparotomy may also be a factor in treatment. About one-third of patients with upper torso disease and negative lymphangiograms will still have microscopic abdominal disease. The lymphangiogram does not delineate nodes in the celiac and porta hepatis areas, and the CT scan is usually negative in this area, since celiac nodes are too small to be detected when the lymphangiogram is negative for disease in the para-aortic nodes. Therefore, it it is necessary to know whether abdominal disease is present, a laparotomy becomes an important staging method for the individual patient.

Results of treatment for stage IIIA Hodgkin's disease also indicate that staging by laparotomy may determine treatment selection for patients with clinically staged disease. These patients have better disease-free survival results when they receive combined modality therapy instead of radiation therapy alone, even when they have stage III_1 disease limited to the celiac axis or spleen (45,46). Therefore, patients with only clinically staged disease should receive both chemotherapy and irradiation to the upper and lower torso.

Radiotherapy Concepts: Upper Torso Presentations

Is Abdominal Radiotherapy Needed for Laparotomy-Staged Disease?

In the 1950s, many patients treated with low-dose involved-field radiotherapy had good responses; however, most developed disseminated disease and died within 5 years. Peters and others, using higher doses of radiation, wider fields, and prophylactic treatment to adjacent areas (47), reported excellent results for patients with stage I disease, but not for those with stage II or III disease (48).

Given these findings, investigators at Stanford began to treat patients with involved- or extended-field therapy in a randomized trial (49). Patients with mediastinal disease had better results when treated with extended fields; however, patients with only cervical or axillary nodal disease had poor results, owing to a high rate of abdominal relapse. This led to the use of total nodal irradiation to encompass potential sites of abdominal relapse in patients with clinically staged disease. Originally, irradiation was restricted to initial sites of involvement and immediately adjacent uninvolved regions for prophylaxis. With development of megavoltage equipment, prophylactic treatment could be expanded to include the mantle technique for patients with upper torso presentations and the inverted-"Y" (50,51).

After the development of the mantle and total nodal irradiation fields, Rosenberg and Kaplan reported a reduction in relapse in the abdomen with inverted-Y prophylaxis for patients with clinically staged disease. Subsequently, these investigators recommended prophylactic abdominal irradiation for patients with not only clinically staged, but also laparotomy-staged upper torso disease (52,53). Optimal doses for treatment to involved original sites of disease were 40–45 Gy, but doses for prophylaxis to involved, adjacent nodal areas were effective at 30–35 Gy (54). Eventually, they omitted pelvic fields for patients with laparotomy-staged IA or IIA disease (55).

Prophylactic irradiation below the diaphragm for laparotomy-staged disease remained the treatment of choice in the United States for many years. However, investigators have questioned the need for prophylactic abdominal radiotherapy in recent years, and convincing evidence has emerged that such treatment is unnecessary. From one study, Farah et al. reported results of treatment of 135 adults and children, with pathologically staged I and II Hodgkin's disease, who received extended mantle radiation, a combination of the standard mantle field and a para-aortic field in one port. Only 12 had pathologically staged IIB disease.

The 10-year disease-free survival and survival rates were 82% and 83%, respectively. However, the number of patients with large mediastinal masses or hilar involvement—known adverse features for relapse in the lung—was not reported. It is unclear how abdominal radiation therapy was of benefit to these patients, and it is possible that these patients may have represented a favorable group with small mediastinal masses.

Other investigators have demonstrated that radiation to the upper abdomen is not required for patients who undergo staging by laparotomy (57–60). However, in all instances, recommendations for mantle radiotherapy alone are based on the presence of favorable prognostic factors: patients selected for mantle irradiation alone may not have large mediastinal masses or other adverse features. From the M. D. Anderson Cancer Center, we have reported results of treatment of patients with laparotomy-staged I or II disease, using either involved-field (IF), mantle, or extended-field (EF) irradiation, to include para-aortic lymph nodes and spleen (57). In this series, patients treated with IF or mantle radiotherapy had 5-year disease-free survival results of 72%, compared with 66% for those treated with EF. The nodal relapse rate in the abdomen was the same for those treated with either IF or EF. Prognostic factor analysis demonstrated that a mediastinal mass larger than 7.5 cm on a chest posteroanterior radiograph, hilar involvement, and B symptoms, all were adverse features. Abdominal radiotherapy did not reduce the risk of relapse in patients with or without these features.

Carde and associates found that patients with laparotomy findings that were negative for disease had similar results when randomized to therapy with EF or mantle radiotherapy; disease-free survival results were 72% and 74%, respectively (58). However, the patients in this group had favorable presentations. Anderson and colleagues treated patients with mantle radiotherapy or the mantle followed by six cycles of MVPP (mechlorethamine, vinblastine, procarbazine, prednisone) (60). In this series, patients with B symptoms or large mediastinal mass had the highest relapse rates. Those with favorable presentations had a relapse rate of only 19% with mantle radiotherapy alone, compared with 75% for those with bulky mediastinal involvement. Results for favorable presentations from these two series are similar to those reported from our institution, suggesting that patients with laparotomy-staged disease do not need abdominal radiotherapy. However, current treatment policies from other investigators may differ, depending upon the reliability of results of staging by laparotomy, capability of performing and interpreting the effectiveness of the lymphangiogram, and experience of the hematopathologist.

Toxicity of Radiation Therapy

There is variability in the radiation dose necessary to cure patients. Kaplan found a high rate of permanent local control with doses above 30 Gy and few local relapses after a total tumor dose of 40 Gy (61). Radiotherapists have usually treated patients with 40 Gy, delivered in 20 fractions over 4 weeks for optimal results. However, because large volumes of disease required large fields, particularly in the mediastinum, treatment with radiotherapy often caused unacceptable complications. Because of these complications, radiotherapists have tried to limit doses and volumes of radiotherapy fields, although no investigators have conclusively demonstrated a reduction in complication rates with their modifications.

CARDIAC DYSFUNCTION. Radiation therapy can induce cardiac damage to all three layers of the heart (62). Although most patients who receive radiation therapy and develop coronary artery disease have pathological changes identical with nonradiation-induced coronary artery disease, some patients may develop total obliteration of the coronary artery (63,64). In one study, more than 50% of patients treated with irradiation had subclinical pericardial or myocardial dysfunction, demonstrated by chest x-ray films, echocardiogram, or radionuclide ventriculogram (65). In patients 35 years of age or younger, myocardial perfusion scintigraphy was normal. However, 24% had abnormalities demonstrated by gaited equilibrium rest and exercise radionuclide ventriculography, and abnormal left ventricular ejection fraction (LVEF) response to exercise, with ventricular dilatation and apical hypokinesis. Twelve percent of patients treated with mantle radiotherapy may develop conduction defects on electrocardiogram (ECG) (66). Others had borderline abnormalities including ST-T changes, prolonged QT intervals, or axis deviation. Other patients had pericardial or valvular thickening, thickening of the aortic or mitral valves, right ventricular dilatation or hypokinesis, or left ventricular dysfunction demonstrated by echocardiography (67). However, echocardiograms for patients whose whole heart volume was within the radiation ports were similar to those for patients who received radiation to only part of the heart, with the left ventricle excluded. There were also no differences in the incidence of ECG abnormalities in patients treated with doses above 35 Gy, compared with patients who received lower doses. There was a lower prevalence of left-sided valvular thickening and right ventricular abnormalities in patients treated with more modern radiation therapy techniques, including equally balanced anterior and posterior radiation fields and doses.

Children and adolescents may also develop cardiac dysfunction following mantle radiation. In one study, 43% had pericardial thickening on echocardiograms, this being more frequent in those followed for more than 6 years (68). Therefore, longer follow-ups may be necessary to determine late complications of cardiac dysfunction. Combined modality therapy might permit lower doses of radiation therapy and might lower the risk. However, since most patients are asymptomatic, treatment with modern mantle radiotherapy alone may still be appropriate for patients with favorable prognostic features.

PULMONARY DYSFUNCTION. Pulmonary dysfunction is generally related to dose and field technique. In the past, when radiation therapy alone was used to treat a large mediastinal mass, it was necessary to irradiate large volumes of lung, resulting in acute radiation pneumonitis, a complication that appeared at intervals up to 6 months after treatment (69). With development of the shrinking-field technique and lung blocks to limit the amount of pulmonary radiation, the incidence of pulmonary complications was significantly reduced. Morgan and colleagues studied the late pulmonary sequelae of radiation therapy for Hodgkin's disease in 18 patients (65). Pulmonary function tests were abnormal in 16, with a 10% reduction of alveolar volume or vital capacity and a 28% reduction in mean diffusing capacity. Patients who receive combined modality therapy were at a higher risk of developing pulmonary complications.

THYROID DYSFUNCTION. Pasqualini et al. reported that radiation therapy produces thyroid dysfunction in 50% of patients receiving radiotherapy, compared with only 27% for those receiving chemotherapy alone (70). In their study, 12 of 51 patients had elevated thyrotropin (TSH) values. Sixteen also had exaggerated TSH responses to thyrotropin-releasing hormone (TRH), with the most abnormal responses seen in patients receiving combined modality therapy. Six patients (27%) who received chemotherapy alone had abnormal TSH basal levels or elevated TSH response to TRH, whereas 13 (50%) of those treated with chemotherapy plus irradiation had abnormal tests. Three of the patients with high TSH levels also had low thyroxine (T_4) levels, and 12 had positive antimicrosomal antibody titers, without evidence of antithyroglobulin antibody. This suggests that patients with lymphoma may be predisposed to autoimmune thyroid disease. Although patients who receive radiation therapy that encompass the thyroid often have elevated TSH levels, clinical hypothyroidism occurs in relatively few such patients. Patients should be followed carefully, since they may not become symptomatic for 5 years or more after therapy (71).

GONADAL DYSFUNCTION. Kinsella and co-workers assessed testicular function following 6–70 cGy of radiation as treatment for patients with pathologically staged Hodgkin's disease (72). They prospectively followed follicle-stimulating hormone (FSH), luteinizing hormone (LH), and testosterone levels, as well as semen analyses. In patients who received 20 cGy or more, serum FSH levels rose, with maximum levels at 6 months posttreatment. All had a return to normal values within 12–24 months. Below 20 cGy, FSH values remained normal. There were no changes in LH or testosterone levels at any dose. Five patients with normal pretreatment sperm counts received <20 cGy and all had normal counts at follow-up evaluation. Of three who received more than 20 cGy, two had transient decrease in sperm counts for 6–18 months, but eventually recovered spermatogenesis. This suggests that seminiferous tubules can be damaged; however, Leydig cell function is not affected by treatment with radiation.

SECOND MALIGNANCIES. Five different solid tumors are seen with increased frequency in patients treated for Hodgkin's disease with radiotherapy: sarcomas, both bone and soft tissue; lung cancer, which occurs in smokers and nonsmokers; squamous carcinoma of the head and neck; melanoma, with the highest risk occurring in patients with the dysplastic nevus syndrome; and breast carcinoma (73). Patients with Hodgkin's disease can also develop non-Hodgkin's lymphoma as a complication of therapy, but the risk is highest when both radiotherapy and chemotherapy are used. The overall risk of this complication was 4.4% in a report from Stanford University (74). The risk for patients treated with combined modality therapy was 15.2% at 10 years. However, the risk of lymphoma was extremely low in patients who received chemotherapy only. Most of these patients had B-cell lymphoma, and the disease tended to originate in the gastrointestinal tract or retroperitoneum.

Reducing Complications of Radiotherapy. Improved tolerance to mantle radiotherapy can be achieved by using the "split-course technique." However, this increases the risk of local relapse (69,75). Another maneuver limits the dose to the heart to 25–30 Gy; however, this may be impossible when treating large mediastinal masses (76). The shrinking-field technique permits reduction in the dose of irradiation to the lung and the heart, but the dose may still be high, particularly with large mediastinal masses extending onto the diaphragm. These improvements have reduced the incidence of radiation pneumonitis and cardiac complications (57,67,77–79), but were associated with an increased local relapse rate, either within the radiotherapy field or as a geographic miss, unless strict treatment policies are followed.

The likelihood of local relapse is related to the experience of the radiotherapist. In one study, Kinzie and associates evaluated portal films to determine the adequacy of fields and their relationship to relapse rate (80). The rate of infield or marginal recurrence varied significantly among radiation oncologists providing therapy for these patients. Inadequate margins were associated with a 54% overall relapse rate, of which 33% were infield or marginal recurrence. However, when the portal films were judged adequate, the total relapse rate was only 14%, with 7% infield or marginal recurrence.

Prognostic Factors for Patients Treated with Radiotherapy

Investigators disagree over the importance of various prognostic features in the treatment of patients with stage I–II Hodgkin's disease. Features considered prognostically important for patients with disease staged by laparotomy include large mediastinal adenopathy, elevated erythrocyte sedimentation rate (ESR), the presence of B symptoms, hilar involvement, and involvement of more than two lymph node sites.

Large Mediastinal Adenopathy

Most investigators agree that the presence of large mediastinal adenopathy is one of the most adverse features predicting relapse. Traditionally, the ratio of the widest diameter of the mediastinum to the widest diameter of the thorax has been predictive of relapse in patients treated with radiotherapy. Others have measured the mediastinal mass directly. At our institution, any mediastinal mass measuring 7.5 cm or larger is an adverse feature. However, measurement of mediastinal mass volumes by CT before and after therapy might be the best way to predict relapse for the patient with a large mediastinal mass (81,82). In one study of patients treated with radiotherapy, those with a mediastinal volume smaller than 200 mL had a mediastinal relapse rate of only 13%, compared with 32% for those with volumes larger than 200 mL. Patients receiving methchlorethamine, vincristine (Oncovin), procarbazine, prednisone (MOPP) also had a lower incidence of mediastinal relapse when they had more than 85% reduction in volume 1–2 months after chemotherapy, compared with patients who had a lower reduction in volume.

RESULTS OF TREATMENT AT M. D. ANDERSON CANCER CENTER. At our institution, patients treated with radiation therapy after staging by laparotomy had excellent results when they did not have a mediastinal mass measuring 7.5 cm or larger in diameter on a chest x-ray film, B symptoms, or hilar involvement (83). Patients with small mediastinal masses and no B symptoms had a 5-year disease-free survival rate of 82%, compared with 50% for those patients with small masses and B symptoms. However, patients without mediastinal disease had a disease-free rate of 79%, compared with 59% for patients with mediastinal involvement, and patients with large mediastinal masses, treated with extended-field radiotherapy, had a 45% disease-free rate. In this last group, hilar involvement was associated with a disease-free rate of only 35%.

The incidence of intrathoracic relapse, especially the lung, was 38% for those with large mediastinal masses and 16% for patients with smaller disease. The incidence of abdominal relapse was low, verifying the effectiveness of the laparotomy in detecting occult abdominal disease. When patients had no mediastinal disease, the disease-free survival rate was 94% when they were treated with mantle radiation. Thus, the mantle is an extremely effective treatment for these patients. However, patients with unfavorable presentations require additional therapy to control the problem of recurrence.

Others have also reported that a mediastinal mass of 7.5 cm or larger in diameter is an adverse prognostic feature. Zagars and Rubin reported results of patients with laparotomy-staged IA or IIA Hodgkin's disease treated with radiation therapy alone (84). The 10-year disease-free survival result for patients with stage IA was 92%, compared with 52% for those with stage IIA, and for patients with stage IIA, a large mediastinal mass was the most adverse feature for disease-free survival. These investigators identified three major groups with low, intermediate, and high risks of relapse: those with stage IA or IIA, with small mediastinal disease < 7.5 cm in diameter with less than 10% relapse; those with stage IIA disease, without mediastinal disease with a 33% relapse rate; and those with stage IIA, with large mediastinal masses measuring 7.5 cm or larger with a relapse rate of 55%. There was an additional small subset of patients with a mediastinal mass larger than 10 cm, all of whom developed progressive disease.

Other investigators have also recommended combined modality therapy for patients with large mediastinal masses. Willett et al. reported treatment of 122 patients with extended-field radiation therapy (85). Five-year disease-free survival results were 75% for the entire group, 86% for patients with stage IA, and 65% for patients with stage IIA. Adverse prognostic features by univariate analysis were more than four sites of involvement at initial presentation, large mediastinal mass, hilar disease, and extension to lung, pleura, or pericardium. The presence of a large mediastinal mass appeared to be the most statistically important feature for disease-free survival results. This group proposed that patients with large mediastinal masses should receive six cycles of chemotherapy before irradiation to improve disease-free survival rates.

RESULTS FROM THE UNIVERSITY OF MINNESOTA AND JOINT CENTER. Not all investigators recommend combined modality therapy for patients with large mediastinal masses. Lee and associates have analyzed the results for curative radiation treatment of patients with surgically staged IA–IIIA Hodgkin's disease (86). They defined two treatment groups: patients receiving mantle irradiation or mantle and the inverted-Y, including the splenic pedicle; and a second group treated with additional irradiation to both lungs and the liver as part of initial radiotherapy. The projected 5-year recurrence-free survival rate for the first group was 58% and, for the second, it was 82%, although survival results were 86% and 89%, respectively. By multivariate analysis, two risk factors—mediastinal involvement and stage IIB disease—were important features predicting disease progression for patients in group 1. They concluded that low-dose irradiation to the lung and liver significantly improved the relapse-free survival results for patients with stages IA–IIIA disease.

From the Joint Center for Radiation Therapy, Leslie et al. reported radiotherapy treatment results of patients with pathologically staged IA and IIB supradiaphragmatic Hodgkin's disease (87). Ten-year freedom from progression and survival rates were 88% and 95% for stage IA patients, and 76% and 93% for patients with stage IIA. For patients with IB and IIB, combined modality therapy yielded a relapse-free rate of 85%, compared with 69% after radiation therapy alone. Patients with large mediastinal masses had significantly worse results than patients with small or no mediastinal masses. They concluded that patients with large mediastinal masses should receive initial combined modality therapy. However, in more recent reports, the same investigators recommended radiotherapy only as possible treatment for patients with laparotomy-staged I–II disease with large mediastinal masses, based on the expectation that CT and MRI of the chest might better delineate radiotherapy fields to lessen the risk of relapse for patients with a high risk of failure (88). They also suggested that chemotherapy could salvage many of these patients at relapse.

Erythrocyte Sedimentation Rate

The ESR is a feature considered important in treatment of patients with advanced Hodgkin's disease in Europe (89,90). Tubiana and co-workers studied the influence of B symptoms and elevated ESRs for patients with clinically staged I or II Hodgkin's disease treated with radiation alone or combined modality therapy (89). Of all the prognostic factors studied, the ESR correlated best with relapse-free survival rates, and was independent of the presence of B symptoms. However, there was a relationship between ESR and presence of B symptoms, with 23% of the patients with B symptoms having an ESR lower than 30, compared with 67% of those without B symptoms. However, the ESR alone had much less prognostic significance for relapse-free survival of patients with clinically staged disease who received combined modality therapy.

Others have reported that the ESR is an important predictor of early relapse. Friedman and collaborators identified two groups of patients with different prognoses, based on posttreatment ESR rates (90). Patients with a low ESR following initial therapy had a good survival rate, regardless of treatment. However, patients had a higher relapse rate when the ESR remained elevated more than 30 mm at 1 hour after the completion of therapy, regardless of the value before treatment. They concluded that patients with a high ESR following completion of treatment for clinically staged I and II Hodgkin's disease should receive additional therapy.

B Symptoms

Although most investigators have demonstrated that B symptoms are important adverse prognostic features for relapse, the type of B symptoms may be important. Crnkovich and colleagues reviewed their experience in pathologically staged IIB Hodgkin's disease (91). Survival and freedom from relapse rates at 10 years were 81% and 74%, respectively, and there were no statistically significant differences in results for patients treated with radiation alone or combined modality. However, the number of B symptoms present was an important prognostic factor for results. The freedom from relapse rate at 8 years for patients with all three B symptoms was only 55%, compared with 87% for patients with only one or two B symptoms. On the basis of this analysis, these investigators recommended total lymphoid irradiation alone for patients with pathologically staged IIB disease and only one or two B symptoms. However, patients with all three B symptoms needed other therapy.

Hilar Involvement

The importance of hilar involvement is controversial, but in some series, it is an important prognostic factor for patients treated with radiotherapy alone (57,86). In our studies, hilar involvement was an adverse feature predicting relapse (57). The 5-year disease-free survival rate for patient with large mediastinal masses without hilar disease was 58%, compared with 35% for those with hilar involvement. The survival rate for this latter group was only 63% and was unaffected by the presence of B symptoms.

Number of Nodal Sites

This prognostic feature has been extensively studied in Europe (59,92,93). However, this adverse feature may be correlated with a higher risk of abdominal relapse specifically. It may also predict the presence of abdominal disease in patients with clinically staged disease, making the likelihood of relapse higher for patients with more nodes when treated with radiation therapy alone.

Tubiana et al. have defined three groups of patients, based on the number of involved lymph nodes in the upper torso: those with stage I disease; those with two nodes, stage II_2; and those with three or more, stage II_3 (93). In their study, approximately 50% of patients with clinically staged I or II Hodgkin's disease and involvement of one or two lymph node sites developed infradiaphragmatic dissemination after treatment with upper torso radiotherapy alone. Most of these patients had relapse in the spleen or para-aortic lymph nodes, indicating that radiotherapy to the upper abdomen might be able to control relapse for some. However, in patients with three or four lymph nodes involved, 50% had relapse in pelvic nodes or extranodal sites. These investigators concluded that this group needed total nodal irradiation.

Specht and co-workers have assessed tumor burden in a unique way, measuring the size of each involved region and calculating the number of regions involved in patients with nodal involvement (94). For patients with pathologically staged I or II disease, multivariate analysis of prognostic factors for disease-free survival confirmed that tumor burden was the most important factor for patients treated with radiation alone or combined modality therapy. Only tumor burden and age were independently significant factors for survival. They were also able to separate patients with pathologically staged I or II disease treated with radiotherapy-only into groups with low, intermediate, and high risks of relapse with 10-year freedom from relapse rates of 90%, 76%, and 40%, respectively. However, for patients treated with combined modality therapy, the 5-year disease-free survival rates were 98%, 95–98%, and less than 95%, respectively, demonstrating the impact of treatment on prognostic factor analysis.

Response to Treatment

The quality of response may also be an important feature determining risk of relapse for patients with mediastinal involvement. Radford and associates have studied residual radiographic changes in the mediastinum after treatment with chemotherapy alone (95). Minimal abnormalities on the chest x-ray films occurred in 64% of all patients after the completion of therapy, but occurred in 83% of those with large mediastinal masses before treatment. There was a 19% relapse rate in patients with residual abnormalities, compared with only 10% for those with normal mediastinal contours. Such patients with a high risk of relapse may need irradiation as consolidation therapy.

Combined Modality Therapy for Laparotomy-Staged Disease

In the past, investigators emphasized overall survival results of patients with Hodgkin's disease, since most who received radiation therapy as initial treatment were easily salvaged with chemotherapy when they developed relapse (96,97). However, because of a high relapse rate for patients with unfavorable presentations, investigators began to study the benefit of adjuvant chemotherapy for all patients treated with radiation therapy. Patients who received adjuvant chemotherapy had disease-free survival results that were better than those for patients treated with radiation therapy alone (57,83). Survival results for these patients, even for most of those with unfavorable presentations, were not statistically different from those for patients who received radiation therapy alone. Most patients received six cycles of adjuvant chemotherapy, and for some investigators, the risk of leukemia, sterility, and neutropenic fever or infection for the entire group outweighed the benefit afforded to the smaller subset of patients with unfavorable presentations. However, in the 1980s, adjuvant chemotherapy became more acceptable as treatment.

Certain patients with relapse after radiation therapy have inferior results after salvage chemotherapy. Roach and associates studied patients with relapse after treatment with radiation therapy (98). Most of these patients received MOPP and, at a follow-up of 8.3 years, the freedom from second relapse was 57%. The extent of disease at the time of relapse was the most important prognostic factor for second relapse, with 90% of those with stage IA and 60% of those with stage II or IIIA disease without relapse at 10 years. However, only 34% of those patients with B symptoms or stage IV disease were free of relapse. Therefore, patients with B symptoms or stage IV disease at relapse should receive high-dose chemotherapy followed by bone marrow transplantation or other chemotherapy regimens at the time of first relapse. In this series, results were not statistically influenced by dose of chemotherapy, perhaps because of the few patients studied.

In addition to improvement in early-relapse rates, adjuvant chemotherapy reduced the risk of late relapse (99). The disease-free result became more important than the survival result, and most investigators now agree that patients with unfavorable mediastinal presentations should receive combined modality treatment (84,87,100,101). Combined modality therapy has also become more attractive because of recent improvement in tolerance to chemotherapy. The MOPP regimen is associated with both early and late complications. Alternative regimens to MOPP including doxorubicin (Adriamycin), bleomycin, vinblastine, dacarbazine (ABVD), may cause fewer long-term complications. In some series, only two or three cycles of MOPP chemotherapy gave results as good as those following six cycles of MOPP, indicating that less chemotherapy may be needed in an adjuvant setting.

Combined Modality Therapy: M. D. Anderson Results for Laparotomy-Staged Disease

At our institution, we compared treatment results for patients who received radiotherapy or combined modality therapy (CMT) for laparotomy-staged I or II disease (99). Patients treated with radiotherapy received extended-field (EF), mantle, or involved-field (IF) radiotherapy; those treated with CMT received IF radiotherapy followed by six cycles of adjuvant MOPP. Five-year disease-free survival (DFS) rates were 55% for those treated with EF, 62% for those receiving IF, and 97% for those treated with CMT. Results for those with large mediastinal masses were 45%, 50%, and 95%, respectively. Patients with large mediastinal masses and hilar disease had a DFS of only 35% following radiotherapy, compared with 95% for similar patients treated with CMT. However, MOPP was associated with sterility and the risk of acute leukemia.

From this experience, we designed a program of radiation therapy for patients with favorable presentations while administering only two cycles of MOPP and radiotherapy for patients who had unfavorable presentations (102). We continued to recommend laparotomy for patients with upper torso presentations and lymphangiograms negative for disease. Radiation fields for all patients included the mantle, for control of upper torso nodal disease, and low-dose lung irradiation to reduce the risk of disease progression in the lungs for patients with large mediastinal or hilar disease. In this study, patients with unfavorable presentations had results that were as good as those for patients with favorable presentations treated with radiation alone. Four-year disease-free survival results for patients with favorable presentations were 79%, compared with 78% for those who had unfavorable presentations. Comparable survivals were 92% and 100%, respectively. Toxicity with this program was acceptable, with four men developing azospermia with MOPP, and two of these recovering their sperm counts. No women who received two cycles of MOPP suffered menstrual abnormalities. One patient in this series developed acute myelogenous leukemia. Thus, two cycles of MOPP and radiotherapy produced results comparable with those obtained with six cycles of MOPP and radiotherapy.

Treatment of Clinically Staged Disease

Over the last 5–10 years, there has been a strong trend among investigators to eliminate the staging laparotomy in treatment of patients with Hodgkin's disease. Most management programs have done this with the addition of adjuvant chemotherapy, to prevent relapse in the abdomen. However, current programs differ in the extent of radiation fields to be employed, the prognostic factors that determine results, and the toxicity that is considered acceptable. One group of investigators even uses radiotherapy alone for patients with favorable presentations, reserving chemotherapy for relapse. In this section, we will compare some of these treatment plans and discuss the benefits and drawbacks of each.

Radiotherapy Alone for Clinically Staged Disease

At the Princess Margaret Hospital, patients have always been treated without staging by laparotomy. In a study of 252 patients with clinically staged I and II Hodgkin's disease, 10-year overall survival and disease-free survival rates were 78% and 61% (103). These investigators defined three groups of patients according to risk of relapse following radiation therapy alone. Group 1 consisted of those with isolated cervical nodes above the thyroid cartilage notch, with a relapse rate of only 8%. Group 2 consisted of patients with stage IA other than those in group 1, patients with stage IIA disease who were younger than 50 years of age, patients with IIA disease who were older than 50 years of age with lymphocyte predominant or nodular sclerosis histology, and those with IB and IIB disease who are younger than 50 years old with lymphocyte predominant or nodular sclerosis histology. Group 3 contained patients with stage IA–IIB disease, over 50 years of age with mixed cellularity or lymphocyte depletion histology, those with IB and IIB disease younger than 50 years with mixed cellularity or lymphocyte depletion histology, and those with IB or IIB disease older than 50 years of age with lymphocyte predominant or nodular sclerosis histology. The relapse rates for patients in groups 2 and 3 were significantly higher than those for patients in group 1, although the relapse rate was low for patients in group 2. Even though mediastinal involvement was not an unfavorable prognostic feature in this series, patients with mediastinal masses measuring larger than 10 cm in diameter had a very high intrathoracic failure rate after radiotherapy alone, whereas those who received chemotherapy and irradiation therapy had a low relapse rate. Given the data from this study, these investigators recommended involved-field radiotherapy for group 1, extended-field radiotherapy for group 2, and combined modality therapy for group 3 or for those with large mediastinal masses.

Combined Modality Therapy for Clinically Staged Disease

Multiple investigators have recommended treatment without laparotomy, but most have used CMT, although the amount of chemotherapy and extent of radiotherapy differ among series. Carde et al. reported their results for patients with clinically staged I or II Hodgkin's disease with therapy tailored according to prognostic factors (58). Patients with unfavorable characteristics included those who had one or more of the following features: age older than 40 years; sedimentation rate higher than 70; mixed cellularity or lymphocyte-depleted histology and clinical stage II disease mediastinal involvement; and favorable histology with stage III disease following staging by laparotomy. These patients were randomized to receive either total or subtotal nodal irradiation therapy alone, or three cycles of MOPP followed by mantle irradiation, followed by three more cycles of MOPP. The relapse-free survival rate was significantly better for the patients who received six cycles of MOPP and radiotherapy, but the overall survival rates were similar.

Zittoun et al. also reported results for patients with CS I–IIIA Hodgkin's disease treated with six cycles of MOPP followed by irradiation (104). Patients with favorable prognostic features received only three cycles of MOPP followed by radiation therapy. Patients with more extensive disease and any adverse feature received six cycles of MOPP and irradiation. Radiation therapy for patients with CS I or II was randomized to extended- or involved-field irradiation. Six-year disease-free survival rates were excellent for most subgroups of patients. However, males and patients over aged 40 with mixed cellularity disease had inferior results when treated with involved fields. Therefore, these authors concluded that treatment with the mantle field is adequate adjuvant therapy following MOPP, except for male patients and those with mixed cellularity disease. Six cycles of MOPP also did not prevent relapse for these latter patients unless they also received extended field irradiation.

Although extended fields may be necessary to prevent abdominal disease, it may not be necessary to use six cycles of chemotherapy to achieve excellent results for CS disease. Andrieu et al. reported treatment of 166 patients with CS IA–IIA disease (92). These patients received three cycles of MOPP, followed by mantle radiotherapy for patients with mediastinal disease, involved-field radiotherapy for patients with upper cervical nodes, and inverted-Y irradiation for those with abdominal involvement. They reported a 5-year survival rate of 93% and a 90% disease-free survival rate for patients entering complete remission. Patients without mediastinal disease did not develop relapse in the mediastinum, and only 4% had abdominal relapse. This rate was much lower than the 20–30% rate expected, since no abdominal radiation was administered. Thus, MOPP can eliminate mediastinal relapse in patients with large mediastinal masses, and laparotomy can be eliminated for patients with clinically staged I–IIA disease, as long as patients receive three cycles of MOPP.

These same investigators have subsequently reported results of a second study in which they treated patients with clinically staged IA–IIIB Hodgkin's disease (105). All patients in this trial received three cycles of MOPP-like chemotherapy, plus supra- and infradiaphragmatic irradiation. This study randomized mantle or inverted-Y radiotherapy and involved-field radiation therapy for CS IA and II_2A disease. Patients with CS III or IB, IIB, or II_3A disease received chemotherapy first, followed by laparotomy. All 64 responding patients who underwent laparotomy had no findings positive for disease in the abdomen. The actuarial disease-free survival of CS IA and II_2A patients was 89%, compared with 83% for patients with CS IB, IIB, and II_3A, and 89% for those with CS IIIA and IIIB. Survival results were 94%, 83%, and 80%, respectively. Also, involved field radiotherapy alone controlled mediastinal relapse. However, there was a 7% infradiaphragmatic relapse rate for patients who underwent laparotomy. Therefore, both the laparotomy and three cycles of chemotherapy were inadequate for total prevention of abdominal relapse. In another of their studies, six cycles of MOPP still did not prevent relapse in the abdomen. These investigators concluded that patients with CS disease should receive adjuvant upper abdominal irradiation, even if they receive adjuvant chemotherapy.

Other investigators have also demonstrated that patients with CS IB–III disease have excellent results when treated with three cycles of MOPP, followed by extended field irradiation (106). In this study, patients received either three or six cycles of MOPP before radiotherapy. Complete remission (CR) rates were 96% following three cycles of MOPP and radiotherapy and 94% after six cycles of MOPP and radiotherapy. The relapse-free survival rates for patients entering CR were also similar for the two treatment arms: 88% for those treated with three cycles of MOPP and 97% for those treated with six cycles of MOPP. The most important finding of this study was that three cycles of MOPP is as efficient as six cycles of MOPP in the control of occult abdominal disease for patients with supradiaphragmatic presentations.

Although CMT may prevent abdominal relapse for patients with CS disease, especially when EF radiotherapy is utilized, the large mediastinal mass may still be an adverse prognostic factor. Ferrant et al. reported treatment results of 182 patients with stage I–IV disease and mediastinal involvement (107). Most patients with CS stage IIB–IIIB received six cycles of MOPP, followed by EF radiotherapy. Patients with stages IA or IIA had three cycles of MOPP before radiation therapy, and patients with stage IV disease had six cycles of MOPP, followed by radiation to the sites of bulky disease as well as 1 year of treatment with maintenance carmustine (BCNU). Patients were divided into two groups, based on whether or not they had large mediastinal masses. The 10-year survival results were 43% for patients with large mediastinal masses and 66% for those with small mediastinal masses; disease-free survivals were 46% and 69%, respectively. Patients with B symptoms had only a 44% survival rate and 47% disease-free survival rate, compared to 79% and 80% without B symptoms. From this study, patients with B symptoms and large mediastinal masses should be treated with alternating chemotherapy regimens as well as radiation therapy, although it is not clear that such patients will have better results when treated with such a program.

Regardless of the method of staging, most patients with large mediastinal adenopathy should receive CMT for optimum disease-free results. Leopold et al. reported their results of treatment of patients with stages IA–IIB Hodgkin's disease and large mediastinal adenopathy (100). In this series, patients received one of three treatment plans: EF radiotherapy alone, after staging by laparotomy; CMT following laparotomy; and CMT without laparotomy. Ninety percent of the patients receiving CMT with no laparotomy received EF radiotherapy, and two-thirds of these received six cycles of MOPP before radiotherapy to the mediastinum. Patients treated with radiotherapy alone had a 12-year freedom from progression rate of 54%, compared with 87% for those treated with laparotomy and CMT, and 91% for those treated with CMT without laparotomy. However, overall survival rates were 87%, 90%, and 87%, respectively. There was a tendency to treat patients with disease entirely above the diaphragm with radiotherapy alone, and patients with B symptoms and extranodal extension often received CMT. This selection process even more strongly supported the use of CMT for patients with unfavorable features. Given these results, most patients with clinically staged IA–IIB disease and large mediastinal adenopathy should receive combination chemotherapy and radiotherapy, without staging by laparotomy. They also suggested that there might be a small group of patients who could receive radiation therapy alone; however, these investigators recommended CT scan and gallium scan for such patients before initial treatment, with management to include laparotomy. Other investigators have made similar recommendations for patients with disease limited to sites above the carina (108).

Chemotherapy Alone for Clinically Staged Disease

Although most investigators recommend CMT for patients with CS disease, other investigators have reported excellent results for patients with favorable disease when they receive intensive chemotherapy, with or without EF radiotherapy (104,109–111). Pavlovsky and associates have treated 277 adults and children with CS I and II disease wth either CVPP (cyclophosphamide, vinblastine, procarbazine, prednisone) or CVPP followed by radiation therapy to nodal areas at diagnosis (109). They defined two groups of patients according to treatment results. Those in the unfavorable group had one or more unfavorable features: age over 45 years, more than two lymph node areas of involvement, and mediastinal mass larger than 10 cm or peripheral lymph nodes 5 cm or larger in diameter. For patients in the favorable group, who had none of the unfavorable features, 7-year freedom from progression results were 77% for patients treated with chemotherapy alone and 70% for those treated with CMT. However, for patients in the unfavorable group, freedom from progression rates were only 34% for those patients treated with chemotherapy alone and 75% for those treated with CMT. Because of these results, these investigators recommended treatment of the favorable group with chemotherapy alone and use of CMT for patients in the unfavorable group.

Other investigators have made similar recommendations based on their experience. Cimino and colleagues studied the randomized treatment of patients with pathologically staged I–IIA disease who received either EF radiotherapy or six cycles of MOPP chemotherapy (111). The disease-free survival rates were 73% for patients treated with chemotherapy and 74% for those treated with radiation therapy. However, the survival for patients who had relapse following radiation was much better than that of those who had relapse following chemotherapy. Patients treated with MOPP alone relapsed more frequently in previously involved nodal sites, whereas for patients treated with radiotherapy, the relapse was outside of the radiation field. Those with extensive or bulky nodal disease had higher relapse rates than those with smaller tumor extent. These investigators suggested that patients with extensive nodal disease or bulky disease might have better results if treated with CMT. They also concluded that MOPP alone should be used to treat patients with early-staged disease. However, none of these patients had B symptoms, and others have reported better results with MOPP in asymptomatic patients. Regardless of results, such therapy places these patients at risk for toxicity with chemotherapy, a factor to consider when choosing treatment for patients with pathologically staged disease.

Special Treatment Considerations: Lower Torso Presentations

Radiotherapy for treatment of abdominal disease has not been well-described in the literature, since Hodgkin's disease presenting in the abdomen is unusual. About 50% of these patients present with extensive abdominal involvement, usually in para-aortic and pelvic nodes, and a laparotomy is often necessary to establish the diagnosis (112–114). Radiotherapy with 40 Gy exceeds the normal kidney and liver dose tolerance, with excessive nausea and vomiting. In a recent review of treatment of patients with disease limited to the abdomen, Krikorian et al. concluded that treatment of this uncommon presentation should depend upon the presence of B symptoms and bulky disease (113). For patients with pathological stage IA, these investigators recommended the inverted-Y, including the splenic pedicle. For patients with stage IIA, total nodal radiotherapy achieved good results, whereas patients with stage IIB required CMT.

At our institution, we limit the dose of radiotherapy to the abdomen to 30 Gy, shielding the kidneys from the beginning treatment and limiting the dose to 18–20 Gy. Such treatment is well tolerated, without hepatitis or significant neurological dysfunction. In a series of patients treated between 1956 and 1987, 60 patients with clinically or laparotomy stage I–II lower torso disease were treated with radiation, with or without MOPP (114). Twenty-two had inguinal or pelvic presentations, and 24 had abdominal disease, all of whom were treated with radiation only. The 5-year freedom from progression rate for the patients with inguinal or pelvic disease was 86%. However, patients with abdominal disease had a disease-free survival rate of only 50%. Fourteen additional patients with abdominal involvement received MOPP before radiotherapy; 11 of these received only two cycles. Their disease-free survival was 92%. These results are equivalent to the best possibly achieved with six cycles of MOPP and radiation therapy, or even with the most favorable upper torso presentations, indicating that lower torso disease need not be a poor prognostic feature in stages I–II, even in patients with B symptoms. Radiation therapy alone appears adequate to control disease in patients who undergo lymphangiography and have involvement of only the pelvis, inguinal, or femoral areas.

New Directions of Treatment for Patients with Clinically Staged Disease

In recent years, there has been development of new programs that eliminate the laparotomy as a staging technique. This eliminates the risks of surgery, and most patients with unfavorable upper torso presentations need chemotherapy anyway. However, patients with favorable presentations present a more complex challenge. Although disease-free survivals for such patients with laparotomy-staged disease treated with mantle radiotherapy alone are good, CMT without laparotomy staging can give equivalent or better results. However, chemotherapy exposes 75–80% of such patients to the risk of myelosuppression and other toxic effects. Finally, although chemotherapy may be able to control abdominal relapse for most patients, many investigators rely upon abdominal radiotherapy to control relapse, even when CMT is used, and particularly with fewer than six cycles of chemotherapy. Clearly, less toxic, but effective, adjuvant chemotherapy is needed for combination with radiotherapy.

The dose and extent of radiation is as important as the type of chemotherapy. A dose of 40 Gy for patients with upper torso disease is considered adequate for control of local disease when radiotherapy is used alone. For patients in partial remission after chemotherapy, who have residual thickening of tissues without obvious nodal enlargement, and for patients who have complete resolution of disease after chemotherapy, lower doses of radiation to areas of initial disease may be as effective as higher doses. At our institution, patients with good response to initial chemotherapy receive at least 30-Gy tumor dose. With modern restaging techniques, radiation fields may be reduced over the pericardium and heart to lessen the likelihood of cardiac complications. Patients with large mediastinal masses may also receive low-dose radiation therapy to the lung, as long as they do not receive bleomycin as part of initial chemotherapy. Patients staged by laparotomy may not require radiotherapy to the abdomen if the treatment is combined modality. A laparotomy may not be necessary for optimal treatment decisions, especially for patients with unfavorable upper torso presentations. However, lower torso radiation may be important, especially when fewer than six cycles of adjuvant chemotherapy are administered. Patients with lymphangiograms and CT scans of the abdomen that are negative for Hodgkin's disease still have a risk of abdominal involvement, except for few with extremely favorable upper torso presentations. For this reason, patients with upper torso stage I–II disease staged by lymphangiography alone should receive radiotherapy to the celiac axis nodes and spleen, although recommendations for doses and fields of irradiation vary among institutions.

Two new treatment regimens have recently been developed to treat patients with early-staged disease. Horning et al. have reported that VBM (vinblastine, bleomycin, methotrexate) is effective treatment in combination with radiotherapy for patients with stages I–IIIA Hodgkin's disease (115). In this study, patients received randomized therapy consisting of subtotal or total lymphoid irradiation versus involved field radiation followed by six cycles of VBM. With a median follow-up of 37 months, 5-year freedom from progression results were 70% after radiation alone and 95% for involved fields followed by VBM, results similar to those expected with adjuvant MOPP. Patients selected for this study were those with favorable, instead of unfavorable, presentations, and yet results were significantly better than those obtained with involved field radiation alone. The authors did not compare the results with those obtained with mantle irradiation alone, since most patients with favorable presentations have received extended-field irradiation. Nevertheless, this randomized study demonstrates that treatment with VBM after irradiation is well tolerated and produces excellent short-term results.

On the basis of our experience in using two cycles of MOPP and radiation therapy, we have recently designed NOVP [Novantrone (mitoxantrone), Oncovin (vincristine), vinblastine, prednisone], a new treatment regimen for patients with unfavorable presentations, to deliver chemotherapy with minimal toxicity before radiation (116). Because chemotherapy is to be administered to these patients, we decided to omit staging laparotomy in patients who appeared to have threatening upper torso presentations with either large mediastinal masses, hilar involvement, or B symptoms. Results for these patients are promising. It is hoped that other regimens will be developed to prevent acute and long-term toxicity in patients who are treated with CMT. Future therapeutic goals will include measures to eliminate staging laparotomy for patients with threatening upper torso disease, deletion of full-mantle radiation, and the use of only involved-field radiation for upper torso presentations.

TREATMENT OF STAGE III HODGKIN'S DISEASE

Management of Hodgkin's disease in patients with nodal involvement, above and below the diaphragm, is controversial. Until recently, patients with stage IIIA have received primarily radiation therapy. However, CMT programs have improved disease-free survival results for most of these patients (42,43,46,117,118). Hence, most recent programs for patients with stage IIIA disease have included chemotherapy. Except for a small subset, patients with stage IIIA disease have survival results similar to those for patients with pathological or clinically staged I or II Hodgkin's disease, even when they receive radiation therapy alone. However, disease-free survival results are less favorable, especially for those with adverse prognostic features. In this section, we will discuss treatment options for stage IIIA disease, prognostic factors that influence treatment decisions, and results of various treatment programs.

The treatment emphasis for patients with stage IIIB is different from that for patients with stage IIIA disease. Results with radiation therapy alone were significantly inferior for stage IIIB, compared with IIIA, and radiation alone was abandoned as treatment (48). Patients with stage IIIB have results similar to those with stage IVB disease, and most investigators combine these two stages when reporting chemotherapy treatment results. However, a subgroup of patients with stage IIIB, as many as 70%, may have a very favorable prognosis when treated with limited chemotherapy and in radiation (118). For patients with extensive disease, it is not clear that adjuvant radiation therapy plays an important role. Limited therapy for patients with a good prognosis, and the significance of radiation therapy in treatment of patients with stage III disease will be discussed.

Factors Influencing Results of Treatment for Patients with Stage IIIA Hodgkin's Disease

Extent of Nodal Involvement in the Abdomen

In a series of patients treated with radiation therapy alone, Stein et al. demonstrated that patients with stage IIIA disease, limited to the upper abdomen (III_1A), had better survival and disease-free survival results than patients who had disease involving the upper abdomen and the para-aortics or pelvis (III_2A) (45). The disease-free survival rates at 5 years were 64% and 32%, respectively. However, patients with stage III_2A who received chemotherapy and radiation therapy had a disease-free survival rate of 84%. Because of this, patients with III_2A disease, according to Stein's definition, should receive CMT or chemotherapy alone.

Number of Splenic Nodules

Investigators at Stanford analyzed their results for treatment of stage IIIA Hodgkin's disease, with a focus on disease extent as a prognostic factor (42). They could not duplicate the significance of Stein's abdominal substaging scheme. This may be due to differences in treatment techniques. Regardless, Hoppe et al. reported 90% 5-year disease-free survival results for patients with fewer than five splenic nodules in the resected specimen, compared with only 30% for patients with five or more splenic nodules. Overall survival rates were good for both groups because of effective salvage chemotherapy.

Size of Nodes at Clinical Staging

Patients with IIIA and IIIB disease staged by lymphangiography who receive chemotherapy and irradiation have results that are significantly better when their abdominal nodes are smaller than 3 cm in diameter, compared with those who have nodes 3 cm or larger in diameter. In the report of Mazza et al., the 5-year survival rate for those with small nodes was 85%, compared with 48% for those with larger nodes (119). There was no difference between patients who had limited nodal involvement and those who had more extensive nodal involvement.

Specht and Nissen have also studied tumor burden in stage III Hodgkin's disease (120). They calculated tumor burden by measuring the size of nodes and the number of specific regions of nodes involved. For patients with stage III disease, tumor burden was the only pretreatment factor of independent prognostic significance for disease-free survival. For overall survival, age and intra-abdominal tumor burden were two independent prognostic features. This method of predicting results should be prospectively tested by other groups of investigators.

Combined Modality Therapy for Patients with Stage IIIA Disease

Patients with IIIA disease have results that are significantly better when they receive chemotherapy with or without radiation therapy. DeVita and associates have recommended CMT as treatment for patients with stage IIIA if they have massive mediastinal disease (101). Chemotherapy alone did not adequately control disease in such patients. They also suggested that patients without B symptoms or early staged disease could receive MOPP alone, avoiding the added toxicity of radiotherapy (121). However, not all investigators agree that radiotherapy adds significant toxicity for these patients.

Results for Stage IIIA at M. D. Anderson Cancer Center

At our institution, the use of CMT for stage IIIA Hodgkin's disease began in 1966, with the use of COP chemotherapy [cyclophosphamide, vincristine (Oncovin), prednisone] to treat patients with stage IIIB disease before radiation. Subsequently, we treated patients with IIIA disease with the same plan. When mechlorethamine (Mustargen) and procarbazine became available, the treatment plan was changed to three cycles of MOPP followed by radiation therapy to all sites of involvement. Chemotherapy was later reduced to two cycles, and radiation fields were modified to limit irradiation of the liver to 1.0–1.5 Gy. In an early analysis, patients with IIIA disease and only porta hepatis or celiac axis nodal or splenic involvement (III_1A) had extremely good results (122). Therefore, in 1981, we deleted pelvic irradiation for stage III_1 disease.

We have recently completed a 10-year analysis of our results for IIIA Hodgkin's disease (118). Outcome was not affected by abdominal substage. One hundred two patients had stage III_1A or III_1B disease, and 73 patients were treated according to the original plan, which required pelvic irradiation. Ten-year survival and freedom from progression results for these 73 patients were 89% and 83%, respectively. Five-year survival and freedom from progression results for the 29 patients treated without pelvic irradiation were 93% and 85%, respectively. Twenty-three patients with stage IIIA disease that included para-aortic and celiac axis involvement, but no pelvic involvement (III_2A) were treated with two cycles of MOPP and irradiation to the abdomen, pelvis, and upper torso sites of involvement. Five-year survival and freedom from progression results were 85% and 79%, respectively. Twenty patients with stage IIIA disease had involvement of the pelvis, usually with involvement of the para-aortics, demonstrated by lymphangiography (III_3A). Five-year survival and freedom from progression results were 82% and 85%, respectively. The number of splenic nodules also did not affect prognosis for patients with stage III_1A or III_1B disease (43). In this series, the only patients who developed acute leukemia were those who had received pelvic irradiation.

Others have also found that stage IIIA disease can be treated with CMT, with low toxicity and better results than those who receive radiation therapy alone. Mauch and associates have treated 54 patients with stage III Hodgkin's disease with radiation therapy and 66 with radiation therapy followed by adjuvant MOPP chemotherapy (46). The 12-year survival rates were 64% and 80%, respectively ($p = 0.026$). Freedom from relapse rates were 83% and 40% ($p < 0.0001$). A subset of patients, who had only stage III_1A disease with fewer than five splenic nodules, had a favorable prognosis, regardless of therapy (123). Only 4 of these 21 patients developed recurrence, and all 21 were alive without disease. These investigators suggested patients might be candidates for mantle and para-aortic irradiation instead of total nodal irradiation or CMT. However, in a subsequent study, 40% of these patients, staged by laparotomy and treated with mantle and para-aortic radiotherapy, developed a recurrence in the pelvis, a relapse rate significantly higher than that for patients who had received more extensive treatment (124). Consequently, these investigators have revised their opinion and recommend total nodal irradiation to treat patients with favorable stage III_1A disease, reserving CMT for all other patients with stage IIIA disease.

Greenberg et al. have also reported that, in pathologically staged IIIA Hodgkin's disease, the 5-year relapse-free survival with radiation and chemotherapy was 76%, compared with only 47% for irradiation alone (117). They recommend CMT for patients with extensive splenic involvement or stage III_2A disease, but radiation alone for patients with less disease.

Management of Stage IIIA Disease: Conclusions

Some investigators recommend radiation therapy alone for patients with stage IIIA disease and no large mediastinal adenopathy, limited splenic disease, and no nodal involvement in the para-aortic or pelvic nodes. However, this group represents fewer than 20% of all patients with stage IIIA disease, and treatment must include irradiation to the pelvis or iliac nodes, which often results in sterility and in bone marrow damage, which would complicate salvage therapy. We have demonstrated that treatment of patients with stage III_1A disease with two cycles of MOPP and irradiation to the mantle and upper abdomen yields excellent results, while avoiding irradiation to the pelvis.

For patients with more extensive abdominal disease, including those with Stein's III_2A disease or the M. D. Anderson stages III_2A and III_3A, and for patients with five or more splenic nodules, chemotherapy is necessary to assure good disease-free survival, regardless of the extent of irradiation. Two cycles of MOPP is adequate treatment, provided it includes mantle, abdominal, and pelvic irradiation. Future studies should address the necessity of irradiation to the pelvis and new radiotherapy fields, the need for radiotherapy to the liver, and the type of chemotherapy to be administered. Treatment programs including ABVD and other less-toxic regimens are currently being studied for these patients (115,116).

Factors Influencing Results of Treatment for Patients with Stage IIIB Hodgkin's Disease

Investigators from Stanford reported poor results for patients treated with radiation alone for stage IIIB Hodgkin's disease because of progression while on therapy or soon after treatment was completed. Therefore, with the development of MOPP, intensive chemotherapy alone became standard therapy for most patients with stage IIIB disease. However, in the series of patients reported by Longo et al., B symptoms were an adverse prognostic feature for patients with stage III or IV Hodgkin's disease treated with MOPP chemotherapy alone, with long-term survival rates of 50–60% (110,121). There was a tendency for patients to develop relapse in previously involved nodal sites, with relapse in nodal sites compared with extranodal sites (125). Because of these relatively low survival rates in comparison with those for patients with stage IIIA disease, investigators attempted to improve these results by treating patients with radiotherapy after intensive chemotherapy. At the National Cancer Institute, radiation therapy after extensive MOPP chemotherapy was too toxic, resulting in the impression that such treatment was unreasonable (126). Others have subsequently treated patients with radiotherapy after chemotherapy with less toxicity than that reported in the NCI series. However, investigators disagree on the number of cycles of chemotherapy needed to treat such patients, the importance of the extent of both mediastinal and abdominal disease, and the effect of B symptoms on results. Other features that may also be important include age of the patient, pathological subtype, and tumor burden, measured by extent of involvement and size of nodes.

Combined Modality Therapy for Patients with Stage IIIB Disease

After the report of poor results using MOPP alone from the NCI, investigators studied the addition of radiotherapy to nodal sites to improve results. Although most investigators used six cycles of chemotherapy and many added total nodal radiotherapy, many patients with stage IIIB disease do not need this much treatment to achieve good results.

Combined Modality Therapy for Stage IIIB at M. D. Anderson

At our institution, patients with stage IIIB treated with two cycles of MOPP and irradiation had 5- and 10-year survival rates of 80% and 72%; freedom from progression rates were 70% and 64%, respectively (118). Patients with stage III_1B disease, limited to the spleen or celiac axis, had 5- and 10-year survival rates of 91%, and freedom from progression rates of 85% and 78%, respectively. For patients with stage III_2B disease, limited to the para-aortic nodes without pelvic involvement, 5- and 10-year survival rates were 83%, and freedom from progression rates were 85%. However, on the other hand, results for patients with stage III_3B disease, with involvement of the para-aortic and pelvic nodes, had survival results at 5 and 10 years of 65% and 45%, and freedom from progression rates were only 44% and 37%. Thus, patients with stages III_1B and III_2B can be treated with only two cycles of chemotherapy, followed by radiation therapy, but patients with stage III_3B should be treated differently, perhaps with more intensive treatment.

Combined Modality Therapy at Other Centers

Other investigators have used adjuvant radiotherapy to improve results for patients with stage IIIB disease. Bonadonna et al. reported results for patients with stages IIB, III, and IV Hodgkin's disease who received either six cycles of MOPP or six cycles of ABVD, with consolidative radiation therapy (127,128). In this randomized study, treatment was eventually modified to include three cycles of chemotherapy, followed by radiation, and three final cycles of chemotherapy. Radiation therapy increased the CR rate for patients treated with MOPP from 66% to 95% and with ABVD from 69% to 94%. In a recent update, the freedom from progression rates following ABVD was 81%, compared with 63% for patients who received MOPP (128). By multivariate analysis, treatment was the most important prognostic feature, followed by extent of nodal disease and age. However, many patients in this series did not complete more than three cycles of chemotherapy for various reasons, and had outcomes similar to those who completed six cycles (129).

Other investigators have reported similar results for stage IIIB using CMT. However, most patients received five or six cycles of chemotherapy in addition to radiotherapy. Prosnitz and associates treated patients with MVVPP (mechlorethamine, vincristine, vinblastine, procarbazine, prednisone) and radiation, with 5-year survival and disease-free survival rates of 88% and 80%, respectively (96). Horning and colleagues have also treated patients with total lymphoid irradiation, followed by MOPP or with MOPP alternating with PAVe (procarbazine, melphalan, vinblastine) followed by total lymphoid irradiation (130). Results were better in patients treated with chemotherapy first followed by irradiation. Mauch and associates have performed similar studies with MOPP, followed by total lymphoid or subtotal lymphoid irradiation, and obtained 12-year projected overall and disease-free survival rates of 76% and 79%, respectively (46).

Management of Stage IIIB Disease: Conclusions

Most investigators recommend chemotherapy for patients with stage IIIB disease, and many recommend radiation therapy as well. These patients should undergo complete staging evaluation, with bone marrow biopsies, careful study of the mediastinum and pulmonary parenchyma for evidence of involvement, and clinical evaluation of the liver, since they do not usually undergo laparotomy. It is not yet clear whether MOPP–ABVD will produce better results than MOPP alone, and radiation therapy may play an important role in preventing nodal relapse. Most investigators recommend a minimum of six cycles of chemotherapy, followed by radiation therapy to involved nodal sites. Our experience suggests that two cycles of chemotherapy and radiation are adequate to treat 75% of these patients with M. D. Anderson stages III_1B and III_2B disease. Future treatment for patients at our institution with B symptoms and pelvic involvement (III_3B) will include intensive chemotherapy for a minimum of six cycles, followed by radiation therapy. Controversial issues are the benefits of treatment with ABVD alone, ABVD and radiation therapy, or MOPP–ABVD alone. Storage of marrow or peripheral stem cells before initiation of radiation should be considered for possible later use as part of salvage therapy with autologous bone marrow transplantation (BMT).

TREATMENT OF STAGE IV HODGKIN'S DISEASE

The presence of B symptoms is an important prognostic factor in treatment outcome of stage IV disease. At the NCI, patients treated with MOPP had significantly lower complete remission (CR) and survival rates if they had B symptoms (121). In a recent report, the dose of vincristine administered was an additional important factor associated with disease-free survival (110). However, we found the extent of disease to be also prognostically important (131). Patients with stage IV disease had a higher CR rate if they had only one extranodal site of involvement, rather than two or more. The likelihood of patients remaining disease-free was better in patients who received adequate doses of mechlorethamine (nitrogen mustard). The presence of B symptoms did not predict inferior

CR or disease-free survival rates. Others have reported bone marrow involvement, hemoglobin level, ESR, and older age to be important prognostic features.

Specht and Nissen calculated tumor burden based on nodal and extranodal extent: the former measurement is based on size of nodes and number of involved sites, and the latter is based on number of sites involved (132). For patients with stage IV disease, factors of independent prognostic significance for disease-free survival by multivariate analysis were gender and lymphocytopenia, but tumor burden was also closely linked to lymphocytopenia. For overall survival, features including age, gender, bone marrow involvement, and elevated serum creatinine were important predictors of survival. Tumor burden was also associated with these features. Therefore, they suggested that tumor burden was indirectly related to results because of its association with lymphocytopenia, and bone marrow involvement.

Some of the differences in results reported by investigators may be related to different patient populations and statistical methods used to study prognostic factors. Despite these inconsistencies, prognostic features for different treatment programs may be helpful for treatment decisions. Next, we will discuss various treatment regimens and their side effects.

Treatment Regimens and Toxicity

MOPP Chemotherapy

More patients have been cured with this regimen than with any other. Information from reported studies is also important for comparisons with newer regimens. In the report by Longo et al., 48% of all patients with stage IV disease were alive and continuously free of disease at 9 years from the end of treatment (110). However, several patients died of treatment complications. Of 188 patients, 84% achieved a CR. The CR rate and survival were higher for patients without B symptoms. The rate of vincristine administration over six cycles was a significant prognostic factor for CR and tumor mortality. The dose of vincristine or other drugs had no influence on the remission duration, although patients who entered complete remission with five cycles of MOPP or fewer had significantly longer remissions than those requiring six or more cycles to achieve complete remission. Of the 150 in CR, 101 patients, or 64% of the 188 patients treated, remained disease-free for more than 10 years from the end of treatment. By multivariate analysis, adverse features for remission duration were the presence of B symptoms, pleural involvement, older age, and number of extranodal sites.

Results of other studies using MOPP in stage IV disease were inferior to those reported by Longo et al. Bonadonna et al. reported that MOPP produced significantly inferior results, compared with those obtained with MOPP–ABVD, with only 36% free of progressive disease at 8 years (133). Our study with

MOPP in 53 patients showed that only the number of extranodal sites was predictive of CR (131). Seventy-five percent of those with one extranodal site entered CR, compared with only 25% of those with two or more ($p < 0.05$). Survival was also affected by this factor: 78% of those with one extranodal site were alive at 5 years, compared with only 17% of those with more than one. The 5-year freedom from progression rate after CR for those who received 80% or more of the planned dose of mechlorethamine in the first three cycles of therapy was 89%, compared with only 39% for those who received lower doses. This treatment-related feature predicted survival: 89% of those receiving higher doses were alive at 5 years, compared with only 45% of those receiving lower doses.

THE IMPORTANCE OF DOSE. Doses of oral medications were not considered in our analysis. Patients often do not carefully follow instructions for prescribed oral medications and calculations of disease-free survival rates based on oral medications may be inaccurate (134). Therefore, when assessing the effect of total dose in studies of patients with Hodgkin's disease, the possibility of patient nonadherence must be considered.

Others have studied the importance of doses of chemotherapy agents in treatment of patients with the MOPP regimen. Van Rijswijk and associates demonstrated that the dose intensity of mechlorethamine, represented by the total dose of mechlorethamine delivered divided by the planned dose, was associated with attainment of CR and with overall survival for patients receiving MOPP as initial therapy (135). The difference between this report and the M. D. Anderson study may be in the definition of CR, and may be one reason why the dose of drug given appears important for attainment of CR in some series and not in others. Regardless, the dose of mechlorethamine is an important determinant of the freedom from progression and survival rates of all patients, not only for those in CR.

TOXICITY OF MOPP. MOPP chemotherapy is associated with significant toxicity. In some series, the cumulative risk of secondary leukemia is as high as 20% for certain subgroups of patients treated with MOPP and irradiation (136). However, others have reported a lower risk of acute leukemia. In the NCI study, the risk of acute leukemia was less than 2% with MOPP, despite the fact that many patients received prolonged maintenance therapy, a feature known to increase the risk of secondary malignancy (137). Patients who received CMT had a 2–3% risk of developing acute leukemia or myelodysplastic syndrome at 20 years. No patient developed this malignancy after 12 years of follow-up. Features that may predict a high risk of developing acute leukemia are (1) older age at start of therapy; (2) addition of radiation therapy to the treatment program, particularly radiation therapy to the abdomen; and (3) the use of prolonged maintenance with MOPP. Most reported series have not contained enough patients to be able to detect differences between risks for various subgroups, and large-scale studies are needed to confirm which risk factors are more important for the development of acute myelogenous leukemia or myelodysplastic syndrome after treatment with any type of chemotherapy, with or without radiation therapy.

Not all the cases of leukemias and myelodysplastic syndromes seen after therapy for Hodgkin's disease are treatment-related; some cases may be associated with the disease itself. Chromosome studies demonstrated a 43% incidence of abnormalities of chromosomes 5 or 7, or both, in patients with therapy-associated leukemia, compared with only 18% in patients with de novo leukemia (138). These specific chromosome abnormalities occurred in 72% to 83% of patients previously treated with chlorambucil, melphalan (Alkeran), mechlorethamine, procarbazine, or nitrosoureas, compared with only 29% of those who received cyclophosphamide-based regimens, 14% of those receiving other chemotherapy, and 29% of those treated with radiation alone. Thus, abnormalities of chromosomes 5 and 7 may be important for establishing the diagnosis of therapy-related leukemia and myelodysplastic syndrome versus disease-associated secondary leukemia.

In a study of 744 patients, van Leeuwen et al., from the Netherlands Cancer Institute, reported a 21% risk of developing second malignancies at 15 years after the diagnosis of Hodgkin's disease (139). The risk was statistically higher than that of the average population for development of lung cancer, non-Hodgkin's lymphoma, and leukemia or myelodysplastic syndrome. Patients were stratified into three groups depending upon their "treatment intensity": patients who received *low intensity* received only limited radiotherapy to one side of the diaphragm. Those with *high intensity* received radiotherapy to both sides of the diaphragm and six cycles of a combination of three or more different cytotoxic drugs. Those with *intermediate intensity* received all other types of therapy. The risk of developing lung cancer was noted only in groups of patients treated with radiotherapy, and all lung cancers arose in irradiated fields. However, patients treated with radiotherapy alone had no increased incidence of secondary lymphomas. Instead, CMT was the most important risk factor for non-Hodgkin's lymphomas, with risks of 0.7% and 6% at 10 and 15 years, respectively. Multivariate analysis indicated that age older than 40 at diagnosis of Hodgkin's disease and chemotherapy, irrespective of intensity, were the most important determinants of secondary lymphoma. Their finding that age had an independent effect on leukemia development is also consistent with other studies (136,137, 140–144). It may be important to consider this finding when administering chemotherapy to patients over aged 40, to avoid the risk of acute leukemia.

Other investigators have suggested that radiotherapy to the abdomen may also be associated with increased risk of leukemia in CMT programs. Andrieu et al. have reported a higher incidence of acute nonlymphocytic leukemia following CMT in 462 patients with clinically staged I–III Hodgkin's disease who received three or six cycles of MOPP, with or without infradiaphragmatic irradiation (145). Ten patients developed leukemia after 34–123 months of follow-up from complete remission, with a 15-year risk of 3.5%. Regression analysis showed that the only important variable for risk of acute leukemia was the extent of irradiation, with only a 2.2% risk following supradiaphragmatic irradiation alone, compared with 9.1% for subtotal or total nodal irradiation ($p < 0.001$).

Variations of MOPP including ChlVPP (chlorambucil, vinblastine, procarbazine, prednisone), MVVPP (mechlorethamine, vincristine, vinblastine, procarbazine, prednisone), C-MOPP (cyclophosphamide, vincristine, procarbazine, prednisone), CVPP (cyclophosphamide, vinblastine, procarbazine, prednisone), and BCVPP [carmustine (BCNU), cyclophosphamide, vincristine, prednisone, procarbazine] have been developed to decrease the acute toxicity of MOPP, especially nausea and vomiting (96,139,146–149). Long-term toxicity including sterility and myelodysplasia and acute leukemia is not likely to be altered by these substitutions, although C-MOPP, CVPP, and ChlVPP have yielded CR rates and overall results similar to those obtained with MOPP. Vose et al. reported a 3% neutropenic fever rate with ChlVPP. There also was no life-threatening gastrointestinal or neurological toxicity (149). Seventy-six percent of patients treated achieved CR with ChlVPP. In a series with longer follow-up, ChlVPP resulted in 5-year disease-free survival of 82% for patients entering CR (148). Another regimen called BCVPP, a combination combining carmustine (BCNU), cyclophosphamide, vinblastine, procarbazine, and prednisone, produced results that were better in one study with a better CR rate and duration of complete remission, compared with those obtained with MOPP (147). However, results following MOPP in this series were inferior to those reported by DeVita et al. (101). Population variations may account for some of the differences in MOPP results in these two studies. Regardless, these regimens, like MOPP, also carry a risk of inducing acute leukemia.

Sterility is a significant complication after MOPP chemotherapy (150). Most males treated with six or more cycles of MOPP will be azospermic or severely oligospermic years after treatment with MOPP. This toxicity is directly related to the cumulative dose of chemotherapy administered, and patients who receive two cycles of MOPP have a better chance of earlier recovery than patients who receive four or more cycles. MOPP chemotherapy causes ovarian dysfunction, the risk of this complication being related to the patient's age. Older patients tend to develop early menopause, whereas younger patients are less affected. Although these considerations seemed previously unimportant, they have become significant in the choice of therapy, now that cure is possible. Studies on possible chromosomal abnormalities of spermocytes and oocytes have not been extensively performed after MOPP therapy, but a higher number of spontaneous abortions and potentially abnormal fetal development might result after such treatment. This complication is rare after two cycles of MOPP, and all children born to patients treated at our institution with two cycles of MOPP have been normal.

Other annoying or undesirable side effects of MOPP are tolerable, since they can often be controlled with appropriate management. These include nausea and vomiting, frequently accompanying administration of mechlorethamine; procarbazine drug allergy; chemical phlebitis associated with mechlorethamine and vincristine; neutropenic fever; and profound weakness.

Alternatives to MOPP for Treatment of Advanced Disease

ABVD

Multiple studies have demonstrated that doxorubicin (Adriamycin)-containing regimens are effective in patients with relapsing Hodgkin's disease, or with untreated early and advanced stages. ABVD, consisting of doxorubicin, dacarbazine (DTIC), vinblastine, and bleomcyin, was first utilized to treat patients with Hodgkin's disease refractory to MOPP (151).

TREATMENT RESULTS. Bonadonna et al. were the first to report long-term treatment results for patients with ABVD, demonstrating its efficacy in treatment of patients with Hodgkin's disease in relapse after MOPP. However, many of the patients initially treated with ABVD may not have had disease that was truly refractory to MOPP. In subsequent reports, only 10–15% of patients with MOPP-refractory disease had long-term disease control with ABVD alone (152–154). Patients who had a response to MOPP initially often had a good response to ABVD, with about 30–40% of the patients entering long-lasting complete remission.

As frontline treatment, Bonadonna and colleagues tested MOPP against ABVD in the initial treatment of patients with advanced Hodgkin's disease (127). In this study, ABVD was equivalent to MOPP in producing CRs, and the percentage of patients alive without recurrent disease was better after ABVD. Other investigators have studied the potential importance of doxorubicin in alternating chemotherapy regimens (155–157). However, MOPP alone has produced results somewhat similar to those reported for the alternating regimen.

More recently, the Cancer and Leukemia Group B (CALGB) have studied MOPP and ABVD as treatment for advanced Hodgkin's disease (158). The CR rate was 47% with MOPP and 83% with ABVD. With further follow-up, patients who received ABVD had a better disease-free survival rate than those who received MOPP. Prognostic factor analyses will be performed to determine comparability of these two groups of patients. Regardless, results with ABVD may be equivalent or superior to those achieved with MOPP.

TOXICITY OF ABVD. Additional factors may make ABVD a better choice for treatment of patients with advanced Hodgkin's disease. The risk of leukemia for patients treated with ABVD is low (159). Other secondary tumors may develop in patients with longer follow-up after receiving ABVD. However, the individual drugs in ABVD have a lower carcinogenic potential, suggesting that secondary malignancies may be less frequent after ABVD than after MOPP (140).

Two potential side effects of ABVD may be important in limiting its use. First, many patients with Hodgkin's disease present wih a mediastinal mass. These patients may require radiation therapy, which can synergize with bleomycin to induce pulmonary toxicity. Doxorubicin may increase the risk of cardiotoxicity (160). In the series reported by Viviani et al., patients treated with ABVD and radiotherapy had a higher likelihood of developing pulmonary dysfunction immediately after discontinuation of therapy (161). Others have also reported a higher risk of pulmonary dysfunction following ABVD and radiotherapy, compared with that seen following MOPP and radiotherapy (160).

Other side effects of ABVD may be troublesome. The degree of myelosuppression and the infection rates are similar following ABVD and MOPP. Both regimens cause phlebitis, nausea, and vomiting. ABVD causes alopecia, a side effect that may be significant for a young patient's self-image. Sterility with ABVD is less frequent than with MOPP. In the study reported by Viviani et al., ABVD caused oligo- or azospermia in 54% of patients, compared with 97% in those patients treated with MOPP (162). It is possible that use of only two or three cycles of ABVD might result in an even lower incidence of sterility.

MOPP–ABVD

After Bonadonna et al. reported the usefulness of ABVD in treatment of patients with recurrent Hodgkin's disease, they began investigating an alternating regimen known as MOPP–ABVD (133). This treatment program induced a higher CR rate and longer duration of CR than did MOPP alone in a randomized study. However, the results following MOPP alone were inferior to those reported by the NCI, and the results of MOPP–ABVD were similar to those reported by DeVita et al. with MOPP alone (101). It is difficult to make such comparisons, since there may have been variations between the groups of patients treated. Nonetheless, the freedom from progression rate at 8 years for patients treated with the MOPP–ABVD regimen was 65%, compared with only 36% for patients treated with MOPP. Overall survival figures were 84% with MOPP–ABVD and 64% with MOPP. Toxicity was similar in the two arms and in terms of development of acute leukemia and the degree of myelosuppression. Prognostic factor analyses of these results have not revealed any subgroups with poor results, including patients with B symptoms, large mediastinal masses, adverse histological subtype, or older age, all of which have been important features in treatment of advanced Hodgkin's disease. In the MOPP group, only 19 of 43 patients (44%) received 80% or more of the planned doses of chemotherapy. In the group receiving MOPP–ABVD, 14 of 22 patients (64%) received at least 80% of the planned doses of each combination. This may account for some of the differences in results between those two regimens. In a recent update, overall survival results were similar with MOPP–ABVD and MOPP (161). The potential use of radiation therapy after treatment of patients with MOPP–ABVD is under investigation.

The CALGB treated patients with MOPP–ABVD, ABVD alone, and MOPP alone (158). Results for both the ABVD and MOPP–ABVD arms were superior to those obtained with the MOPP arm, with 83% and 76% of patients entering CR, respectively, and 57% and 66% projected free of progressive disease at 5 years, respectively, compared with only 47% CR and a 47% disease-free survival result for patients treated with MOPP alone.

In a study performed by the Eastern Cooperative Oncology Group (ECOG), 232 patients with advanced Hodgkin's disease received six cycles of MOPP plus bleomycin (163). Patients responding to treatment were randomized to consolidation with either ABVD or low-dose radiaton therapy to sites of involvement. The CR rate with induction chemotherapy was only 59%, but 63% of the patients in PR obtained CR with consolidation therapy, 62% with ABVD and 64% with radiation therapy. Patients who received ABVD also had an 8-year survival rate of 81%, compared with 67% for those receiving radiation therapy. Overall survival results were also better following ABVD compared with radiation therapy. Freedom from progression rates were 62% for ABVD and 44% with radiation therapy ($p = 0.06$). These authors concluded that ABVD can be used to treat patients in CR or PR following MOPP, with better results than those obtained with low-dose radiation therapy. Radiation therapy also did not improve results expected with MOPP alone, in contrast with the report by Prosnitz et al. (96).

MOPP–ABV Hybrid

This regimen, reported by Connors and Klimo from Canada, has produced survival and relapse-free survival rates similar to MOPP–ABVD for patients with advanced disease (164). MOPP–ABV is similar to MOPP–ABVD, except that no dacarbazine is administered. One of the proposed benefits of this regimen is that patients receive all seven of these drugs every month, rather than receiving only four drugs each month in an alternating fashion. Of the 76 patients treated, 74 were evaluable for response, with a 96% CR rate. No presenting feature affected response. With a median follow-up of 35 months, 86% of the 74 patients were alive without relapse. The combination of large mediastinal mass and B symptoms was predictive of relapse. Toxicity with MOPP–ABV was very low, with nonfatal infections requiring hospitalization in only 8% of the patients. In this study, all patients were previously untreated, and only 13 were over aged 50. These investigators are now comparing MOPP–ABV with MOPP–ABVD in a multicenter trial.

Combined Modality Therapy for Stage IV Hodgkin's Disease

At the NCI, radiation therapy did not improve results for patients treated with MOPP, mainly because of toxicity. Other investigators have administered radiation therapy without significant toxicity, but the potential benefit of adjuvant radiation therapy is difficult to demonstrate without randomized studies. Patients without mediastinal masses may not require radiation therapy after achieving CR with chemotherapy. Also, the presence of abdominal disease may not be equivalent to mediastinal disease as a prognostic factor. The extent of both nodal and extranodal tumor burden may play a role in determining the extent of radiation therapy. For these reasons, many studies of patients with advanced Hodgkin's disease now include radiation therapy for residual masses, although no proof exists for such benefit.

Andrieu and associates treated 20 patients with six cycles of MOPP, followed by total nodal irradiation or subtotal nodal irradiation (165). This treatment resulted in a CR rate of 85%, with a 20% 5-year relapse rate, results similar to those seen with MOPP alone. However, they found that CR rates and sites of relapse were similar if patients were treated with only three cycles of MOPP, followed by irradiation. Consequently, they instituted a trial for stage IV disease using three cycles of ABVD, followed by total nodal irradiation or subtotal nodal irradiation, including the spleen, with low-dose irradiation to the lung, bone, or liver. After treating 28 patients, the CR rate was 89%, the 5-year survival 75%, and the 5-year relapse rate of CR patients only 20%, with a median follow-up of 30 months. From these early trials, it appears that radiation therapy may increase the CR rate of patients treated with MOPP or ABVD and may reduce the relapse rate.

These investigators have also reported results for 32 patients, with marrow involved by Hodgkin's disease, who received chemotherapy plus radiation or chemotherapy alone (166). The 5-year disease-free survival rate for 12 patients in CR treated with chemotherapy only was only 42%, compared with 100% for 9 patients treated with chemotherapy followed by 40-Gy irradiation. Five-year survival results were 42% and 76%, respectively. All relapses occurred in previously involved lymph node areas and none in the bone marrow. In this study, bone marrow disease was not an adverse prognostic feature, whereas eradication of Hodgkin's disease in nodes with chemotherapy alone was not more difficult to achieve with chemotherapy alone.

What Is the Best Treatment for Patients with Stage IV Hodgkin's Disease?

Following reports of its initial effectiveness, MOPP–ABVD became standard therapy in the oncology community, especially in the United States, even though it had not been adequately tested. In Europe, ABVD became a popular regimen.

Investigators from the CALGB have performed a three-way randomized study comparing MOPP alone with MOPP–ABVD and ABVD alone in treatment of 369 patients with advanced Hodgkin's disease (158). Both MOPP–ABVD and ABVD produced better results than MOPP alone. However, by cycle 3 of treatment with MOPP, only 44% of the patients were actually receiving full doses of mechlorethamine (nitrogen mustard). However in the alternating regimen, it was possible to give 74% of the patients full doses of mechlorethamine. Doses of chemotherapy agents are known determinants of results; for this reason alone, alternating regimens or ABVD may be better treatment. Although associated with low risks of sterility and leukemia, ABVD can produce pulmonary and cardiac complications. In combined modality treatment programs, ABVD may not be the optimal treatment choice, since cardiopulmonary complication rates may be higher if radiation therapy is administered.

Investigators have not yet developed the ideal regimen for treatment of advanced Hodgkin's disease. Some have treated patients with regimens that employ etoposide (VP-16), vinblastine, and doxorubicin. Mitoxantrone may also be useful in treatment of patients with this disease. Presently, doxorubicin-containing regimens should be employed in the treatment of patients with advanced disease, and alternating regimens or single combination regimens containing doxorubicin produce the best results. Adjuvant radiation therapy should also be considered for treatment of patients with residual mediastinal masses. New studies should address these questions.

Side effects will occur with any treatment program; however, our goal is to minimize these side effects and improve long-term quality of life and decrease toxicity. Patients treated for Hodgkin's disease often have long-term psychosocial problems (167). This disease affects adolescents and young adults who often find difficulty in work because of job discrimination, obtaining life or health insurance, and dealing with educational, physical, and psychological problems, including the threat of recurrence. Further studies should assess better ways of assisting these patients in adjusting to future problems. One goal in cancer therapy, particularly in a highly curable disease, is to attempt to improve the quality of life and minimize toxicity, without compromising the cure potential.

REFERENCES

1. Hodgkin T: On some morbid appearances of the absorbant glands and spleen. *Med Chir Trans* 1932; 17:68–114.
2. Reed DM: On the pathologic changes in Hodgkin's disease with special reference to its relationship to tuberculosis. *Johns Hopkins Hosp Rep* 1902; 10:133–196.
3. Maksen JA, Hassan MO, Carter JR: The ultrastructural heterogeneity of the Reed–Sternberg cell and its resemblance to monocyte macrophage differentiation in vivo. *Ultrastruct Pathol* 1983; 4:379–389.

4. Rappaport H: Tumors of the hematopoietic system. In, *Atlas of Tumor Pathology*, Sect 3, Fasc 8. Washington, DC, US Armed Forces Department of Pathology, 1983; pp 97–161.
5. Hsu S, Jaffe ES: Leu-M1 and peanut agglutinin stain the neoplastic cells of Hodgkin's disease. *Am J Clin Pathol* 1984; 92:29–32.
6. Meis JM, Osborne BM, Butler J: A comparative marker study of large cell lymphomas, Hodgkin's disease and true histiocytic lymphoma. *Am J Clin Pathol* 1986; 86:591–599.
7. Sherbarri B, Battiflora H, Burke JS, Rappaport H: Leu-M1 antigens in human neoplasms: An immunologic study of 400 cases. *Am J Surg Pathol* 1986; 10:227–236.
8. Stein H, Uchanska-Ziegler G, Gerdes J, et al: Hodgkin's and Sternberg–Reed cells contain antigens specific to late cells of granulopoiesis. *Int J Cancer* 1982; 29:283–290.
9. Lukes RJ, Butler JJ: The pathology and nomenclature of Hodgkin's disease. *Cancer Res* 1966; 26:1063–1081.
10. Lukes RJ, Carver LF, Hall TC, et al: Report of the nomenclature committee. *Cancer Res* 1966; 26:1311.
11. Buyssens N, Bourgeois N: The Sternberg-Reed cell: Mononuclear, multinucleated or multilobulated. *Virchows Arch Pathol Anat* 1980; 385:334–335.
12. Cross RM: Hodgkin's disease: Histological classification and diagnosis. *J Clin Pathol* 1969; 22:165–182.
13. Lukes RJ: Criteria for involvement of lymph node, bone marrow, spleen, and liver in Hodgkin's disease. *Cancer Res* 1971; 31:1755–1767.
14. Butler JJ: Natural history of Hodgkin's disease and its classification. In, Bernard CW, Rebuck JW, Abell MR (eds): *The Reticuloendothelial System*. Int Acad Pathol Monogr 1975; 16:184–212.
15. Pinkus GS, Said JW: Hodgkin's disease, lymphocyte predominance type, nodular—a distinct entity? *Am J Pathol* 1985; 118:1–6.
16. Stein H, Hansmann ML, Lennert K, et al: Reed–Sternberg and Hodgkin cells in lymphocyte-predominant Hodgkin's disease of nodular subtype contain J chain. *Am J Clin Pathol* 1986; 86:292–297.
17. Chittal SM, Caveriviere P, Schwarting R, et al: Monoclonal antibodies in the diagnosis of Hodgkin's disease. The search for a rational panel. *Am J Surg Pathol* 1988; 12:9–21.
18. Hall PA, D'Ardenne AJ, Stansfeld AG: Paraffin section immunohistochemistry. II. Hodgkin's disease and large cell anaplastic (Ki-1) lymphoma. *Histopathology* 1988; 13:161–169.
19. Abdulaziz Z, Mason DY, Stein H, et al: An immunohistological study of the cellular constituents of Hodgkin's disease using a monoclonal antibody panel. *Histopathology* 1988; 8:1–25.
20. Regula DP Jr, Hoppe RT, Weiss LM: Nodular and diffuse types of lymphocyte predominance Hodgkin's disease. *N Engl J Med* 1988; 318:214–219.
21. Borg-Grech A, Radford JA, Crowther D, et al: A comparative study of the nodular and diffuse variants of lymphocyte-predominant Hodgkin's disease. *J Clin Oncol* 1989; 7:1303–1309.

22. Colby TV, Hoppe RT, Warnke RA: Hodgkin's disease: A clinicopathological study of 659 cases. *Cancer* 1982; 49:1848–1858.
23. Ben-Yehuda-Salz D, Ben-Yehuda A, Polliack A, et al: Syncytial variant of nodular sclerosing Hodgkin's disease. A new clinicopathologic entity. *Cancer* 1990; 65:1167–1172.
24. MacLennan KA, Bennett MH, Tu A, et al: Relationship of histopathologic factors to survival and relapse in nodular sclerosing Hodgkin's disease. *Cancer* 1989; 64:1686–1693.
25. Wijlhuizen TJ, Vrints LW, Jairam R, et al: Grades of nodular sclerosis (NSI–NSII) in Hodgkin's disease. Are they of independent value? *Cancer* 1989; 63:1150–1153.
26. Gartner HV, Wehrman M, Iniger R, Steinke B: Nodular sclerosing Hodgkin's disease: Prognostic relevance of morphologic parameters. First International Symposium on Hodgkin's Lymphoma, Cologne, 1987.
27. Kant JA, Hubbard SM, Longo D, et al: The pathologic and clinical heterogeneity of lymphocyte depletion Hodgkin's disease. *J Clin Oncol* 1986; 4:284–294.
28. Hoppe RT, Coleman CN, Cox RS, et al: The management of stage I–II Hodgkin's disease with radiation alone or combined modality therapy: The Stanford experience. *Blood* 1982; 59:455–465.
29. Fuller LM, Gamble JF, Butler JJ, Gehan EA: Prognostic factors and localized Hodgkin's disease treated with regional radiation. *Radiology* 1971; 98:641–645.
30. Ibrahim ME, Fuller LM, Gamble JF, et al: Stage I Hodgkin's disease: Comparison of surgical staging with incidence of new manifestations in lymphogram- and prelymphogram-studied patients. *Radiology* 1972; 104:145–151.
31. Castellino RA, Hoppe RT, Blank N, et al: Computed tomography, lymphography, and staging laparotomy: Correlations in initial staging of Hodgkin's disease. *AJR* 1984; 142:37–41.
32. Glatstein E, Guernsey JM, Rosenberg SA, Kaplan HS: The value of laparotomy and splenectomy in the staging of Hodgkin's disease. *Cancer* 1969; 24:709–718.
33. Castellino RA, Dunnick NR, Goffinet DR, et al: Predictive value of lymphography for sites of subdiaphragmatic disease encountered at staging laparotomy in newly diagnosed Hodgkin's disease and non-Hodgkin's lymphoma. *J Clin Oncol* 1983; 1:532–536.
34. Stevens SO, Harher GH, Dempsey JA, Handly CK: Evaluation of staging procedures for abdominal involvement. *Med J Aust* 1979; 1:424–426.
35. Larson RA, Ultmann JE: The strategic role of laparotomy in staging Hodgkin's disease. *Cancer Treat Rep* 1982; 66:767–774.
36. De La Cruz, GA, Cardenes H, Otero J, et al: Individual risk of abdominal disease in patients with stages I and II supradiaphragmatic Hodgkin's disease. A rule index based on 341 laparotomized patients. *Cancer* 1989; 63:1799–1803.
37. Hagemeister FB, Fuller LM, Martin RG: Staging laparotomy: Findings and applications to treatment decisions. In, Fuller LM, Hagemeister FB, Sullivan MP, Velasquez WS (eds): *Hodgkin's Disease and Non-Hodgkin's Lymphomas in Adults and Children*. New York, Raven Press, 1988, pp 170–185.
38. Mauch P, Larson D, Osteen R, et al: Prognostic factors for positive surgical staging in patients with Hodgkin's disease. *J Clin Oncol* 1990; 8:257–265.

39. Kaplan HS, Dorfman RF, Nelson TS, Rosenberg SA: Staging laparotomy and splenectomy in Hodgkin's disease: Analysis of indications in 285 consecutive, unselected patients. *NCI Monogr* 1973; 36:291–301.
40. Beretta G, Spinelli P, Rilke F, et al: Sequential laparoscopy and laparotomy combined with bone marrow biopsy in staging Hodgkin's disease. *Cancer Treat Rep* 1978; 60:1231–1237.
41. Levi JA, Wiernik PH: Therapeutic implications of splenic involvement in stage IIIA Hodgkin's disease. *Cancer* 1977; 39:2158–2165.
42. Hoppe RT, Cox RS, Rosenberg SA, Kaplan HS: Prognostic factors in pathologic stage III Hodgkin's disease. *Cancer Treat Rep* 1982; 104:145–151.
43. Henkelmann GC, Hagemeister FB, Fuller LM: Two cycles of MOPP and radiotherapy for stage III_1A and stage III_1B Hodgkin's disease. *J Clin Oncol* 1988; 6:1293–1302.
44. Lister TA, Crowther D, Sutcliffe SB, et al: Report of a committee convened to discuss the evaluation and staging of patients with Hodgkin's disease: Cotswolds meeting. *J Clin Oncol* 1989; 7:1630–1636.
45. Stein RS, Golomb HM, Wiernik PH, et al: Anatomic substages of stage IIIA Hodgkin's disease: Follow-up of a collaborative study. *Cancer Treat Rep* 1982; 66:733–742.
46. Mauch P, Goffman T, Rosenthal DS, et al: Stage III Hodgkin's disease. Improved survival with combined modality therapy as compared with radiation therapy alone. *J Clin Oncol* 1985; 3:1166–1173.
47. Peters MV: A study of survivals of Hodgkin's disease treated radiologically. *AJR* 1950; 63:299–311.
48. Peters MV: Prophylactic treatment of adjacent areas of Hodgkin's disease. Symposium: Obstacles to the Control of Hodgkin's Disease. *Cancer Res* 1966; 26:1232–1243.
49. Kaplan HS, Rosenberg SA: Current status of clinical trials: Stanford experience, 1962–1972. *NCI Monogr* 1973; 36:363–371.
50. Page V, Gardner A, Karzmark CJ: Physical and dosimetric aspects of the radiotherapy of malignant lymphoma. I. The mantle technique. *Radiology* 1970; 96:609–618.
51. Page V, Gardner A, Karzmark CJ: Physical and dosimetric aspects of the radiotherapy of malignant lymphoma. II. The inverted Y technique. *Radiology* 1970; 96:619–626.
52. Rosenberg SA, Kaplan HS: Hodgkin's disease and other malignant lymphomas. *Calif Med* 1970; 113:23–38.
53. Fuller LM, Hutchinson GB: Collaborative clinical trial for stage I and II Hodgkin's disease: Significance of mediastinal and nonmediastinal disease of laparotomy and nonlaparotomy-staged patients. *Cancer Treat Rep* 1982; 66:775–787.
54. Nixon JJ: Hodgkin's disease clinical trial. *Cancer Res* 1966; 26:1279–1283.
55. Rosenberg SA, Kaplan HS: The evolution and summary results of the Stanford randomized clinical trials for the management of Hodgkin's disease: 1962–1984. *Int J Radiat Oncol Biol Phys* 1985; 11:5–22.
56. Farah R, Ultmann J, Griem M, et al: Extended mantle radiation therapy for pathologic stage I and II Hodgkin's disease. *J Clin Oncol* 1988; 6:1047–1052.

57. Hagemeister FB, Fuller LM, Sullivan JA, et al: Treatment of stage I and II mediastinal Hodgkin disease. A comparison of involved fields, extended fields, and involved fields followed by MOPP in patients staged by laparotomy. *Radiology* 1981; 141:783–789.
58. Carde P, Burgers JMV, Henry-Amar M, et al: Clinical stages I and II Hodgkin's disease: A specifically tailored therapy according to prognostic factors. *J Clin Oncol* 1988; 6:239–252.
59. Tubiana M, Henry-Amar M, Carde P, et al: Toward comprehensive management tailored to prognostic factors of patients with clinical stages I and II in Hodgkin's disease. The EORTC lymphoma group controlled clinical trials: 1964–1987. *Blood* 1989; 73:47–56.
60. Anderson H, Deakin DP, Wagstaff J, et al: A randomised study of adjuvant chemotherapy after mantle radiotherapy in supradiaphragmatic Hodgkin's disease PS IA–IIB: A report from the Manchester lymphoma group. *Br J Cancer* 1984; 49:695–702.
61. Kaplan HS: Evidence for a tumoricidal dose level in the radiotherapy of Hodgkin's disease. Symposium: Obstacles to the Control of Hodgkin's disease. *Cancer Res* 1966; 26:1221–1224.
62. Fajardo LF, Steward JR: Pathogenesis of radiation-induced myocardial fibrosis. *Lab Invest* 1973; 29:224–256.
63. McReynolds RA, Gold GL, Roberts WC: Coronary heart disease after mediastinal irradiation for Hodgkin's disease. *Am J Med* 1976; 60:39–45.
64. Mittal B, Deutsch M, Thompson M, Dameshek HL: Radiation-induced accelerated coronary arteriosclerosis. *Am J Med* 1986; 81:183–184.
65. Morgan GW, Freeman AP, McLean RG, et al: Late cardiac, thyroid, and pulmonary sequelae of mantle radiotherapy for Hodgkin's disease. *Int J Radiat Oncol Biol Phys* 1985; 11:1925–1931.
66. Watchie J, Coleman CN, Raffin TA, et al: Minimal long-term cardiopulmonary dysfunction following treatment for Hodgkin's disease. *Int J Radiat Oncol Biol Phys* 1987; 13:517–524.
67. Perrault DJ, Levy M, Herman JD, et al: Echocardiographic abnormalities following cardiac radiation. *J Clin Oncol* 1985; 3:546–551.
68. Green DM, Gingell RL, Pearce J, et al: The effect of mediastinal irradiation on cardiac function of patients treated during childhood and adolescence for Hodgkin's disease. *J Clin Oncol* 1987; 5:239–245.
69. Carmel RJ, Kaplan HS: Mantle irradiation in Hodgkin's disease: Analysis of technique, tumor eradication, and complications. *Cancer* 1976; 37:2813–2825.
70. Pasqualini T, Iorcansky S, Gruneiro L, et al: Thyroid dysfunction in Hodgkin's disease. *Cancer* 1989; 63:335–339.
71. Schimpff SC, Diggs CH, Wiswell JG, et al: Radiation related thyroid dysfunction: Implications for the treatment of Hodgkin's disease. *Ann Intern Med* 1980; 92:91–98.
72. Kinsella TJ, Trivette G, Rowland J, et al: Long-term follow-up of testicular function following radiation therapy for early-stage Hodgkin's disease. *J Clin Oncol* 1989; 7:718–724.

73. Bookman MA, Longo DL: Concomitant illness in patients treated for Hodgkin's disease. *Cancer Treat Rev* 1986; 13:77–111.
74. Krikorian JG, Burke JS, Rosenberg SA, et al: Occurrence of non-Hodgkin's lymphoma after therapy for Hodgkin's disease. *N Engl J Med* 1979; 300:452–458.
75. Thar TL, Million RR, Hausner RJ, McKetty MHB: Hodgkin's disease, stage I and II: Relationship of recurrence to site of disease, radiation alone, and number of sites involved. *Cancer* 1979; 43:1101–1105.
76. Mauch P, Goodman R, Halman S: The significance of mediastinal involvement in early stage Hodgkin's disease. *Cancer* 1978; 42:1029–1045.
77. Ali MK, Khalil KG, Fuller LM, et al: Radiation related myocardial injury: Management of two cases. *Cancer* 1976; 38:1941–1946.
78. Nickson JJ, Hutchinson GB: Extensions of disease, complications of therapy and death in localized Hodgkin's disease: Preliminary report of a clinical trial. *Am J Roentgenol Radiat Nucl Med* 1972; 3:564–573.
79. Stewart M, Cohn JR, Fajardo KE, et al: Radiation induced heart disease: A study of 25 patients. *Radiology* 1967; 89:302–310.
80. Kinzie JJ, Hanks GE, Maclean CJ, Kramer S: Patterns of care study: Hodgkin's disease relapse rates and adequacy of portals. *Cancer* 1983; 52:2223–2226.
81. Rostock RA, Siegelman SS, Lenhard RE, et al: Thoracic CT scanning for mediastinal Hodgkin's disease: Results and therapeutic implications. *Int J Radiat Oncol Biol Phys* 1983; 9:1451–1457.
82. Willett CG, Linggood RM, Leong JC, et al: Stage IA to IIB mediastinal Hodgkin's disease: Three-dimensional volumetric assessment of response to treatment. *J Clin Oncol* 1988; 6:819–824.
83. Hagemeister FB, Fuller LM, Sullivan JA, et al: Treatment of patients with stages I and II nonmediastinal Hodgkin's disease. *Cancer* 1982; 50:2307–2313.
84. Zagars G, Rubin P: Laparotomy-staged IA versus IIA Hodgkin's disease. A comparative study with evaluation of prognostic factors for stage IIA disease. *Cancer* 1985; 56:864–873.
85. Willett CG, Linggood RM, Meyer J, et al: Results of treatment of stage IA and IIA Hodgkin's disease. *Cancer* 1987; 59:1107–1111.
86. Lee CKK, Aeppli DM, Bloomfield CD, Levitt SH: Hodgkin's disease: A reassessment of prognostic factors following modification of radiotherapy. *Int J Radiat Oncol Biol Phys* 1987; 13:983–991.
87. Leslie NT, Mauch PM, Hellman S: Stage IA to IIB supradiaphragmatic Hodgkin's disease. Long-term survival and relapse frequency. *Cancer* 1985; 55:2072–2078.
88. Mauch P, Tarbell N, Weinstein H, et al: Stage IA and IIA supradiaphragmatic Hodgkin's disease: Prognostic factors in surgically staged patients treated with mantle and paraaortic irradiation. *J Clin Oncol* 1988; 6:1576–1583.
89. Tubiana M, Henry-Amar M, Burgers MV, et al: Prognostic significance of erythrocyte sedimentation rate in clinical stages I–II of Hodgkin's disease. *J Clin Oncol* 1984; 2:194–200.
90. Friedman S, Henry-Amar M, Cosset JM, et al: Evaluation of erythrocyte sedimentation rate as predictor of early relapse in post-therapy early-stage Hodgkin's disease. *J Clin Oncol* 1988; 6:596–602.

91. Crnkovich MJ, Hoppe RT, Rosenberg SA: Stage IIB Hodgkin's disease: The Stanford experience. *J Clin Oncol* 1986; 4:472–479.
92. Andrieu JM, Montagnon B, Asselain B, et al: Chemotherapy–radiotherapy association in Hodgkin's disease, clinical stages IA, II_2A: Results of a prospective clinical trial with 166 patients. *Cancer* 1980; 46:2126–2130.
93. Tubiana M, Henry-Amar M, Hayat M, et al: Prognostic significance of the number of involved areas in the early stages of Hodgkin's disease. *Cancer* 1984; 54:885–894.
94. Specht L, Nordentoft AM, Cold S, et al: Tumor burden as the most important prognostic factor in early stage Hodgkin's disease. Relations to other prognostic factors and implications for choice of treatment. *Cancer* 1988; 61:1719–1727.
95. Radford JA, Cowan RA, Flanagan M, et al: The significance of residual mediastinal abnormality on the chest radiograph following treatment for Hodgkin's disease. *J Clin Oncol* 1988; 6:940–946.
96. Prosnitz LR, Farber LR, Kapp DS, et al: Combined modality therapy for advanced Hodgkin's disease. Long-term follow-up data. *Cancer Treat Rep* 1982; 66:871–880.
97. DeVita VT: Hodgkin's disease. The salvage of radiation treatment failures. *Int J Radiat Oncol Biol Phys* 1976; 17:252.
98. Roach M III, Brophy, N, Cox R, et al: Prognostic factors for patients relapsing after radiotherapy for early-stage Hodgkin's disease. *J Clin Oncol* 1990; 8:623–629.
99. Hagemeister FB, Fuller LM, Velasquez WS, et al: Stage I and II Hodgkin's disease: Involved-field radiotherapy versus extended-field radiotherapy versus involved-field radiotherapy followed by six cycles of MOPP. *Cancer Treat Rep* 1982; 66:789–798.
100. Leopold KA, Canellos GP, Rosenthal D, et al: Stage IA–IIB Hodgkin's disease: Staging and treatment of patients with large mediastinal adenopathy. *J Clin Oncol* 1989; 7:1059–1065.
101. DeVita VT, Longo DL, Glatstein, et al: A randomized comparison of radiotherapy (RRX) versus primary treatment with MOPP chemotherapy (M-CRX) in early stage Hodgkin's disease. *Proc Int Conf Adjuvant Ther Cancer* 1990; 6:57.
102. Fuller LM, Hagemeister FB, North LB, et al: The adjuvant role of two cycles of MOPP and low-dose lung irradiation in stage IA through IIB Hodgkin's disease: Preliminary results. *Int J Radiat Oncol Biol Phys* 1988; 14:683–692.
103. Sutcliffe SB, Gospodarowicz MK, Bergsagel DE, et al: Prognostic groups for management of localized Hodgkin's disease. *J Clin Oncol* 1985; 3:393–401.
104. Zittoun R, Audebert A, Hoerni B, et al: Extended versus involved fields irradiation combined with MOPP chemotherapy in early clinical stages of Hodgkin's disease. *J Clin Oncol* 1985; 3:207–214.
105. Andrieu JM, Coscas Y, Cramer P, et al: Chemotherapy plus radiotherapy in clinical stage IA to IIIB Hodgkin's disease. Results of the H 77 trial (1977–1980). In, Cavalli F, Bonadonna G, Rozenczweig M (eds): *Lymphomas and Hodgkin's Disease: Experimental and Therapeutic Advances*. Boston, Martinus Nijhoff Publishing, 1985, pp 353–361.

106. Ferme C, Teillet F, d'Agay MF, et al: Combined modality in Hodgkin's disease. Comparison of six versus three courses of MOPP with clinical and surgical restaging. *Cancer* 1984; 54:2324–2329.
107. Ferrant A, Hamoir V, Binon J, et al: Combined modality therapy for mediastinal Hodgkin's disease. Prognostic significance of constitutional symptoms and size of disease. *Cancer* 1985; 55:317–322.
108. Hoppe RT: The management of stage II Hodgkin's disease with a large mediastinal mass: A prospective program emphasizing irradiation. *Int J Radiat Oncol Biol Phys* 1985; 11:349–355.
109. Pavlovsky S, Maschio M, Santarelli MT, et al: Randomized trial of chemotherapy versus chemotherapy plus radiotherapy for stage I–II Hodgkin's disease. *JNCI* 1988; 80:1466–1473.
110. Longo DL, Young RC, Wesley M, et al: Twenty years of MOPP therapy for Hodgkin's disease. *J Clin Oncol* 1986; 4:1295–1306.
111. Cimino G, Biti GP, Anselmo AP, et al: MOPP chemotherapy versus extended-field radiotherapy in the management of pathological stages I–IIA Hodgkin's disease. *J Clin Oncol* 1989; 7:732–737.
112. Fuller LM: Results of large volume irradiation in the management of Hodgkin's disease and malignant lymphomas originating in the abdomen. *Radiology* 1966; 87:1058–1064.
113. Krikorian J, Portlock C, Mauch P: Hodgkin's disease presenting below the diaphragm. A review. *J Clin Oncol* 1986; 4:1551–1562.
114. Givens SS, Fuller LM, Hagemeister FB, Gehan EA: Treatment of lower torso stages I and II Hodgkin's disease with radiation with or without adjuvant mechlorethamine, vincristine, procarbazine, and prednisone. *Cancer* 1990; 66:69–74.
115. Horning SJ, Hoppe RT, Hancock SL, Rosenberg SA: Vinblastine, bleomycin, methotrexate: An effective adjuvant in favorable Hodgkin's disease. *J Clin Oncol* 1988; 6:1822–1831.
116. Hagemeister FB, Cabanillas F, Velasquez WS, et al: NOVP, a novel chemotherapy regimen with minimal toxicity for treatment of Hodgkin's disease. *Semin Oncol* 1990; 16:34–40.
117. Greenberg P, Parker RG, Northrop MF, Simko TG: Treatment of pathologically staged IIIA Hodgkin's disease. *Am J Clin Oncol* 1986; 9:416–419.
118. Hagemeister FB, Fuller LM, Velasquez WS, et al: Two cycles of MOPP and radiotherapy: Effective treatment for stage IIIA and IIIB Hodgkin's disease. *Ann Oncol* 1990; 2:25–32.
119. Mazza P, Miniaci G, Lauria F, et al: Prognostic significance of lymphography in stage III_s Hodgkin's disease (HD). *Eur J Cancer Clin Oncol* 1984; 20:1393–1399.
120. Specht L, Nissen NI: Prognostic factors in Hodgkin's disease stage III with special reference to tumour burden. *Eur J Haematol* 1988; 41:80–87.
121. DeVita VT, Simon RM, Hubbard SM, et al: Curability of advanced Hodgkin's disease. *Ann Intern Med* 92:587–595.
122. Rogers RW, Fuller LM, Hagemeister FB, et al: Reassessment of prognostic factors in stage IIIA and IIIB Hodgkin's disease treated with MOPP and radiotherapy. *Cancer* 1981; 47:2196–2203.

123. Powlis WD, Mauch P, Goffman T, Goodman RL: Treatment of patients with "minimal" stage IIIA Hodgkins disease. *Int J Radiat Oncol Biol Phys* 1987; 13:1437–1442.
124. Mauch P: Presented at Educational Symposium for Hodgkin's Disease. American Society Hematology Annual Meeting, December 1988.
125. Young R, Canellos G, Chabner B, et al: Patterns of relapse in advanced Hodgkin's disease treated with combination chemotherapy. *Cancer* 1978; 42:1001–1007.
126. Kun LI, DeVita VT, Young RC, Johnson RE: Treatment of Hodgkin's disease using intensive chemotherapy followed by irradiation. *Int J Radiat Oncol Biol Phys* 1976; 1:619–626.
127. Bonadonna G, Santoro A, Zucoli R, Valagussa PM: Improved 5-year survival in advanced Hodgkin's disease by combined modality approach. *Cancer Clin Trials* 1979; 2:217–226.
128. Valagussa P, Santoro A, Boracchi P, et al: 9-Year results of two randomized studies with MOPP and ABVD in Hodgkin's disease (HD): Multiple regression analysis. *Proc Am Soc Clin Oncol* 1989; 8:250.
129. Valagussa PM: Presented at the First Meeting of the International Database for Hodgkin's Disease. Paris, France, 1989.
130. Horning SJ, Hoppe RT, Rosenberg SA: The Stanford Hodgkin's disease trials 1968–1984: Results of combined modality therapy in PSI, II and III. In, Salmon SE, Jones SE (eds). *Adjuvant Therapy of Cancer IV*. New York, Grune & Stratton, 1984, pp 633–642.
131. Pillai G, Hagemeister F, Velasquez W, et al: Prognostic factors for stage IV Hodgkin's disease (HD) treated with MOPP with or without bleomycin. *Cancer* 1985; 55:691–697.
132. Specht L, Nissen NI: Prognostic factors in Hodgkin's disease stage IV. *Eur J Haematol* 1988; 41:359–367.
133. Bonadonna G, Valagussa P, Santoro A: Alternating non–cross-resistant combination chemotherapy or MOPP in stage IV Hodgkin's disease. A report of 8-year results. *Ann Intern Med* 1986; 104:739–746.
134. Lebovits AH, Strain JJ, Schleifer SJ, et al: Patient noncompliance with self-administered chemotherapy. *Cancer* 1990; 65:17–22.
135. van Rijswijk REN, Haanen C, Dekker AW, et al: Dose intensity of MOPP chemotherapy and survival in Hodgkin's disease. *J Clin Oncol* 1989; 7:1776–1782.
136. Coltman CA Jr, Dixon DO: Second malignancies complicating Hodgkin's disease. A Southwest Oncology Group 10-year follow-up. *Cancer Treat Rep* 1982; 66:1023–1034.
137. Glicksman AS, Pajak TF, Gottlieb A, et al: Second malignant neoplasms in patients successfully treated for Hodgkin's disease. Cancer and Leukemia Group B study. *Cancer Treat Rep* 1982; 66:1025–1044.
138. Kantarjian HM, Keating MJ, Walters RS, et al: Therapy-related leukemia and myelodysplastic syndrome: Clinical, cytogenetic, and prognostic features. *J Clin Oncol* 1986; 4:1748–1757.
139. van Leeuwen FE, Somers R, Taal BG, et al: Increased risk of lung cancer,

non-Hodgkin's lymphoma, and leukemia following Hodgkin's disease. *J Clin Oncol* 1989; 7:1046–1058.

140. Valagussa P, Santoro A, Fossati-Bellani F, et al: Second acute leukemias and other malignancies following treatment for Hodgkin's disease. *J Clin Oncol* 1986; 4:830–837.
141. Tucker MA, Coleman CN, Cox RS, et al: Risk of second cancers after treatment for Hodgkin's disease. *N Engl J Med* 1988; 318:76–81.
142. Coleman C, Kaplan HS, Cox R, et al: Leukaemias, non-Hodgkin's lymphomas and solid tumors in patients treated for Hodgkin's disease. *Cancer Surv* 1982; 1:733–744.
143. Pedersen-Bjergaard J, Larson SO: Incidence of acute non-lymphocytic leukemia, preleukemia and acute myeloproliferative syndrome up to 10 years after treatment of Hodgkin's disease. *N Engl J Med* 1982; 307:965–971.
144. Henry-Amar M: Second cancers after radiotherapy and chemotherapy or early stages of Hodgkin's disease. *JNCI* 1981; 71:911–916.
145. Andrieu JM, Dana M, Desprez-Curely JP, et al: MOPP chemotherapy plus irradiation for Hodgkin's disease, stages IA to IIB. Long-term results of the prospective trial H72 (1972–1976, 334 patients). *Hematol Oncol* 1985; 3:219–231.
146. Bloomfield CD, Weiss RB, Fortuny I, et al: Combined chemotherapy with cyclophosphamide, vinblastine, procarbazine, and prednisone (CVPP) for patients with advanced Hodgkin's disease. *Cancer* 1976; 38:42–48.
147. Bakemeier RF, Anderson JR, Costello W, et al: BCVPP chemotherapy for advanced Hodgkin's disease. Evidence for greater duration of complete remission, greater survival, and less toxicity than with a MOPP regimen. Results of the Eastern Cooperative Oncology study. *Ann Intern Med* 1984; 101:447–456.
148. Druker BJ, Rosenthal DS, Canellos GP: Chlorambucil, vinblastine, procarbazine, and prednisone. An effective but less toxic regimen than MOPP in advanced-stage Hodgkin's disease. *Cancer* 1989; 63:1060–1064.
149. Vose J, Armitage J, Weisenburger D, et al: ChlVPP—An effective and well-tolerated alternative to MOPP therapy for Hodgkin's disease. *Am J Clin Oncol* 1988; 11:423–426.
150. daCunha MF, Meistrich ML, Samaan NA: Gonadal toxicity from chemotherapy and radiotherapy for lymphomatous diseases in Hodgkin's disease. In, Fuller LM, Hagemeister FB, Sullivan MP, Velasquez WS (eds): *Hodgkin's Disease and Non-Hodgkin's Lymphomas in Adults and Children*. New York, Raven Press, 1988; pp 186–200.
151. Bonadonna G, Santoro A: ABVD chemotherapy in the treatment of Hodgkin's disease. *Cancer Treat Rev* 1982; 9:21–35.
152. Piga A, Ambrosetti A, Todeschini G, et al: Doxorubicin, bleomycin, vinblastine, and dacarbazine (ABVD) salvage of mechlorethamine, vincristine, prednisone and procarbazine (MOPP)-resistant advanced Hodgkin's disease. *Cancer Treat Rep* 1984; 68:947–951.
153. Krikorian JG, Portlock, CS, Rosenberg SA: Treatment of advanced Hodgkin's disease with Adriamycin, bleomycin, vinblastine, and imidazole carboxamide (ABVD) after failure of MOPP therapy. *Cancer* 1978; 41:2107–2111.

154. Sutcliffe SB, Wrigley PFM, Stansfeld AG, et al: Adriamycin, bleomycin, vinblastine, and imidazole carboxamide (ABVD) therapy for advanced Hodgkin's disease resistant to Mustine, vinblastine, procarbazine, and prednisone (MVPP). *Cancer Chemother Pharmacol* 1979; 2:209–213.
155. Glick J, Tsiatis A, Chen M, et al: A randomized ECOG trial of alternating MOPP/ABVD vs BCVPP vs BCVPP plus radiotherapy (RT) for advanced Hodgkin's disease (HD). *Proc Am Soc Clin Oncol* 1988; 7:223.
156. Jones SE, Haut A, Weick JK, et al: Comparison of Adriamycin-containing chemotherapy (MOP–BAP) with MOPP, bleomycin in the management of advanced Hodgkin's disease. *Cancer* 1983; 51:1339–1347.
157. Gams RA, Omura GA, Velez-Garcia E, et al: Alternating sequential combination chemotherapy in the management of advanced Hodgkin's disease. *Cancer* 1986; 58:1963–1968.
158. Anderson JR, Canellos GP, Propert KJ, et al: MOPP vs ABVD vs MOPP alternating with ABVD as treatment for advanced Hodgkin's disease: Results at a median follow-up of 4 years. Fourth International Conference on Malignant Lymphoma. Lugano Switzerland, June 6–9, 1990.
159. Papa G, Mauro FR, Anselmo AP, et al: Acute leukemia in patients treated for Hodgkin's disease. *Br J Haematol* 1984; 58:43–52.
160. Cosset JM, Henry-Amar M, Thomas JS, et al: Increased pulmonary toxicity ABVD on the arm of the EORTC H6-U trial. *Proc Am Soc Clin Oncol* 1989; 8:253.
161. Viviani S, Bonadonna G, Santoro A, et al: Alternating vs hybrid administration of MOPP–ABVD in Hodgkin's disease. *Proc Am Soc Clin Oncol* 1990; 9:254.
162. Viviani S, Santoro A, Ragni G, et al: Gonadal toxicity after combination chemotherapy for Hodgkin's disease. Comparative results of MOPP and ABVD. *Eur J Cancer Clin Oncol* 1985; 21:601–605.
163. Glick J, Tsiatis A, Rubin P, Bennett J: Improved survival with sequential Bleo-MOPP followed by ABVD for advanced Hodgkin's disease (HD): 8-year results. *Blood* 1987; 70:245a.
164. Connors JM, Klimo P: MOPP/ABV hybrid chemotherapy for advanced Hodgkin's disease. *Semin Hematol* 1987; 24:35–40.
165. Colonna P, Andrieu JM, Ghouadni R, et al: Advanced Hodgkin disease (Clinical Stages IIIB and IV): Low relapse rate after brief chemotherapy followed by high-dose total lymphoid irradiation. *Am J Hematol* 1989; 30:121–127
166. Andrieu JM, Cramer P, Asselain B, et al: Chemotherapy–radiotherapy versus chemotherapy in Hodgkin's disease with bone marrow involvement. *Acta Haematol* 1981; 66:217–225.
167. Wasserman AL, Thompson EI, Wilimas JA, Fairclough DL: The psychological status of survivors of childhood/adolescent Hodgkin's disease. *Am J Dis Child* 1987; 141:626–631.

9

Malignant Lymphomas

Fernando Cabanillas

University of Texas
M. D. Anderson Cancer Center
Houston, Texas

Two fundamental requirements for the management of lymphomas are the appropriate pathological classification and a good understanding of the natural history of the various cell types. The malignant lymphomas are a group of heterogeneous disorders that cover a wide range of clinical behaviors. During the past 15 years, many pathological classifications have been proposed both in Europe and North America. This has led to confusion because there was no clear indication of which nomenclature was superior. The National Cancer Institute (NCI) organized a task force of renowned hematopathologists to evaluate the existing classifications. As a result, a consensus classification, known as the *Working Formulation,* was devised with the purpose of establishing a common language that would enable pathologists and clinicians around the world to communicate (1) (Table 1). This formulation has gained acceptance in America. In Europe, some pathologists have embraced it, whereas others still prefer to use the Kiel classification. Throughout this chapter, the Working Formulation will be used when applicable.

GENERAL CONCEPTS

Staging and Restaging

The Ann Arbor staging system (Table 2) was originally devised for Hodgkin's disease, but has been indiscriminately applied to the lymphomas. Its obvious shortcomings have prompted several investigators to challenge it. The major drawback of this system is its neglect of tumor bulk and tumor burden as

Table 1 Working Formulation of Non-Hodgkin's Lymphoma for Clinical Use[a]

Type	Histologic cell type	Rappaport equivalent
A.	Malignant lymphoma, small lymphocytic: consistent with chronic lymphocytic leukemia; plasmacytoid	(DWDLL)
B.	Malignant lymphoma, follicular, predominantly small cleaved cell	(NPDL)
C.	Malignant lymphoma, follicular, mixed small cleaved and large cell: diffuse areas; sclerosis	(NMxL)
D.	Malignant lymphoma, follicular, predominantly large cell: diffuse areas; sclerosis	(NHL)
E.	Malignant lymphoma, diffuse, small cleaved cell: sclerosis	(DPDL)
F.	Malignant lymphoma, diffuse, mixed, small and large cell: Sclerosis; epithelioid cell component	(DMxL)
G.	Malignant lymphoma, diffuse, large cell: cleaved cell; noncleaved cell; sclerosis	(DHL)
H.	Malignant lymphoma, large cell, immunoblastic: plasmacytoid, clear cell; polymorphous; epithelioid cell component	(DHL)
I.	Malignant lymphoma, lymphoblastic: convoluted cell; nonconvoluted cell	(DPDL)
J.	Malignant lymphoma, small noncleaved cell: Burkitt's follicular areas	(DUL)

[a]Recommendations of an expert international panel.

Table 2 Ann Arbor Staging Classification for Malignant Lymphomas[a]

Stage I: Involvement of a single lymph node (I) or of a single extralymphatic organ or site (I_E)

Stage II: Involvement of two or more lymph node regions on the same side of the diaphragm (II) or solitary involvement of an extralymphatic organ or site and of one or more lymph node regions on the same side of the diaphragm (II_E)

Stage III: Involvement of lymph node regions on both sides of the diaphragm (III), which may also be accompanied by involvement of the spleen (III_S) or by solitary involvement of an extralymphatic organ or site (III_E) or both (III_{SE})

Stage IV: Multiple or disseminated foci of involvement of one or more extralymphatic organs or tissue, with or without associated lymph node involvement

[a]Each stage is subdivided into

A: without systemic effects of disease.

B: with systemic effects of disease.

Table 3 Staging Procedures

Physical examination
Blood tests: CBC, chemistry profile (to include LDH), protein electrophoresis, β_2-microglobulin
Bone marrow aspirate and biopsy (bilateral in low-grade lymphoma)
CT scan of abdomen and pelvis (depending on clinical presentation, CT chest or head and neck might be necessary)
Lymphangiogram
Bone scan (only if symptoms suggest bone involvement)
Upper gastrointestinal and small bowel series in GI lymphomas and Waldeyer's ring lymphomas (frequency of GI involvement and is high in the latter)
Gallium scan ? (see text)

important prognostic features. Consider, for example, a patient with an intermediate-grade lymphoma with a large mediastinal mass and a large (>7 cm) supraclavicular mass. He or she would be assigned a stage II, whereas another patient with smaller adenopathy, but with a small pulmonary metastasis would be considered a stage IV. Even though the Ann Arbor system would assign a poorer prognosis to the latter patient, we know nowadays that he or she actually stands a better chance of achieving a complete response (CR) and cure than the patient with stage II disease who has a larger tumor burden.

The use of the tumor burden concept, as well as other criteria, as the basis for staging will be discussed under the sections for each histological grade. In addition to serving as a prognostic indicator, the baseline staging should provide all the necessary information to delineate the extent of the disease before treatment is initiated. Thus, an adequate baseline staging should include certain essential tests, in addition to others that might be necessary according to the clinical presentation (Table 3).

It is of utmost importance to identify all areas initially involved by the lymphoma to be able to adequately assess the response to treatment. *Restaging* can be defined as the process by which all tests initially positive are repeated after therapy to classify the quality of response to treatment as complete, partial, or failure. The frequency of restaging will depend on the treatment protocol, but

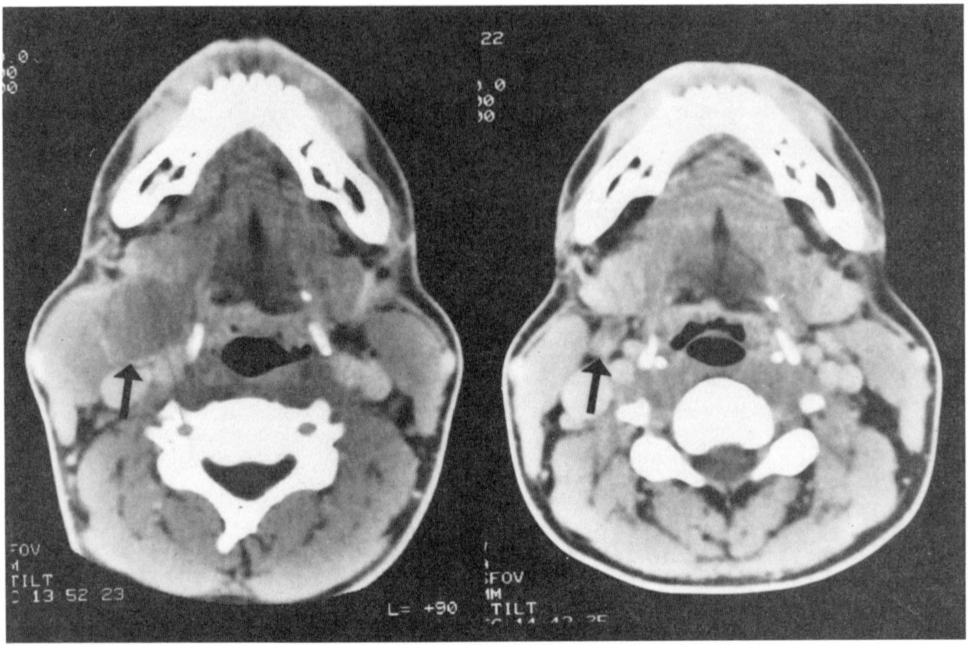

Figure 1 Left panel is a CT scan of the head and neck showing a large tumor mass (see arrow) diagnosed as large-cell lymphoma. Right panel shows the appearance after chemotherapy with the presence of a small residual abnormality in the area where there was previously a large mass. The patient remains free of recurrence for over 2 years.

in general, it should be carried out approximately every 6 weeks initially and eventually every 3–4 months for the first 2 years.

The introduction of modern equipment, such as single-photon emission computed tomography (SPECT) radionuclide imaging, which is a direct extension of the computed tomography (CT) radiologic technique, has created a resurgence of interest in gallium scanning. The major application of gallium scanning is in the evaluation of posttherapy residual abnormalities (2). Most patients who present with large abdominal, head and neck, or mediastinal masses after treatment will still show evidence of residual abnormalities that usually consist of a fibronecrotic mass with no viable tumor (3, 4) (Fig. 1). The gallium scan, however, has been shown by investigators at the Dana–Farber Institute to be capable of discerning viable residual tumor from a fibrotic mass (2). If this can be confirmed by other investigators, the gallium scan will become an essential test for restaging.

LOW-GRADE LYMPHOMA

The three cell types that constitute the group of disorders known as low-grade lymphoma (LGL) (see Table 1) are characterized by several common features: (1) usually the disease is widespread at the time of diagnosis; (2) it usually responds to chemotherapy; (3) patients with the most advanced stage IV presentations manifest a continuous relapse pattern after they achieve CR; (4) in spite of the disseminated nature of the disease and its tendency to relapse, the median survival usually is approximately 8 years.

These cell types are also known as the *indolent lymphomas* and, in the past, have also been designated with the unfortunate term "favorable lymphoma." In view of the unfavorable trend for late and continuous relapses, this term should be avoided. Recently, we have recognized a variant of small lymphocytic lymphoma that is associated with the t(11;14) cytogenetic abnormality. This variant type usually pursues a more aggressive clinical course and should be separated from the rest of the indolent lymphomas, because its treatment should be more intensive than what is normally recommended (5).

A good staging classification should allow discrimination of prognosis among the various stages. One of the drawbacks of the Ann Arbor staging system is that the vast majority of cases of low-grade lymphoma present with stage III–IV disease. Even though it is capable of identifying patients with good prognosis, such as stage I–II, these are, nevertheless, relatively rare. If surgical staging is carried out with laparotomy and splenectomy, these very early stages are even more unusual. In an effort to devise a more effective way of staging patients with low-grade lymphoma, Litam and associates studied the correlation of the serum beta$_2$-microglobulin (β2M) level with time to treatment failure (TTF) in 80 cases of LGL (6). This measurement proved to be the single most important variable that correlated with TTF. It was capable of discriminating patients with favorable prognosis within the stage IV presentations. Patients with serum levels $\geq$3.0 had the highest rate of treatment failure.

Management of Ann Arbor Stage I–II Presentations of Low-Grade Lymphoma

Even though the current thinking is that LGL are incurable disorders, the unusual stage I–II presentations constitute a well-recognized exception to this rule. Two large series each have described 10-year relapse-free survival rates of 31% and 54% with radiotherapy alone (7, 8). This approach would require the use of aggressive staging, including laparotomy and splenectomy if limited x-ray therapy (XRT) is going to be used or more aggressive (total nodal radiation) if less extensive staging is desirable. An alternative has been to utilize a combined modality approach with chemotherapy and radiotherapy. At M. D. Anderson Cancer Center (MDACC), the use of such combined approach has been associated with a long-term relapse-free survival of 64%, compared with 31% for radiation alone (7). No relapses have been seen beyond 4 years in the combined modality group, although the number of patients followed for longer than 4 years is limited. The optimum chemotherapy regimen to be utilized in combination with radiotherapy is not known, but recently, we have used COP-Bleo [cyclophosphamide, vincristine (Oncovin), prednisone, bleomycin] (9). Also, it is not known whether chemotherapy alone can achieve the same results as combined modality.

Management of Ann Arbor Stage III Low-Grade Lymphoma

Most investigators have managed patients with stage III LGL with the same approach as that for stage IV, mainly either single-agent chemotherapy or close observation, without any treatment. However, several centers have reported the potential curability of these patients when treated with either radiation alone or CHOP-Bleo (cyclophosphamide, doxorubicin, vincristine, prednisone, bleomycin) chemotherapy plus irradiation. Cox and Paryani have each reported relapse-free survival (RFS) rates at 5 years of 61% and 40%, respectively, with aggressive radiotherapy alone (10, 11). More recently, McLaughlin reported on 74 patients treated with CHOP-Bleo and "sandwich XRT" to involved fields (12). At 5 years, the RFS was 64% for responders and 52% for all patients. A plateau in the RFS was observed at 4 years, suggesting a potential for cure for patients with this stage.

Management of Ann Arbor Stage IV Low-Grade Lymphoma

One of the greatest areas of controversy in the field of lymphomas involves the management of the stage IV LGL. Most of these patients are staged as IV, based on bone marrow involvement. Management of these patients has ranged from the "watch-and-wait" approach, promoted by the Stanford group, to the most aggressive intervention with high-dose chemotherapy and autologous bone marrow transplantation (ABMT) currently being investigated at several centers, including Stanford (13). Single-agent treatment with chlorambucil (Leukeran) has been used for years now and is considered by many to be the mainstay of treatment for these patients. This is based on a study carried out at Stanford in which patients were randomized to either chlorambucil, CVP (cyclophosphamide, vincristine, prednisone), or whole body irradiation (WBI) (14). The total number of patients randomized in this study was 51 (17 in each arm). Furthermore, the group was not homogeneous, because it contained patients with both stage III and IV. The survival of patients treated with CVP at 4 years was 90%, for WBI 95%, and for single agents 57%. With such a few patients on each arm, it is not surprising that the statistical power of the study was not high enough to detect any statistical significance. This absence of statistical significance has been incorrectly interpreted as being equivalent to no difference between the single-agent arm and the other two arms. In spite of this survival advantage in favor of CVP, there was no difference in the RFS of the three arms at 4 years. However, the small number of patients in each arm and the smaller number followed beyond 3 years make these results uninterpretable.

Mild combination regimens such as CVP, COP-Bleo, and COPP (cyclophosphamide, vincristine, procarbazine, prednisone) have been evaluated by several investigators. Jones et al. in a randomized study conducted by the Southwestern Oncology Group (SWOG), have compared COP-B (cyclophosphamide, vincristine, prednisone, bleomycin) against CHOP-B (15). The CR rate was similar, 71% and 72%, respectively. At 3 years, 28% of patients were relapse-free in the COP-B arm, compared with 39% in the CHOP-B arm. The survival was 55% and 65%, respectively, for each arm. Because these differences were not statistically significant, the conclusion was reached that both arms are equivalent. One of the most successful regimens has been the COPP combination reported by Ezdinli from ECOG (16). In a randomized study, it was associated with a RFS of 57% at 5 years, compared with 22% for cyclophosphamide and prednisone, and 26% for BCVP [carmustine, cyclophosphamide, (BCNU), vincristine, prednisone]. This difference was statistically significant, but the overall survival was essentially the same at 6 years for the three arms, probably reflecting the initial effectiveness of doxorubicin-based salvage treatment for patients failing cyclophosphamide and prednisone and BCVP, as well as the indolent nature of these disorders.

Peterson et al. reported the results of a randomized trial conducted by the Cancer and Leukemia Group B (CALGB) in patients with stage III–IV LGL. They compared-single agent cyclophosphamide with CAVPB [cyclophosphamide, doxorubicin (Adriamycin), vincristine, prednisone, bleomycin] (17). No difference in CR rate or failure-free survival was observed between the two arms. The median follow-up was only 2.5 years.

In an effort to resolve the controversy over the watch-and-wait approach, a study was designed at the NCI to test this approach in a randomized setting against the intensive ProMACE (prednisone, doxorubicin, cyclophosphamide, etoposide, methotrexate, leukovorin)–MOPP regimen plus total nodal irradiation in patients with stage III–IV LGL (18). At a median follow-up of 50 months, 44% of patients in the watch-and-wait arm have required therapy, whereas only 43% of these have been able to attain a CR. Of those who did achieve a CR, 71% are still in CR. On the other hand, of those treated with ProMACE–MOPP at the onset, 78% have reached CR and 86% of those remain in CR. Even though survival, so far, has not been different for these two groups, the quality of life of the patients treated with ProMACE–MOPP has been superior, because most of them have been able to complete the planned therapy and are in continuous CR, off treatment, whereas many of those in the watch-and-wait approach who required treatment have been on continuous therapy because of their suboptimal response once they needed treatment.

At MDACC, for the last 15 years, we have used combination regimens based on doxorubicin (Adriamycin) to treat advanced stages of LGL. We have persisted in using doxorubicin-based regimens because of our poor experience with the COP regimens (19). In our hands, the CR rate for COP has been 53%, versus 83% for CHOP (19). Survival also has been significantly better for CHOP, when compared with previous experience with COP.

Nevertheless, the use of CHOP-Bleo in stage IV LGL has not been associated with a cure potential. The median duration of CR has been 30 months and the median survival 8 years (20). In view of the single-agent activity of interferon in these disorders, in 1982 we initiated a trial of CHOP-Bleo chemotherapy followed by 2 years of maintenance interferon therapy for complete responders. The initial results reveal that at 4-years follow-up, 63% of complete responders continue in remission, compared with 42% of the historical controls treated with CHOP-Bleo alone ($p=0.03$) (20). A slight, but not yet statistically significant, advantage in survival is emerging at 4 years for the interferon group, of which 82% are alive, compared with 73% of the controls. Although it is not yet clear whether interferon is going to result in cures, it already has changed the natural history of these disorders by significantly prolonging the duration of CR, which, in the past, has ranged from only 1.5 to 3 years in practically all published studies.

INTERMEDIATE-GRADE LYMPHOMAS

The disorders known as the intermediate-grade lymphomas constitute a somewhat heterogeneous group (see Table 1). The most common of these, by far, are the diffuse large-cell lymphomas (DLCL) which compose approximately 33% of all lymphomas. Most of these (90%) are of B-cell phenotype. The follicular large-cell lymphomas (FLCL) are also intermediate grade, although they can behave in a slightly more indolent fashion than their diffuse counterpart. There is general consensus that these two disorders are curable, even in their advanced presentations. If a patient with DLCL is able to maintain a CR for more than 3 years, the probability is high that he or she is cured because relapses occur infrequently beyond that point. In FLCL, that figure has to be extended to 4 years because there is a trend for relapses to occur later than in DLCL. Although immunoblastic lymphoma, a more aggressive variant of LCL, belongs in the high-grade category, most investigators treat it similarly to large-cell lymphoma, and the results are practically identical.

The other two disorders included in the category of intermediate-grade lymphoma, diffuse mixed (DMxL) and diffuse small cleaved cell lymphoma

(DSCCL), occur less frequently. Most of these are of T-cell phenotype in our experience, and can be included within the broad category of peripheral T-cell lymphoma (21). Lennert's lymphoma is a variant of either DMxL or DSCCL, which shows an abundant content of large epithelioid histiocytes, with a tendency to arrange themselves into granulomalike formations (22). The diffuse mixed cell lymphoma and DSCCL of T-cell type are more unfavorable in their prognosis, and their potential for cure is low when treated with standard CHOP-type regimens (23, 24). Currently, the experience with these disorders is so poor, especially in their advanced stage III–IV presentations, that some investigators are currently treating them with megadose chemotherapy plus autologous bone marrow transplantation (ABMT) at the onset (25). Unfortunately, because of their low frequency, little experience has been gathered with the use of the newer third-generation regimens; accordingly, the best management for these neoplasms remains uncertain.

Before embarking on therapy for the LCLs, it is important to first classify them according to their prognostic features. The current Ann Arbor staging system is not adequate for this purpose. Several studies have confirmed that clinical features such as lactate dehydrogenase (LDH), tumor bulkiness, tumor burden, performance status, number of extranodal sites, and number of nodal sites correlate well with clinical outcome in the LCLs. Many of these factors are tightly interrelated. For example, most patients with poor performance status have high tumor burden. We have devised a clinical staging system that utilizes both tumor burden and serum LDH level to determine the stage (26). Tumor burden is calculated by determining the number of bulky sites and the number of extranodal sites (Fig. 2, Table 4). By adding the scores assigned for tumor burden and serum LDH level, the patients can be divided into four stages: A,B,C,D, with correspondingly lower 10-year survival rates (Table 5).

Table 4 Criteria for Extensive Nodal Involvement

Site	Criteria
Waldeyer's ring	T3–T4 tumor (TNM AJC)
Neck–axilla	Nodal mass >7 cm
Mediastinal involvement	Any mediastinal mass
Abdomen	Any palpable mass Organ displacement Para-aortic and pelvic nodal involvement Nodal tumor mass >7 cm

Table 5 Correlation of M.D. Anderson Cancer Center Staging System and Survival

Tumor burden	Serum LDH	M.D. Anderson Cancer Center stage	10-yr survival (%)
Low	Normal	A	82
Low	High	B	65
Intermediate	Normal	B	
Intermediate	High	C	44
High	Low	C	
High	High	D	0

Treatment of Stage I–II Large-Cell Lymphoma

In spite of the inadequacy of the Ann Arbor staging system, most of the studies in the literature have used this system to report the results. One of the most common stage I–II presentations involves extranodal sites, of which Waldeyer's ring and stomach predominate, but other sites, such as bone, skin, and, recently, central nervous system (CNS), also are seen. The earlier studies relied on radiotherapy alone to manage patients with stage I–II LCL. Depending on the extensiveness of the staging procedures, which can range from clinical to surgical, results ranged from 20–75% cure rates (27–30). In general, however, the results were suboptimal, with usually fewer than 50% of patients cured. More recently, the trend has been to combine chemotherapy with radiation (29, 31, 32). Most investigators utilize chemotherapy first, followed by radiotherapy as consolidation. Chemotherapy alone has also been utilized successfully (33, 34). Monfardini and co-workers have compared a combination of cyclophosphamide, vincristine, and prednisone (COP) to BACOP (bleomycin, doxorubicin, cyclophosphamide, vincristine, prednisone) in a randomized study for stage I–II LCL (31). Chemotherapy was followed by radiation after three courses and, subsequently, chemotherapy was resumed. At 5 years, 77% of patients treated with BACOP, versus only 57% treated with COP, were still in remission. Another study by Mauch and colleagues compared XRT alone to XRT plus chemotherapy with CHOP-type regimens (35). With XRT alone, 45% of patients survived, compared with 75% with chemoradiotherapy. In a study using CHOP chemotherapy without XRT, we observed 82% disease-free survivors at 10 years in 11 stage I patients and

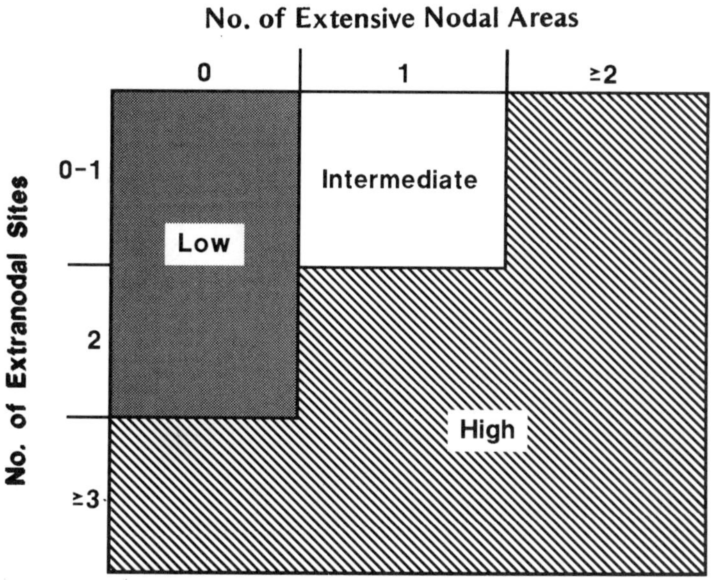

Figure 2 Diagram illustrating the criteria used at M. D. Anderson Cancer Center to determine the extent of tumor burden for large-cell lymphoma.

64% in 28 patients with stage II (34). In a larger series consisting of 147 patients with prolonged follow-up treated with CHOP-Bleo followed by radiation, 79% of stage I patients and 57% of those with stage II were alive at 10 years (36). The role of XRT is still not clear in the management of these disorders, but several investigators feel that its use is important as consolidation to chemotherapy, particularly in patients with bulky, albeit early-stage, presentations.

Connors and associates have recently attempted a short chemotherapy program consisting of three courses of CHOP, followed by radiation (37). The aim was to reduce the toxicity of protracted chemotherapy while maintaining the high cure rate. In 78 cases with stage I–II nonbulky presentations (<10 cm) and no constitutional symptoms, slightly over 80% of patients were cured (37). Even more recently, they have used a 6-week "ACOB" (doxorubicin, cyclophosphamide, vincristine, bleomycin) regimen consisting of weekly doses of chemotherapy followed by radiation. The preliminary results are comparable with three cycles of CHOP (38).

Stage III–IV Large-Cell Lymphoma

Most investigators treat patients with stage III and IV with chemotherapy alone. Others have added radiation sandwiched with chemotherapy. Very little difference exists in results between stages III and IV, which points out one of the deficiencies of the Ann Arbor system. One of the first successful combinations for advanced LCL was the CHOP regimen (39). In spite of the 58% CR rate described initially, only 30% of all patients treated with CHOP in the SWOG study actually were cured after long follow-up (40). The CHOP-Bleo regimen used at MDACC, which added bleomycin, 15 units on days 1 and 5, was associated with slightly over 50% cures in 55 patients with stage III–IV disease (41). In a larger series also from MDACC, 105 patients were treated with CHOP-Bleo but only one dose of bleomycin was given at 5 units/m^2. Also, radiation was given to patients with stage III presentations. At 10 years, 42% of patients were alive (42).

At Dana–Farber, high-dose methotrexate 3 g/m^2, with leucovorin rescue, was incorporated into a combination known as M-BACOD (methotrexate, bleomycin, doxorubicin, cyclophosphamide, vincristine, dexamethasone) (43). At 2 years, 59% of patients were disease-free. Later on, the methotrexate dose was reduced from 3 g/m^2 to 200 mg/m^2 on days 8 and 15, with oral leucovorin rescue. No difference was observed in the results between these two regimens, although there was significantly more mucositis with the latter regimen (44).

A series of recent combinations, which have come to be known as the third-generation regimens, have been associated with a higher cure rate, in the neighborhood of 66% (Table 6). These regimens have in common one of two features: either the use of multiple agents given in sequence according to the patient's response (regimens A,B,C; see Table 6) or the use of intensive combinations given in a unique schedule (regimens D,E; see Table 6).

The general strategy used in regimens A–C (45–47) is to exploit the maximum benefit of one particular combination (e.g., CHOP or ProMACE) and, at the time of plateau in the response, the treatment is changed to a second or third non–cross-resistant combination (HOAP-Bleo, IMVP-16, or MOPP) (see Table 6). For a CR, patients also receive the alternate combination as consolidation. Recently, the SWOG has unsuccessfully attempted to confirm the results of the ProMACE–CytaBOM (cytarabine, bleomycin, vincristine, methotrexate) regimen. In their hands, it is not superior to CHOP (48).

In regimens D–E, the emphasis is on delivering maximal doses of chemotherapy in an intensive schedule (48, 49). The MACOP-B regimen utilizes weekly doses of chemotherapy with myelosuppressive agents (doxorubicin, vincristine), alternating with nonmyelosuppressive agents (methotrexate plus leucovorin, vincristine, bleomycin) (48). Prednisone is given continuously throughout the 12 weeks. Several attempts at reproducing the results of this study have not been successful (50–52).

The COP–BLAM regimen relies heavily on bleomycin, which is given at high doses (49). The most recent of the series of COP–BLAM regimens utilizes

Table 6 Third-Generation Drug Combinations for Treatment of Stage III–IV Large-Cell Lymphoma

Regimen	Acronym/ institution	Drugs[a]	N	%CR	% Disease-free >2 yr
A	CHOP–HOAP-Bleo–IMVP-16/ MDACC	CHOP: Ctx, Adria, Oncovin, Pred HOAP–Bleo: Adria, Oncovin, Ara-C, Pred, bleomycin IMVP-16: Ifos, Mtx, VP-16	56	81	62
B	ProMACE–MOPP/ NCI	ProMACE: Pred, Mtx, Adria, Ctx, VP-16 MOPP: Mustard, Oncovin, Procarb, Pred	79	74	65
C	Pro-MACE–CytaBOM/NCI	ProMACE: See above CytaBOM: Ara-C, Bleo, Oncovin, Mtx	73	79	60
D	COP–BLAM/ Cornell	Ctx, Oncovin, Pred, Bleo CI × 5 days (in alternating cycles), Adria, Matulane	43	86	70
E	MACOP–B/ Vancouver	Mtx, Adria, Ctx, Oncovin, Pred, Bleo	116	85	66

[a]Drug codes: Ctx, cyclophosphamide; Adria, doxorubicin (Adriamycin); Oncovin, vincristine; Pred, prednisolone; Ara-C, cytarabine; Bleo, bleomycin; Ifos, ifosfamide; Mtx, methotrexate; VP-16, etoposide; mustard, mechlorethamine; Procarb, procarbazine; CI, continuous infusion; Matulane, procarbazine.

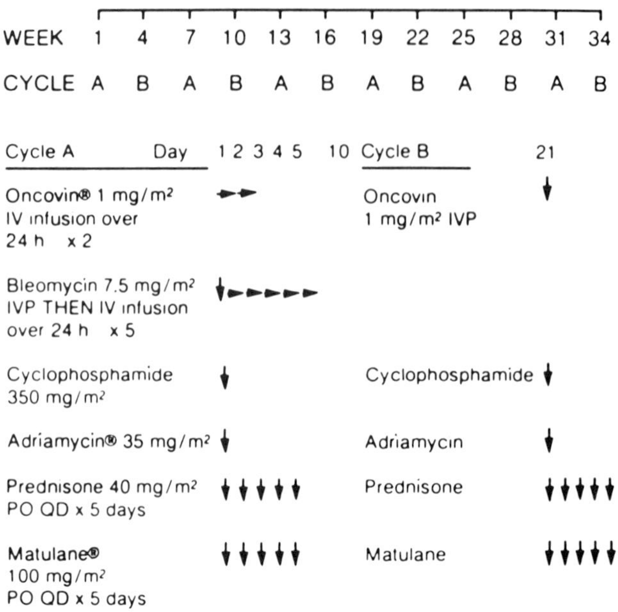

Figure 3 Schema illustrating the COP–BLAM regimen originated by Coleman et al. (49).

continuous infusion of bleomycin at 7.5 units/m^2 daily for 5 days, after a loading dose of 7.5 units/m^2 (Fig. 3).

At this point, all of the third-generation regimens can be considered more effective than CHOP, but their effectiveness remains unconfirmed outside of the single institutions from which they are derived. Whether the explanation for this lies in improper use of the regimen or in patient selection remains largely unknown.

Currently, at MDACC, we are investigating the usefulness of a triple-therapy regimen, which consists of three different non–cross-resistant drug combinations, given in an alternating sequence. The first combination consists of ASAP [doxorubicin (Adriamycin), methylprednisolone (Solu-Medrol), cytarabine (ara-C), cisplatin (Platinol)] followed 21–25 days later by M-BACOS (methotrexate with leucovorin rescue, bleomycin, doxorubicin, cyclophosphamide, vincristine, methylprednisolone) and 21 days later by MINE [mesna, ifosfamide, minoxantrane (Novantrone), etoposide]. The sequence is repeated for a total of nine cycles.

Diffuse Mixed and Diffuse Small Cleaved Cell Lymphoma

Within the Working Formulation, these two entities are considered as intermediate-grade lymphomas. They can be of either B- or T-cell phenotype. In our experience at MDACC, the vast majority of these two disorders are of T-cell derivation and would be considered within the spectrum of the peripheral T-cell lymphomas (PTCL) (21). Most of these tumors are of mature T-cell type: CD4-, CD2-, CD5-positive, and Tdt-negative.

The natural history of these PTCL is usually that of an aggressive malignancy, which frequently presents in elderly patients with widespread adenopathy and constitutional symptoms. Commonly affected areas include bone marrow involvement (30%), in addition to skin (30–50%) and lung (20%) (53, 54). In contrast with the lymphoblastic lymphomas, which is a malignancy of immature T cells, the PTCLs involve the mediastinal nodes in only approximately 10% of patients, compared with 66% of the former. Polyclonal hypergammaglobulinemia is seen in as many as 50% of the patients. The disorder known as angioimmunoblastic lymphadenopathy, formerly thought to be a benign condition with a fatal outcome, is now recognized by most expert hematopathologists as diffuse mixed lymphoma of T-cell type.

The prognosis of both DMxL and DSCCL has generally been very unfavorable, particularly when they present with advanced disease (Ann Arbor stage III–IV). With standard chemotherapy regimens, such as CHOP, the cure rate for those patients who present with advanced disease is extremely poor, with the median survival in the range of only 1 to 1.5 years (23, 24).

Recently, 17 patients with PTCL, who had experienced a relapse after front-line treatment, were treated with high-dose chemotherapy plus ABMT (25). The 59% CR rate and 35% DFS in this preliminary report from the University of Nebraska are very encouraging and suggest that these disorders might be amenable to intensive chemotherapy. At MDACC, we currently manage these patients with alternating therapy using a similar strategy as that for patients with unfavorable presentations of intermediate-grade lymphoma.

HIGH-GRADE LYMPHOMAS

This particular category includes three disorders: diffuse small noncleaved (both Burkitt's and non-Burkitt's), lymphoblastic, and immunoblastic lymphomas. As previously discussed, the latter, in spite of its more aggressive behavior and high S phase, should be considered as a variant of diffuse large-cell lymphoma and treated as such. The management of the two remaining high-grade disorders should rely, with few exceptions, exclusively on chemotherapy. Because of the exquisite sensitivity to chemotherapy of these disorders and because of their high S phase and frequent bulky presentations, particular care must be taken to prevent the serious complications that arise from tumor lysis syndrome. Aggressive hydration and urine alkalinization must precede chemotherapy. Allopurinol and IV sodium bicarbonate should be started before chemotherapy and continued for at least 5 days; for the first 96 hours, close monitoring of renal function, as well as serum electrolyte, calcium, and phosphorus concentrations is mandatory. This syndrome is characterized by rapid breakdown of tumor-derived DNA, which results in massive production of xanthine, hypoxanthine, and uric acid. These metabolites are more soluble in an alkaline urine, but if their concentration is massive, they can still precipitate and give rise to renal failure. Levels of potassium and phosphorus, primarily intracellular ions, can rise rapidly in serum. Hemodialysis should be rapidly instituted at the first sign of hyperkalemia or renal dysfunction. If properly managed, this syndrome is fully reversible and transitory.

Diffuse Small Noncleaved Cell Lymphoma

Of all the lymphomas, the DSNCCL is the fastest growing neoplasm. For this reason, treatment should be instituted as rapidly as feasible, even if baseline-staging procedures are not completed. This disorder has been divided by pathologists into two forms: Burkitt's and non-Burkitt's. Biologically, however, these two variants, which are extremely similar morphologically, do not differ at all. Both of these are associated with a very high S phase (16–50%) and with the same cytogenetic abnormality t(8;14)(q24;q32) or one of its variants (55, 56). Both forms also have been associated with a high frequency of central nervous system (CNS) and marrow involvement, both at diagnosis and relapse. Whenever relapses occur, these tend to happen early, usually between 6 and 12 months after initiation of treatment. This phenomenon probably reflects the high S phase of this tumor. Consequently, disease-free survival beyond this period is usually tantamount to cure.

This disorder can occur at any age, but is more common in the pediatric-age group. With the acquired immune deficiency syndrome (AIDS) epidemic, its incidence has increased considerably, and it is the impression of some investigators, that it is increasing in parallel in patients not exposed to the human immunodeficiency virus (HIV) (Hagemeister FB, unpublished data). Most of the literature related to DSNCCL is derived from pediatric patients. As usual, results in children are more favorable than in adults and, thus, not always applicable. Several staging classifications have been used for pediatric Burkitt's lymphoma, including Ziegler's and Murphy's systems (57, 58). These systems have emphasized the presence of intra-abdominal disease (Ziegler) or abdominal–mediastinal disease (Murphy) and deemphasized visceral disease as a poor prognostic indicator, with the exception of CNS and marrow disease. We have not found this system to be any better in adults than dividing patients into two basic groups: those with only lymph node-based disease and those with visceral disease. In our experience, patients with only lymph node involvement have an excellent prognosis, whereas those with visceral disease have a much less favorable outcome (59).

Straus and co-workers, at Memorial Sloan–Kettering Cancer Center (MSKCC), have utilized an acute lymphoblastic leukemia-type regimen, based on a multitude of drugs, given in a rotating schedule, with emphasis on CNS prophylaxis through an Ommaya shunt (60). Their cure rate in 20 patients was 58% and, in an additional 9 patients who had AIDS it was 30%.

At MDACC, we have utilized a rotating schedule of three combinations to treat 44 patients, of which 12 had AIDS (59). The three alternating combinations consisted of M-COAP (methotrexate at intermediate dose, with leucovorin rescue; cyclophosphamide; vincristine; one dose of high-dose cytarabine; and prednisone), HOAP-Bleo (doxorubicin, vincristine, cytarabine, prednisone, bleomycin), CMED (cyclophosphamide, methotrexate intermediate dose, etoposide, dexamethasone). The intermediate doses of methotrexate, cytarabine, and dexamethasone were aimed at providing systemic CNS prophylaxis, which was supplemented with intrathecal doses of methotrexate and cytarabine. Radiotherapy was not used as CNS prophylaxis. At 5 years, 57% of HIV-negative cases were disease-free, compared with 36% of HIV-positive. However, many of the HIV-positive cases developed other AIDS-related complications, such as Kaposi's sarcoma, and died of these, in spite of the fact that they were free of their lymphoma. Ninety-one percent of the 23 patients whose disease was limited to lymph nodes are disease-free, compared with 24% for 21 patients with visceral disease (59).

Lymphoblastic Lymphoma

A typical presentation of this tumor type would consist of a young male, with a symmetric mediastinal mass associated with superior vena cava syndrome (SVCS). Bone marrow involvement, which is frequently diffuse, is common and, when prominent, can lead to a leukemic presentation that is equivalent to T-cell acute lymphoblastic leukemia (ALL). Meningeal and testicular involvement are also common at diagnosis or relapse. Kidneys, liver, and breasts can be involved, but in contrast with Burkitt's lymphoma, the gastrointestinal tract is not frequently seen as an involved site. Lymphoblastic lymphoma (LBL), which is usually a T-cell disorder, constitutes only 5% of all lymphomas seen in adults, whereas it is one of the most common cell types in children younger than 15 years of age.

Management of this disorder should include intensive systemic chemotherapy, with emphasis on CNS prophylaxis. Whenever superior vena cava syndrome is present, prompt chemotherapy should be instituted. This particular problem is discussed under the section Management of Complicated Situations.

Because LBL is biologically the same disorder as T-cell ALL, with the exception that it presents with primarily extramedullary disease, its treatment should be essentially the same. For practical purposes, when LBL presents with >25% lymphoma cells in the bone marrow, it should be considered as ALL, by definition. Therapy with regimens, such as CHOP-Bleo, that can cure 40–50% of cases of large-cell lymphoma, are usually not successful in LBL. Rosen et al., in a series of 12 cases, described survival over 2 years in only 2 cases (61); Nathwani et al., in their retrospective series, describe a median survival of only 17 months (62). These patients were not uniformly treated, but they were managed with lymphoma-type regimens before it was generally recognized that the disease was equivalent to T-cell ALL.

At Memorial Sloan-Kettering, this disorder has been treated with the same protocols that they have used for adult ALL. These protocols have evolved throughout the past 15 years, but basically, they share the same basic strategy: an intensive induction strategy, an aggressive consolidation phase, intensive CNS prophylaxis by Ommaya shunt, and a prolonged maintenance phase, lasting 3 years. The outcome was essentially the same for leukemic as well as nonleukemic cases in this series (63). Forty-five percent of 51 cases were alive at 5 years. Care should be exercised in interpreting data for ALL and LBL, as late relapses can occur in some patients.

Because of the low frequency of this disorder in adults, the available data are rather limited, and the published series include few patients. A series by Coleman et al. from Stanford University included 13 patients treated with CHOP for the induction phase, followed by high-dose systemic methotrexate with intrathecal prophylaxis (64). Maintenance consisted of 6-mercaptopurine plus methotrexate for a total of 1 year. At 3 years, 50% of patients were disease-free. Of 4 relapses, 3 were in the CNS, which prompted the authors to recommend earlier use of CNS prophylaxis during induction.

Another series by Levine et al. comprised 15 patients who received a similar induction phase, but CNS prophylaxis as well as mediastinal radiation, were instituted early during induction. Also, additional CNS prophylaxis was delivered later during consolidation, with the inclusion of brain radiation. The chemotherapy consolidation phase included cytarabine (ara-C), 6-thioguanine, L-asparaginase, and lomustine (CCNU). Although they did not observe any CNS relapses, their 3-year survival was 40% and their disease-free survival was even lower, suggesting that cranial radiation and mediastinal radiation might prevent relapses in those areas, but do not alter the systemic relapse rate.

MANAGEMENT OF COMPLICATED SITUATIONS

Superior Vena Cava Syndrome

The clinical manifestations of the superior vena cava syndrome (SVCS) can range from subtle puffiness of the upper extremities, face, and neck, to extreme

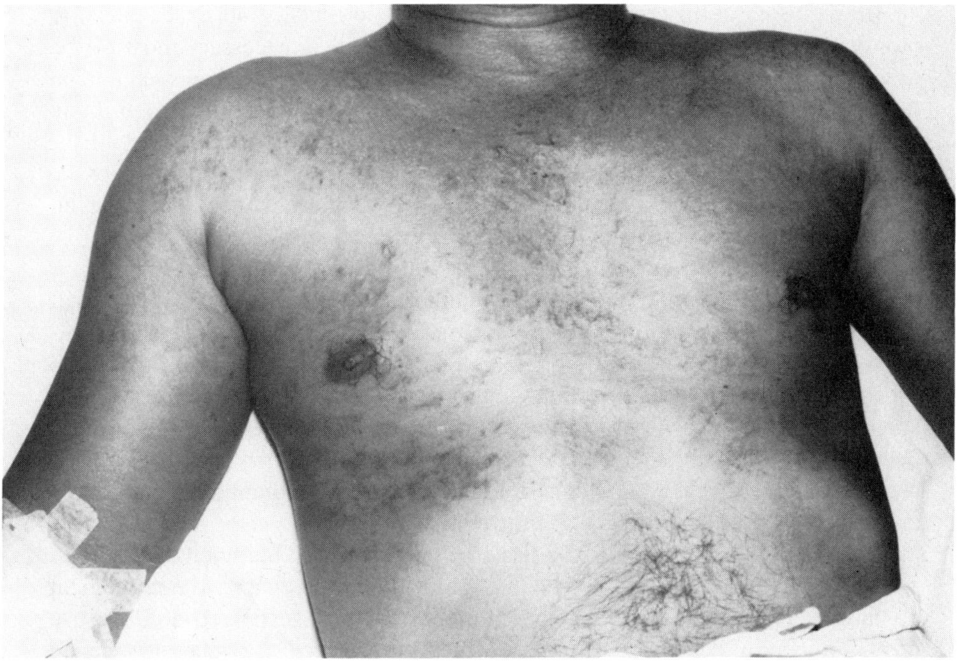

Figure 4 Extensive telangiectasias over chest wall of a patient with severe superior vena cava syndrome (SVCS). This abnormality is almost always present in patients with SVCS.

swelling of these areas, with a plethoric face in addition to severe neurological manifestations. One sign that is practically always present and that should alert the physician to suspect this complication is the presence of dilated veins over the chest wall, which usually takes the form of telangiectasias. In the most extreme cases, these are striking in their appearance, but can be more subtle in mild cases (Fig. 4). Their appearance is due to collateral venous circulation that develops in an attempt to bypass the SVC obstruction.

In the past, this complication has been managed as a serious emergency because it can lead to severe neurological sequelae. In our experience, we have never observed any of these serious neurological complications in lymphoma. Because of the belief that this syndrome should be handled as an emergency, management in the past consisted of immediate radiation, without a diagnostic biopsy. Nowadays, this is not considered appropriate, because SVCS can arise as a complication of various different tumors, including lung cancer, lymphoma, and sarcoma. Benign conditions such as tuberculosis, fibrosis, and venous thrombosis can occasionally give rise to this syndrome.

The first step in managing this complication is to establish its exact cause. A biopsy of the mediastinal mass, when one is present, is necessary most of the time. Whenever a peripheral lymph node is present, a biopsy specimen should be taken from this instead, because it is simpler and safer. Occasionally, a bone marrow examination might reveal the diagnosis. The major obstacle to establishing a diagnosis is the surgeon's unwillingness to perform a thoracotomy because of the tendency to bleed excessively owing to the venous obstruction. In such an event, a useful alternative is to biopsy the right supraclavicular space where most of the time the tip of the mediastinal mass will project through, even though it might not be palpable because of the edema. A CT scan of the chest will frequently reveal the presence of such a mass. In the absence of this, a compromise solution we have used is to initiate treatment with mild chemotherapy with a broad-spectrum CHOP-like combination and arrange for an early thoracotomy as soon as the first sign of subsidence of the syndrome is observed. This usually occurs soon within the first 48–72 hours. An early biopsy can still reveal characteristic features of the tumor. Another alternative is to initiate radiotherapy and proceed to a thoracotomy shortly thereafter.

The SVCS should be approached as an urgent situation, but not necessarily as an emergency unless it is so severe that it already has given rise to neurological complications, such as seizures, or respiratory problems, such as stridor. The use of chemotherapy designed specifically for the tumor type has been associated with excellent results (65) and is preferable to the blind use of radiotherapy, without a diagnosis, which, even though effective in alleviating the edema and obstruction, interferes with the proper selection of specific systemic chemotherapy.

Spinal Cord Compression

In contrast with SVCS, spinal cord compression (SCC) is a very serious emergency, requiring prompt action, otherwise, permanent loss of function of lower extremities, in addition to bowel and bladder incontinence, can result. Fortunately, fewer than 5% of all cases of lymphoma present with cord compression as the first manifestation of the disease. Management of this complication requires, in the first place, that the signs and symptoms be recognized. The usual constellation of findings includes back pain, loss of strength and paresthesia in lower extremities, a discrete sensory level, bladder incontinence and constipation, followed later by loss of bowel control. These symptoms can progress very fast or gradually, depending on the aggressiveness of the lymphoma.

The diagnosis depends on the specific circumstances. In a patient with a known diagnosis of lymphoma, the presence of any of these signs should immediately lead to a series of tests to rule out this complication. The simplest test is a plain x-ray film of the thoracic or lumbosacral spine, depending on the level of the abnormalities. In many cases of cord compression, accompanying radiological bone abnormalities can be seen in these plain films. The most conclusive x-ray examination would be either an MRI of the spine or a myelogram. If the diagnosis is strongly suspected, these should be ordered on an emergency basis. Once a characteristic mass is confirmed in this area in a patient with known lymphoma, therapy should be immediately instituted without need for a biopsy. The earlier the treatment is initiated the better is the chance for recovery. Once the paraparesis has been present for several days, the condition is mostly irreversible.

In patients who have not previously had lymphoma diagnosed, and who do not have peripheral adenopathy for biopsy, surgery is mandatory to diagnose the cause of the cord compression. In those instances, in addition to performing a biopsy, the neurosurgeon should simultaneously do a laminectomy for decompression of the cord.

The traditional management of SCC has consisted of radiotherapy to the spine. An interesting retrospective study from the Royal Marsden Hospital, however, has shown that after surgical decompression, patients can be effectively treated with chemotherapy, without the need for radiation (66). This offers the additional benefit of providing systemic therapy that would have to be delayed if radiation is used as the primary modality of treatment. There are no data on the use of chemotherapy as the first treatment for patients who have not been surgically decompressed. However, it is quite clear that chemotherapy is effective in the treatment of cord compression in patients who have been previously radiated and who have recurred in an area of the spine that cannot receive more radiation (67). In view of the demonstrated effectiveness of chemotherapy in this circumstance, it is logical to conclude that it should be also effective in the primary therapy of cord compression.

Central Nervous System Lymphoma

The problem of CNS lymphoma can assume three forms: (1) primary CNS lymphoma, which has become more common after the AIDS epidemic; (2) recurrent lymphoma, which is the most common type; (3) simultaneous CNS and systemic disease at the time of presentation.

Interestingly, primary CNS lymphoma has become more common not only in HIV-positive patients, but also its prevalence is increasing in the general population (69). Typically, it appears with one or more parenchymal masses distributed around the ventricles (Fig. 5). The most frequent sites are paraventricular areas, basal ganglia, thalamus, and corpus callosum (68). Most of the time meningeal disease is not present. The histological diagnosis is almost always LCL. Currently, there is no proved effective treatment for this disorder. it is widely known that radiotherapy, as the only modality of therapy, is ineffective, with fewer than 20% of cases being cured (69). This is somewhat paradoxical because this disease tends to be a localized process. Death usually ensues from local recur-

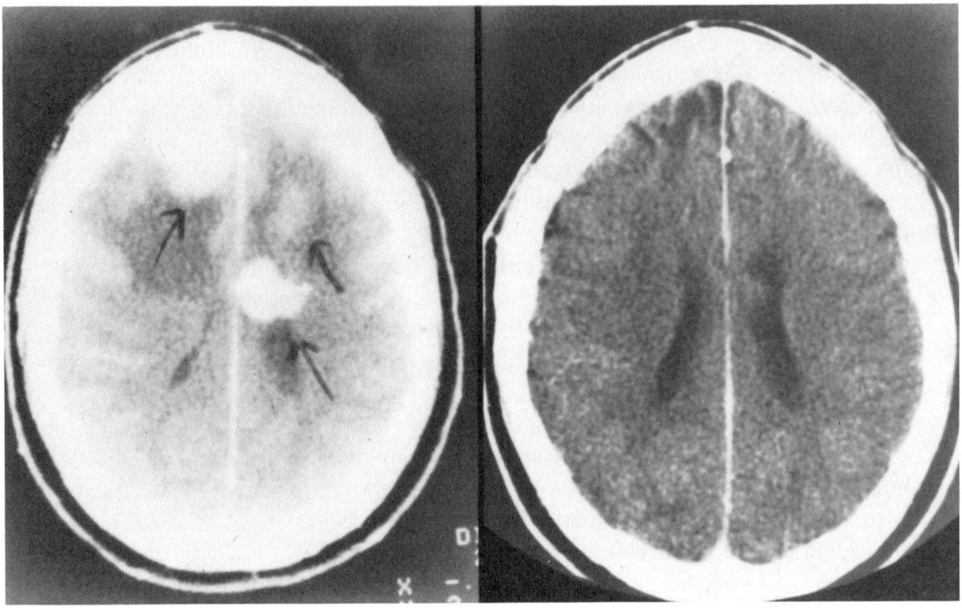

Figure 5 Left panel shows a CT scan of the brain in a patient with multicentric primary brain large-cell lymphoma with several areas of contrast enhancement. Right panel is the same patient after chemotherapy.

rence in the brain, even after intensive radiation. In view of this, we have recently administered chemotherapy first and radiation later as consolidation (70). The preliminary results are encouraging when compared with radiation alone. Of four patients treated this way, using DHAP (dexamethasone, high-dose cytarabine and cisplatin), which contains agents that penetrate the blood–brain barrier, two are disease-free at 18+ and 22+ months. At this point, however, this approach remains investigational.

Secondary or recurrent CNS lymphoma tends to occur most frequently as meningeal disease, especially in lymphoblastic and Burkitt's lymphoma. Parenchymal masses occur mostly with large-cell lymphoma, although simultaneous meningeal involvement also occurs frequently in those cases. A CT scan of the brain is recommended to rule out the presence of a parenchymal mass before performing a spinal tap. Once it is clear that a mass is not present, it is safe to proceed with a lumbar puncture with little risk of herniation. Management of secondary CNS lymphoma will depend largely on the pattern of involvement. Patients with parenchymal brain disease have been treated with radiation, which is usually effective in controlling the disease. Before instituting radiation, steroids should be initiated to prevent brain edema. Dexamethasone, 40 mg daily, which can be tapered gradually after 2–3 weeks, is a commonly used schema. Should there be any evidence of meningeal seeding, an Ommaya shunt should be placed for intraventricular treatment. We use triple therapy with methotrexate 15 mg, cytarabine 100 mg, and hydrocortisone 100 mg, simultaneously. In the absence of parenchymal brain disease, we have relied on intraventricular chemotherapy alone, without radiation. In the occasional patient who fails chemotherapy, we have then utilized radiation. In most patients, the disease in the CNS can be controlled, but unfortunately, the disease will later progress in the vast majority, with few exceptions. Most of the time, progression of the disease takes place outside of the CNS, which has led us to think that CNS recurrences are just the first indication of a systemic relapse (71). This hypothesis has been substantiated by Recht et al. from MSKCC who showed, in postmortem studies, that 52% of the patients with CNS lymphoma were free of disease in the CNS, yet died of systemic disease instead (72). Consequently, we also recommend a change in the systemic chemotherapy to prevent, or at least delay, the appearance of a systemic relapse, which usually occurs within 3 months. In spite of intensive treatment, the median survival in most series has been only 4 months.

Simultaneous CNS and systemic lymphoma at the time of diagnosis occurs infrequently. We have observed it mostly in Burkitt's and lymphoblastic lymphoma. The management should be similar to the situation with recurrent CNS lymphoma discussed in the foregoing. Even though the prognosis is unfavorable when CNS lymphoma is present at diagnosis, there is still a potential for cure (about 25%), and it should be treated aggressively (72). Some investigators have used ABMT successfully to treat this complication in Burkitt's lymphoma (73).

Central Nervous System Prophylaxis

In spite of all measures, the prognosis for recurrent CNS lymphoma remains unfavorable. It is much more convenient to prevent it than to deal with it at recurrence. Nevertheless, CNS lymphoma occurs in only approximately 5% of all cases of lymphoma (71); therefore, CNS prophylaxis in all patients is not justified. It has become clear that only certain histological types of lymphoma are associated with an increased incidence of CNS recurrence. Burkitt's and lymphoblastic lymphoma are, by far, the most frequent histological types associated with CNS relapse. We recommend that patients with these cell types receive routine CNS prophylaxis, preferably with a regimen that contains both systemic high-dose methotrexate and cytarabine, as well as intrathecal therapy. If the bone marrow is involved in these tumor types, the risk of CNS relapse is even higher. Patients with low-grade histologies seldom, if ever, relapse in the CNS, unless they transform to a large-cell lymphoma, which is a phenomenon that occurs usually after several years of disease. Of the intermediate-grade lymphomas,

DLCL is the cell type more frequently associated with CNS relapse. However, less than 10% of patients with DLCL will develop this complication. Consequently, not all patients with this cell type need to receive CNS prophylaxis. When DLCL presents in the bone marrow, the risk of CNS relapse increases substantially and, in these cases, prophylaxis is necessary. We have also found that serum LDH elevation is associated with CNS relapse as well as with poor prognosis (74). Every single case of CNS relapse in DLCL we observed had a high serum LDH level at diagnosis of the lymphoma.

There is no fixed rule for which method of CNS prophylaxis is superior. At MSKCC, Ommaya shunts have been installed routinely for prophylaxis of lymphoblastic lymphoma (63). We have relied on the use of alternating systemic chemotherapy regimens, which contain high-dose methotrexate and cytarabine, but also recommend the simultaneous use of intrathecal chemotherapy with these drugs on the same day as the systemic high doses are given (59). At least three to four intrathecal doses of chemotherapy have been used as part of this CNS prophylaxis regimen. We do not recommend radiotherapy as prophylaxis because of the known complications that occur, especially when used in conjunction with intrathecal methotrexate.

Recurrent and Refractory Lymphoma

Any discussion of the management of recurrent and refractory lymphoma has to start by defining these terms. In the past, these terms have been utilized as synonyms, leading to considerable confusion. Not all refractory lymphomas are necessarily recurrent, and not all recurrent lymphomas are necessarily refractory. For instance, a patient with lymphoma that fails to respond to front-line chemotherapy clearly has refractory lymphoma, but not recurrent, because it never responded. A patient with lymphoma that has recurred after achieving a CR and remaining off treatment for more than 1 year has recurrent lymphoma, but most likely it is not refractory, because it probably will respond again to the same drugs utilized in front-line treatment. Evidently, the latter situation is easier to manage than the former. Therefore, when describing the results of salvage treatment, it is imperative to describe how many patients were treated for refractory disease and how many for nonrefractory. Intermediate situations also occur, such as cases that respond to front-line treatment, but progress while still receiving treatment. These cases should be considered as "acquired refractoriness."

Before embarking on treatment for recurrent lymphoma, the clinician should establish with certainty the presence of disease. Several benign disorders can mimic recurrent or persistent lymphoma, among which can be counted osteoporotic vertebral fractures, Paget disease of bone, reactive lymphadenopathy, chronic seromas in sites of prior lymphoma node biopsy, pulmonary infections, radiotherapy-induced pulmonary changes, and residual posttherapy

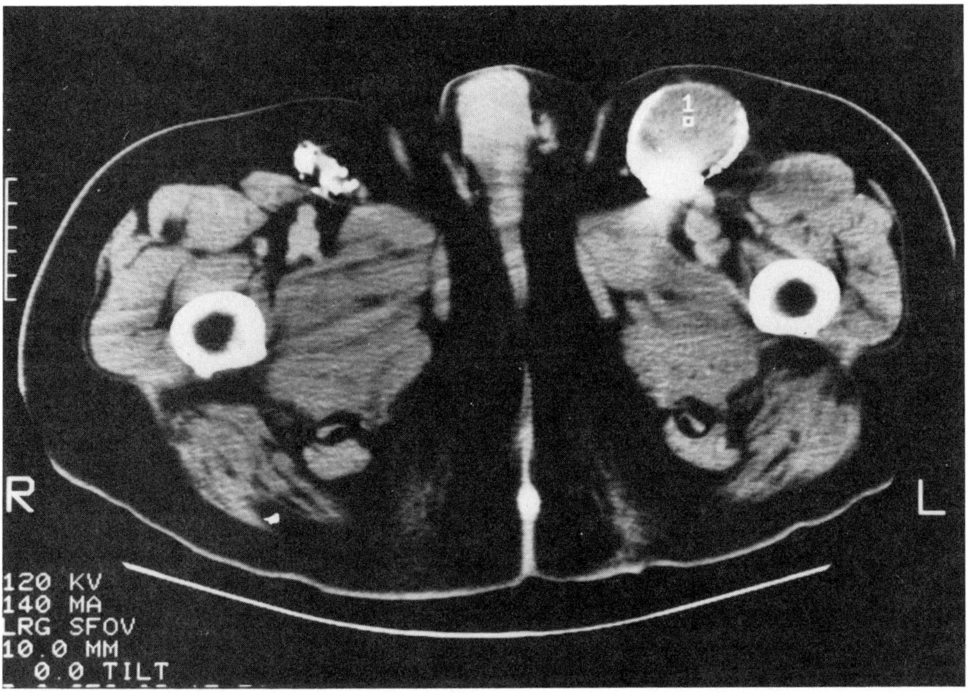

Figure 6 A CT scan at the level of the inguinal areas in a patient with a persistent firm mass in the left groin. Prior biopsy had revealed a low-grade lymphoma, but by physical examination, the disease was manifesting refractoriness to chemotherapy. A lymphangiogram had been performed before this CT scan. Aspiration of this cystic-looking mass showed serous fluid and no evidence of lymphoma. The diagnosis of refractory lymphoma was thus discarded.

fibronecrotic masses in sites at which large tumoral masses were initially present (Fig. 6).

Which modality of salvage treatment to choose is an important consideration because, in spite of all the advances in the last 10–15 years, there still remains from 33 to 50% of cases of intermediate- and high-grade lymphomas, and an even higher proportion of low-grade lymphomas, that will require second-line treatment. Currently, this issue has not been resolved, and the management of recurrent and refractory lymphomas remains largely an investigational endeavor. We do not pretend to exhaustively cover this complex issue in this chapter.

The two major options now available consist of either megadose chemotherapy, with ABMT, or standard-dose chemotherapy salvage regimens. Even though the use of high-dose chemotherapy and ABMT has been associated with

20% long-term disease-free survival (>2 years), whereas standard-dose chemotherapy has only yielded 7% disease-free survival, the patients treated in these studies are widely different (75, 76). The ABMT studies have traditionally selected patients with good performance status, younger age, and no marrow involvement. Consequently, it remains unclear which of the two modalities is superior. An ongoing study comparing standard-dose chemotherapy with DHAP (see later discussion) versus two courses of DHAP, followed by ABMT, should throw more light on this question in the near future (Philip T, personal communication).

A series of salvage regimens have been tested during the last decade at MDACC. The first series of regimens were developed using ifosfamide and etoposide (VP-16) as the backbone. The largest of these was the MIME regimen (Table 7), which was used to treat 208 patients (77). The results are summarized in Table 8.

More recently, the synergism between high-dose cytarabine and cisplatin has been exploited in the DHAP regimen (Table 9) (78). This combination has yielded results that are very similar to MIME, although it appears to be more active than MIME in the low-grade lymphomas (see Tables 7 and 10).

In spite of the fact that CR can be obtained in 25–30% of cases, most of these do relapse. The long-term outcome is favorable in only about 7% of all cases treated or in 25% of all intermediate-grade lymphomas who achieve CR.

Current investigations at MDACC involve the study of a new ifosfamide–etoposide regimen to which we have added Mitoxantrane (Novantrone) (MINE = mesna, ifosfamide, Novantrone, etoposide), which is later consolidated with cytarabine–cisplatin-based regimen, ESAP [etoposide, methylprednisolone (Solu-Medrol), cytarabine, (ara-C), cisplatin (Platinol)].

NEW HISTOLOGICAL ENTITIES

Ki-1 Lymphoma

Stein et al. recently described a new entity that they called Ki-1 large-cell lymphoma (79). It consists of a subset of patients whose lymphoma cells stain

Table 7 Doses of MIME

Drug	Dose
Methylguazone (methyl gag)	500 mg/m^2 IV days 1 and 14
Ifosfamide	1000 mg/m^2 IV days 1–5
Methotrexate	30 mg/m^2 day 3
Etoposide (VP-16)	100 mg/m^2 days 1–3

Table 8 MIME Salvage Regimen Response Rate Related to Histological Type

Diagnosis[a]	Type	Total No. of Patients	CR(%)	PR(%)
DLCL (DHL)	Aggressive	94	31(33)	27(29)
FLCL (NHL)	Aggressive	6	1(17)	3(50)
FSCC (NPDL)	Indolent	27	3(11)	14(52)
DSCC (DPDL)	Aggressive	13	3(23)	7(54)
SNCL (DUL)	Aggressive	4	1(25)	2(50)
SLL (DWDL)	Indolent	9	0	2(22)
Lymphoblastic	Aggressive	6	3(50)	0
FML (NML)	Indolent	13	4(31)	3(23)
Other[b]	Indolent	36	3(8)	17(47)
Total		208	49(24)	75(60)

[a]Abbreviations: DLCL, diffuse large-cell lymphoma; FLCL, follicular large-cell lymphoma; FSCC, follicular small cleaved cell lymphoma; DSCC, diffuse small cleaved cell lymphoma; SNCL, small noncleaved cell lymphoma; FML, follicular mixed lymphoma; DHL, diffuse histiocytic lymphoma; NHL, nodular histiocytic lymphoma; NPDL, nodular poorly differentiated lymphocytic lymphoma; DPDL, diffuse poorly differentiated lymphocytic lymphoma; DUL, diffuse undifferentiated lymphoma; DWDL, diffuse well-differentiated lymphocytic lymphoma; NML, nodular mixed lymphoma.
[b]Consists of 31 FSCC transformed to DLCL and 5 miscellaneous.

Table 9 Treatment Scheme

Drugs	Dose	Route	Duration	Day
Full dose				
Cisplatin	100 mg/m^2	IV	CI × 24 hr	1
Cytarabine	2 g/m^2	IV	3 hr, q12 h	2
Dexamethasone	40 mg	IV	15 min	1–4

Table 10 Treatment Results

Diagnosis	Evaluable patients	CR(%)	PR(%)
Low grade[a]	13	4 (31)	4 (31)
Intermediate grade:			
DLCL: De novo	43	12 (28)	11 (26)
Transformed	15	5 (33)	3 (20)
FLCL	5	2 (40)	2 (40)
DMCL	5	3 (60)	0
High grade[b]	5	1 (25)	1 (20)
Miscellaneous[c]	3	1 (33%)	1 (33%)
Total	90	28 (31%)	22 (24%)

[a]Low-grade lymphoma includes follicular small cleaved cell lymphoma and follicular mixed cell lymphoma.
[b]High-grade lymphoma includes diffuse small noncleaved cell and lymphoblastic lymphoma.
[c]Miscellaneous includes two patients with mycosis fungoides and one patient with diffuse lymphoma, cell type undetermined.
CR, complete remission; PR, partial remission; DLCL, diffuse large-cell lymphoma; FLCL, follicular large-cell lymphoma; DMCL, diffuse mixed cell lymphoma.

positively with the Ki-1 monoclonal antibody. This antibody was originally raised against Reed–Sternberg cells, with the hope that it would serve as a specific marker for Hodgkin's disease. Later on, it was found to also positively stain the malignant cells of a small subset of large-cell lymphomas. The typical Ki-1 large-cell lymphoma patient presents with spontaneously regressing skin lesions, which frequently will lead to confusion with a benign disorder. Pathologically, the tumor consists of anaplastic large cells, easily confused with the malignant cells of other disorders such as melanomas, sarcomas, and carcinomas. Frequently, in the past, this disorder has been mislabeled as malignant histiocytosis, because Ki-1-positive large-cell lymphoma frequently will express histiocytic markers. Most Ki-1 lymphomas are of T-cell origin, but some have been identified as arising from B cells. Sometimes, Hodgkin's disease can also be confused with Ki-1 large-cell lymphoma, especially in those patients in whom Reed–Sternberg-like cells are present, which is a common finding. Most cases of Ki-1 large-cell lymphoma, however, stain positively for leukocyte common antigen and negative for Leu-M1, whereas the opposite is true of Hodgkin's disease.

In the original description of this entity, the clinical course was characterized as aggressive, with a poor prognosis. However, the clinical experience has been very limited because its recent description. A recent series of six pediatric patients revealed that when treatment with combination chemotherapy was used from the onset, the outcome was favorable, in contrast with those treated with radiation at diagnosis (80).

FUTURE PERSPECTIVES

Polymerase Chain Reaction

The definition of cure as well as CR is difficult. Because there is no serum tumor marker available for lymphoma that can be used to define total eradication of the disease, the clinician cannot guarantee that a patient is cured, except in retrospect and, even then, there are instances of relapses that occur beyond 2 years, which has been the landmark used to define cure (81). If a reliable blood tumor marker were available to follow the response of the disease, this would enable the clinician to treat until objective evidence of a plateau and to change therapy at that point until total eradication of tumor was attained.

After the introduction of the polymerase chain reaction (PCR) technique, it was adapted by Lee et al. at MDACC to enable amplification of the DNA sequences present in t(14;18), which is seen in 85% of follicular lymphomas and 20–40% of LCL (82). This permitted detection of 1 : 100,000 circulating cells with this translocation. The method proved successful in detecting the presence of circulating tumor cells in practically all pretreatment samples of early, as well as late, stages of patients bearing tumors with this translocation (83). Furthermore, even patients with DLCL who had been in CR for years still showed evidence of circulating tumor cells (83). This knowledge has prompted us to propose the hypothesis that to obtain a cure, it is not necessary to eradicate all tumor cells. It is conceivable that the host's immune system is able to maintain a small number of persistent tumor cells under control as long as that number is below a certain threshold. That threshold, however, has yet to be defined. Because the PCR technique is not quantitative, it has not yet been possible to define this point. Another possible explanation for the persistent abnormal cells in these patients in long-term CR is that the circulating tumor cells might not be clonogenic. Studies are presently underway to study further these two hypotheses. The availability of a quantitative PCR assay would have tremendous advantages in managing patients in the future.

Multidrug Resistance

It has long been known that cell lines rendered resistant to certain drugs, such as vinca alkaloids, will simultaneously manifest resistance to other unrelated drugs, such as the antitumor antibiotics, doxorubicin and dactinomycin (actinomycinD). This phenomenon was designated *multidrug resistance* (MDR), and recently Ling et al. identified a 170-Da membrane glycoprotein, known as GP170, that is associated with this phenomenon (84). The gene responsible for this protein has been cloned. The mechanism of action of this protein is analogous to that of a pump that excludes the drugs as soon as they enter the tumor cell. It is now known that this protein occurs normally in certain cells, particularly those of the gastrointestinal tract and liver. It probably exists as a mechanism for cells to defend themselves against normally occurring environmental toxins. Tumors that express this protein are usually resistant to all drugs derived from natural sources, such as plants and fungi.

Studies conducted at the University of Arizona in Tucson have revealed that this protein is seldom expressed in lymphoma cells at diagnosis. However, treatment appears to select out MDR-positive cells so that at relapse MDR positivity is very common (85). This has led to a search for MDR-inhibiting agents. Drugs such as the calcium channel blocker, verapamil, as well as others, such as cyclosporine have been identified as potent inhibitors of MDR (86, 87). Results from a small series of patients with lymphoma treated with VAD (vincristine, doxorubicin (Adriamycin), dexamethasone) plus verapamil have shown promise (85). Future studies along these lines, as well as additional insights into other mechanisms of drug resistance, will be very important in delineating the rational management of patients with relapsed and refractory lymphomas.

CONCLUSIONS

In spite of a recent study from the Southwest Oncology Group indicating otherwise, most single-institution studies point toward a consistent improvement in prognosis of intermediate- and high-grade lymphomas during the past decade. A better understanding of the natural history, as well as the increasing knowledge about the biology of these disorders, should guide future efforts in managing them. The HIV-related lymphoma remains an area for which new ideas are needed. The opportunistic infections frequently seen in these patients when treated with chemotherapy, especially in patients whose absolute T4 lymphocyte count is fewer than 100, are a formidable challenge for their management (88). Also, the occurrence of Kaposi's sarcoma in patients who have been cured of their lymphoma continues to plague us.

Currently, however, the most pressing challenge is the treatment of patients with stage IV low-grade lymphoma in whom the natural history of the disease is characterized by a steady and continuous relapse pattern. The great sensitivity to chemotherapy shown by these disorders gives us hope that with more intensive regimens it will also soon join the ranks of the curable lymphomas.

REFERENCES

1. National Cancer Institute Sponsored Study of Classification of Non-Hodgkin's Lymphomas: Summary and description of a Working Formulation for clinical usage. The non-Hodgkin's lymphoma pathologic classification project. *Cancer* 1982; 49:2112–2135.
2. Anderson KC, Leonard RC, Canellos GP, et al: High-dose gallium imaging in lymphoma. *Am J Med* 1983; 75:327–331.
3. Lewis E, Bernardino ME, Salvador PG, et al: Post-therapy CT-detected mass in lymphoma patients: Is it viable tissue? *J Comput Assist Tomogr* 1982; 6:792–795.
4. Surbone A, Longo DL, DeVita VT Jr, et al: Residual abdominal masses in aggressive non-Hodgkin's lymphoma after combination chemotherapy: Significance and management. *J Clin Oncol* 1988; 6:1832–1837.
5. Rodriguez M, Pugh W, Ince C, et al: Clinical and histologic characteristics of lymphomas with the translocation (11;14) (q13;q32). *Proc Am Soc Clin Oncol* 1989; 8:256.
6. Litam P, Swan F, Tucker S, et al: Beta$_2$-microglobulin (β2M) is the best predictor of prognosis in low grade lymphoma (LGL). *Proc Am Soc Clin Oncol* 1989; 8:275.
7. McLaughlin P, Fuller LM, Velasquez WS, et al: Stage I–II follicular lymphoma. Treatment results for 76 patients. *Cancer* 1986; 58:1596–1602.
8. Paryani SB, Hoppe RT, Cox RS, et al: Analysis of non-Hodgkin's lymphomas with nodular and favorable histologies, stages I and II. *Cancer* 1983; 52:2300–2307.
9. McLaughlin P, Fuller L, Hagemeister FB, et al: Combination chemotherapy (CT) and radiotherapy (XT) for stage I–II low-grade lymphoma (LGL). *Blood* 1989; 74:377a.
10. Cox JD, Komaki R, Kun LE, et al: Stage III nodular lymphoreticular tumors (non-Hodgkin's lymphoma): Results of central lymphatic irradiation. *Cancer* 1981; 47:2247–2252.
11. Paryani SB, Hoppe RT, Cox RS, et al: The role of radiation therapy in the management of stage III follicular lymphomas. *J Clin Oncol* 1984; 2:841–848.
12. McLaughlin P, Fuller LM, Velasquez WS, et al: Stage III follicular lymphoma: Durable remissions with a combined chemotherapy–radiotherapy regimen. *J Clin Oncol* 1987; 5:867–874.
13. Hornings SJ, Rosenberg SA: The natural history of initially untreated low-grade lymphomas. *N Engl J Med* 1984; 311:1471–1475.
14. Hoppe RT, Kushlan P, Kaplan HS, et al: The treatment of advanced stage favorable histology non-Hodgkin's lymphoma: A preliminary report of a randomized trial comparing single agent chemotherapy, combination chemotherapy, and whole body irradiation. *Blood* 1981; 58:592–598.
15. Jones SE, Grozea PH, Miller TP, et al: Chemotherapy with cyclophosphamide, doxorubicin, vincristine and prednisone alone or with levamisole or with levamisole plus BCG for malignant lymphoma: A Southwest Oncology Group study. *J Clin Oncol* 1985; 3:1318–1324.
16. Ezdinli EZ, Anderson JR, Melvin F, et al: Moderate versus aggressive chemotherapy of nodular lymphocytic poorly differentiated lymphoma. *J Clin Oncol* 1985; 3:769–775.

17. Peterson BA, Frizzera G, Anderson JR, et al: Response of low grade lymphomas to cyclophosphamide (CTX) or cyclophosphamide, Adriamycin, vincristine, prednisone and bleomycin (CAVPB). *Proc Am Soc Clin Oncol* 1985; 4:211.
18. Young RC, Longo DL, Glatstein E, et al: The treatment of indolent lymphomas: Watchful waiting v aggressive combined modality treatment. *Semin Hematol* 1988; 25:11–16
19. Cabanillas F, Freireich EJ: Intensive treatment of nodular non-Hodgkin's lymphoma. In, Wiernik PH (ed): *Controversies in Oncology*. New York, John Wiley & Sons, 1981, pp 31–43.
20. McLaughlin P, Hagemeister FB, Romaguera J, et al: CHOP-Bleo plus α-interferon (IFN) for stage IV low grade lymphoma. *Proc Am Soc Hematol* 1988; 72:165a.
21. Waldron JA, Leech LH, Glick AD, et al: Malignant lymphoma of peripheral T-lymphocyte origin: Immunologic, pathologic, and clinical features in six patients. *Cancer* 1977; 40:1604–1617.
22. Feller AC, Griessee GH, Mak TW, Lennert K: Lymphoepithelioid lymphoma (Lennert's lymphoma) is a monoclonal proliferation of helper/induced T-cells. *Blood* 1986; 68:663–667.
23. Riggs SA, Hagemeister FB: The clinical and pathologic spectrum of peripheral T cell lymphomas. In, Fuller LM, Hagemeister FB, Sullivan MP, Valasquez WS (eds): *Hodgkin's Disease and Non-Hodgkin's Lymphomas in Adults and Children*. New York, Raven Press, 1988, pp 381–401.
24. Swan F, Cabanillas F, Velasquez W, et al: The adverse prognostic significance of the peripheral T-cell lymphoma (PTCL) as defined by both the histology and the immunophenotype. *Proc Am Soc Clin Oncol* 1987; 6:195.
25. Bierman P, Peterson C, Vose J, et al: Autologous bone marrow transplantation (ABMT) for patients (pts) with T-cell non-Hodgkin's lymphoma (T-NHL). *Proc Am Soc Clin Oncol* 1989; 8:255.
26. Velasquez WS, Cabanillas F, Salvador P, et al: Effective salvage therapy for lymphoma with cisplatin in combination with high-dose ara-C and dexamethasone (DHAP). *Blood* 1988; 71:117–122.
27. Fuller LM, Banker FL, Butler JJ, Gamble JF: The natural history of non-Hodgkin's lymphomas stages I and II. *Br J Cancer* 1975; 32:270–285.
28. Fuks Z, Kaplan HS: Recurrence rates following radiation therapy of nodular and diffuse malignant lymphomas. *Radiology* 1973; 108:675–684.
29. Lester JN, Fuller LM, Conrad FG, et al: The roles of staging laparotomy, chemotherapy, and radiotherapy in the management of localized diffuse large cell lymphoma: A study of 75 patients. *Cancer* 1982; 49:1746–1753.
30. Levitt SH, Lee CKK, Bloomfield CD, Frizzera G: The role of radiation therapy in the treatment of early stage large cell lymphoma. *Hematol Oncol* 1985; 3:33–37.
31. Monfardini S, Banfi A, Bonadonna G, et al: Improved 5-year survival after combined radiotherapy–chemotherapy for stage I–II non-Hodgkin's lymphomas. *Int J Radiat Oncol Biol Phys* 1980; 6:125–134.
32. Nissen NI, Ersboll J, Hansen HS, et al: A randomized study of radiotherapy versus radiotherapy plus chemotherapy in stage I–II non-Hodgkin's lymphomas. *Cancer* 1983; 52:1–7.

33. Miller TP, Jones SE: Chemotherapy of localized histiocytic lymphoma. *Lancet* 1980; 1:358–360.
34. Cabanillas F: Chemotherapy as definitive treatment of stage I–II large cell and diffuse mixed lymphomas. *Hematol Oncol* 1985; 3:25–31.
35. Mauch P, Leonard R, Skarin A, et al: Improved survival following combined radiation therapy and chemotherapy for unfavorable prognosis stage I–II non-Hodgkin's lymphomas. *J Clin Oncol* 1985; 3:1301–1307.
36. Velasquez WS, Fuller LM, Kong JS, Jagannath S: Diffuse large-cell lymphomas: Stages I and II in adults. In, Fuller LM, Hagemeister FB, Sullivan MP, Velasquez WS (eds): *Hodgkin's Disease and Non-Hodgkin's Lymphomas in Adults and Children*. New York, Raven Press, 1988, pp 319–345.
37. Connors JM, Klimo P, Fairey RN, et al: Brief chemotherapy and involved field radiation therapy for limited-stage, histologically aggressive lymphoma. *Ann Intern Med* 1987; 107:25–30.
38. Connors JM, Fairey R, Klimo P, et al: ACOB: 6 week chemotherapy and involved field radiotherapy (IFRT) for limited stage large cell lymphoma, initial results. *Proc Am Soc Clin Oncol* 1988; 7:224.
39. Gottlieb JA, Gutterman JU, McCredie KB, et al: Chemotherapy of malignant lymphoma with Adriamycin. *Cancer Res* 1983; 33:3024–3028.
40. Coltman CA, Dahlberg S, Jones SE, et al: CHOP is curative in thirty percent of patients with large cell lymphoma: A twelve year Southwest Oncology Group follow-up. In, Skarin AT (ed): *Advances in Cancer Chemotherapy*. New York, Park Row, 1986; pp 71–78.
41. Lee R, Cabanillas F, Bodey GP, Freireich EJ: A 10-year update of CHOP-Bleo in the treatment of diffuse large-cell lymphoma. *J Clin Oncol* 1986; 4:1455–1461.
42. Velasquez WS, Jagannath S, Tucker S, et al: Prognostic factors for stage III and stage IV diffuse large cell lymphoma: Long-term follow-up. In, *Hodgkin's Disease and Non-Hodgkin's Lymphoma: New Perspectives in Immunopathology Diagnosis and Treatment*. New York, Raven Press, 1984; pp 357–376.
43. Skarin AT, Canellos GP, Rosenthal DS, et al: Improved prognosis of diffuse histiocytic and undifferentiated lymphoma by use of high dose methotrexate alternating with standard agents (M-BACOD). *J Clin Oncol* 1983; 1:91–98.
44. Skarin A, Canellos GP, Rosenthal DS, et al: Moderate dose methotrexate (m) combined with bleomycin (B), adriamycin (A), cyclophosphamide (C), Oncovin (O) and dexamethasone (D), m-BACOD, in advanced diffuse histiocytic lymphoma. *Proc Am Soc Clin Oncol* 1983; 2:220.
45. Cabanillas F, Burgess MA, Bodey G, Freireich EJ: Sequential chemotherapy and late intensification for malignant lymphomas of aggressive histologic type. *Am J Med* 1983; 74:382–388.
46. Fisher RI, DeVita VT Jr, Hubbard SM, et al: Diffuse aggressive lymphomas: Increased survival after alternating flexible sequences of ProMACE and MOPP chemotherapy. *Ann Intern Med* 1983; 98:304–309.
47. Longo D, DeVita VT, Duffey P, et al: Randomized trial of ProMACE–MOPP (day 1,d8) vs ProMACE–CytaBOM in stage II–IV aggressive non-Hodgkin's lymphoma. *Proc Am Soc Clin Oncol* 1987; 6:206.

48. Klimo P, Connors J: MACOP-B chemotherapy for the treatment of diffuse large-cell lymphoma. *Ann Intern Med* 1985; 102:596–602.
49. Laurence J, Coleman M, Allen SL, et al: Combination chemotherapy of advanced diffuse histiocytic lymphoma with the six-drug COP–BLAM regimen. *Ann Intern Med* 1982; 97:190–195.
50. Kath R, Gunzel K, Overkamp F, et al: Results of the MACOP-B regimen in patients with high-grade malignant lymphoma. *Proc ECCO* 1989; 5:0–0369.
51. Lowenthal DA, White A, Koziner B, et al: MACOP-B for advanced diffuse intermediate and high grade non-Hodgkin's lymphoma (NHL): Preliminary results of the Memorial Hospital experience. *Proc Am Soc Clin Oncol* 1987; 6:201.
52. Reynoso EE, Sobrevilla PJ, Lara FU, Bares JP. MACOP-B for advanced intermediate and high grade non-Hodgkin lymphomas (NHL) with poor prognostic features. Preliminary experience of the Instituto Nacional de Cancerologia Mexico. *Proc Am Soc Clin Oncol* 1988; 7:238.
53. Weis LW, Winter MW, Phyliky RL, Banks PM: Peripheral T-cell lymphomas: Histologic, immunohistologic and clinical characterization. *Mayo Clin Proc* 1986; 61:411–426.
54. Greer JP, York JC, Cousar JB, et al: Peripheral T-cell lymphoma: A clinicopathologic study of 42 cases. *J Clin Oncol* 1984; 2:788–798.
55. Srigley J, Barlogie B, Butler J, et al: Heterogeneity of non-Hodgkin's lymphoma probed by nucleic acid cytometry. *Blood* 1985; 65:1090–1096.
56. Aisenberg AC: New genetics of Burkitt's lymphoma and other non-Hodgkin's lymphomas. *Am J Med* 1984; 77:1083–1090.
57. Ziegler J, Magrath I: Burkitt's lymphoma. In, Ioachim HL (ed): *Pathology Annual.* New York, Appleton-Century-Crofts, 1974, pp 129–142.
58. Murphy SB: Childhood non-Hodgkin's lymphoma. *N Engl J Med* 1978; 299:1446–1448.
59. Lopez T, Hagemeister F, Velasquez W, McLaughlin P, et al: Alternating chemotherapy regimens are effective in adult small noncleaved cell lymphoma (SNCCL) both HIV+ and HIV–. *Proc Am Soc Cancer Oncol* 1989; 8:274.
60. Straus DJ, Oppenberg J, Filippa DA, et al: Small non-cleaved cell lymphoma (undifferentiated lymphoma—Burkitt's type) is curable in 50% of American adults. *Blood* 1988; 72:258a.
61. Rosen PJ, Feinstein DI, Pattengale PK, et al: Convoluted lymphocytic lymphoma in adults. A clinicopathology entity. *Ann Intern Med* 1978; 89:319–324.
62. Nathwani BN, Diamond LW, Winberg CD, et al: Lymphoblastic lymphoma: A clinicopathologic study of 95 patients. *Cancer* 1981; 48:2347–2357.
63. Slater DE, Mertlesmann R, Koziner B, et al: Lymphoblastic lymphoma in adults. *J Clin Oncol* 1986; 41:57–67.
64. Coleman CN, Cohen JR, Burke JS, Rosenberg SA: Lymphoblastic lymphoma in adults: Results of a pilot protocol. *Blood* 1981; 57:679–684.
65. Perez-Soler R, Cabanillas F, McLaughlin P, et al: Clinical features and results of management of superior vena cava syndrome (SVCS) secondary to lymphoma. *J Clin Oncol* 1984; 2:260–266.
66. Eeles R, O'Brien P, Brada M: Functional outcome following treatment of non-

Hodgkin's lymphoma (NHL) presenting with spinal cord compression (SCC). *Proc ECCO* 1989; P-0402.
67. Oviatt DL, Kirshner HS, Stein RS: Successful chemotherapeutic treatment of epidural compression in non-Hodgkin's lymphoma. *Cancer* 1982; 49:2446–2448.
68. Grote TH, Grosh WW, List AF, et al: Primary lymphoma of the central nervous system. A report of 20 cases and a review of the literature. *Am J Clin Oncol* 1989; 12:93–100.
69. Murray K, Kun L, Cox J: Primary malignant lymphoma of the central nervous system. *J Neurosurg* 1986; 65:600.
70. McLaughlin P, Velasquez WS, Redman JR, et al: Chemotherapy with dexamethasone, high-dose cytarabine, and cisplatin for parenchymal brain lymphoma. *JNCI* 1988; 80:1408–1412.
71. Litam J, Cabanillas F, Smith T, et al: Central nervous system relapse in malignant non-Hodgkin's lymphoma: Risk factors and implications for prophylaxis. *Blood* 1979; 54:1249–1257.
72. Recht L, Straus DJ, Cirrincione C, et al: Central nervous system metastases from non-Hodgkin's lymphoma: Treatment and prophylaxis. *Am J Med* 1988; 84:425–435.
73. Philip T, Pinkerton R, Hartmann O, et al: The role of massive therapy with autologous bone marrow transplantation in Burkitt's lymphoma. *Clin Haematol* 1986; 15:205–217.
74. Perez-Soler R, Smith TL, Cabanillas F: Central nervous system prophylaxis with combined intravenous and intrathecal methotrexate in diffuse lymphoma of aggressive histologic type. *Cancer* 1986; 57:971–977.
75. Philip T, Armitage JO, Spitzer G, et al: High dose therapy and autologous bone marrow transplantation in 100 adults with intermediate or high grade non-Hodgkin's lymphoma. *N Engl J Med* 1987; 316:1493–1498.
76. Cabanillas F: Experience with ifosfamide combinations in malignant lymphomas. *Semin Oncol* 1989; 16:78–81.
77. Cabanillas F, Hagemeister FB, McLaughlin P, et al: Results of MIME salvage regimen for recurrent or refractory lymphoma. *J Clin Oncol* 1987; 5:407–412.
78. Velasquez WS, Cabanillas F, Salvador P, et al: Effective salvage therapy for lymphoma with cisplatin in combination with high-dose ara-C and dexamethasone (DHAP). *Blood* 1988; 71:117–122.
79. Stein H, Mason DY, Gerdes J, et al: The expression of the Hodgkin's disease associated antigen Ki-1 in reactive and neoplastic lymphoid tissue: Evidence that Reed–Sternberg cells and histiocytic malignancies are derived from activated lymphoid cells. *Blood* 1985; 66:848–858.
80. Kadin ME, Sako D, Berliner N, et al: Childhood Ki-1 lymphoma presenting with skin lesions and peripheral lymphadenopathy. *Blood* 1986; 68:1042–1049.
81. Cabanillas F, Velasquez WS, Hagemeister FB, et al: Clinical, biological and histological features of late relapses (LR) in diffuse large cell lymphoma (DLCL). *Proc Am Soc Hematol* 1989;
82. Lee MS, Chang KS, Cabanillas F, et al: Detection of minimal residual cells carrying the t(14;18) by DNA sequence amplification. *Science* 1987; 237:175–178.

83. Lee M, Cabanillas F, Chang KS, et al: Detection of minimal circulating cells carrying the t(14;18) by the polymerase chain reaction (PCR) technique. *Blood* 1987; 70:217a.
84. Kartner N, Riordan JR, Ling V: Cell surface P-glycoprotein associated with multidrug resistance in mammalian cell lines. *Science* 1983; 221:1285.
85. Miller TP, Grogan TM, Spier CM, et al: High dose verapamil infusion added to chemotherapy reverse drug resistance in lymphoma patients in relapse. *Proc Am Soc Clin Oncol* 1989; 8:252.
86. Tsuruo T, Iida H, Tsukagoshi S, Sakurai Y: Overcoming of vincristine resistance in P388 leukemia in vivo and in vitro through enhanced cytotoxicity of vincristine and vinblastine by verapamil. *Cancer Res* 1981; 41:1967–1972.
87. Slater LM, Sweet P, Stupecky M, Gupta A: Cyclosporin A reverses vincristine and daunorubicin resistance in acute lymphatic leukemia in vitro. *J Clin Invest* 1986; 77:1405.
88. Kaplan LD, Abrams DI, et al: AIDS-associated NHL in San Francisco. *JAMA* 1989; 261:719–724.

10

Supportive Care of the Patient with Hematological Malignancy

Ralph Wallerstein, Jr., and Kenneth McCredie

University of Texas
M. D. Anderson Cancer Center
Houston, Texas

Supportive care of the patient with hematological malignancy consists of measures to diminish treatment- and disease-related morbidity and mortality. Increased sophistication of supportive care has permitted the intensification of therapy for many diseases, which has resulted in improved long-term disease-free survival. With this increased likelihood of prolonged survival and cure, the need to prevent early deaths becomes even more important. For each of the hematological malignancies, it is possible to identify specific complications, and periods of high risk for these complications, that identify areas for rigorous supportive care.

In acute leukemia, for example, the period of initial diagnosis and treatment initiation is one such high-risk period. Complications at diagnosis and during induction therapy are related to high blast counts, bleeding from disseminated intravascular coagulation (DIC), and tumor lysis syndrome. Another period of high risk occurs during profound pancytopenia after induction, consolidation, or intensification therapy. Death at these times is due to acute bacterial infection, fungal superinfections, opportunistic infections, bleeding owing to refractory thrombocytopenia, and, less commonly, to hepatic, cardiac, or pulmonary failure. Death due to leukemic relapse may represent a supportive care failure if treatment-related complications (e.g., hepatic candidiasis) have precluded further consolidations or allogeneic transplant. Thus, the goals of supportive care for the patient with acute leukemia and other hematological malignancies are to prevent death at initial diagnosis and during treatment initiation, control infection and bleeding at nadir, and preserve normal organ function to permit ongoing treatment. In addition to preventing death and facilitating curative therapy, an additional goal of supportive care is to maximize the patient's quality of life during and after treatment.

SUPPORTIVE CARE AT PRESENTATION

Leukostasis

Patients with acute leukemia who present which blast counts higher than 100,000/μL are at risk for pulmonary and cerebral leukostasis, acute respiratory distress syndrome (ARDS), and acute renal failure. The occurrence of hyperviscosity and vessel occlusion related to high counts is a function of cell type and number. Leukostasis is relatively uncommon in chronic lymphocytic leukemia (CLL) or chronic-phase chronic myelogenous leukemia (CML), despite very high white cell counts. In acute myelogenous leukemia (AML) or CML in blast crisis, leukostasis generally occurs with blast counts over 100,000/μL and, in ALL, with counts over 200,000–250,000/μL. The signs and symptoms of leukostasis are primarily pulmonary and neurological, with dyspnea, hypoxia, blurred vision, altered mental status and, occasionally, acute cerebral hemorrhage. Although laboratory evaluation may show pseudohypoxia and pseudohypoglycemia caused by in vitro metabolism by the blasts after the blood is drawn, the majority of patients have true hypoxia caused by sludging of blasts in the pulmonary capillaries, with ventilation/perfusion mismatching. In a patient with relapsing acute leukemia, these complications may develop rapidly over hours. Patients with rapidly rising blast counts should be treated or referred without delay. The treatment of leukostasis in a patient with hyperleukocytosis is prompt cytoreduction. This may be accomplished with hydroxyurea, 6–12 g/day in divided doses. With this approach, however, the rapid lysis of enormous numbers of blasts releases tremendous quantities of intracellular contents that the body is unable to handle.

Tumor Lysis Syndrome

Administration of chemotherapy or radiation to a patient with a high tumor burden of a treatment-sensitive tumor (primarily acute leukemia and intermediate- or high-grade lymphoma) can release intracellular potassium, phosphate, and nucleic acids, resulting in acute hyperkalemia, hyperphosphatemia with secondary hypocalcemia, and hyperuricemia with crystallization in the urine, causing acute renal failure. The metabolic consequences of tumor lysis syndrome can be prevented or diminished by aggressive hydration, alkalinization, the use of allopurinol, and careful laboratory and clinical monitoring. One specific approach uses a 5% dextrose/water solution (D5W) with 3 ampules of sodium bicarbonate per liter (which results in 150 mEq $NaHCO_3$ per liter) infused as rapidly as the patient can safely tolerate cardiovascularly (generally 150–250 mL/hr). The patient should be given allopurinol, 300 mg PO every 12 hours, preferably starting as soon as the diagnosis is made, but at least 12–24 hours before the chemotherapy. The allopurinol is generally continued throughout the period of cytoreduction, about 7 days, and then stopped, since it can cause rash and agranulocytosis. With the foregoing hydration regimen, the urine pH should ideally be 7 or higher before chemotherapy is started. If not, additional sodium bicarbonate can be ordered as 1 ampule IV q4h until the pH exceeds 7. While the patient is receiving hydration at this rate, accurate hourly input and output and daily weight measurements should be taken and frequent auscultation of the heart and chest performed (twice per shift by the nurses and twice a day by the physician). Electrolyte concentrations, including sodium, potassium, bicarbonate, and magnesium, should be measured every 8 hours, and IV fluids adjusted appropriately. In addition, the blood urea nitrogen (BUN) and creatinine levels should be monitored daily, and early nephrology consultation for hemodialysis obtained as soon as the creatinine level starts to increase, since the release of intracellular potassium in the setting of acute renal failure can be rapidly fatal. Finally, coagulation tests, even if normal at presentation, should be performed daily during induction therapy to detect the development of DIC.

Despite these measures, when tumor lysis syndrome is severe, hyperkalemia, hyperuricemia, acute renal failure, and respiratory failure may still occur. If a blood cell separator is available, the preferred approach to the initial treatment of patients with leukostasis or hyperleukocytosis is leukopheresis which physically removes the blasts from the circulation, rather than allowing them to lyse in vivo. Generally, a large-bore, rigid double-lumen catheter (e.g., Quinton catheter) is placed into the subclavian or femoral vein for venous access. The normal soft Silastic central venous catheters are not suitable for apheresis because the intake side will collapse from the negative pressure, and the soft tip of the return line may be torn loose within the subclavian vein by the high pressure. Generally, chemotherapy is started immediately after the leukopheresis, to prevent a rapid rebound in counts. Red cell transfusions should not be given prior to leukopheresis in the patient with hyperleukocytosis and leukostasis because the blood volume and relative viscosity are already substantially increased. Generally, leukopheresis is repeated daily for 1 or 2 more days until the absolute blast count is fewer than 10,000/μL. An additional advantage of the apheresis approach is that for those patients with evidence of DIC, a partial plasma exchange can be performed simultaneously by discarding the plasma from the plasma-return line from the centrifuge and infusing the patient with fresh-frozen plasma and cryoprecipitate.

Disseminated Intravascular Coagulation

Acute promyelocytic leukemia (APL) is frequently associated with DIC at the time of diagnosis. The DIC may be dramatically accelerated by induction chemotherapy, presumably because of release of intracellular granules containing tissue thromboplastic material that activates the coagulation cascade. In contrast with the low-grade DIC associated with solid tumors, the DIC of acute leukemia occurs primarily as a bleeding diathesis. The concurrent decreased production thrombocytopenia and presence of plasminogen activators (present in the granules of the leukemic blasts of some patients with APL) contribute to the bleeding. Feinstein (1) has recently reviewed the data on the value of heparin to prevent or treat the DIC of APL. At our institution, Kantarjian et al. (2) have identified four risk factors for hemorrhagic death in APL: thrombocytopenia, absolute blast count, aged 50 or older, and a hemoglobin level less than 11 g/dL. Patients with no more than two risk factors had a 5% death rate with heparin administration, versus 6% without, and those with more than two risk factors had a 67% death rate with administration of heparin, versus 45% without. This suggests that patients at low risk do not need heparin, and those at high risk are not helped, and may even be hurt, by the use of heparin. This may account for some of the differences between studies, since bleeding will be uncommon, regardless of treatment, when few high-risk patients are involved. These findings were also confirmed by Goldberg et al. (3) in their own study and in reviewing the literature on DIC and heparin administration in APL. In addition, some investigators feel that DIC with clinically significant bleeding is less common with APL in relapse than at initial diagnosis. This may be due to the generally lower tumor burden at relapse in a patient who is being carefully followed. In a recently reported retrospective review of 268 patients with APL treated at 29 Italian centers with either heparin, antifibrinolytics [tranexamic acid, ϵ-aminocaproic acid (EACA), or aprotinin], or supportive care alone, the overall incidence of early hemorrhagic deaths was 9.4%, with no difference among the groups (4). In this study, a blast count of more than 10,000/μL at diagnosis was the only significant predictive variable for early hemorrhagic death.

Our present management of DIC in acute leukemia is based on the four predictive variables of blast count, platelet count, patient age, and fibrinogen and the rate of consumption of platelets and fibrinogen. Patients who have blast counts of more than 10,000/μL and DIC initially receive leukopheresis. Cryoprecipitate is given if the fibrinogen concentration is less than 100 mg/dL, fresh-frozen plasma if the partial thromboplastin time (PTT) or prothrombin time (PT) are prolonged, and platelets if the platelet count is fewer than 50,000/uL. Platelet count, PT, PTT, and fibrinogen are repeated 1 and 6 hours later. If there is a less than expected increment following transfusion or if there is significant consumption of fibrinogen or platelets at the 6-hour follow-up, patients receive plasma exchange with cryoprecipitate and fresh frozen-plasma replacement. This plasma exchange not only allows large-volume replacement of factors, but also removes fibrin and fibrinogen degradation products, which are potent anti-coagulants, from the circulation. Leukopheresis is performed daily until the blast count is fewer than 10,000/μL. Leukopheresis and plasma exchange are performed simultaneously, and leukopheresis is continued until the absolute blast count is fewer than 10,000/μL, and plasma exchange is continued until the DIC resolves. Platelet transfusions are given (sometimes as often as every 8–12 hours) to maintain a platelet count above 50,000/μL. Cryoprecipitate is given, as needed, to keep the fibrinogen concentration above 100 mg/dL, and preferably, above 200 mg/dL. The DIC usually worsens within the first 24 hours from the start of chemotherapy, persists for 4–5 days, and resolves by day 7 among patients receiving cytarabine (cytosine arabinoside) and anthracycline induction.

SUPPORTIVE CARE AFTER THERAPY

The two major causes of death after intensive treatments for hematological malignancies are infection and bleeding. Prevention of these problems actually begins before treatment, if time permits. Dental consultations should be obtained routinely before beginning intensive treatments, and abscessed teeth should be extracted. Sinus films and consultation with an otolaryngologist should be obtained to detect and treat chronic sinusitis, since in some geographic regions, fungal sinusitis may serve as a nidus for systemic fungal dissemination during intensive treatment.

In addition to the cell counts, differentials, coagulation tests, and chemistry profiles, patients should have human leukocyte antigen (HLA) typing done before starting therapy. This is helpful should HLA-matched platelet transfusions be required at nadir and to search for HLA-matched related or unrelated donors, in the event that an allogeneic transplant is required. Serologic tests should be performed for cytomegalovirus (CMV), herpes simplex, toxoplasmosis, human immunodeficiency virus (HIV), human T-cell lymphotropic virus (HTLV-1), and hepatitis A, B, and C.

Venous access is achieved by the percutaneous introduction of a soft Silastic double-lumen central venous catheter into the subclavian vein percutaneously. With rigorous attention to wound care and dressing changes, the incidence of infection is not significantly increased, compared with central venous catheters inserted through a subcutaneous tunnel in the operating room (e.g., Hickmann). In addition, percutaneous subclavian catheters are easier and less expensive to place and easier to change or remove if the catheter becomes infected.

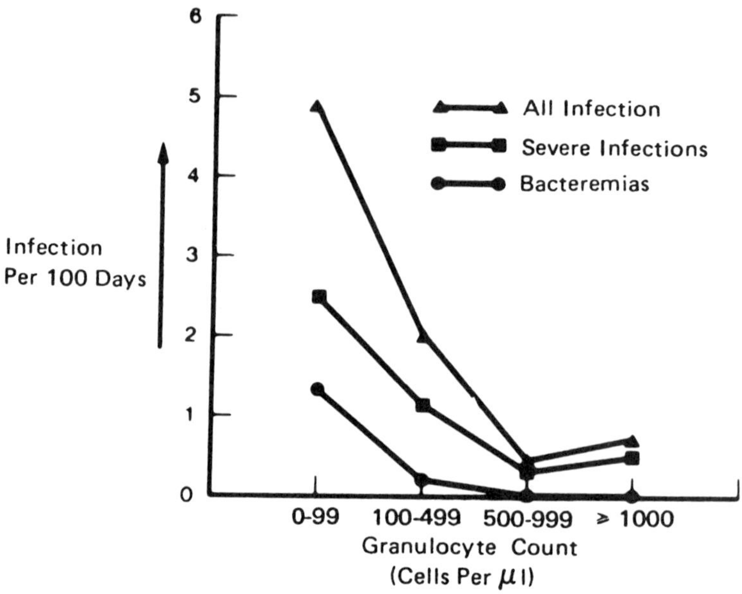

Figure 1 Relationship between neutrophil count and infection. (From Ref. 32 with permission.)

INFECTION

Prevention of death due to infection has two aspects: prophylaxis and aggressive empiric therapy. The incidence of infection is a function of the absolute neutrophil count and the duration of the neutropenia. The incidence of infection begins to increase when the absolute neutrophil count falls below 500/uL (Fig. 1). With a neutrophil count below 100/uL, the incidence of infection becomes extremely high. Older studies with regular surveillance cultures of hospitalized patients with acute leukemia showed that 80% of infections were caused by organisms colonizing the skin and gastrointestinal tract, many of which were nosocomially acquired (5). Thus, one means of decreasing the incidence of infection is to prevent colonization with pathogenic bacteria and fungi.

Prophylaxis Against Infection

Total decontamination of the patient can be approximated by preparing the patient with cutaneous antiseptics and oral gentamicin, vancomycin, nystatin (GVN) solution and then placing the patient into a sterile room with laminar air flow through high-efficiency particulate air (HEPA) filters (6). These filters remove particles larger than 0.3 μm in diameter, which includes fungal spores, bacteria, and even some viruses. All items entering the room are sterilized, including food, medicine, linen, and clothing. Although such protective environments do decrease the incidence of infection, particularly that of fungal infection from airborne fungi such as *Aspergillus* (7), they are very expensive, they limit physician access for careful physical examination, they are psychologically stressful because of the isolation, and they are limited by gastrointestinal intolerance of the oral solutions. Most importantly, it has been very difficult to reproducibly demonstrate a survival advantage for the use of total protective environments.

An alternative approach is selective antimicrobial suppression. The theory of this approach is to reduce the number of aerobic gram-negative rods that cause acute onset of fever with septic shock, but leave the anaerobic flora intact. The use of antibiotics with activity against aerobic gram-negative rods, but not anaerobes [e.g., trimethoprim–sulfamethoxazole, norfloxacin (8), or ciprofloxacin (9)] preserves the relatively nonpathogenic anaerobic flora of the intestine as a "colonization resistance" to prevent overgrowth by pathogenic aerobic gram-negative organisms. In a prospective randomized, placebo-controlled, and double-blind study in patients with acute leukemia, norfloxacin delayed the onset of fever, was associated with a more rapid resolution of fever, a lower incidence of gram-negative bacteremia and hypotension at the onset of fever, and did not increase the incidence of resistant organisms. Ciprofloxacin may be associated with a higher incidence of fungal overgrowth because of its broader spectrum of antibacterial activity than norfloxacin. Trimethoprim–sulfamethoxazole may cause nausea and vomiting or rash in some patients and, in higher doses, may delay myeloid recovery (10). One advantage of trimethoprim–sulfamethoxazole is that it provides prophylaxis against *Pneumocystis carinii* pneumonitis, which is a not uncommon complication in patients with acute lymphocytic leukemia, Hodgkin's disease, or intermediate- and high-grade lymphoma, who are undergoing intensive chemotherapy or combined chemoradiation therapy. On the other hand, trimethoprim–sulfamethoxazole appears to be as effective given 3 days a week as it is when given daily for the prevention of pneumocystis infection, and this intermittent schedule is associated with a lower incidence of fungal superinfection (11). Alternatively, inhaled pentamadine, once every 3 weeks, can be given for pneumocystis prophylaxis, thereby avoiding the systemic toxicities of trimethoprim–sulfamethoxazole. Unfortunately, both the fluoroquinalones and trimethoprim–sulfamethoxazole have poor activity against α-hemolytic streptococci and coagulase-negative staphylococci, which have emerged as major pathogens in neutropenic patients. Currently, we are using prophylactic vancomycin, 1 g IV every 24 hours, and trimethoprim–sulfamethoxazole, 1 double-strength tablet twice daily, while developing new strategies to address these organisms.

Without antifungal prophylaxis, most neutropenic patients receiving broad-spectrum antibiotics will develop candidal overgrowth in the mouth or esophagus, which is not only painful, but also, if untreated, can result in systemic (including liver) dissemination. Hepatic candidiasis, once established, is difficult to eradicate and may preclude further intensive chemotherapy. Our practice is to administer clotrimazole troches five times daily starting when the patient begins prophylactic antibiotics. Although ketoconazole, 400 mg/day, could also be used, it requires an acidic pH in the stomach, and many of our patients are taking prophylactic antacids or H_2-blockers. In addition, ketoconazole can occasionally induce adrenal suppression, testosterone suppression, and hepatic dysfunction. Despite prophylactic clotrimazole, systemic candidal infection remains a problem. Whether prophylactic fluconazole or other new antifungals will be effective for systemic prophylaxis, without unacceptable toxicity, is currently under evaluation. Pulmonary aspergillosis prophylaxis is now primarily limited to environmental measures to limit inhalation of spores. Patients with acute leukemia and documented invasive aspergillosis during a prior course of therapy may benefit from prophylactic amphotericin B started before or concurrently with further intensive therapy.

Cytomegalovirus (CMV) pneumonia occurs in 15% of patients after allogeneic bone marrow transplantation and has historically been associated with a mortality in excess of 85%. Many patients with hematologic malignancies may become candidates for an autologous or allogeneic transplant at some point in the course of their disease. Hence, every effort should be made to prevent the acquisition of CMV infection among the 20% of the population that is CMV-seronegative at diagnosis. Exclusive use of CMV-seronegative blood products with prophylactic intravenous immunoglobulin has prevented CMV infection in bone marrow transplant patients (12). Application of this strategy to all new acute leukemia patients is hampered by the limited supply of CMV-negative blood, the potential for false-negative CMV serologic test results in donors, and the logistics of ensuring proper control against accidental transfusion of CMV-positive blood products in patients who will receive many blood products or pooled random donor platelets. Furthermore, because of the limited availability of CMV-negative blood in some geographic areas, blood banks may limit its use to CMV-negative allogeneic transplant patients. Several reports have suggested that leukocyte depletion of blood products may significantly decrease the risk of CMV transmission (13–16). Given the limited availability of CMV-negative blood and the desire to prevent CMV transmission, we have adopted the policy of leukocyte-filtering all blood products given to new leukemic patients who are CMV-seronegative. Patients who have recently received intravenous immunoglobulin may be falsely positive for CMV antibody and, in such cases when question arises, it would seem prudent to provide CMV-negative or filtered blood. For patients who are CMV-seropositive, studies with prophylactic ganciclovir and foscarnet are currently in progress.

Patients who are seropositive for herpes simplex virus frequently have reactivation of the virus after high-dose chemotherapy. Although this reactivation may take the form of a classic "fever blister," many patients simply experience severe mucositis, which can be due to chemotherapy, herpes virus, *Candida*, or CMV. Without a biopsy or culture, it can be clinically impossible to discern the etiology of the mucositis. Prophylactic acyclovir after high-dose therapy in those patients who are seropositive for herpes is thus a reasonable approach to prevent at least one of the treatable causes of mucositis (17,18). After both autologous and allogeneic transplantations there is also a high incidence of herpes zoster. Prophylactic oral acyclovir, 200 mg twice daily, decreases the incidence of both herpes simplex and varicella–zoster reactivation (19).

Prophylactic Immunoglobulin

Intravenous immunoglobulin is indicated for CMV-seronegative patients in combination with the use of CMV-negative blood in the setting of an allogeneic transplant (2). A dose of 400 mg/kg IV every 3 weeks should also be given to patients with chronic lymphocytic leukemia (and probably multiple myeloma) who have significant hypogammaglobulinemia or recurrent bacterial infections (21).

Empiric Antibiotic Therapy

The second major concept in preventing death from infection is aggressive empiric antibiotic therapy for the febrile neutropenic patient. Site- and organism-specific therapy is difficult in neutropenic patients because many or all of the classic signs of infection (erythema, swelling, heat, tenderness) may be absent without neutrophils. Neutropenic patients with pneumonia may have few or no physical findings and may have a clear chest radiograph. Awaiting the results of culture to direct specific therapy is limited by the substantial risk of septic shock and death, which may occur within hours of the first fever and, also, by the failure of cultures to reliably identify organisms in this setting. Accordingly, early and aggressive empiric antibiotic therapy is now the standard of care in a neutropenic patient with a fever. Historically, these antibiotics have been administered intravenously. Recent studies have explored the possibility that a very selective group of clinically stable patients with fever and neutropenia could be treated with oral clindamycin and ciprofloxacin. If they remained perfectly stable under observation in the emergency room for 8–12 hours, they were treated on an outpatient basis and evaluated daily. Hospital admission and intravenous antibiotics were required for any clinical deterioration (22). In general, however, the standard practice involves a prompt careful physical examination, including fundi (for signs of fungal or viral infection), ears, skin (particularly around catheter sites), and anus. Blood cultures are obtained from the peripheral blood and from each lumen of any central venous catheter. Urine, throat, and any oral lesions are cultured for bacteria, as well as herpes simplex and CMV, if appropriate. A chest radiograph is generally obtained, particularly if there are signs or symptoms of pulmonary infection. The empiric intravenous antibiotics should cover the organisms specific to the patient's geographic region. In many centers, there is now a significant incidence of methicillin-resistant *Staphylococcus epidermidis* and *Staph. aureus*—particularly in patients with central venous catheters—which are capable of causing septic shock and DIC (23). Very recently, we and others (24) have observed the appearance of highly virulent strains of *Streptococcus* that may cause the sudden onset of septic shock and respiratory distress, at times even before the patient is severely neutropenic, which may even be fatal, despite prompt administration of antibiotics to which the organism is sensitive in vitro. Therefore, we have chosen to use empiric vancomycin, 1 g IV q12h with a third-generation cephalosporin (e.g., ceftazidime 2g IV q8h) or imipenem plus cilastatin (500 mg IV q6h), which provide excellent broad-spectrum coverage. Because of its anaerobic spectrum, imipenem plus cilastatin is preferred over ceftazidime, if there is necrotizing oral mucositis or perirectal tenderness. If infection with a gram-negative organism is strongly suspected, an aminoglycoside should be added to one of the foregoing combinations (25).

Because of the high frequency of fungal superinfection in patients taking broad-spectrum antibiotics who remain profoundly neutropenic for more than a few days, the difficulty in establishing a prompt diagnosis of invasive fungal infections, and the high mortality associated with delayed institution of therapy for fungal infections, empiric antifungal treatment is indicated for the neutropenic patient who remains febrile without a source. We and others (27) add IV antifungal treatment if the patient remains febrile for 4 days while receiving broad-spectrum antibiotics. The choice of empiric IV antifungal treatment is currently in a state of flux. Amphotericin has been the traditional agent for empiric treatment. We customarily give a 1-mg test dose in 50 mL of D5W over 20–30 minutes. Unless there is a severe reaction, we proceed to give 0.5 mg/kg (1 mg/kg if there is an infiltrate on chest radiograph) in a 1 mg/10 mL dilution (may be given in a 1 mg/5 mL dilution by a central line) of D5W, 4 hours after the test dose. Although amphotericin has customarily been given over 4 hours, we and others have found that it can be safely given over 1 hour, with no increase in side effects. We do not routinely add hydrocortisone because we are almost always using a central venous catheter and do not need to prevent superficial venous phlebitis. Although hydrocortisone is quite effective at suppressing the rigors, chills, and fevers often seen with amphotericin, the steroids increase the already substantial immune suppression. Therefore, in those patients who have rigors with the amphotericin we pretreat with intravenous meperidine, 25 mg, ½ hour before the amphotericin and repeat 25 mg of meperidine IV every hour for two or three more doses (75- to 100-mg total). In those patients who have severe reactions despite the meperidine, we will pretreat with hydrocortisone, 25–100 mg IV ½ hour before subsequent doses. When amphotericin is started empirically for persistent fever without a source while the patient is receiving broad-spectrum antibiotics, we continue it until the absolute neutraphil count (ANC) is ≥ 500. For patients in whom fungal pneumonia is diagnosed or suspected, we use 1 mg/kg per day of amphotericin and continue it to a full course of 1–2 g. While receiving amphotericin, patients must be monitored daily for potassium and magnesium depletion, renal tubular acidosis, and nephrotoxicity. The combination of amphotericin with an aminoglycoside antibiotic is particularly nephrotoxic and potassium wasting, and may require a continuous IV infusion of 10–20 mEq/hr of KCl. The addition of a potassium-sparing diuretic (aldactone or triamterine) may facilitate potassium repletion. The major problems with amphotericin administration are its nephrotoxicity and relatively poor activity against aspergillus pneumonia in patients with persistent severe neutropenia. In patients who are not critically ill, amphotericin is withheld when the creatinine concentration reaches 3 mg/dL, or it is administered on an alternate-day schedule.

Fluconazole, which has recently been approved by the FDA, is much less nephrotoxic than amphotericin and has excellent activity against *Candida* in vitro and in clinical studies to date (29). It has not shown clinical activity in doses of 400 mg/day against aspergillus pneumonia in neutropenic patients. In a situation in which *Candida* is known to be the infecting agent or if the suspicion of aspergillus infection is low (e.g., in the total protective environment), 400 mg/day of IV fluconazole appears to be as effective as, and much less toxic than, amphotericin. In our experience, if fluconazole has been started as empiric antifungal therapy and the patient remains febrile, switching to amphotericin has sometimes rendered the patient afebrile (no hydrocortisone was given with the amphotericin).

New antifungal agents (e.g., Schering 39304), with better activity against *Aspergillus* species, and exploration of higher doses of fluconazole are the subject of current clinical trials.

Because of the emergence of superinfection with *Pseudomonas (Xanthomonas) maltophilia,* a gram-negative rod resistant to ceftazidime and imipenem, but sensitive to trimethoprim–sulfamethoxazole (26), we add empiric trimethoprim–sulfamethoxazole for persistent fever with the foregoing antibacterial and antifungal therapy, or if a patient who has become defervescent on the aforementioned regimen subsequently becomes septicemic.

Persistent Fever and Neutropenia

Neutropenic patients who remain febrile with administration of vancomycin, imipenem, amphotericin, fluconazole, conventional-dose trimethoprim–

sulfamethoxazole, or acyclovir, may have an abscess or localized intravascular source (e.g., an infected central venous catheter), resistant fungal infection (especially with *Aspergillus*), cytomegalovirus infection, pseudomembranous colitis, infection with resistant gram-negative rods, legionnaires' disease, tuberculosis, pneumocystis infection, drug fever, or occasionally infection with parasites (28).

In a febrile neutropenic patient who develops bilateral interstitial infiltrates, seen on a chest radiograph, prompt bronchoscopy with lavage is indicated, with the empiric institution of erythromycin, 500 mg IV q6h (by a central line to prevent phlebitis and pain); high-dose trimethoprim–sulfamethoxazole, 5 mg/kg IV q6h; full-dose antifungal treatment (e.g., 1 mg/kg per day of amphotericin); and possibly ganciclovir.

As discussed earlier, members of the mold family including *Aspergillus, Mucor,* and *Fuserium* are often fairly resistant to fluconazole, ketoconazole, nystatin, and even amphotericin, unless there is neutrophil recovery. Careful examination of the skin, fundi, and nasal mucosa should be performed, and radiographs of the sinuses should be obtained.

Patients who are CMV-seropositive often have reactivation of CMV in the setting of depressed T-cell immunity. Although CMV pneumonia has been recognized primarily after an allogeneic transplant, with increasing treatment intensity, CMV infection and pneumonia are being observed with autologous bone marrow transplantation, and even with intense conventional-dose chemotherapy. In addition to pneumonitis, CMV reactivation may also cause fever, anorexia, nausea, headache, mild hepatitis, oral and esophageal mucositis, gastrointestinal bleeding, rash, retinitis (particularly in patients with AIDS), and, in some cases, may cause delayed myeloid recovery or graft rejection. Following intensive treatments requiring stem cell support, CMV cultures and immunofluorescent staining of urine and blood buffy coat should be performed weekly. Specimens for cultures, immunofluorescent staining, and in situ DNA probes for CMV should be obtained from any suspicious lesions or from endoscopy or bronchoscopy.

Ganciclovir has substantially altered the acute mortality of CMV pneumonia. Intravenous immunoglobulin, 500 mg/kg every other day, with ganciclovir, 2.5 mg/kg IV every 8 hours for 21 days, has reduced the acute mortality from more than 85% to 48% (55, 56). It appears that both the immunoglobulin and the ganciclovir together are both required to lower the acute mortality, possibly because the ganciclovir prevents further viral replication, whereas the IgG binds to the viral antigens present on the surface of the infected cells and prevents the host immune system from attacking and damaging these cells, similar to the situation in acute viral hepatitis. Early diagnosis of CMV or empiric treatment are necessary for a successful outcome. Patients with diffuse "whiteout" on chest radiograph, and who have severe pulmonary compromise requiring intubation and ventilation with high inspired oxygen concentrations, are unlikely to recover. Therefore, patients at risk for CMV pneumonia, who develop bilateral chest infiltrates and persistent fever, despite antibacterial and antifungal therapy, should be strongly considered for empiric ganciclovir after bronchoscopy. Because ganciclovir itself frequently causes neutropenia, the addition of granulocyte–macrophage colony-stimulating factor (GM-CSF) if the absolute neutrophil count is falls below 1000/uL may permit continued administration without dose reduction, which could increase efficacy. Our preliminary experience suggests that it is important to start the GM-CSF before the absolute neutrophil count falls to extremely low levels. Unfortunately, even after recovery from CMV pneumonia when treated with ganciclovir and IgG, there appears to be an increased incidence of death caused by fungal and bacterial infections over the next several months.

Patients who develop herpes zoster are generally admitted for intravenous acyclovir, 12.5 mg/kg or 500 mg/m^2 every 8 hours for 3–5 days, to prevent dissemination, then discharged on an oral high-dose acyclovir regimen, 800 mg orally five times daily to complete a 10-day course, or until the lesions have healed over. Unfortunately, acyclovir treatment does not prevent postherpetic neuralgia.

The presence of diarrhea or tenderness on deep palpation of the cecum or distal left colon and sigmoid raises the possibility of pseudomembranous colitis. Although this classically presents with five or more loose stools a day, it may occasionally occur as a localized inflammation of the cecum with minimal diarrhea or as a hectic fever without diarrhea (30). Stools should be sent to test for *Clostridium difficile* toxin. If diarrhea is present, examination for ova and parasites (particularly those of *Strongyloides* and *Cryptosporidium*) and culture for enteric pathogens including *Yersinia* and *Campylobacter* should be performed. In a severely neutropenic patient, we do not perform sigmoidoscopy, but in a patient with adequate neutrophils and platelets, endoscopy can sometimes immediately establish the diagnosis if the appearance is classic. Since the assay for *C. difficile* toxin is not 100% sensitive and since the results may not be available for several days, if the clinical suspicion is high, one can consider an empiric trial of oral vancomycin, 125 mg PO four times per day, or metronidazole. Antiperistaltic drugs, such as the combination of atropine and diphenoxylate (Lomotil) and loperamide (Imodium) should be avoided if the clinical suspicion of pseudomembranous colitis is high.

Drug fever is often difficult to diagnose. Although, classically, the onset of drug fever occurs 7–10 days after starting the offending drug, the onset may be sooner in patients with previous exposure and may be delayed beyond 10 days owing to the immunosuppressive effects of the hematological disease and its treatment (31). In the presence of rash, eosinophilia, or fever occurring regularly in relationship to drug infusion, the diagnosis is straightforward. Often, however, one must stop or change all nonessential medications, particularly cephalosporins and penicillins, to see if the patient's fever abates.

Although still uncommon, tuberculosis infection has increased in prevalence in immunocompromised patients, particularly in communities with large populations of refugees or patients with AIDS.

Infected central venous catheters can be a source of persistent infection without any other source. Removal of a central venous catheter is indicated (1) if positive fungal cultures are obtained; (2) if bacteremia persists, despite appropriate antibiotic coverage; (3) if there is a progressive exit site infection; or (4) if there is persistent fever without a source.

Granulocyte Transfusions

Like many new treatments, granulocyte transfusions underwent an initial phase of popularity, then fell from favor, and now have found renewed application for specific indications. Because of the relationship between the absolute neutrophil count and infection shown by Bodie et al. (32) in 1966, it was logical to try prophylactic granulocyte transfusions to prevent infection. Several prospective randomized studies showed a decreased incidence of infection, but no survival advantage for the use of prophylactic granulocytes. With more powerful antibiotics, improved strategies for empiric antibiotic use, and improved induction chemotherapy achieving a higher immediate complete response rate (thereby avoiding reinduction at week 3 or 4 with a resulting prolonged period of absolute neutropenia), it became more difficult to show an advantage for the addition of granulocyte transfusions. Indeed, the prospective study of Winston et al., published in 1982 (33), was unable to confirm the benefit of granulocyte transfusions shown in earlier studies. The granulocytes used in the early studies were often obtained by passing blood over nylon filters to which the granulocytes adhered and were subsequently eluted. This undoubtedly resulted in damage and activation of the neutrophils, which contributed to the toxicity, particularly pulmonary, in the earlier literature on granulocyte transfusions. With the availability of blood cell separators, current administration of granulocyte transfusions is much better tolerated. Currently, granulocyte transfusions are indicated for severely neutropenic patients who are not expected to recover granulocytes for 1 week, who have (1) persistent positive blood cultures, despite appropriate antibiotics to which the organism is sensitive in vitro, and who do not have an intravascular source (e.g., a CVC) that can be removed; (2) a progressive local infection (e.g., cellulitis or perirectal abscess), despite antibiotic therapy; or (3) fungal infection progressing on appropriate antifungal therapy. Once begun, granulocyte transfusions are given daily for 1 week (and then the patient is reevaluated) or until the granulocyte count recovers or the patient is off antibiotics and afebrile for 48–72 hours.

PREVENTION AND TREATMENT OF BLEEDING COMPLICATIONS

Two categories of bleeding disorders commonly complicate the treatment of acute leukemia. The occurrence of DIC at presentation or upon initiating chemotherapy for acute myeloid and monocytic and, particularly, acute promyelocytic leukemia has already been discussed. The other major problem is bleeding caused by thrombocytopenia during chemotherapy-induced nadirs. It is important to understand the relationship between platelet number and function and the bleeding time (34) (Fig. 2). As the platelet count falls below 100,000/μL, there is a gradual and linear prolongation of the bleeding time. When the platelet count is below 10,000/μL, owing to decreased production, the bleeding time will virtually always be longer than 30 minutes. In immune thrombocytopenia purpura (ITP), in which there is accelerated autoantibody-mediated platelet destruction, partially compensated by accelerated production of young hemostatically vigorous platelets, for any given platelet count the bleeding time will be shorter than in states of decreased production, such as acute leukemia, in which all of the circulating platelets are older and less effective hemostatically. In addition, single-donor platelets obtained by plateletpheresis and transfused as soon as possible will be more physiologically active, will shorten the bleeding time more, and will prevent and treat bleeding more effectively than 5-day old platelets. In older studies, it was found that if the platelet count was kept above 20,000/μL by prophylactic platelet transfusions, cerebral hemorrhage was uncommon. In our own experience, those patients who have cerebral bleeding with platelet counts over 20,000/μL usually have had leukemic infiltration of cerebral blood vessels, disseminated fungal infections that invade and infarct cerebral vessels, or a concurrent bleeding diathesis (e.g., DIC). During induction therapy for acute promyelocytic leukemia with DIC, we attempt to keep the platelet count above 50,000/μL.

Prevention of Bleeding

As with infection, prevention of death by bleeding involves both prevention and treatment. Prevention of bleeding involves giving prophylactic platelet transfusions two to three times per week or daily, if necessary, whenever the platelet count is below 20,000/μL. In addition, all drugs that can induce a qualitative platelet defect should be avoided. Patients should be told not to take aspirin or nonsteroidal medications. A major limitation to prophylactic platelet transfusions, particularly for patients who undergo repeated cycles of intensive therapy, is the development of antibodies, which can preclude clinically significant posttransfusion increments.

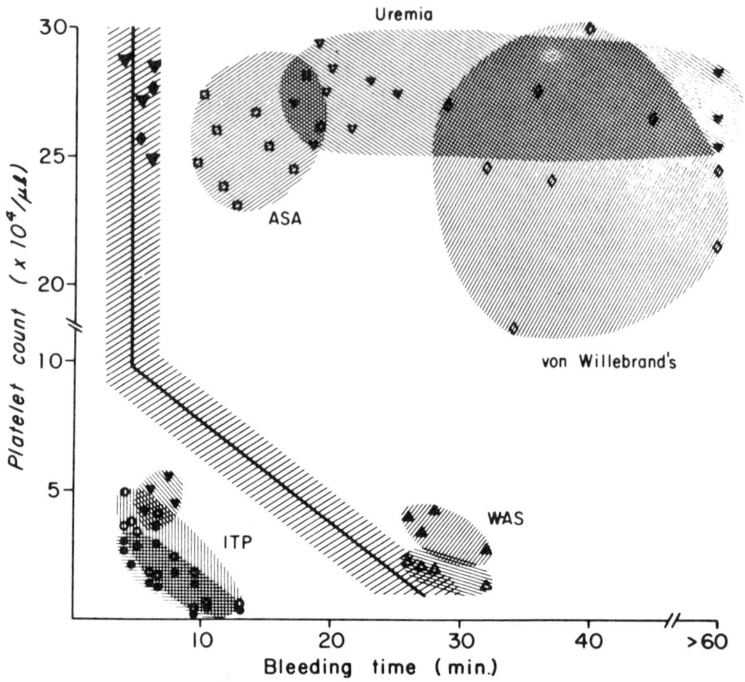

Figure 2 Relationship between platelet number and function and the bleeding time. More than predictable shortening of the bleeding time for normal platelets by young platelets, as found in patients with ITP (●) or rapidly returning bone-marrow function after chemotherapy (▼).

Bleeding times remain short even after adjustment for the increase in platelet volume (○). Impaired platelet plug formation is reflected as bleeding times longer than predicted by the platelet count as shown by 3 g of ASA daily (□) and von Willebrand's disease (◇), which corrects with cryoprecipitate infusion (◆). In uremia platelets have marked dysfunction in the untreated state (▼), which improves after hemodialysis (▽) and reverses to normal with peritoneal dialysis (▼). The modestly disparate bleeding times in Wiscott–Aldrich syndrome (WAS) (▲) become appropriate after adjustment for the small platelet volume (△). (From Ref. 34, reprinted by permission.)

Prevention of Platelet Alloimmunization

One new approach to this problem is prevention of the development of alloimmunization in the first place. It appears that platelets, by themselves, will not result in the development of antibodies because they carry only class I HLA antigens and platelet-specific antigens. The development of alloimmunization requires the presence of class I antigens together with class II antigens, which, in the case of transfused blood, are provided by monocytes, lymphocytes, and dendritic cells. Although not yet rigorously proved, it now appears that if the number of leukocytes can be reduced to fewer than 10^6/bag of platelets and red cells, that alloimmunization to platelets can be markedly delayed or possibly even totally prevented (35–37). Single-donor platelets obtained by apheresis using the Cobe Spectra blood cell separator have between 10^6 and 10^7 white cells per bag depending on the counts of the donor and the skill of the operator. This is significantly fewer than the $0.5–1 \times 10^8$ white cells in a unit of platelets concentrated from whole blood. Even though reducing the number of leukocytes below 10^8 will prevent chill and fever reactions, it is necessary to remove another 2 logs to significantly prevent alloimmunization. This can be accomplished using a leukocyte-depletion filter, either at the time the platelets are collected and before storage, or at the time of administration by filtering either in the blood bank or at the bedside. Considerations of the efficiency of leukocyte removal (significant differences in the number of logs of leukocyte removal exist between the different filters), the extent of platelet loss, ease of use, and cost should determine the choice of filter.

Another approach to preventing alloimmunization is to use ultraviolet irradiation of the blood products (38). Unlike gamma radiation, which is used to damage the DNA of the lymphocytes to prevent transfusion-induced graft-versus-host disease, ultraviolet irradiation is an investigational procedure that appears to modify surface membrane antigens, rendering the cells nonimmunogenic, without altering function. Unfortunately, special bags and ultraviolet irradiators are necessary because of the limited penetration into standard storage bags.

Despite the exclusive use of leukocyte-depleted blood products in all patients with newly diagnosed hematological malignancies, some women at diagnosis will have some degree of alloimmunization from earlier pregnancies. In these patients, leukocyte filtration may prevent worsening of the alloimmunized state and, usually, one or more single donors can be found empirically or by partial HLA matching who can serve as effective donors. After every platelet transfusion, a 10-minute to 1-hour posttransfusion blood sample should be drawn for platelet count and another sample obtained 24 hours later (39). A poor increment (fewer than $10{,}000 \cdot \mu L^{-1} \cdot m^{-2}$ of body surface area per unit of platelets) at 1 hours is seen with splenomegaly or alloimmunization. On the other hand, a good 1-hour posttransfusion count that returns to baseline by 24 hours is much less specific and can be seen with bleeding, infection, poor quality platelets, or any cause of accelerated platelet consumption, including some drugs.

All blood products given to severely immunocompromised patients should be treated with 1500–2500 rad to prevent viable lymphocytes from engrafting in the recipient and causing graft-versus-host disease. Recently, it was reported that designated donor transfusions from first-degree relatives may cause fatal graft-versus-host disease, even in recipients who are not severely immunocompromised (40). Since there is no clinical evidence that blood irradiation is harmful, and since most patients with hematopoietic neoplasms, particularly when undergoing chemotherapy or radiation are immunocompromised to some extent, it would seem prudent to irradiate all blood products, if that is feasible. For patients with Hodgkin's and non-Hodgkin's lymphoma and acute lymphocytic leukemia who are undergoing intensive chemotherapy, irradiation of blood products should be standard practice. In practice settings at which blood irradiators are not available, leukocyte filtration may diminish the risk by decreasing the number of lymphocytes transfused.

Management of the Patient with Platelet Alloimmunization

Occasionally, patients who have become alloimmunized may be supported with partially HLA-matched platelets or completely matched platelets if HLA-identical siblings are available. Often, if several different single donors are tried, one will empirically find a donor whose platelets are less rapidly destroyed. An alternative approach for patients who have recovered from a cycle of therapy during which they demonstrated platelet refractoriness, is to collect and cryopreserve autologous platelets while the patient is in remission (41). Although there is loss of cell number and function (42) as a result of the freezing and thawing, this technique can still permit platelet transfusion increments and clinical hemostasis, even in patients totally refractory to allogeneic platelets. In one severely alloimmunized patient in whom we had cryopreserved autologous platelets during remission, we were unable to get significant platelet count increments, even with these autologous platelets, leading us to suspect an autoantibody. After plasmapheresis daily for a few days we were able to get a significantly improved platelet increment from transfusion.

Some patients will become refractory even to HLA-matched platelets. Although this may occur from antibodies to platelet-specific antigens, one should also consider the possibility of a drug-induced immune thrombocytopenia [for example, this has recently been reported with vancomycin (43)] or the development of an autoantibody. Although small randomized studies have shown no general benefit, high-dose intravenous immune globulin (400 mg/kg daily for 5 days) will occasionally permit better platelet increments in platelet-refractory patients (44,45). Possibly, those patients who benefit have a different mechanism of accelerated platelet destruction than the usual alloimmunized patient. In the absence of a way to prospectively identify those who will benefit, and given the minimal disadvantages of intravenous immunoglobulin other than cost, and since there are few alternative approaches, an empiric trial of IgG seems reasonable for severely thrombocytopenic platelet-refractory patients, especially if they are bleeding.

Despite the moderate success of using HLA-matched platelets and the occasional success with IgG and plasmapheresis, the development of platelet alloimmunization remains a serious life-threatening problem. In extreme cases when a patient gets no increment to transfused platelets, is bleeding, and all of the foregoing measures have been tried, one can use oral tranexamic acid mouth wash (46) to control oral mucosal bleeding or, if there is no evidence of DIC, systemic intravenous ϵ-aminocaproic acid (24 g/day as a continuous infusion or in divided doses every 4 hours). This agent should not be given for the control of upper tract genitourinary bleeding because it can result in ureteral obstruction. Because of the dangers of thrombosis, EACA should be used for as short a time as possible.

OTHER COMMON PROBLEMS

Mucositis

Oral and esophageal mucositis is a frequent occurrence after intensive chemotherapy. The differential diagnosis includes toxicity from chemotherapy or infection caused by *Candida,* herpes simplex, or CMV. For some chemotherapeutic agents, such as methotrexate, mucositis occurs with conventional doses and schedules. For others, mucositis is schedule-dependent (e.g., 5-fluorouracil and doxorubicin when given by continuous infusion). For a third group of agents, mucositis is dose-dependent. High-dose therapy with cytarabine, etoposide, mitoxantrone, thiotepa, or methotrexate frequently causes severe mucositis. Currently, the management of chemotherapy-induced mucositis consists of intravenous hyperalimentation, analgesia, and the prevention of further damage. For distal esophagitis, intravenous H_2-blockers may prevent aggravation of the mucositis by acid reflux. Although oral sucralfate (Carafate) solution, 1 g every 6 hours, may have some value, most patients with severe mucositis are unable to tolerate it because of pain and nausea. If oral bleeding is a major problem, tranexamic acid mouthwash may help maintain hemostasis, particularly in thrombocytopenic patients. Both G-CSF and GM-CSF have been reported to decrease the incidence and severity of oral mucositis when given after high-dose therapy to accelerate myeloid recovery. Whether this is simply related to acceleration of neutrophil recovery or whether there is a protective effect, independent of neutrophil count, is not yet clear. Clinical trials of recombinant epidermal growth factor to accelerate mucosal healing are planned.

For patients with dysphagia, but without lesions in the mouth, there are two approaches. If a skilled endoscopist is available, esophagoscopy with a pediatric endoscope can be performed with culture or brushings taken to test for *Candida,* herpes, and CMV, with specific therapy dictated by the appearance of the lesions and the results of stains and culture. Alternatively, one can treat empirically for the common and treatable pathogens—*Candida* and herpes—with fluconazole or low-dose amphotericin (15 mg/day) and intravenous acylcovir (250 mg/m^2 IV every 8 hours). Because candidal esophagitis can cause local life-threatening hemorrhage or serve as a source for systemic and hepatic (through the portal vein) dissemination, clotrimazole (Mycelex) or ketoconazole (because of the unreliable absorption especially when the patient is receiving H_2 blockers) is not adequate empiric therapy for an immunocompromised neutropenic patient with dysphagia. Candidal abscesses in the liver are suggested by persistent fever, abdominal symptoms, and an increased alkaline phosphatase level. The characteristic hypodense or targetlike lesions on abdominal ultrasound or computerized tomography may be absent in the neutropenic patient, and repeated scans or liver biopsy may be required to establish the diagnosis (47). Even with neutrophil recovery and full-dose amphotericin, it has been difficult to totally eradicate hepatic candidiasis, once microabscesses have formed. Thus, prompt aggressive therapy for dysphagia is imperative.

Nausea and Vomiting

From a supportive care viewpoint, it is important to consider that "nausea and vomiting are *not* due to chemotherapy until proven otherwise." The emetic stimulus from most chemotherapeutic agents is gone by 24 hours, with the exception of cisplatin, which may cause delayed nausea and vomiting for up to 7 days. In any patient with nausea and vomiting persisting for longer than 24 hours after chemotherapy (except cisplatin) or with nausea and vomiting out of proportion to the agent being used, one must consider the differential diagnosis (see Table 1). Hypercalcemia occurs commonly with uncontrolled multiple myeloma. The earliest symptoms are generally polyuria, polydipsia, constipation, and anorexia, but nausea and vomiting commonly follow as the calcium increases. Many medications can cause nausea and vomiting, particularly oral trimethoprim–sulfamethaxazole and intravenous imipenem. Infiltration of the leptomeninges with tumor cells (common in ALL, intermediate- and high-grade lymphoma, and the late stages of multiple myeloma) may cause cranial nerve palsies, altered mental status, focal neurological deficits, seizures, or simply anorexia and nausea. Space-occupying lesions of the parenchyma of the brain can be caused by intermediate- and high-grade lymphoma, toxoplasmosis, or fungal abscesses (after systemic fungemias during profound myelosuppression). Infectious meningitis with opportunistic organisms, such as *Listeria, Cryptococcus, Toxoplasma,* or *Mycobacterium tuberculosis* may occur in patients with Hodgkin's and non-Hodgkin's lymphoma and ALL undergoing intensive treatment. Chemotherapy-induced mucositis, in its mildest forms, may simply present as nausea or postprandial vomiting occurring several days after the acute (first 24 hours) chemotherapy-induced nausea and vomiting resolve. Diarrhea,

Table 1 Causes of Nausea and Vomiting in Patients with Hematological Malignancy

Metabolic:	hypercalcemia, hyponatremia, adrenal insufficiency, renal failure
Gastrointestinal:	Mucositis caused by chemotherapy or radiation, CMV infection, pseudomembranous colitis, paralytic ileus, bowel obstruction, hepatitis
Renal failure:	Hypercalcemia, uric acid, amyloidosis, hydronephrosis, interstitial nephritis, hyperviscosity, light chain nephropathy, infection, tumor infiltration, chemotherapy (cisplatin, methotrexate), drug effect (cyclosporine, amphotericin, aminoglycoside), prerenal
CNS:	Infiltration of leptomeninges, parenchymal metastasis, infectious meningitis or encephalitis
Drugs:	Trimethoprim–sulfamethoxazole, cilastin–imipenem (Primaxin), narcotics
Chemotherapy:	Within 24 hours of chemotherapy, except for cisplatin, which may last for 7 days

oral mucositis, and abdominal cramps or pain may or may not be present, depending on the agent and the severity of the mucositis. Many patients have nausea and vomiting during radiation therapy or as a delayed effect as a result of gastrointestinal mucositis or hepatitis. Lymphomas may cause bowel obstruction from involvement of mucosal-associated lymphoid tissue (MALT) or from adenopathy causing external compression. Nausea and vomiting are commonly caused by infection of the esophagus, stomach, small bowel, or colon by herpes, *Candida,* CMV, *C. difficile,* common enteric pathogens, parasites such as *Strongyloides,* or opportunistic infectious agents such as *Cryptosporidium.* Vinblastine and vincristine can cause a paralytic ileus, with abdominal pain, constipation, distension, nausea, and vomiting. Nausea and vomiting may be caused by inflammation or disturbance of the liver. Hepatitis may be caused by infection with hepatitis A, B, or C, cytomegalovirus, or candidal microabscesses. Chemotherapy, radiation, tumor infiltration, drug effects (e.g., cyclosporine or androgens), or veno-occlusive disease of the liver after an autologous or allogeneic transplant may also cause altered hepatic function with nausea and vomiting. Acute renal failure presenting with nausea and vomiting may be due to chemotherapy (e.g., cisplatin or high-dose methotrexate), interstitial nephritis caused by drugs (e.g., cephalosporins), uric acid nephropathy, hypercalcemia, tubular damage from myeloma light chains, amyloidosis (e.g., in myeloma), hyperviscosity in Waldenstrom's macroglobulinemia or in multiple myeloma, hydronephrosis caused by retroperitoneal lymphadenopthy, tumor infiltration of the kidney, radiation, or urinary tract infection. Hyponatremia after vincristine or high-dose cyclophosphamide or in patients with substantial cerebral or pulmonary disease can cause nausea and vomiting. Iatrogenic Addison's disease is not uncommon in patients with hematological malignancies, owing to long-term steroid treatment, particularly of low-grade B-cell neoplasms, and can present as nausea and vomiting or with hyponatremia. Thus, nausea and vomiting more than 24 hours after chemotherapy demands an explanation. One should check the medications the patient is receiving, order an electrolyte and chemistry panel, examine the abdomen, evaluate the character of the stools (culture and *C. difficile* toxin analysis ordered if loose stool or frequent bowel movements), perform lumbar puncture and CT brain scan if appropriate, and obtain a cosyntropin (Cortrosyn)-stimulation study for adrenal reserve in patients who have been receiving long-term steroid treatment.

Bone Pain

The consequences of pathological fracture of a weight-bearing bone, particularly the femur, are debilitating and difficult to treat. Patients with multiple myeloma should have a complete radiographic skeletal survey (not a bone scan) at diagnosis and at regular intervals when in relapse to detect impending pathological fractures so that radiation therapy can be given prophylactically. In addition to regular surveillance of asymptomatic patients at diagnosis and in relapse, one should obtain radiographs for any focal bone pain in patients with myeloma, lymphoma, or Hodgkin's disease.

Back pain in a patient with hematological malignancy always demands consideration for the possibility of spinal cord compression. The extent of neurological recovery with emergency radiation therapy for cord compression decreases with the severity of the neurological deficit at the time treatment starts. Hence, it is imperative that cord compression be considered, appropriate confirmatory studies performed, and therapy instituted before neurological deficits develop. Whereas cord compression from breast and lung cancer almost always occurs by metastasis to the vertebral body followed by posterior extension, with hematological malignancies (especially lymphoma and late-stage myeloma), extradural nonosseous lymphomas, plasmacytomas, or chloromas may cause cord compression with a normal scan and plain films. In a patient with hematological malignancy and back pain, and any signs or symptoms of motor, sensory, or autonomic disturbance (e.g., bowel or bladder dysfunction), an MRI scan of the spine or a myelogram is indicated.

Dyspnea and Tachypnea

New onset of dyspnea or tachypnea in a patient with hematological malignancy should be regarded as extremely serious and demand immediate evaluation

Table 2 Causes of Dyspnea and Tachypnea in Patients with Hematological Malignancies

Clear chest radiograph	
	Anemia
	Bacterial or fungal pneumonia in a neutropenic patient
	Pneumocystis carinii
	Viral pneumonia (e.g., respiratory syncytial virus (54)
	Impending sepsis
	Congestive heart failure
	Recurrent pulmonary emboli
	Malignant pericardial effusion
	Superior vena cava syndrome
	Chemotherapy pulmonary toxicity
	Radiation pneumonitis
	Hyperleukocytosis syndrome
	Anaphylaxis
Abnormal chest radiograph	
	Pleural effusion
	Pneumonia
	Mediastinal mass with tracheal or bronchial compression
	Radiation pneumonitis
	Congestive heart failure
	Pericardial effusion

(Table 2). Several life-threatening conditions may present as dyspnea on exertion *with a normal chest radiograph*. Impending sepsis is often heralded by dyspnea, tachypnea, and mild confusion. A neutropenic patient with these symptoms should be presumed to have impending sepsis and be examined, specimens take for culture, and started on antibiotic therapy (if he or she is already receiving antibiotics, strongly consider empirically adding or changing antibiotics). Because patients who initially appear stable can rapidly develop septic shock and severe hypoxia with cardiac and respiratory arrest, frequent monitoring of vital signs, monitoring of arterial blood gases or trancutaneous oxygen saturation with a pulse oxymeter should be initiated. Malignant pericardial effusions often present with dyspnea or arrhythmias. The chest radiograph may or may not show an enlarged cardiac shadow, depending on the extent of pericardial infiltration with tumor, which limits compliance and may permit clinically critical symptoms without obvious radiographic changes. Anaphylaxis from asparaginase or parenteral iron dextran, or as a reaction to foreign proteins in plasma and platelets may be heralded by tachypnea and may require administration of epinephrine, steroids, diphenhydramine, and even fluid volume replacement and intubation. Pulmonary emboli, commonly associated with adenocarcinomas, may occur in hematological malignancies when lymphadenopathy is causing vena cava, internal iliac, or femoral venous compression. Pulmonary vessel occlusion and endothelial cell damage with adult respiratory distress syndrome may also occur from hyperleukocytosis with dyspnea and hypoxia, but a clear chest film. Mediastinal masses may cause superior vena cava syndrome, bronchial obstruction, or tracheal compression. Large mediastinal masses will generally be seen on a chest radiograph, but small masses within the cardiac shadow may require a CT scan for diagnosis. Pleural effusions causing dyspnea will be seen on chest films, but in the absence of neutrophils, bacterial and fungal pneumonias, particularly early on, may not. *Pneumocystis carinii,* CMV, and other viral pneumonias, even in the nonneutropenic patient, may be difficult to detect early in their course. Hypoxia on an arterial blood gas determination or a positive gallium lung scan in a patient at risk for pneumocystis infection would indicate the need for a bronchoscopy with empiric treatment with high-dose trimethoprim–sulfamethoxazole, pending the results of staining and culture. In a patient who has been receiving prophylactic pentamidine or trimethoprim–sulfamethoxazole, the staining results of the bronchoscopy specimen may be negative, even in the presence of pneumocystic infection. Radiation-induced constrictive effusive pericarditis, which occurs after mantle radiation for Hodgkin's disease was more common in the past when anterior-weighted ports were used, but should still be considered in the differential of new onset of dyspnea and may require a cardiac catheterization to document. Congestive heart failure may occur as a function of cumulative anthracycline dose; but may also occur after high-dose cyclophosphamide, particularly in combination with other agents in high dose (48). Anemia is a common cause of dyspnea in the hematological malignancies. Systematic consideration should be given to the etiology of the anemia, particulary if there has been an acute worsening (49). For example, sudden exacerbation of anemia may be due to bleeding, autoimmune hemolytic anemia (common in chronic lymphocytic leukemia and low-grade lymphomas), or microangiopathic hemolytic anemia (for example, with DIC or after mitomycin).

Hematopoietic Growth Factors

Several reviews on the role of the hematopoietic growth factors in cancer treatment have recently appeared (50–53). Erythropoietin can decrease the transfusion requirement of patients with the anemia of advanced cancer; the anemia of chemotherapy, including that caused by cisplatin; and the anemia associated with myelodysplasia. Both G-CSF and GM-CSF can increase neutrophil counts in most patients with myelodysplasia and in many with aplastic anemia. They can accelerate neutrophil recovery after standard and high-dose chemotherapy, although this is primarily an acceleration of the rate of recovery once an ANC of 100/μL is reached. Both seem to decrease the incidence of mucositis, the antibiotic requirement, the extent of creatinine and bilirubin rise, and length of hospital stay after high-dose chemotherapy. GM-CSF can stimulate the proliferation of leukemic blasts and, in some cases, may accelerate the conversion from myelodysplasia to acute leukemia, primarily when there are greater than 10–20% marrow blasts. Trials are underway to turn this into a therapeutic advantage by stimulating the leukemic stem cells into cycle with GM-CSF just before administering induction chemotherapy. GM-CSF can salvage graft failures after autologous or allogeneic bone marrow transplantation (defined as absence of neutrophil recovery by day 28 after marrow infusion or 1 week with an ANC below 500/μL after 1 week with an ANC over 500/μL) in a significant proportion of patients. GM-CSF or G-CSF can also be used to correct the neutropenia of hairy cell leukemia, permitting the safe institution of interferon alpha therapy. GM-CSF may permit the continued administration of ganciclovir for life-threatening CMS infections.

CONCLUSION

The rational use of supportive care requires a knowledge of the major causes of death and disability and the periods of greatest risk for specific problems. Rigorous attention to subtle signs and symptoms, and aggressive, often empiric, supportive care are essential for the patient's survival. This is particularly important as therapies become more aggressive and the goal of achieving long-term disease-free survival and cure for many of the hematological malignancies is realized.

REFERENCES

1. Feinstein DI: Treatment of disseminated intravascular coagulation. *Semin Thromb Hemost* 1988; 14:351–362.
2. Kantarjian HM, Keating MJ, Walters RS, et al: Acute promyelocytic leukemia. *Am J Med* 1986; 80:789.
3. Goldberg MA, Ginsburg D, Mayer RJ, et al: Is heparin administration necessary during induction chemotherapy for patients with acute promyelocytic leukemia? *Blood* 1987; 69:187.
4. Rodeghiero F, Avvisati G, Castaman G, et al: Early deaths and anti-hemorrhagic treatments in acute promyelocytic leukemia. A GIMEMA retrospective study in 268 consecutive patients. *Blood* 1990; 75:2112–2117.
5. Schimpff SC, Young VM, Greene WH, et al: Origin of infection in acute non-lymphocytic leukemia: Significance of hospital acquisition of potential pathogens. *Ann Intern Med* 1972; 77:707–714.
6. Walsh TJ, Schimpff SC: Prevention of infection among patients with cancer. *Eur J Cancer Clin Onol* 1983; 19:1333–1344.
7. Sherertz RJ, Belani A, Kramer BS, et al: Impact of air filtration on nosocomial aspergillus infections. *Am J Med* 1987; 83:709–718.

8. Karp JE, Merz WF, Hendricksen C, et al: Oral norfloxacin for prevention of gram-negative bacterial infections in patients with acute leukemia and granulocytopenia. *Ann Intern Med* 1987; 106:1–7.
9. Dekker AW, Rozenberg-Arska M, Verhoef J: Infection prophylaxis in acute leukemia: A comparison of ciprofloxacin with trimethoprim–sulfamethoxazole and Colistin. *Ann Intern Med* 1987; 106:7–12.
10. Rubin M, Hathorn JW, Pizzo PA: Controversies in the management of febrile neutropenic cancer patients. *Cancer Invest* 1988; 6:167–184.
11. Hughes WT, Rivera GK, Schell MJ, et al: Successful intermittent chemoprophylaxis for *Pneumocystis carinii* pneumonitis. *N Engl J. Med* 1987; 316:1627–1632.
12. Bowden RA, Sayers M, Flournoy N, et al: Cytomegalovirus immune globulin and seronegative blood products to prevent primary cytomegalovirus infection after marrow transplantation. *N Engl J Med* 1986; 314:1006–1010.
13. Verdonck LF, Graan-Hentzen YCE, Dekker AW, et al: Cytomegalovirus seronegative platelets and leukocyte-poor red blood cells from random donors can prevent primary cytomegalovirus infection after bone marrow transplantation. *Bone Marrow Transplantation* 1987; 2:73–78.
14. de Graan-Hentzen YC, Gratama JW, Mudde GC, et al: Prevention of primary cytomegalovirus infection in patients with hematologic malignancies by intensive white cell depletion of blood products. *Transfusion* 1989; 29:757–760.
15. Brady MT, Milam JD, Anderson DC, et al: Use of deglycerolized red blood cells to prevent posttransfusion infection with cytomegalovirus in neonates. *J Infect Dis* 1984; 150:334–339.
16. Bowden RA, Sayers M, Slichter SJ, Meyers JD: Use of leukocyte-poor transfusions to prevent transfusion-associated cytomegalovirus (CMV) infection after marrow transplant. Abstr. *Am Assoc Blood Banks,* November 1989; p. 67.
17. Dorsky DI, Crumpacker CS: Drugs five years later: Acyclovir. *Ann Intern Med* 1987; 107:859–874.
18. Wade JC, Newton B, Flournoy N, Meyers JD: Oral acyclovir for prevention of herpes simplex virus reactivation after marrow transplantation. *Ann Intern Med* 1984; 100:823–828.
19. Ljungman P, Lonnqvist B, Gahrton G, et al: Clinical and subclinical reactivations of varicella–zoster virus in immunocompromised patients. *J Infect Dis* 1986; 153:840–847.
20. Berkman SA, Lee ML, Gale RP: Clinical uses of intravenous immunoglobulins. *Semin Hematol* 1988; 25:140–158.
21. Cooperative Group for the Study of Immunoglobulin in Chronic Lymphocytic Leukemia: Intravenous immunoglobulin for the prevention of infection in chronic lymphocytic leukemia. *N Engl J Med* 1988; 319:902–907.
22. Rubenstein E, Rolston K, Moreland B, et al: Ambulatory treatment of febrile episodes in neutropenic patients. *Proc Am Soc Clin Oncol* 1990; 9:321.
23. Martin AM, Pfaller MA, Wenzel RP: Coagulase-negative staphylococcal bacteremia. *Ann Intern Med* 1989; 110:9–16.
24. Reed E, Arneson M, Vaughan W, Armitage J: *Streptococcus viridans:* A significant cause of neutropenic fever that caused death in some patients not empirically treated for gram-positive bacteria. *Proc Am Soc Clin Oncol* 1990; 9:321.

25. The EORTC International Antimicrobial Therapy Cooperative Group: Ceftazidime combined with a short or long course of amikacin for empirical therapy of gram negative bacteremia in cancer patients with granulocytopenia. *N Engl J Med* 1987; 317:1692–1698.
26. Marshall WF, Keating MR, Anhalt JP, Steckelberg JM: *Xanthomonas maltophilia:* An emerging nosocomial pathogen. *Mayo Clin Proc* 1989; 64:1097–1104.
27. EORTC International Antimicrobial Therapy Cooperative Group: Empiric antifungal therapy in febrile granulocytopenic patients. *Am J Med* 1989; 86:668–672.
28. Wong B: Parasitic disease in immunocompromised hosts. *Am J Med* 1984; 76:479–486.
29. Dismukes WE: Azole antifungal drugs: Old and new. *Ann Intern Med* 1988; 109:177–179.
29a. Conti DJ, Tolkoff-Rubin NE, Baker GP, et al: Successful treatment of invasive fungal infection with fluconazole in organ transplant recipients. *Transplantation* 1989; 48:692–694.
30. Silva J: Update on pseudomembranous colitis. *West J Med* 1989; 151:644–648.
31. Mackowiak PA, LeMiastre CF: Drug fever: A critical appraisal of conventional concepts. *Ann Intern Med* 1987; 106:728–733.
32. Bodey GP, Buckley M,. Sathe YS, et al: Quantitative relationships between circulating leukocytes and infection in patients with acute leukemia. *Ann Intern Med* 1966; 64:328–340.
33. Winstone DJ, Ho WG, Gale RP: Therapeutic granulocyte transfusions for documented infections. *Ann Intern Med* 1982; 97:509–515.
34. Harker LA, Slichter SJ: The bleeding time as a screening test for evaluation of platelet function. *N Engl J Med* 1972; 287:155–159.
35. Andreu G, Dewailly J, Leberre C, et al: Prevention of HLA immunization with leukocyte-poor packed red cells and platelet concentrates obtained by filtration. *Blood* 1988; 72:964–969.
36. Murphy MF, Metcalfe P, Thomas H, et al: Use of leukocyte-poor blood components and HLA-matched-platelet donors to prevent HLA alloimmunization. *Br J Haematol* 1986; 62:529–534.
37. Sniecinski I, O'Donnell MR, Nowicki B, Hill LR: Prevention of refractoriness and HLA-alloimmunization using filtered blood products. *Blood* 1988; 71:1402–1407.
38. Deeg HJ: Ultraviolet irradiation in transplantation biology. *Transplantation* 1988; 5:845–851.
39. Daly PA, Schiffer CA, Aisner J, Wiernik PH: Platelet transfusion therapy, one-hour posttransfusion increments are valuable in predicting the need for HLA-matched preparations. *JAMA* 1980; 243:435–438.
40. Transfusions and graft-versus-host disease. *Lancet* 1989; 1:529–530.
41. Schiffer CA, Aisner J, Wiernik PH: Frozen autologous platelet transfusion for patients with leukemia. *N Engl J Med* 1978; 299:7–12.
42. Dullemond AC, Prooijen HC, Riemens MI, Akkerman JWN: Cryopreservation disturbs stimulus-response coupling in a platelet subpopulation. *Br J Haematol* 1987; 67:325–333.
43. Christie DJ, Buren N, Lennon SS, Putnam JL: Vancomycin-dependent antibodies

associated with thrombocytopenia and refractoriness to platelet transfusion in patients with leukemia. *Blood* 1990; 75:518–523.
44. Zeigler ZR, Shadduck RK, Rosenfeld CS, et al: High-dose intravenous gamma globulin improves responses to single-donor platelets in patients refractory to platelet transfusion. *Blood* 1987; 70:1433–1436.
45. Lee EJ, Norris D, Schiffer CA: Intravenous immune globulin for patients alloimmunized to random donor platelet transfusion. *Transfusion* 1987; 27:245–247.
46. Sindet-Pederson S, Ramstrom G, Bernvil S, Blomback M: Hemostatic effect of tranexamic acid mouthwash in anticoagulant-treated patients undergoing oral surgery. *N Engl J Med* 1989; 320:840–843.
47. Thaler M, Pastakia B, Shawker TH, et al: Hepatic candidiasis in cancer patients: The evolving picture of the syndrome. *Ann Intern Med* 1988; 108:88–100.
48. Kupari M, Volin L, Suokas A, et al: Cardiac involvement in bone marrow transplantation: Electrocardiographic changes, arrhythmias, heart failure and autopsy findings. *Bone Marrow Transplantation* 1990; 5:91–98.
49. Wallerstein RO: Laboratory evaluation of anemia. *West J Med* 1987; 146:443–451.
50. Andreeff M, Welte K: Hematopoietic colony-stimulation factors. *Semin Oncol* 1989; 16:211–229.
51. Groopman JE, Molina J, Scadden DT: Hematopoietic growth factors. *N Engl J Med* 1989; 321:1449–1459.
52. Laver J, Moore MAS: Clinical use of recombinant human hematopoietic growth factors. *JNCI* 1989; 81:1370–1382.
53. Metcalf D: The colony stimulating factors. *Cancer* 1990; 65:2185–2206.
54. Englund JA, Sullivan CJ, Jordan MC, et al: Respiratory syncytial virus infection in immunocompromised adults. *Ann Intern Med* 1988; 109:203–208.
55. Reed EC, Bowden RA, Dandliker PS, et al: Treatment of cytomegalovirus pneumonia with ganciclovir and intravenous cytomegalovirus immunoglobulin in patients with bone marrow transplants. *Ann Intern Med* 1988; 109:783–788.
56. Emanuel D, Cunningham I, Jules-Elysee K, et al: Cytomegalovirus pneumonia after bone marrow transplantation successfully treated with the combination of ganciclovir and high-dose intravenous immune globulin. *Ann Intern Med* 1988; 109:777–782.

11

Infections in Hematological Malignancies

Nancy Khardori and Gerald P. Bodey

University of Texas
M. D. Anderson Cancer Center
Houston, Texas

The substantial improvement in the management of patients with hematological malignancies can be attributed only in part to the discovery of more effective chemotherapeutic regimens. Equally important has been the discovery of more potent and broad-spectrum antimicrobial agents that have successfully controlled many of the infections in these patients. However, despite these improvements, infection remains a common complication. New therapeutic modalities cause greater impairments in host defense mechanisms and more severe ulceration of the gastrointestinal mucosa. The widespread use of long-term indwelling venous catheters has been associated with the frequent occurrence of gram-positive bacteremias and, to a lesser extent, fungemia. Extensive use of prophylactic and therapeutic antibiotics has resulted in selection of nosocomial pathogens that are resistant to multiple antibiotics.

FACTORS PREDISPOSING TO INFECTION

There are many components to the host's defense against infection, ranging from an intact integument, to circulating antibodies and neutrophils. Each component protects against infection by specific pathogens, and each hematological malignancy is characteristically associated with a deficiency in a specific component of host defenses. Thus, if the physician is aware of the specific deficiencies present in a patient, he or she can focus diagnostic efforts on those organisms

Table 1 Risk of Infection Related to Type of Leukemia

Type of Leukemia	Usual primary deficiency	Risk of duration	Infection
Acute myelogenous	Neutropenia	Prolonged	High
Acute lymphocytic	Neutropenia	Short	Moderate
Chronic myelogenous, stable	Impaired neutrophil function	Prolonged	None
Chronic myelogenous, blastic	Neutropenia	Prolonged	High
Chronic lymphocytic stable	Impaired antibody production	Prolonged	Moderate
Chronic lymphocytic, advanced	Neutropenia	Prolonged	High
Hairy cell	Neutropenia, monocytopenia	Prolonged	High

most likely to be the cause of infection in that malignancy. Unfortunately, in many instances, multiple deficiencies are present simultaneously, especially if the patient is receiving chemotherapy. Table 1 lists the hematological malignancies and major deficiency in host defenses likely to be associated with it.

Deficiencies in Neutrophil Number and Function

The level of circulating granulocytes is the single most important determinant of susceptibility to bacterial and fungal infections. The relationship between granulocytopenia and infection has been studied most extensively in acute leukemia, for granulocytopenia is especially common and severe in patients with this disease. Both the incidence and severity of infection are inversely related to the level of circulating granulocytes in patients with acute leukemia (Fig. 1). Virtually every patient whose granulocyte count is fewer than 100/μL for longer than 3 weeks will develop an infection. Although the frequency of severe infection decreases sharply with increasing levels of circulating granulocytes, no further reduction occurs at granulocyte counts above 1000/μL.

Neutropenic patients often fail to develop the characteristic signs and symptoms of infection because they are unable to mount an adequate inflammatory response (1). For example, purulent sputum and pyuria is seen in a minority (8–11%) of granulocytopenic patients with pneumonia and urinary tract infection, respectively. Neutropenic patients who develop pneumonia may not have

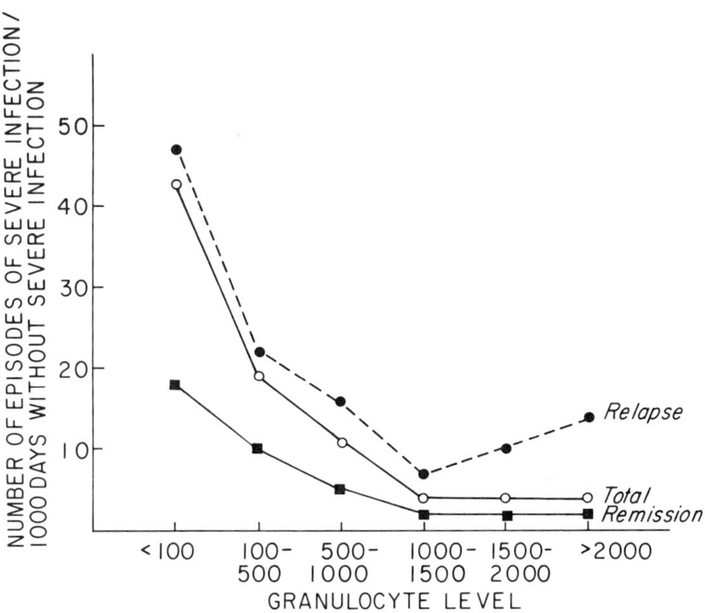

Figure 1 The frequency of infectious episodes related to the granulocyte level. The number of episodes of severe infection 1000 days without severe infection is plotted for granulocyte level.

pulmonary infiltrates shown on chest roentgenograms or may fail to demonstrate meningismus when they develop meningitis. Infection disseminates widely and rapidly in patients with neutropenia. Nearly all episodes of bacteremia and disseminated fungal infection complicating malignant disease arise in patients with granulocyte counts of fewer than 500/μL.

The failure rate for most severe infections is related to the patient's ability to respond with an increased production of neutrophils. Neutropenic patients who respond to their infection with an increased number of circulating granulocytes have a cure rate of 70%, compared with 45% for patients whose granulocyte count fails to increase during the first week of severe infection.

Patients with adequate granulocyte counts may be susceptible to infection owing to impaired neutrophil function secondary to their disease or its therapy. Deficiencies observed include inability to migrate to sites of inflammation, impaired phagocytosis, and reduced killing of ingested organisms. The frequency of infection in acute leukemia is higher among patients whose granulocytes have reduced bactericidal capacity in vitro, compared with patients whose granulocytes function normally. Some of the apparent defects in neutrophil function are related to deficiencies in serum factors, which can be corrected when the neutrophils are incubated in normal serum.

Defects in Cell-Mediated Immunity

Cell-mediated immunity refers to the complex interaction between T lymphocytes, monocytes, and macrophages. Infection may be a consequence of deficiencies in number or function of these cells. It is difficult to quantitate the number of these cells because the number circulating in the bloodstream is not an adequate reflection of the total number in the body. Defects in monocyte function include decreased adherence, phagocytosis, chemotaxis, and production of colony-stimulating factors (CSFs). Lymphocyte dysfunction is characterized by decreased response to mitogens, decreased antibody-dependent cellular cytotoxicity, and cutaneous anergy. Macrophages are responsible for the phagocytosis and killing of some bacterial and fungal pathogens. Knowledge concerning the interactions between these cells and their effects on host defenses is rapidly expanding and beyond the scope of this discussion.

Deficiencies in Immunoglobulins

Deficiency in normal immunoglobulins occurs in patients with chronic lymphocytic leukemia, multiple myeloma, Waldenstrom's macroglobulinemia, and occasional patients with lymphoma. Encapsulated organisms such as the pneumococcus, meningococcus, and *Haemophilus influenzae,* require opsonization before they can undergo phagocytosis by neutrophils. Both antibody and the products of complement activation by antigen–antibody complexes are effective opsonins. Additionally, antibody present in γ-globulin can neutralize endotoxin produced by gram-negative bacilli.

Defective Integumentary and Mucosal Surfaces

An intact skin and gastrointestinal mucosa are an important defense against invasion by potentially pathogenic organisms. The insertion of an indwelling intravenous catheter provides a direct entry from the skin into the bloodstream. Extravasation of vesicant chemotherapeutic agents causes necrosis and ulceration of the skin, facilitating invasion by organisms. Ulceration of the oropharyngeal and gastrointestinal mucosa is a common side effect of many antitumor agents and results not only in local infection, but the possibility of invasion into the bloodstream.

Microbial Colonization

There is no evidence that antibiotics enhance susceptibility to infection. Antibiotics can suppress the normal microbial flora of the host and permit overgrowth by resistant bacteria and fungi. Broad-spectrum oral antibiotics and antibiotics with substantial biliary excretion have the greatest impact on the endogenous flora of the gastrointestinal tract. Other factors in addition to antibiotic therapy affect colonization. Several studies have demonstrated that first admission to the hospital is associated with colonization by nosocomial gram-negative bacteria. Recent years have witnessed the reemergence of gram-positive organisms as a significant cause of infections in granulocytopenic patients. Prolonged hospitalization for the management of the underlying malignancy and its complications and broad-spectrum antimicrobial prophylaxis and therapy cause a shift in the patients' microbial flora, allowing overgrowth of gram-positive and resistant gram-negative bacteria and fungi.

Patients with hematological malignancies, especially those with chronic lymphocytic leukemia, multiple myeloma, lymphomas, and those receiving immuno-suppressive therapy after bone marrow transplantation, develop deficiencies of both humoral and cell-mediated immune mechanisms. These deficiencies render them susceptible to specific infections, especially those caused by encapsulated organisms, intracellular bacteria, systemic fungi, and viruses.

INFECTIONS TYPICALLY FOUND IN HEMATOLOGICAL MALIGNANCIES

Infections in Patients with Acute Leukemia

Patients with acute leukemia generally have a higher prevalence of infections than those with other malignancies. The incidence of infection with acute leukemias varies with the type of leukemia and the intensity of the chemotherapy administered (2). Patients with acute myelogenous leukemia (AML) generally have a higher prevalence of infection because of the uniformly myelosuppressive chemotherapy administered for this disease. The infection rate is more variable in children with acute lymphocytic leukemia (ALL). Children with ALL treated on the most aggressive chemotherapy regimens have infection rates similar to those seen in children with AML. Adults with ALL are generally treated with intensive myelosuppressive chemotherapy and, hence, are at risk of developing the same infections as patients with AML.

The most important factor predisposing patients with acute leukemia to infection is neutropenia. This is primarily due to deficient production of neutrophils by the bone marrow, but is aggravated by myelosuppressive chemotherapy. Because of bone marrow failure, neutropenia is usually severe and prolonged. Consequently, these patients are highly susceptible to repeated infections caused by gram-positive cocci, aerobic gram-negative bacilli, and certain fungi, especially *Candida* spp. and *Aspergillus* spp.

The relationship between lymphopenia and infection has been studied in patients receiving chemotherapy for acute leukemia. Generally, lymphopenia is not as severe as neutropenia, and patients with lymphopenia usually have normal lymph node architecture. The frequency of infection is inversely proportional to the number of circulating lymphocytes, and more severe infections are associated with more prolonged lymphopenia. However, most patients with lymphopenia also have neutropenia, which is of greater significance.

Lymphopenia caused by chemotherapy interferes with antibody production, especially to new antigens. Patients with acute leukemia have lower levels of antibody to the core glycolipid of *Enterobacteriaceae* than patients without cancer (3). The antibody levels decrease further in patients receiving antileukemic therapy. Patients who develop gram-negative bacteremias have lower levels of antibody than those in whom infection does not develop.

Impaired cellular immunity also plays a role in predisposing to some infections. Disseminated viral infections alone or in association with other coexistent pathogens are responsible for more than 50% of deaths in children with ALL during remission (4). Infections caused by varicella–zoster virus, cytomegalovirus, herpes simplex virus, and *Pneumocystis carinii* represent a significant proportion of infections in children with ALL, especially during periods of maintained remission. Varicella may be more severe, and healing of lesions delayed more than in normal children. For children on maintenance therapy, the risk of dissemination correlates with the severity of the underlying defect in cellular immunity. Children with absolute lymphopenia (fewer than 500/μL) at the time of varicella infection are at a greater risk of dissemination. Herpes zoster frequently occurs within 1 year of irradiation to the nerve root of the corresponding dermatome. This may imply the suppression of local immune responses by irradiation. Measles in children with acute leukemia can be severe and fulminant. The complications of cutaneous and visceral bleeding, secondary bacterial pneumonia, and otitis media are increased in these patients. Disseminated disease causing hepatitis, encephalitis, and nephritis can also occur (5).

The organisms that cause infections in neutropenic patients are listed in Table 2. Gram-negative bacilli still remain frequent causes of infection in neutropenic patients. The most common offenders are *Escherichia coli, Klebsiella* spp., and *Pseudomonas aeruginosa*. Their relative frequency varies considerably from hospital to hospital. Other gram-negative organisms, such as *Enterobacter* spp., *Acinetobacter* spp., and other *Pseudomonas* spp. are emerging as important pathogens. Often these organisms are resistant to multiple antibiotics, including extended-spectrum penicillins and third-generation cephalosporins. Many of these latter organisms predominantly cause superinfections in patients already receiving antibiotic therapy.

Gram-positive organisms have reemerged as significant pathogens in recent years. The use of indwelling vascular catheters is the major factor responsible for increase in infections caused by gram-positive organisms, but other factors,

Table 2 Organisms that Cause Infection in Patients with Neutropenia

Frequent	Occasional
Gram-negative bacilli	Gram-negative bacilli
Escherichia coli	*Enterobacter* spp.
Klebsiella spp.	*Acinetobacter* spp.
Pseudomonas aeruginosa	*Pseudomonas* spp.
Serratia marcescens	*Aeromonas hydrophila*
Gram-positive cocci and bacilli	Gram-positive cocci and bacilli
Staphylococcus aureus	*Enterococcus*
S. epidermidis	α-Hemolytic streptococci
Corynebacterium jeikeium	*Clostridium perfringens*
Bacillus spp.	*C. septicum*
C. difficile	
Fungi	Fungi
Candida spp.	*Zygomycetes*
Aspergillus spp.	*Trichosporon beigelii*
	Fusarium spp.

including antimicrobial prophylaxis and severe mucositis play an important role in these infections. Gram-positive organisms have become the most common isolates in some institutions (6). *Staphylococcus aureus* causes about 25% of infections in neutropenic patients. *Staphylococcus epidermidis,* once considered a contaminant, has emerged as an important pathogen in patients with indwelling vascular catheters (7). Enterococci are also emerging as nosocomial pathogens in neutropenic patients, particularly with the widespread use of broad-spectrum empiric antimicrobial therapy with no or poor activity against these organisms. alpha-Hemolytic streptococci, *Bacillus* spp. and *Corynebacterium,* including the multiple–drug-resistant *C. jeikeium,* also cause serious infections in neutropenic patients (8,9).

Opportunistic fungal pathogens especially *Candida* spp. and *Aspergillus* spp. cause most of the fungal infections in neutropenic patients. Currently, they account for 20–40% of fatal infections in patients with acute leukemia. The increasing frequency of these infections during the period of initial remission induction chemotherapy is especially disturbing. *Candida* spp. are the most common fungal pathogens, but *Aspergillus* spp. are more prevalent in some cancer centers. *Candida* spp. cause a variety of superficial infections of the skin, oropharynx, and esophagus, which are usually amenable to topical or systemic therapy. However, if not treated promptly, they may lead to disseminated candidiasis, which is difficult to treat.

Infections caused by *Aspergillus* spp. usually present as pneumonia and, less frequently, as rhinocerebral infection. Occasionally, primary cutaneous infection or disseminated infection occurs. Recently, *Fusarium* spp., *Curvularia* spp., *Altenaria* spp., and *Trichosporon beigelii* have been recognized as pathogens in neutropenic patients (10). These organisms are more likely to cause disseminated disease.

Infections in Patients with Chronic Leukemia

Patients with chronic myelogenous leukemia (CML) have impaired neutrophil function. However, during the stable phase of CML, impairment of neutrophil function is compensated for by the increased number of neutrophils. These patients are not at a high risk for developing infections. During the blastic phase, patients with CML experience prolonged periods of neutropenia and are at a risk of developing the same infections as patients with acute leukemia.

Patients with stable chronic lymphocytic leukemia (CLL) have an increased risk of infection if their disease results in impaired antibody production. Hypogammaglobulinemia has been reported to occur in up to 67% of patients with CLL, with 10% of these patients having immunoglobulin levels of less than 200 mg/dL (11). The antibody deficiency predisposes these patients to infections by encapsulated organisms, such as the pneumococcus, meningococcus, and *H. influenzae*.

Defects in cell-mediated immunity have also been described in patients with CLL. Many of these patients have a reduced ability to respond to new antigens such as dinitrochlorobenzene (DNCB), but have good recall to common bacterial antigens, such as purified protein derivative (PPD). Patients with CLL have approximately a 10% incidence of herpes zoster. Other infections associated with depressed cellular immunity that have been noted in patients with CLL include histoplasmosis, nocardiosis, cryptococcosis, and legionnaires' disease.

Patients with advanced CLL are at high risk of developing infections because of neutropenia secondary to the disease as well as chemotherapy. The spectrum of infections in these patients is similar to that seen in patients with acute leukemia.

INFECTIONS IN HAIRY CELL LEUKEMIA

Hairy cell leukemia causes both neutropenia and cell-mediated immune deficiency. In addition to the infections associated with neutropenia, these patients are susceptible to pathogens for which cell-mediated immune mechanisms form the primary defense. Several defects in cell-mediated immunity have been described in this disease. Both monocytopenia and defects in monocyte function may occur. Defects in monocyte function include a decrease in adherence, phagocytosis, chemotaxis, and production of colony-stimulating factors (12,13).

Lymphocyte dysfunction is characterized by decreased responses to mitogens, decreased antibody-dependent cellular cytotoxicity, and decreased cutaneous anergy (13). Because of multiple defects in host defense mechanisms, many types of infections are observed in patients with hairy cell leukemia. Infections with enteric gram-negative bacilli are the most common, occurring in 50–60% of patients (14). Infections caused by opportunistic pathogens have been emphasized in the recent years. Organisms causing infections because of deficiency in cell-mediated immunity have included nontuberculous mycobacteria, *Mycobacterium tuberculosis, Histoplasma capsulatum, Cryptococcus neoformans,* herpes simplex, herpes zoster, cytomegalovirus, *Toxoplasma gondii, Pneumocystis carinii, Strongyloides stercoralis, Legionella pneumophila,* and *Listeria monocytogenes* (15).

Infections in Patients with Hodgkin's Disease and Lymphoma

Patients with Hodgkin's disease have a relatively low overall incidence of infection because of usual rapid response to therapy. Since fewer patients with malignant lymphoma achieve a complete remission, intensive chemotherapy regimens are employed leading to a much higher incidence of infection (16). The spectrum of infection is similar in the two groups. The most important predisposing factor to infection in patients with lymphoma is defective cell-mediated immunity. The organisms that cause infection in patients with lymphoma owing to defective cell-mediated immune responses are listed in Table 3. Cellular immune defects in Hodgkin's disease occur simultaneously with the onset of disease, are aggravated by treatment, and may persist for as long as 10–12 years after successful therapy. Abnormalities in cellular immunity are less common in

Table 3 Organisms Causing Infection in Patients with Lymphoma Secondary to Defective Cell-Mediated Immunity

Bacteria	Viruses
Mycobacterium spp., especially *M. tuberculosis*	Herpes simplex virus
Listeria monocytogenes	Varicella–zoster
Brucella spp.	Cytomegalovirus
Salmonella spp.	
Nocardia spp.	
Fungi	Parasites
Cryptococcus neoformans	*Toxoplasma gondii*
Histoplasma capsulatum	*Pneumocystis carinii*
Coccidioides immitus	*Strongyloides stercoralis*

malignant lymphoma. Patients with Hodgkin's disease are especially susceptible to infections caused by facultative intracellular pathogens, including Mycobacteria, Brucellae, *Listeria monocytogenes, T. gondii, C. neoformans,* and *Histoplasma capsulatum.*

Patients with Hodgkin's disease appear to be particularly susceptible to infections caused by herpes zoster virus (17). Herpes zoster develops in 15–30% of patients, usually within 8–10 months after completion of radiation therapy. Most cases occur in the lower cervical, thoracic, lumbar, or sacral dermatomes, depending upon the anatomical area irradiated. Dissemination of herpes zoster, although uncommon during initial therapy, is more likely to occur in the patient with recurrent Hodgkin's disease. Herpes zoster is less frequent in patients with non-Hodgkin's lymphoma (8–10%), perhaps owing to the use of chemotherapy alone (without radiation therapy) (18).

Since intensive myelosuppressive and immunosuppressive therapy is employed more often in malignant lymphoma and fewer patients achieve a complete remission, the prevalence of serious infection is higher than in patients with Hodgkin's disease. In a review of 360 patients treated with various forms of combination chemotherapy, bacteria caused 77% of the microbiologically documented infections. Gram-negative bacilli were the most frequent pathogens: *E. coli, K. pneumoniae,* and *P. aeruginosa* accounted for 83% of these organisms. (18) The most frequent gram-positive organism was *Staph. aureus,* and 30% of infections were caused by a single gram-positive organism. During chemotherapy 32% of the patients with Hodgkin's disease and 79% with malignant lymphoma developed infection.

Infections in Patients with Multiple Myeloma and Macroglobulinemia

Patients with multiple myeloma are much more prone to develop infection than those with macroglobulinemia. The most important risk factor in these patients is the reduced levels of normal circulating antibodies that develop early in the course of the disease. A population of circulating monocytes in these patients has been found to suppress the synthesis of immunoglobulin by normal plasma cells (19). An RNA-containing factor released from plasma cell tumors has been postulated to impair the immunological responsiveness of lymphocytes and to stimulate suppressor macrophages that, in turn, inhibit normal antibody production. Serum from patients with multiple myeloma has a defect in the activation of the third component of complement (C3), which may contribute to deficient opsonization of encapsulated bacteria. Defective antibody production and complement activation render these patients susceptible to infections by encapsulated organisms. Some patients also have neutropenia and poor neutrophil adherence, which may contribute to increased susceptibility to infection.

During initial therapy of multiple myeloma, the risk of developing a bacterial infection is increased, even though neutropenia is uncommon in this phase. Elevated serum creatinine levels, immunoglobulin deficiency, advanced age, and advanced clinical stages are predictors of increased risk of infection. The lungs and urinary tract are most common sites of infection. Although pneumococcal pneumonia was previously the most frequently reported infection in multiple myeloma, recent reports have emphasized the significance of gram-negative infections in these patients. Gram-negative bacilli have been reported to cause over 70% of all infections in this disease (20). The therapeutic regimens for multiple myeloma in relapse are highly myelosuppressive, rendering these patients susceptible to infections similar to those in other neutropenic patients, especially gram-negative bacterial and opportunistic fungal infections. Bacterial infections have been documented in up to 55% and candidal infection in up to 24% of multiple myeloma patients at autopsy (21).

Infections in Bone Marrow Transplant Recipients

Patients who receive allogeneic bone marrow transplantation have different major abnormalities in host defense mechanisms at various stages. The common infecting organisms at different stages of bone marrow transplantation are listed in Table 4. Potential bone marrow transplant recipients may be infected before the procedure, as a consequence of neutropenia or immunosuppressive effects of their underlying disease or its previous therapy. Such infections are related to the patient's status at the time the conditioning regimen is begun and are common in patients receiving marrow transplantation as salvage therapy for relapsed acute leukemia. Patients with acute leukemia in remission may also be actively infected, and the transplant can be delayed until the infection resolves with appropriate therapy.

Neutropenia and mucosal damage are the major risk factors for infection in bone marrow recipients immediately following the conditioning treatments with intensive chemotherapy, with or without radiation therapy. Mucositis develops concomitant with the decline in the peripheral leukocyte count and platelet count. Herpes simplex and *Candida albicans* are the most common pathogens causing oral infection associated with bone marrow transplantation (22). During the neutropenic phase, bone marrow transplant recipients are susceptible to infections caused by gram-negative bacilli, *Staph. epidermidis,* streptococci, and opportunistic fungi. Long-term venous access devices increase the incidence of infections, especially those caused by gram-positive organisms. A syndrome of sudden onset of shock, pneumonia (resembling adult respiratory distress syndrome), encephalopathy without meningitis, with or without palmer desquamation, has been described in association with viridans streptococcal bacteremia. These infections may develop early in the posttransplantation period, before the

Table 4 Organisms Causing Infections in Bone Marrow Transplant Recipients

Preengraftment infections	Postengraftment infections
Bacterial	Bacterial
Gram-positive organisms	Gram-positive organisms
Staphylococcus epidermidis	*Streptococcus pneumoniae*
S. aureus	*Staphylococcus aureus*
Viridans streptococci	*S. epidermidis*
Corynebacterium jeikeium	β-Hemolytic streptococci
Listeria monocytogenes	
Nocardia spp.	
Gram-negative organisms	Mycobacteria
Pseudomonas aeruginosa	*Mycobacterium tuberculosis*
Escherichia coli	*M. kansasii*
Klebsiella spp.	*M. fortuitum*
M. avium complex	
Fungal	Fungal
Candida spp.	*Candida* spp.
Aspergillus spp.	*Cryptococcus neoformans*
Mucor and *Rhizopus* spp.	*Histoplasma capsulatum*
Fusarium spp.	
Trichosporon beigelii	
Viral	Viral
Herpes simplex virus	Varicella–zoster virus
Cytomegalovirus	
Adenoviruses	
Papovaviruses	
Parasitic	
Pneumocystis carinii	
Toxoplasma gondii	
Strongyloides stercoralis	
Giardia lambia	

development of mucositis or prolonged neutropenia. Central venous catheters, oral herpes simplex virus ulcerations, and the possibility of contaminated marrow have been suggested as the sources of these organisms.

After the engraftment stage, dysfunction of cellular and humoral immune mechanisms become prominent. Most infections that occur between engraftment and up to 100 days posttransplantation are due to opportunistic organisms that had been latent and are reactivated after transplantation. These include cytomegalovirus, varicella–zoster virus, adenoviruses and papovaviruses, *P. carinii,* and *T. gondii*. Nonbacterial interstitial pneumonitis is an important syndrome during this phase, although all cases are not due to infectious agents.

Infections caused by *M. tuberculosis* and nontuberculous mycobacteria (*M. avium* complex, *M. kansasii,* and *M. fortuitum*) (23) have been reported.

The occurrence of infections 6 months or later after transplantation suggest the presence of persistent immunodeficiency in bone marrow transplant recipients. The defects in host defense mechanisms at this stage are caused by graft-versus-host disease or its therapy. Bacterial infections of the upper respiratory tract, skin, and lungs are common, especially those caused by *Streptococcus pneumoniae*. Infections that are due to other gram-positive organisms, such as *Staph. aureus* and *Staph. epidermidis,* are also common, especially in patients with indwelling vascular catheters. Antibody response to pneumococcal antigens may be normal by 6–8 months following transplantation, and the use of pneumococcal vaccine at this stage may be advisable. Reactivated varicella–zoster infections and blood product-related hepatitis are also seen in the late posttransplant period.

Infections Following Splenectomy

Splenectomy has been an accepted practice for the staging of Hodgkin's disease. Some patients with CLL who develop hemolytic anemia and some patients with myelodysplastic syndromes require this procedure. The monocyte–macrophage system of the spleen is important for the clearance of opsonized encapsulated organisms. A study of infectious complications resulting from splenectomy in patients with chronic leukemia over a 22-year period, showed a significant number of serious infections (65% versus 35% in patients without splenectomy). Fatal overwhelming sepsis occurred in 22% of patients after splenectomy, but in only 7% of patients who did not undergo splenectomy.

These patients are most susceptible to overwhelming infection caused by *Strep. pneumoniae,* meningococcus, and *H. influenzae*. These infections present as septic shock, meningitis, or pneumonia and may be rapidly fatal. Other organisms that are capable of causing serious infections in these patients include *Nocardia* spp., *Plesiomonas shigelloides,* the DF-2 bacillus, and *Babesia*. Recent studies in adults and children suggest that the outlook for the splenectomized patient has been improved by the use of pneumococcal vaccine, prophylactic antibiotics, and earlier recognition of this syndrome by clinicians.

INFECTING ORGANISMS

The types of bacteria causing infection in patients with hematological malignancies have changed dramatically during the past four decades. Before antibiotics were available, pneumococcal and streptococcal infections were prevalent. After the introduction of penicillin G, resistant strains of *Staph. aureus* emerged as the predominant cause of fatal infection in this patient population. At that time, erythromycin and chloramphenicol became available, but they proved to be of limited value because they were predominantly bacteriostatic agents. The introduction of methicillin represented a milestone in the management of bacterial infections because of its activity against penicillin-resistant staphylococci. Before this antibiotic became available *Staph. aureus* was responsible for over 30% of all fatal infections occurring in patients with acute leukemia (24). After methicillin was incorporated into routine antibacterial regimens, fewer than 5% of fatal infections were due to this organism.

During the early 1960s, gram-negative bacilli emerged as the most common cause of serious infections in the immunocompromised host, especially in neutropenic patients. Predominant organisms were *E. coli, Klebsiella* spp., and *P. aeruginosa,* with *P. aeruginosa* being especially common as a cause of infection in neutropenic patients. Cephalosporins were effective in curing infections caused by *E. coli* and *Klebsiella* spp. Neither the polymyxins nor the aminoglycosides with antipseudomonal activity were reliable in eradicating pseudomonal infections in neutropenic patients, and the only patients who survived these infections were those whose neutrophil count recovered during therapy. Another milestone in the therapy of infection in neutropenic patients was the introduction of the antipseudomonal penicillin, carbenicillin. Subsequent to its introduction, the cure rate for serious pseudomonal infections increased to 75%, even in patients with persistent neutropenia (25).

Since the late 1970s, gram-positive organisms have reemerged as important pathogens. This has been due to several factors, including the widespread use of indwelling intravascular catheters, the administration of prophylactic antibiotics, and the widespread use of therapeutic antibiotic regimens with limited gram-positive activity. Approximately 60% of all documented infections in neutropenic patients are currently caused by gram-positive organisms. The predominant infection is *S. epidermidis* bacteremia. Although many of these infections appear to arise from an intravascular catheter, some most likely have their origin in the gastrointestinal tract. *Staphylococcus aureus, C. jeikeium,* and *Bacillus* spp. are also important causes of infection. A disturbing feature of these gram-positive infections is that many of the organisms are resistant to the antistaphylococcal penicillins and susceptible only to vancomycin.

Because of the widespread use of broad-spectrum antibiotic regimens, many nosocomial infections are caused by organisms that are resistant to multiple antibiotics. *Enterobacter* spp., *P. aeruginosa, Serratia marcescens,* and *Citrobacter* spp. are especially adept at developing resistant to commonly utilized antibiotics. *Acinetobacter* spp., *Xanthomonas maltophilia,* and other *Pseudomonas* spp. have also emerged as important pathogens at some institutions. These organisms are frequently a cause of catheter-associated bacteremias, but may also cause other serious infections. They also are frequently resistant to most of the commonly utilized antibiotics.

The availability of effective antibiotic regimens to control many of the bacterial infections occurring in neutropenic patients has led to the increasing frequency of infections caused by fungi. Other factors that have facilitated the increased frequency of fungal infections include the use of more intensive chemotherapeutic regimens that cause extensive mucositis and prolonged neutropenia and the widespread use of intravascular catheters that facilitate the development of fungemia. The most common fungal infections are candidiasis and aspergillosis. In the past, these infections occurred almost exclusively in patients with far-advanced malignancies that were no longer responsive to chemotherapy. Unfortunately, in recent years, these infections complicate initial remission-induction chemotherapy. Indeed, in one study, fatal fungal infection was responsible for 40% of failures to initial remission-induction chemotherapy for acute leukemia (26). Major obstacles in diagnosis and therapy have prevented the successful management of fungal infection. These infections often present with fever as the only manifestation, and diagnostic procedures fail to reveal the infecting organism. Currently available antifungal agents are seldom effective in controlling systemic fungal infections, unless the patient's neutrophil count recovers.

Viral infections are also common in patients with hematological malignancies. The DNA viruses have emerged as important pathogens in these patients. Viral infections account for the greatest proportion of infections seen in children with ALL in remission and are equally as common as bacterial infections during relapse. Herpesviruses, particularly herpes simplex virus, varicella–zoster virus, and cytomegalovirus cause most viral infections. Cytomegalovirus infections are seen particularly in patients undergoing bone marrow transplantation and may cause hepatitis, pneumonitis, enterocolitis, or retinitis in these patients. Herpes simplex virus is commonly associated with ulcerations of the oropharynx in patients receiving antineoplastic chemotherapy and in bone marrow transplant recipients. These lesions can extend to the esophagus, with signs and symptoms suggesting candidal esophagitis. Accurate diagnosis requires invasive procedures, such as endoscopy, to obtain a biopsy specimen for histological examination and culture. Dissemination to visceral organs, such as liver, spleen, lungs, and kidneys, occur rarely. The incidence of herpes simplex encephalitis seems to be no greater than that in immunocompetent individuals. However, antiviral therapy may need to be continued for as long as 21 days. Both varicella (chickenpox) and herpes zoster (shingles) are classic opportunistic infections in children with ALL or lymphoma, particularly during chemotherapy. Children who develop chickenpox while undergoing chemotherapy have a visceral dissemination rate of 32% and mortality rate of 7%. Deaths are uniformly associated with varicella pneumonia. Cutaneous dissemination and secondary bacterial infections of the skin following herpes zoster occur in up to 50% of children with acute leukemia. However, visceral dissemination and mortality are low with this type of infection. In contrast, visceral dissemination following zoster can occur in about 15% of bone marrow transplant recipients, and a mortality rate of up to 5% has been reported. Infections caused by adenoviruses have also been reported in patients with hematological malignancies. Human polyomaviruses, JC and SV40-PML, cause a rare subacute and progressive demyelinating disease of the central nervous system in patients with lymphocytic leukemia and lymphoma.

Among RNA viruses, measles virus represents the major viral pathogen encountered in childhood leukemias. Measles can be a severe and fulminant infection in children with leukemia. The complication of cutaneous and visceral dissemination and the incidence of bacterial superinfection and otitis media are increased in children undergoing chemotherapy. Other RNA viruses that have been important causes of morbidity in children with leukemia are parainfluenza, rhinovirus, respiratory syncytial virus, and enteroviruses. Infections caused by hepatitis B virus and non-A, non-B hepatitis (hepatitis C virus) are also frequent complications in patients with leukemia undergoing remission induction therapy and in patients receiving bone marrow transplantation.

SITES OF INFECTION

Central Nervous System

Acute bacterial meningitis is an uncommon infection in patients with hematological malignancies. It is most likely to occur in asplenic or neutropenic patients or in patients with Ommaya shunts. The asplenic patient is most susceptible to infection caused by the pneumococcus *(Streptococcus pneumoniae)*, meningococcus *(Neisseria meningitidis)*, or *Haemophilus influenzae*. Meningitis in neutropenic patients is most likely to be caused by gram-negative bacilli. The most common organism causing infections associated with Ommaya reservoirs is *Staph. epidermidis*. Meningitis in neutropenic patients is often manifested only as fever, headache, and a clouded sensorium. Since these patients are unable to mount an adequate inflammatory reaction, the characteristic clinical features of meningitis are usually absent. Few inflammatory cells may be present in the cerebrospinal fluid. Candidal meningitis occurs in about 20% of neutropenic patients with disseminated infection.

Cryptococcus neoformans is the most common cause of meningitis in patients with impaired cell-mediated immunity. The infection may arise suddenly or insidiously, and the patient usually presents with fever, headache, and impaired mental function. Occasionally, meningitis may be a manifestation of disseminated histoplasmosis or coccidioidomycosis. Bacterial pathogens causing meningitis in patients with impaired cell-mediated immunity include *Listeria monocytogenes, Salmonella* spp., and *M. tuberculosis*.

The brain is often involved in disseminated infections caused by nonbacterial pathogens. *Nocardia* spp. and *Toxoplasma gondii* infections occur preponderantly in patients with impaired cell-mediated immunity. The brain is the most common nonrespiratory organ involved in cases of disseminated aspergillosis. Aspergillosis or zygomycosis should be considered as a likely cause of stroke in a patient with prolonged neutropenia, because these organisms invade blood vessels, causing thrombosis and infarction. Cytomegalovirus occasionally causes a meningoencephalitis. Multifocal leukoencephalopathy is a rare infection caused by a polyomavirus that may occur in patients with lymphoma or chronic lymphocytic leukemia. These patients develop progressive neurological defects that terminate in death.

Sinus Infections

There is no evidence to suggest that acute bacterial sinus infections are especially prevalent in neutropenic patients. A serious form of sinusitis caused by gram-negative bacteria has been described in patients with prolonged nasogastric intubation. This infection may be overlooked because of the patient's underlying critical condition. Occasionally, *P. aeruginosa* causes chronic sinusitis, otitis externa, otitis media, or mastoiditis in neutropenic patients, especially in children. Most sinus infections in neutropenic patients are caused by *Aspergillus* spp. or zygomycetes. These infections are especially dangerous because the organisms are able to penetrate through fascial planes, cartilage, and bone. The infection may erode through the base of the skull and into the brain, causing thrombosis and infarction. Alternatively, ulcerations may arise in the palate or in the nose and cause facial disfigurement. The initial manifestation of this form of aspergillosis is often periorbital swelling. Usually, the eye is not involved, and eyesight is unimpaired, although the patient may develop diplopia.

Oropharyngeal Infection

Most oropharyngeal infections occur as a consequence of chemotherapy-induced mucositis. If the chemotherapy also induces neutropenia, this further enhances the invasion of the damaged mucosal surfaces by microorganisms. Furthermore, if the patient has been exposed to broad-spectrum antibiotics, many of the organisms composing the normal flora of the oropharynx are eliminated, facilitating colonization by resistant gram-negative bacilli and *Candida* spp. Infection is further facilitated in thrombocytopenic patients by hemorrhage into the oropharyngeal tissues that may occur as a consequence of trauma arising during chewing or inflicted by dentures. Several studies have demonstrated that careful attention to dental hygiene effectively reduces the frequency of infection. About 10% of leukemic patients develop bacterial infections of the oropharynx that present as gingivitis, dental abscess, pericoronitis, pharyngitis, or gangrenous stomatitis. Most of these infections are caused by aerobic gram-negative bacilli. The role of anaerobic organisms in the pathogenesis of these infections is unknown; however, *Capnocytophaga* spp., an anaerobic gram-negative bacillus, that inhabits the oropharynx has been recognized as a cause of bacteremia in neutropenic patients who develop mucositis.

A common oral infection in patients with hematological malignancies is thrush. The majority of these infections are caused by *Candida albicans*. Most of these infections cause only superficial involvement and respond to topical antifungal agents. Occasional infections are more deep-seated and require systemic antifungal therapy. It is reasonable to assume that some cases of disseminated candidiasis arise from these oropharyngeal infections, although the actual frequency with which this occurs is unknown. It is unlikely that dissemination is a common event from the oropharynx, considering the frequency of thrush in these patients.

Herpes simplex virus causes infections of the lips and oropharynx. These occur most commonly in transplant recipients but also in neutropenic patients. Most likely, they represent reactivation of latent infection. The initial manifestation of infection is localized vesicular lesions of the lip or oropharynx, which may then progress to large hemorrhagic and necrotic ulcerations. Rarely, infection disseminates to involve internal organs including the trachea, lung, liver, and central nervous system. Infection may be especially severe and chonic in bone marrow transplant recipients. Bacterial superinfection, especially with *Staph. aureus,* is a potentially serious complication of oral cutaneous herpetic infection. There is some evidence to suggest that herpes simplex plays an important role in the ulcerations associated with chemotherapeutic agents, but it is not certain that all patients with chemotherapy-induced mucositis from whom herpes simplex is cultured are actually infected with this virus.

Pneumonitis

Pneumonitis is the most frequent serious infectious complication that occurs in patients with hematological malignancies. Frequently, the identity of the infecting organism cannot be determined, making the selection of appropriate therapy difficult. Furthermore, even when the organism causing infection is known, the response to appropriate therapy is often suboptimal. Consequently, pneumonia in these patients is associated with a high mortality. The usual approach to the diagnosis of bacterial pneumonia is the collection of an adequate sputum specimen and blood specimens for culture. Unfortunately, neutropenic patients are unable to produce adequate sputum, and often, blood cultures are not positive. Furthermore, an organism isolated from a blood culture may not be the cause of the pneumonitis. Bronchoscopy with bronchoalveolar lavage has been useful for determining the cause of many cases of pneumonitis in patients with impaired host defense mechanisms other than neutropenia, but in neutropenic patients, this procedure seldom provides the diagnosis. Even an open-lung biopsy provides the diagnosis in only 40–60% of the cases. Furthermore, invasive prodecures may entail too great a risk in some patients who have a bleeding diathesis or who have severely compromised respiratory function. Pulmonary infection may occur as a consequence of inhalation of infectious material, such as the spores of *Aspergillus* spp., by aspiration, or from hematogenous dissemination, as occurs in candidiasis.

Clues to the possible cause of pneumonitis can be derived from determination of the deficiency in host defenses, history of exposure, presenting signs and symptoms, extrapulmonary findings, and appearance of the chest roentgenogram. Pulmonary infection caused by *Aspergillus* spp. and *Phycomycetes* may present with symptoms of an acute pulmonary embolism, since these organisms invade blood vessels, causing thrombosis and infarction. Patients who present with the early onset of dyspnea on exertion and cyanosis, but have few abnormalities on chest auscultation, most likely are infected with *Pneumocystis carinii* or cytomegalovirus. Diagnoses such as cryptococcosis, listeriosis, or toxoplasmosis should be considered in patients who have central nervous system symptoms in association with their pneumonia. The possibility of cytomegalic inclusion disease or toxoplasmosis should be considered in patients with concomitant myocarditis or hepatitis.

The chest roentgenogram may provide helpful clues to suggest the cause of pneumonitis. The presence of new hilar or mediastinal lymphadenopathy might indicate recurrence of the underlying malignancy, but if associated with pneumonitis might also suggest the possibility of infectious processes such as histoplasmosis, coccidioidomycosis, cryptococcosis, or tuberculosis. The earliest radiological indication of pulmonary aspergillosis is the development of single or multiple round densities or a wedge-shaped infiltrate. Gram-negative bacillary pneumonia often appears as a necrotizing pneumonitis on chest roentgenogram. Abscess formation is characteristic of infection caused by *Staph. aureus* or *Nocardia* spp. Unfortunately, in many cases, the chest roentgenogram shows only a bilateral diffuse pneumonitis that, in the neutropenic patient, could be caused by bacteria, fungi, viruses, or protozoa. Although empiric therapy may be necessary because of the precarious condition of the patient, nevertheless, a vigorous approach to establishing the diagnosis is critically important wherever possible. Inappropriate delays can be disastrous because of the fulminant nature of many of these infections in the immunocompromised patient.

Gastrointestinal Infections

Esophagitis is a relatively common infection that presents as pain on swallowing and retrosternal discomfort. Barium contrast x-ray examination demonstrates ulceration, spasm, and a moth-eaten appearance to the esophageal mucosa, but this appearance does not assist in determining the organism causing the infection. The diagnosis can also be determined by esophagoscopy which reveals the presence of white patches and hemorrhagic ulcerations and also permits the collection of material for microscopic examination and culture. Most esophagitis is caused by *C. albicans* or herpes simplex, but occasional cases are caused by cytomegalovirus and bacteria. Since, in the neutropenic patient, *Candida* spp. are the most likely cause of esophagitis, it is reasonable to attempt a therapeutic trial with an antifungal agent and, if that is not successful, to proceed with esophagoscopy.

Increasingly, colitis caused by *Clostridium difficile* is being recognized in patients with hematological malignancies. Although it is likely that most of these cases are associated with the administration of antibiotics, in some instances, the antineoplastic chemotherapy appears to be the predisposing factor. This organism can be a nosocomial pathogen and, unless adequate housecleaning procedures are followed, can be transmitted to the next patient who occupies the same room. There is no definitive evidence to suggest that Samonella infections occur more frequently in patients with hematological diseases, but when salmonellosis occurs, it is more likely to involve other sites besides the gastrointestinal tract.

Neutropenic patients frequently are found to have candidiasis involving the stomach or small and large intestine at autopsy examination. This gastrointestinal infection is seldom associated with notable symptoms and, consequently, remains clinically unrecognized. It is an important infection, however, because of the potential for causing disseminated candidiasis. *Aspergillus* spp. can also cause infection of the gastrointestinal tract, manifested as acute abdominal pain from vascular thrombosis and infarction. Rarely, the Budd–Chiari syndrome may arise as a consequence of this infection.

Gastrointestinal tract infection with cytomegalovirus can be serious and even result in fatality, especially in children. Cases of protracted severe diarrhea resulting in severe electrolyte imbalance have been observed. Patients have developed ulcerations associated with severe hemorrhage or perforation. Strongyloidiasis occasionally is diagnosed in patients with lymphomas and transplant recipients. It may cause recurrent septicemia from enteric organisms or a hyperacute infection with pulmonary involvement.

Neutropenic patients are especially susceptible to typhlitis, which is an inflammatory disease usually limited to the cecum and terminal ileum (27). In some patients, it may involve the entire intestine or even the entire gastrointestinal tract. It is characterized by well-demarcated ulcers, hemorrhage, and masses of organisms in the bowel wall, with a paucity of inflammatory cells. The usual presenting signs and symptoms of this disease are fever, right lower quadrant pain and tenderness, watery or bloody diarrhea, abdominal distention, and decreased or absent bowel sounds. There is an association between this disease and severe stomatitis, suggesting that the initiating effect may be damage to the mucosa by antitumor agents. Septicemia occurs in about 70% of patients and is usually caused by gram-negative bacilli, especially *P. aeruginosa*. Some cases have been associated with *Clostridium septicum* septicemia. Initial therapy should consist of nasogastric suction, intravenous fluids, analgesics, and broad-spectrum antibiotic regimens that provide adequate coverage against aerobic gram-negative bacteria, especially *P. aeruginosa,* and anaerobes. Surgical exploration may be indicated in occasional patients with localized disease, but should be considered only when the patient is failing to respond to conservative measures. Indications for surgery include severe gastrointestinal hemorrhage, perforation, and a rapidly deteriorating condition. The mortality rate from this disease is high unless the patient's neutrophil count recovers.

Perirectal infections are a potentially serious complication, especially in patients with neutropenia (28). They have been described in 5–10% of patients with hematological diseases and are especially common in patients with acute monocytic and acute myelomonocytic leukemia. Infection often begins at the site of a hemorrhoid or fissure and may progress into the rectum causing extensive necrosis. The infection usually causes fever, pain, and local tenderness. Abscess formation is infrequent because of the patient's neutropenia. Most of the infections are caused by aerobic gram-negative bacilli, especially *P. aeruginosa* and *E. coli,* which often cause associated septicemia. There is also some evidence to suggest that anaerobic bacteria play a role in these infections. Symptomatic therapy consist of sitz baths, warm compresses, stool softeners, and analgesics. Broad-spectrum antibiotic regimens that provide coverage against aerobic gram-negative bacilli and anaerobes should be administered. There are conflicting reports concerning the role of surgery in these cases, but some studies suggest that incision and drainage is beneficial in relieving discomfort and facilitating healing, even when a clearcut abscess is not identified. These patients may respond to initial antibiotic therapy only to become superinfected with a more resistant gram-negative bacillus and ultimately die of septic shock. In most series, the mortality rate has varied from 10–35%. It is of critical importance for those patients who recover from these infections and achieve a remission, that their underlying rectal problem (hemorrhoid or fissure) be corrected to avoid further infection, should their malignancy recur.

Cutaneous Infections

Cellulitis is a common occurrence in patients with hematological malignancies for several reasons. These patients require multiple venipunctures and bone marrow aspirations, and they receive frequent intravenous medications facilitating the development of infection. Some antitumor agents are vesicants and can cause extensive tissue necrosis if they extravasate. Most cases of cellulitis are caused by *Staph. aureus, Staph. epidermidis, Strep. pyogenes,* or gram-negative bacilli. Gram-negative bacilli that are especially likely to cause cellulitis include *Enterobacter* spp., *P. aeruginosa,* and *Aeromonas hydrophila*. The latter organism is frequently a nosocomial pathogen, but it also contaminates fresh water streams and lakes and can cause infection in patients who abrade their skin while engaged in water-related sports activites. Recently, several series of aspergillar skin infections have been reported. In some instances, these have been associated with occlusive dressings that have been contaminated with aspergillus spores and, in other instances, they have occurred at sites of indwelling catheters. Neutropenic patients have developed pulmonary aspergillosis as a direct extension from a skin infection at a subclavian catheter site. Aspiration and biopsy of cellulitis should be performed in an effort to culture the pathogen, but, frequently, it is not recovered from this material.

Herpes simplex causes infection of the lips and surrounding face, but can also cause infection on the hands. Females may develop extensive vulvo-vaginal infection that is disfiguring and painful. Genital condylomas may also occur in females with hematological malignancies. Often these lesions are difficult to eradicate by conventional methods. Herpes zoster occurs in up to 25% of patients undergoing therapy for Hodgkin's disease. Most of these cases will have occurred within the first year after completion of therapy. Although zoster is generally a reactivation of latent infection, there have been microepidemics in susceptible populations that suggest the possibility of exogenous infection. Zoster tends to occur at sites of previous radiotherapy or adjacent to sites at which tumor has been in close association with nerve roots. Cutaneous dissemination occurs in 20–40% of patients, but visceral dissemination occurs infrequently. Intravenous acyclovir probably should be administered to all patients with hematological malignancies who develop zoster to avoid dissemination, facilitate healing, and prevent postherpetic neuralgia.

Catheter-Associated Infections

The wide acceptance of the use of intravascular catheters for the administration of chemotherapeutic agents has resulted in a variety of infectious complications. Depending upon the device utilized, the frequency of infectious complications has been as high as 20–30%, especially in neutropenic patients. Infection may be manifested as a localized cellulitis or tunnel infection, an uncomplicated bacteremia, septic thrombophlebitis, or bacterial endocarditis. The majority of these infections are caused by skin commensals such as *Staph. epidermidis, Corynebacterium* spp. (especially *C. jeikeium*), *Bacillus* spp., and *Staph. aureus*. Gram-negative bacteria associated with catheter infections include *Enterobacter* spp., *Pseudomonas* spp., *Acinetobacter* spp., and *X. maltophilia*. An increased frequency of fungemia caused by *Candida* spp., especially *C. tropicalis,* and *Torulopsis glabrata* have been associated with catheters. Local aspergillar infections have occurred at catheter sites from deposition of spores during the surgical insertion of the device or to impregnation of spores into adhesive dressings. Many of the gram-positive infections are caused by organisms that are susceptible only to vancomycin.

If the patient is suffering from a gram-positive bacteremia, without evidence of local infection, it can usually be treated successfully with antibiotics, without removing the catheter. However, the catheter should be removed if there is evidence of local cellulitis, tunnel infection, or metastatic infection. Other indications for catheter removal include persistent fever or bacteremia, despite appropriate antibiotic therapy, or recurrent infection when therapy is discontinued. If the infection is caused by a gram-negative bacillus or a fungus, then the catheter should always be removed. It is never appropriate to simply remove a catheter without administering specific antimicrobial therapy. This practice had been advocated in the past in cases of candidemia, but the recognition of a high frequency of tissue invasion has abrogated that policy.

PROBLEM ORGANISMS FOR PATIENTS WITH HEMATOLOGICAL MALIGNANCIES

Many organisms are capable of causing serious or fatal infections in patients with hematological malignancies. However, there are certain organisms that represent special problems for this patient population. Included among these are bacteria, fungi, viruses, and protozoa. Consequently, the unique features of some of these infections will be discussed.

Pseudomonas aeruginosa

With the availability of potent antipseudomonal antibiotics, the frequency of these infections has diminished. Nevertheless, *P. aeruginosa* remains one of the most common causes of gram-negative infection in neutropenic patients. It is a ubiquitous organism, colonizing fresh fruits and vegetables, sinks, and showers. The organism has the capability of developing resistance to multiple antibiotics and, therefore, is a common nosocomial pathogen. Several studies have demonstrated that neutropenic patients are exposed to this organism while in the hospital, become colonized, and then, subsequently, develop infection (29).

The lung is the most frequent site of pseudomonal infection. The usual chest roentgenogram appearance is that of a diffuse bronchopneumonia, with nodular infiltrates and small areas of radiolucency. Infection usually involves the lower lobes, sparing the apices. Lesions consist of firm, well-defined, hemorrhagic nodules, with necrotic centers, frequently located subpleurally.

Skin lesions occur in about 20% of cases of bacteremia. The most characteristic skin lesion is ecthyma gangrenosum, usually found in the groin or axilla. It begins as a red macule, becomes pustular, and later develops a central area of hemorrhagic necrosis, at which time it has a characteristic bluish-purple center surrounded by an erythematous halo. These lesions may arise anywhere on the body, including the forehead, eyelid, and tongue. Occasional patients may develop many small lesions suggesting emboli, but endocarditis is an exceedingly rare complication of pseudomonal infection. The organism usually can be cultured from skin lesions, and biopsy reveals an acute vasculitis, with extensive bacterial colonization of the vessel walls. Other types of skin lesions associated with pseudomonal infection include hemorrhagic necrotic cellulitis, painful inflamed vesicles with an erythematous base, and painful subcutaneous nodules.

Pseudomonas may cause serious infections of the head and neck. Occasional patients develop blepharitis or conjunctivitis. This can be a serious infection because of the possibility of progression to an enophthalmitis. Otitis externa and otitis media, sinusitis, mastoiditis, and meningitis can be caused by this organism. Rarely, it is a cause of necrotizing pharyngitis. Therapy usually consists of an aminoglycoside plus an antipseudomonal β-lactam antibiotic; however there are some studies suggesting that β-lactams alone are equally effective if given at the proper dose and schedule.

Salmonellosis

Since most Salmonella infections occur as epidemics of gastroenteritis, there is little evidence to indicate that patients with hematological malignancies are more likely to develop these infections. During the past few years, several areas in the United States, especially New England, have experienced epidemics of infection with *Salmonella enteritidis,* from ingestion of contaminated eggs. However, 15–25% of serious Salmonella infections occur in cancer patients, particularly those with hematological malignancies. *Salmonella typhimurium* is the most common species of this organism causing serious infection in immunocompromised patients, whereas it seldom causes more than gastroenteritis in normal hosts (30). *Salmonella* spp. may cause pneumonia, urinary tract infection, peritonitis, osteomyelitis, or meningitis, and about 30% of cancer patients with Salmonella infections develop bacteremia. *Salmonella* organisms may be difficult to eradicate completely from patients with lymphoma; consequently, these patients develop repeated episodes of infection. Ampicillin or a broad-spectrum cephalosporin are the most appropriate therapies for Salmonella infection.

Listeriosis

Listeria monocytogenes is a gram-positive bacillus that may be confused with diphtheroids. It causes meningitis, encephalitis, and septicemia, especially in patients with lymphoma (31). Most of these patients are undergoing chemotherapy when they become infected. Whereas type 4b *L. monocytogenes* causes nearly 70% of infections in the general population, type 1 causes most infections in cancer patients. Meningitis accounts for over 60% of infections and septicemia without meningitis for 30%. Rarely, other sites, such as pleural effusions and septic arthritis, are found. Examination of the cerebrospinal fluid may reveal a pleocytosis with either neutrophils or mononuclear cells predominating, but, in some instances, the cerebral spinal fluid may be normal. Meningitis can be rapidly fatal, and 20% of these patients die within 48 hours of the onset of symptoms. Appropriate therapy consists of ampicillin or trimethoprim–sulfamethoxazole. These organisms are not susceptible to cephalosporins.

Clostridial Infections

Occasional patients with acute leukemia develop infection with *Clostridium perfringens*. Over 90% of infections are associated with bacteremia, but occasional patients may have progressive gas gangrene. Clinical features of septicemia include an alert sensorium with irritability, tachycardia out of proportion to fever, hypotension with oliguria, and nausea and vomiting. Abdominal pain and distention may be present in some cases. The onset of symptoms is usually sudden, with rapid progression and deterioration. Jaundice, intravascular hemolysis, or gas gangrene with localized crepitation may be present. The mortality in leukemic patients is exceptionally high, despite the prompt administration of appropriate antibiotics. Appropriate therapy consists of penicillin G, administered at a dose of 20 million units daily. Occasional strains may be resistant to this antibiotic.

Clostridium septicum has been identified as one of the organisms causing typhlitis in neutropenic patients. This infection is usually associated with septicemia. Clinical features include fever, shock, abdominal pain, and vomiting. Intravascular hemolysis does not accompany these infections. The fatality rate in neutropenic patients is high, especially if associated with typhlitis.

The toxins that are produced by *C. difficile* are the cause of antibiotic-associated colitis. This pseudomembraneous colitis causes diarrhea that may be profuse and associated with fever and abdominal pain. The diagnosis is established by identifying the presence of toxin in the stool. Therapy should be instituted with oral vancomycin or metronidazole. Intravenous administration of antibiotics is likely to be ineffective. Because of the high frequency of this infection in patients with hematological malignancies, therapy should be instituted empirically if the patient has symptoms of serious infection.

Tuberculosis

Tuberculosis is no more common in patients with acute leukemia than in the general population. However, when infection occurs, it is likely to disseminate widely and rapidly. It is more common in patients with Hodgkin's disease and chronic lymphocytic leukemia. With the effective control of tuberculosis, the frequency has been reduced from 20% to 1–2% of patients with Hodgkin's disease. Unfortunately, in recent years, the incidence of tuberculosis in the general population has increased, and this is likely to be reflected in an increased frequency in patients with hematological diseases in the future. The presence of tuberculosis in patients with Hodgkin's disease is often difficult to recognize because the usual manifestations of fever, weight loss, pulmonary infiltrates, and hepatosplenomegaly are also manifestations of the underlying malignancy. These patients are usually anergic to the tuberculin skin test. Furthermore, fever may be the only manifestation of miliary tuberculosis. Fulminant tuberculous pneumonia has also been described in patients with lymphoma and is associated with a high mortality. Since reactivation of prior tuberculous infection can occur, it is advisable to administer isoniazid prophylactically to patients over aged 65 years, patients with evidence of old tuberculous infection, or patients who are at high risk of having been exposed to this infection in the recent past. Therapy of active tuberculosis consists of the administration of pyrazinamide for 2 months and isoniazid and rifampin for 6–9 months.

Nocardiosis

Nocardia spp. are an occasional cause of infection in patients with lymphoma (32). The lungs are involved in 70% of cases, and infection may present as lobar pneumonia, multiple nodules, miliary abscesses, or cavitation. Pulmonary infection may be associated with empyema or pleural effusion. Brain abscesses occur in about 30% of cases, and skin infection occurs in about 20%. Infection may disseminate to involve multiple organs, including the lungs, skin, brain, kidneys, spleen, liver, heart, and gastrointestinal tract. In patients with central nervous system infection, results of the cerebrospinal fluid examination are normal in about 20%, and the organism usually cannot be cultured. *Norcardia* spp. can be identified in infected material, using an acid-fast stain, as a finely branching organism. It grows slowly aerobically and often is not identified because of overgrowth by other organisms. Infection should be treated with sulfonamides, with or without trimethoprim, and must be continued for prolonged periods. Central nervous system infection is a serious complication and often fails to respond to appropriate therapy.

Candidiasis

Candida spp. are common pathogens in patients with hematological malignancies and may cause either local or systemic infection (33). Although *C. albicans* is the most common pathogenic species, *C. tropicalis* and other *Candida* spp. are emerging as important pathogens. Oropharyngeal candidiasis (thrush) is an extremely common complication of patients receiving antitumor chemotherapy. Lesions appear as white or greyish white plaques surrounded by an erythematous halo. The plaques are viable with a freely bleeding base. The lesions may be difficult to differentiate from a necrotic mucosa caused by antitumor agents. A

KOH preparation of scrapings of the lesion and culture establish the diagnosis of thrush. *Candida* spp. may infect any portion of the gastrointestinal tract and esophagitis is becoming increasingly common. The infection is characterized by ulceration and pseudomembrane formation. Candidal esophagitis may be present, with or without oral candidiasis. The diagnosis can be firmly established only by esophagoscopy and biopsy. Although oral therapy is effective in many patients, parenteral amphotericin B is dramatically effective in within 24–48 hours for patients who fail oral therapy.

Disseminated candidiasis occurs in about 2% of patients with lymphoma and 30–40% of patients with acute leukemia (34). Two patterns of organ involvement have been described. In one, presumably arising from the gastrointestinal tract, the liver, spleen, gastrointestinal tract, and lungs are the predominant organs of involvement. In the second form, presumably arising from hematogenous dissemination through indwelling catheters, the heart, kidney, and lungs are the predominant sites of infection.

Most patients with disseminated candidiasis do not develop any characteristic signs or symptoms to suggest this diagnosis. The most common presentation is persistent fever, without any signs of localized infection, that fails to respond to broad-spectrum antibacterial antibiotics. Some of these patients will have diffuse pulmonary infiltrates. As the infection progresses, the patient becomes increasingly debilitated, with deterioration of liver and renal function. Occasional patients with candidemia develop acute hypotension suggestive of endotoxin shock. Ophthalmitis has been described in patients with adequate neutrophil counts, but is seldom seen in neutropenic patients. Characteristic skin lesions occur in about 10% of patients with disseminated candidiasis. The lesions are nontender, subcutaneous nodules, with a pinkish-purplish color, that may arise anywhere on the body. They are usually discreet but can become confluent. Often the lesions are diffuse, but they may be localized to a small area. Occasional patients develop a myositis that causes muscle tenderness and pain on movement. Most of these patients also have the characteristic skin lesions. The central nervous system is involved in about 20% of cases with disseminated candidiasis. Patients may develop candidal meningitis and present with focal neurological defects. A more common type of nervous system infection is a diffuse cerebritis. These patients present with confusion and lethargy. Candidal endocarditis is a rare complication in patients with indwelling vascular catheters. Candidal pneumonia is usually a manifestation of hematogenous dissemination, but occasionally, may occur as a consequence of aspiration of infected oropharyngeal secretions. There are no characteristic findings on chest roentgenogram to suggest this diagnosis.

Successful management of systemic candidiasis has been hampered by the inability to diagnose many of these infections antimortem. Positive blood cultures are obtained from only 30–50% of patients with disseminated candidiasis.

Serologic tests to detect circulating antigen have been unreliable. Since colonization by *Candida* spp. is common in patients receiving antibacterial antibiotics, the identification of these organisms from body orifices is not a reliable indication of infection. An exception to this general principle may be the isolation of *C. tropicalis* from surveillance cultures, which has been associated with subsequent infection in about 60% of patients.

Transient fungemia is a well-recognized complication associated with intravascular catheters. However, in immunocompromised patients, 70–80% have evidence of tissue invasion at autopsy examination. Consequently, all patients with hematological malignancies who develop positive blood cultures should be treated for disseminated infection. The results of treatment of systemic candidiasis in patients with hematological malignancies are disappointing. Although amphotericin B is considered the drug of choice, only about 25% of patients survive their infection. The major prognostic factor is the patient's neutrophil count. Patients with neutropenia seldom respond to any therapy, unless their neutrophil count recovers.

Recently, a new syndrome of chronic systemic (hepatosplenic) candidiasis has been described, preponderantly in patients with acute leukemia (35). Typically, the patient develops prolonged fever unresponsive to antibacterial antibiotics while neutropenic. Subsequently, the patient achieves remission of the underlying hematological malignancy, and the blood counts recover. Despite the improvement in hematological status, fever persists, and the patient has persistent anorexia and debilitation. Other symptoms may develop, including right upper quadrant pain and pleuritic pain. Some patients develop palpable hepatosplenomegaly. Characteristically, the alkaline phosphatase is elevated, and other liver function tests may also be abnormal. At this time, an ultrasound examination or computed tomography will reveal multiple abscesses in the liver and spleen. Although biopsy may demonstrate the organisms on histopathological examination, they are seldom cultured. Therapy with amphotericin B is often ineffective and, in these patients, the infection persists for many months. Recently, encouraging results have been obtained with liposomal preparations of amphotericin B and fluconazole.

Aspergillosis

Aspergillosis is increasing in frequency in recent years and, at some institutions, has become as common as candidiasis. The most common predisposing factors are severe prolonged neutropenia and chronic adrenal corticosteroid therapy. *Aspergillus fumigatus* is the most common pathogen, but infections caused by *A. flavus, A. niger,* and other species are also increasing in frequency. Infection is usually acquired by inhalation of spores, which are deposited in the paranasal sinuses or lungs. Microepidemics of aspergillosis have been reported from several hospitals and usually occur when there is construction within the hospital or at adjacent sites, or the ventilation system within the hospital is contaminated or defective. The frequency of *Aspergillus* spp. can be greatly reduced in susceptible patient populations by placing them in rooms with HEPA filters.

Over 60% of aspergillar infections are localized to the lungs (36). Pulmonary infection may be manifested as necrotizing bronchopneumonia, hemorrhagic pulmonary infarction, solitary or miliary lung abscesses, or lobar pneumonia. The classic clinical presentation is the sudden onset of pleuritic chest pain, with fever, hemoptysis, and a pleural friction rub suggestive of pulmonary embolus and infarction. Unfortunately, this classic syndrome occurs in fewer than 30% of patients, and the most common clinical presentations are not diagnostic of this infection. Often, the only evidence of infection is prolonged fever, with noncharacteristic pulmonary infiltrates that fail to respond to antibacterial therapy. Not uncommonly, the only manifestation of infection may be fever, with normal physical and chest x-ray examinations. A few patients will develop exsanguinating pulmonary hemorrhage early in the course of their infection.

The earliest typical abnormality on chest x-ray examination is the appearance of single or multiple rounded densities. Patients with symptoms of pulmonary infarction may develop typical wedge-shaped lesions. If the patients predisposing factors are not corrected, the infection will progress to involve the lungs in a diffuse process. Patients whose infection is controlled usually develop cavities, with or without fungus balls. Although pulmonary aspergillosis may be suspected by the clinical presentation, it is usually difficult to isolate the infecting organism. *Aspergillus* spp. are cultured from fewer than 25% of cases. Bronchoscopy and bronchoalveolar lavage have not improved the yield of positive cultures. Tissue biopsy is usually not an option, because most patients are thrombocytopenic and at risk of hemorrhage. The isolation of *Aspergillus* spp. from the respiratory secretions of a susceptible patient generally indicates the presence of infection in either the lung or sinuses. Serological tests for detection of antigens to *Aspergillus* in serum have had varying success. No standard test is available for routine application.

About 15% of cases of invasive aspergillosis in patients with hematological malignancies involve the sinuses. Approximately half of these patients will develop disseminated infection. The earliest manifestation of sinusitis is crusting at the inferior turbinate or adjacent part of the cartilagenous septum. Early symptoms consist of fever, nasal obstruction, and rhinorrhea. As the infection progresses, the patient develops local pain or headache. Since *Aspergillus* spp. are capable of invading across all natural barriers, infection originating in the sinus may erode both cartilage and bone, causing ulcerations of the hard or soft palate or along the nose just below the eye. The periorbital structures may become involved in this process, causing swelling and erythema of the eyelids, ptosis, and retroorbital pain. The organism may also erode through the base of the brain, causing thrombosis and infarction. Aspergillar sinusitis is usually easy to diagnose by biopsy and culture.

Disseminated infection may involve any organ of the body. Often, the brain is a predominant site of disseminated aspergillosis. Patients are asymptomatic until they experience a sudden onset of a stroke, resulting in either major neurological defects or coma, progressing to death. Aspergillosis can present with myocardial infarction, gastrointestinal hemorrhage, Budd–Chiari syndrome, or characteristic necrotic skin lesions.

Amphotericin B is the only antifungal agent with activity against *Aspergillus* spp. Unfortunately, few patients respond to therapy unless their underlying predisposing factors can be corrected. There is anecdotal experience to suggest that the addition of flucytosine (5-fluorocytosine) may enhance the activity of amphotericin B in some patients.

Cryptococcosis

Patients with Hodgkin's disease are especially susceptible to infection caused by *Cryptococcus neoformans* (37). This infection occurs in about 10% of these patients and accounts for 25% of fungal infections. The organism is ubiquitous in animals and soil specimens; consequently, infection is acquired prior to hospitalization. Since *Cryptococcus* is a respiratory pathogen, infection begins in the lungs, where it may remain asymptomatic. Dissemination is frequent in patients with lymphoma, and central nervous infection is a regular feature. Other organs involved in disseminated infection include the lymph nodes, liver, kidneys, spleen, adrenals, bone, and skin.

Infection may be acute, subacute, or chronic, and may arise suddenly or insidiously. Symptoms of meningitis include headache, vertigo, and nausea and vomiting, and physical findings include fever, meningismus, stupor, and focal neurological deficits. Examination of the cerebrospinal fluid reveals a leukocytosis, with a preponderance of lymphocytes, decreased glucose concentration, and an elevated protein concentration. Organisms can be identified in the cerebrospinal fluid with an India ink preparation. The only abnormality in some patients is an elevated protein concentration. The availability of the cryptococcal antigen test for blood and cerebrospinal fluid has facilitated the diagnosis of this infection. Therapy for cryptococcosis is the combination of amphotericin B plus flucytosine, but it is uncertain that flucytosine adds to the efficacy of amphotericin B in lymphoma patients. This drug may delay recovery from the myelosuppressive effects of chemotherapy. It may be necessary to administer amphotericin B intrathecally, at least during the early period of therapy.

Cytomegalic Inclusion Disease

Active infection with cytomegalovirus is primarily a problem in children with acute leukemia and in bone marrow transplant recipients. Infection may be due to acquisition of the virus through infected blood transfusions or by reactivation of latent infection. Transplant recipients may also acquire the infection from infected donor cells. The frequency of infection can be reduced by screening donors of blood products.

About 30% of patients with viremia have clinical symptoms indicative of cytomegalic inclusion disease. Serious manifestations of cytomegalovirus infection are pneumonia, myocarditis, colitis, hepatitis, encephalitis, and retinitis. Pulmonary infection may be acute or chronic, and the patient usually presents with fever, dyspnea on exertion, and cyanosis. Auscultation of the lung reveals fine moist rales over involved areas. The chest x-ray film generally reveals a diffuse pneumonitis that may be unilateral or bilateral and, generally, involves the subpleural areas of the lower lobes. Cytomegalovirus may cause infected gastrointestinal ulcerations, leading to intractable diarrhea or uncontrollable gastrointestinal hemorrhage. Patients have developed myocarditis, leading to cardiac arrhythmias or acute congestive heart failure. Renal failure and adrenal insufficiency have resulted from infection of these organs.

The diagnosis can be established by the demonstration of typical inclusion cells in the urine, sputum, gastric washings, cerebrospinal fluid, bone marrow, or organ biopsy specimens. The virus may be cultured from urine, saliva, sputum, bronchial washings, or peripheral blood cells. Although isolation of the virus from body fluids is not always indicative of disease, the presence of inclusion cells does indicate the diagnosis of active infection. The availability of DNA probes has facilitated rapid diagnosis of cytomegalovirus infection. The only antiviral agent with demonstrable efficacy in treating cytomegalic inclusion disease is ganciclovir. The efficacy of this agent may be enhanced by the concomitant administration of intravenous γ-globulin.

Varicella–Zoster

Varicella is a potentially serious infection in children undergoing cancer chemotherapy. It is a highly contagious infection and epidemics have occurred on pediatric cancer services. Children with hematological malignancies can develop serious complications during varicella infection. In patients with thrombocytopenia, the vesicles become hemorrhagic and necrotic. About 10% of children develop bacterial superinfection. Visceral dissemination may occur and cause widespread pneumonia and focal necrosis of the liver, pancreas, and adrenal glands. Occasional patients develop fulminating encephalitis.

The administration of zoster immune globulin within 72 hours after exposure will prevent or modify the infection. Studies indicate that only 20% of children receiving zoster immune globulin after exposure developed varicella, whereas, 40–90% of children receiving no prophylaxis or pooled γ-globulin developed the disease. If infection has occurred, it should be treated with acyclovir. A live-attenuated varicella virus vaccine is available for immunization of susceptible patients.

Herpes zoster infection occurs in 3–15% of patients with lymphoma, multiple myeloma, and chronic lymphocytic leukemia (38). Over 50% of these patients have a definite history of previous varicella infection, and about 20% have had recent exposure to this virus. In 20% of patients, herpes zoster arises initially at sites where tumor is in close proximity to a nerve trunk. In an additional 20%, infection first appears at sites of recent radiotherapy. Herpes zoster infections disseminate cutaneously in 20–40% of lymphoma patients. Visceral dissemination occurs infrequently and may involve the gastrointestinal tract, liver, pancreas, adrenal glands, lungs, and the brain. Intercurrent bacterial pneumonia is common, whereas herpes zoster pneumonia is infrequent. Complications of zoster infection in these patients include postherpetic scarring, postherpetic neuralgia, deafness, keratitis, and neuropathy. Although many zoster infections remain localized and resolved spontaneously, it is probably advisable to administer acyclovir to all immunocompromised patients with this infection.

Pneumocystis carinii Pneumonia

Infection with *P. carinii* is limited to the lungs, although rare cases with involvement of liver, spleen, lymph nodes, and bone marrow have been described. This infection occurs in patients with impaired cell-mediated immunity and, occasionally, in patients with hypogammaglobulinemia. Before trimethoprim–sulfamethoxazole was used as prophylaxis, a substantial number of infections occurred in children with acute leukemia who were in remission and receiving intensive consolidation therapy. Pneumocystis pneumonia may represent reactivation of latent infection or may be a newly acquired infection.

Pneumonia may be insidious in onset or rapidly progressive. The initial symptoms of infection are unexplained fever and chronic nonproductive cough. As the disease progresses, the patient characteristically develops dyspnea on exertion, cyanosis, and tachycardia. Auscultatory findings are usually minimal, except in advanced disease. The chest roentgenogram often reveals more extensive pulmonary involvement than is suggested by the clinical findings. The usual abnormality on chest x-ray examination is interstitial granular haziness of the perihilar areas, which progresses to generalized irregular patches of consolidation surrounded by translucent areas of emphysema. A variety of chest roentgenogram abnormalities have been found, and occasional patients may even have a normal chest roentgenogram. These patients may demonstrate hypoxemia after exercise as a clue to the correct diagnosis. A gallium scan may also indicate the presence of infection in patients with pneumocystis pneumonia. The organism can be detected in induced sputum specimens of some patients, but often bronchoscopy and bronchoalveolar lavage are necessary to establish the diagnosis. Occasionally, only tissue biopsy will establish this diagnosis.

The recommended therapy for pneumocystis pneumonia is trimethoprim–sulfamethoxazole. Patients failing to respond to this therapy can be treated with pentamidine isethionate. It is advisable to place infected patients in isolation to prevent the spread of this infection to other susceptible patients.

Toxoplasmosis

Toxoplasma gondii is an obligate intracellular parasite that causes occasional infections in patients with impaired cell-mediated immunity. This infection may represent reactivation of latent infection or a newly acquired infection. It can be acquired by the ingestion of improperly cooked meat products and may also be transmitted by blood transfusion. Cats have been identified as an important vector in transmission of this infection.

A variety of clinical syndromes have been described, including atypical pneumonia, chorioretinitis, myositis, myocarditis, hepatitis, or encephalitis. About 60% of patients with lymphoma who develop toxoplasmosis have central nervous system disease, although multiple organs may be infected (39). Central nervous system infection presents as a nonspecific encephalopathy, diffuse meningoencephalitis, or a space-occupying lesion. The usual signs and symptoms include drowsiness, disorientation, acute toxic psychosis, headache, vomiting, cranial nerve palsies, and paresis. Examination of the cerebrospinal fluid reveals pleocytosis, predominantly with lymphocytes, elevated protein concentration, and normal or decreased glucose concentration. *Toxoplasma gondii* organisms are rarely identified in the cerebrospinal fluid.

The most reliable method for determining the diagnosis of toxoplasmosis in patients with hematological malignancies is identification of organisms in specimens. The organisms cannot be grown in culture medium, but can be transmitted to mice. The detection of rising antibody titers is not always reliable in patients with hematological malignancies, since they may have extensive infection, without developing notably elevated antibody titers. Toxoplasmosis can be treated successfully with sulfadiazine and pyrimethamine, but the prognosis in these patients is poor, especially if they have central nervous system infection.

Other Parasitic Infections

Sporadic cases of hyperinfection of *Strongyloides stercoralis* have been reported in patients with chronic lymphocytic leukemia and lymphoma. Although the parasite exists in the gut of normal hosts, without causing severe disability, patients with impaired host defenses may develop a serious disease. Large numbers of rhabditiform larvae may mature to filariform larvae and invade the walls of the gastrointestinal tract, causing ulceration. The symptoms of hyperinfection include nausea and vomiting, diarrhea, fever, abdominal pain, malabsorption, and shock. The larvae may migrate to the lungs, causing a diffuse alveolar pulmonary infiltrate in association with pulmonary insufficiency. Patients with hyperacute infection may develop recurrent septicemia caused by enteric organisms, which is a clue to the diagnosis of stronglylodiasis. Therapy with thiabendazole is indicated in these patients.

Babesiosis is a disease, caused by protozoa, that occurs in patients who have undergone splenectomy. It is transmitted to humans by the *Ixodidae* tick, with mice, voles, and deer serving as the intermediate host. Infections in the United States have occurred in the eastern New England coastal area. Infection may also be transmitted by blood transfusion. The human infection ranges from asymptomatic infection, to prolonged severe illness, characterized by the gradual onset of fever, chills, myalgia, and malaise. Splenectomized patients usually develop a moderate to severe hemolytic anemia. The recommended treatment for this infection is quinine and clindamycin.

THERAPY OF INFECTIONS IN HEMATOLOGIC MALIGNANCY

The introduction of newer broad-spectrum antibacterial agents has made a substantial contribution to the improved outcome of infections in hematological malignancy. However, such use has also been associated with the emergence of resistant nosocomial bacterial and fungal pathogens. The development of effective, nontoxic antifungal agents has lagged behind that of antibacterial agents. However, newer potentially effective antifungal agents are being evaluated in patients with hematological malignancy. The diagnosis of fungal infections is often difficult to establish in these patients, and the response to therapy depends on the early and aggressive use of antifungal agents. The availability of antiviral agents has enabled effective treatment of some of the viral infections in these patients.

Antibacterial Therapy

The β-lactam antibiotics, which include penicillins, cephalosporins, monobactams, and carbapenems, are the mainstay of antibiotic therapy, especially in neutropenic patients. The antibacterial activity of β-lactams is related to the inhibition of cell wall synthesis in susceptible bacteria. Variations in the composition of bacterial cell wall components account for some of the differences in susceptibility of individual bacterial strains to a particular β-lactam. Differences in the binding of specific β-lactams to target sites, the penicillin-binding proteins, also contribute to differences in activity. The most important mechanism of bacterial resistance to β-lactams is enzymatic hydrolysis of the β-lactam ring by β-lactamases, resulting in loss of antibacterial activity of the molecule. Some organisms are resistant because the β-lactam fails to reach its receptor site, a mechanism more likely to occur in gram-negative bacteria.

Extended Spectrum Penicillins

Fewer than 20% of cancer patients who developed pseudomonal septicemia responded to polymixin B or colistin (the only antipseudomonal agent available in the 1950s), and a mortality rate of 90% was reported for patients with acute leukemia. Thus, the availability of the carboxypenicillins, carbenicillin and ticarcillin, with activity against *P. aeruginosa* marked a milestone in the treatment of infections in neutropenic patients. Carbenicillin also has activity against most strains of *Proteus* spp. and *E. coli,* but *Klebsiella* spp., *Serratia* spp., and *Citrobacter* spp. are resistant. A response rate of 58–91% was noted in cancer patients treated with carbenicillin for various gram-negative infections (25). The frequency of *P. aeruginosa* as a cause of fatal infection in adults with leukemia was reported to have decreased from 31% to 8% following the regular use of this antibiotic (40).

Ticarcillin, compared with carbenicillin, has increased in vitro activity against *P. aeruginosa* and, therefore, can be given at a lower dose. Consequently, the risk of side effects, such as volume overload, hypokalemia, and coagulation dysfunction, are reduced. Carbenicillin and ticarcillin demonstrate in vitro synergy with aminoglycosides against most strains of *P. aeruginosa.*

The acylureidopenicillins, mezlocillin and azlocillin, and the piperazine penicillin, piperacillin, are considered extended-spectrum penicillins because they inhibit a wide variety of aerobic and anaerobic organisms, including *P. aeruginosa, Klebsiella* spp., enterococci, and *Bacteroides fragilis.* Like the carboxypenicillins, they are hydrolyzed by staphylococcal β-lactamases and are not reliable for treating staphylococcal infections. Although extended-spectrum penicillins alone were found to be adequate against some infections in myelosuppressed patients, their use as single agents in empiric therapy is not recommended.

Broad-Spectrum Cephalosporins

The era of the broad-spectrum cephalosporins as empiric therapy for presumed infection in cancer patients began with the introduction of moxalactam. Moxalactam was an attractive agent because of it broad-spectrum of activity that included *Staph. aureus,* most enteric gram-negative bacilli, and *P. aeruginosa.* Unfortunately, it caused coagulation defects that made it undesirable. Subsequently, cefoperazone and ceftazidime became available. Cefoperazone has somewhat greater activity against gram-positive organism, whereas ceftazidime has somewhat greater activity against *P. aeruginosa.*

These agents exhibited serum bactericidal levels exceeding those obtained with standard combinations (41). In one study, cefoperazone alone was as effective as cefoperazone plus amikacin in febrile cancer patients. Response rates were equivalent for ceftazidime alone or in combination with tobramycin against gram-negative bacillary infections (42). Response rates for gram-positive infections were lower than those for gram-negative infections; hence vancomycin plus ceftazidime was subsequently evaluated and found to be effective. Ceftazidime has been effective for the treatment of gram-negative bacillary infections in neutropenic patients; however, its usefulness as a single agent for initial therapy in febrile neutropenic patients remains uncertain (43).

Carbapenems

Imipenem, a stabilized derivative of thienamycin, was the first carbapenem. It is combined with cilastatin, an enzyme inhibitor with no intrinsic antibacterial activity, to prevent degradation by naturally occurring renal dehydropeptidase (44). Imipenem has a broad-spectrum of activity that includes most gram-positive cocci, gram-negative bacilli, and anaerobes. The drug has minimal side effects, although occasional patients with renal impairment or CNS disease develop seizures. About 20% of *P. aeruginosa* strains acquire resistance to imipenem during therapy, which occasionally results in treatment failure (46,46). Imipenem-resistant isolates of *P. aeruginosa* that emerge during therapy with this drug remain susceptible to other broad-spectrum β-lactam agents. As initial therapy, imipenem–cilastatin (Primaxin) produced an overall response rate of 77%, comparable with results with β-lactam plus aminoglycoside, double β-lactam, and vancomycin plus β-lactam regimens at the same institution (47). The response rate was lower when imipenem was used as secondary versus initial therapy (69% versus 94%) of gram-negative infections.

Monobactams

Aztreonam is a synthetic monobactam antibiotic, with a broad-spectrum of in vitro activity against gram-negative bacilli, but it has no activity against anaerobes and gram-positive organisms. The two major advantages of aztreonam are its minimal side effects and lack of cross-allergenicity with other β-lactam antibiotics. Aztreonam has been compared with aztreonam plus amikacin (both in combination with vancomycin for gram-positive coverage) for the empiric treatment of febrile episodes in neutropenic cancer patients. Aztreonam alone was as effective as aztreonam plus amikacin against gram-negative bacillary infections.

β-Lactamase Inhibitors

A major mechanism for resistance to β-lactam antibiotics is the ability of some organisms to produce β-lactamases that inactivate these antibiotics. Recently, several compounds have been discovered that bind irreversibly to many β-lactamases and, thereby, convert resistant organisms to sensitive ones. Clavulanic acid and sulbactam are currently available. Clavulanic acid has been combined with amoxicillin and ticarcillin, whereas sulbactam has been combined with ampicillin. Since ticarcillin is the only one of these antibiotics with anti-pseudomonal activity, this combination has been studied in neutropenic patients. Ticarcillin plus clavulanic acid (Timentin®) has activity against most gram-negative bacilli, gram-positive cocci, and anaerobes. This combination was used alone for the treatment of febrile episodes in neutropenic patients and produced an overall response rate of about 75% (48).

Aminoglycosides

The aminoglycosides have a broad-spectrum of antimicrobial activity that includes gram-positive cocci and most gram-negative bacilli. They act by binding to ribosomal subunits and cause a misreading of mRNA, thereby inhibiting protein synthesis. All anaerobic organisms are resistant to aminoglycosides, but the activity of these agents against some gram-positive organisms is inadequate. Although all aminoglycosides share a similar antibacterial spectrum against gram-negative aerobic organism, there are differences in the resistance patterns at different institutions.

Gentamicin was the first aminoglycoside evaluated extensively in patients with malignancies. A response rate of 51% was observed when it was used as the only active agent against infections in cancer patients (49). Gentamicin was very effective in patients who had adequate neutrophil counts or who responded to their infection with an increased production of neutrophils. However, only 22% of infections occurring in patients with severe neutropenia responded, and the response rate was even less in patients who had persistent neutropenia. These findings were in contrast with those with penicillins, that are often effective even in severely neutropenic patients. Nephrotoxicity occurred in 30% of patients with normal renal function at the onset of gentamicin therapy. This higher rate of nephrotoxicity, compared with that of 12% reported in general patient populations, was thought to be due to several reasons unique to cancer patients. Some of the patients had received repeated courses of therapy with other potentially nephrotoxic antibiotics and anti-cancer agents before receiving gentamicin. Ototoxicity was a significant side effect only in patients with compromised renal function.

Tobramycin resembles gentamicin closely in its antimicrobial and pharmacokinetic properties. Two recognized differences are its greater activity against *P. aeruginosa* and lower nephrotoxicity. Amikacin is a semisynthetic aminoglycoside the major advantage of which lies in its resistance to aminoglycoside-inactivating enzymes, making it useful against organisms resistant to other aminoglycosides. Netilmicin, another semisynthetic agent, is effective against some of the organisms resistant to other aminoglycosides, and it may be somewhat less toxic.

The reasons for inadequate response to aminoglycosides in patients with neutropenia are unclear. One reason might be inadequate serum concentrations with intermittent schedules of drug administration. Two studies suggested improved response rates to these agents when they are administered by continuous infusion (50). The incidence of nephrotoxicity was no higher than that previously noted with aminoglycosides given by intermittent injection to similar patient populations.

Quinolones

Although nalidixic acid, the first quinolone, was described in 1960, it was only after the synthesis of norfloxacin that this class of drugs became important. Quinolones act by inhibiting the enzyme DNA gyrase, which is an important component of the bacterial, but not mammalian, DNA replication system. The antibacterial spectrum of the new quinolones includes *Staph. aureus,* coagulase-negative staphylococci, *Enterobacteriaceae,* and *P. aeruginosa*. Activity against streptococci varies, with ciprofloxacin being much more active than norfloxacin, perfloxacin, or enoxacin. Ciprofloxacin is also active against intracellular pathogens such as *Chlamydia, Mycoplasma, Legionella, Brucella,* and *Mycobacterium*. Anaerobic organism are resistant to ciprofloxacin and other currently available quinolones. The availability of an oral formulation provides the option of beginning treatment with an oral agent or changing after initial parenteral therapy (51). Currently, there is very limited clinical experience with ciprofloxacin in neutropenic patients. In a randomized study of febrile neutropenic patients, ciprofloxacin plus netilmicin and piperacillin plus netilmicin produced similar overall response rates (59% and 62%, respectively) (52). In another study of 34 neutropenic patients with 46 febrile episodes, ciprofloxacin plus vancomycin produced an overall response rate of 86% (51). Adverse reactions were minimal and mainly related to vancomycin.

Antistaphylococcal Agents

The development of penicillinase-resistant semisynthetic penicillins marked a milestone in the therapy of infections caused by *Staph. aureus*. Immediately after the introduction of methicillin, the number of fatal infections caused by *Staph. aureus* decreased from about 25% to fewer than 5% (24). Thereafter, for many years, methicillin or cephalothin were routinely incorporated into empiric antibiotic regimens, and *Staph. aureus* infections became uncommon in neutropenic patients at many institutions, until recently.

Vancomycin, a narrow-spectrum bactericidal antibiotic was introduced in 1956 because of its effectiveness against penicillin-resistant staphylococci. However, because of its toxicity, it was used infrequently after methicillin became available. With the emergence of coagulase-negative staphylococci, resistant to antistaphylococcal penicillins and cephalosporins, as frequent pathogens in neutropenic patients, vancomycin has assumed an important role in antibiotic therapy. Vancomycin is also the drug of choice for therapy of infections caused by nosocomial pathogens, such as *C. jeikeium, Bacillus* spp. and some α-hemolytic streptococci. Since vancomycin is completely unrelated immunologically to β-lactam agents, it is the drug of choice for infections caused by gram-positive organisms in patients with serious hypersensitivity reactions to β-lactams. The most important adverse reaction to vancomycin is ototoxicity. Nephrotoxicity is now uncommon because of the availability of purer preparations, but nephrotoxicity has been reported when vancomycin and aminoglycosides are administered concomitantly (53).

Whether vancomycin should be included in the initial antibiotic regimen or added only after the causative organism has been identified is controversial (54). In one study, all patients received ticarcillin plus gentamicin and were randomly assigned to vancomycin or placebo as initial therapy for fever in neutropenic patients (55). None of the patients assigned to vancomycin, but 70% of patients assigned to placebo, subsequently developed gram-positive infections. However, in another study, the addition of vancomycin to the initial antibiotic regimen was necessary in fewer than 15% of the febrile episodes in neutropenic patients (43).

Newer drugs, including the glycopeptide complex teicoplanin, active against gram-positive organisms, are undergoing clinical evaluation. The spectrum of activity of teicoplanin includes essentially all strains of *Staphylococcus* spp., *Streptococcus* spp., *Enterococcus* spp., *C. jeikeium, Listeria monocytogenes, Clostridium difficile, C. perfringens,* anaerobic gram-positive cocci, and *Propionibacterium* spp. (56–58). The pharmacokinetic properties of teicoplanin permit once daily intravenous or intramuscular administration. Clinical studies suggest that the efficacy and adverse effects of teicoplanin are similar to those of vancomycin (59,60).

Selection of Empiric Antibacterial Therapy for Neutropenic Patients

In recent years, the selection of empiric therapy for the febrile neutropenic patient has required a reappraisal because of changes in the spectrum of pathogens causing infection and the introduction of potent, broader-spectrum antibiotics. Gram-negative bacilli are still one of the major causes of death and account for up to 50% of proved infections in cancer patients. *Escherichia coli, Klebsiella* spp., and *P. aeruginosa* are the most common gram-negative pathogens. Infections caused by gram-positive organisms have increased in frequency in recent years and have become the most common infections in some institutions (61). Some of these organisms are susceptible only to vancomycin. Some gram-negative organisms, such as *Aeromonas* spp. and *Pseudomonas* spp. other than *P. aeruginosa,* that are being reported as a cause of infection in neutropenic patients may also not respond to many of the conventional regimens used for initial empiric therapy.

β-Lactam antibiotics form the cornerstone of antibacterial therapy in neutropenic patients. Combination therapy with an aminoglycoside plus a β-lactam has been considered to be standard therapy for fever in neutropenic patients. However, the availability of several new broad-spectrum antibiotics has provided other alternatives. The most important goal of empiric therapy is to ensure broad-spectrum coverage against the majority of potential pathogens. Antibiotic selection should address the increasing significance of gram-positive organisms and the emergence of new pathogens. In addition, it is important to recognize that the predominant microbial flora and susceptibility patterns can vary considerably in different hospitals.

Several in vitro studies have shown synergistic interaction between β-lactams and aminoglycosides against selected gram-negative bacilli. The impact of antibiotic synergism has been evaluated in animal models of infection, with variable results. This potential for synergistic interaction has supported the selection of β-lactam plus aminoglycoside combinations as the most appropriate regimen for initial empiric therapy in neutropenic patients. However, with the availability of new, more potent, broader-spectrum β-lactams, the concept has required a reassessment. Several clinical studies have shown that synergism is not a significant prognostic factor, as long as the therapeutic regimen contains a potent β-lactam that is active against the infecting organism (62).

Another factor to be considered in the selection of empiric therapy for neutropenic patients is the side effects of the agents used and other therapies being administered to the patient concomitantly, to avoid agents with similar toxic profiles. The use of aminoglycosides is associated with potential ototoxicity and nephrotoxicity that may be accentuated by prior or coadministration of other therapeutic agents, such as diuretics, other antibiotics (vancomycin, amphotericin B), or antineoplastic agents (cisplatin). The β-lactams have a very favorable ratio of therapeutic to toxic effects. Their high therapeutic index and bactericidal activity renders them particularly beneficial for neutropenic patients.

Aminoglycosides-Containing Regimens

The conventional approach to empiric therapy of infections in neutropenic patients has involved an aminoglycoside in combination with a broad-spectrum β-lactam agent. The rationale for such therapy has been to provide broad-spectrum bactericidal activity against the most likely pathogens, the potential for synergistic activity, and the reduced likelihood of emergence of resistance. In an early, comparative study there were no overall differences in response rates among febrile, granulocytopenic patients with the use of carbenicillin plus cephalothin versus gentamicin plus carbenicillin or cephalothin. A subset of patients with infections caused by *E. coli* had a lower response rate to carbenicillin plus cephalothin, because some nosocomial strains were resistant to both of these drugs (63). Many recent clinical trials have failed to demonstrate a higher response rate for aminoglycoside-containing regimens in comparison with new broad-spectrum β-lactams. The risk of aminoglycoside-induced nephrotoxicity and ototoxicity may be increased in neutropenic patients because of concomitant drug therapy and other factors. The need for frequent monitoring of serum levels and renal function parameters also renders aminoglycosides less than ideal.

The results of clinical trials do not provide clear-cut direction for selection of a particular aminoglycoside for neutropenic patients. No differences in clinical outcome nor in the incidence of nephrotoxicity or ototoxicity were observed in patients randomized to receive either gentamicin, amikacin, or netilmicin, each in combination with ticarcillin (64). The study demonstrated that a significant number of patients will exhibit toxic responses. In a comparative trial of gentamicin, amikacin, and sisomicin, each in combination with carbenicillin (50), no significant difference was observed in the overall response rate. The selection of an aminoglycoside is often governed by cost, but amikacin may be preferable in hospitals having a high prevalence of infection caused by gentamicin- and tobramycin-resistant gram-negative bacilli.

Double β-Lactam Regimens

The concept of using two β-lactam agents in the therapy of infections in neutropenic patients was first reported with the use of carbenicillin and cephalothin (65). Because of the proved efficacy of β-lactams in neutropenic patients, it was felt that a broad-spectrum penicillin plus a cephalosporin would be at least as effective as an aminoglycoside-containing combination. The combination of carbenicillin plus cephalothin was comparable with that of carbenicillin plus kanamycin as empiric therapy of infections in neutropenic cancer patients. Ticarcillin in combination with cephalothin or gentamicin for empiric therapy of infections in neutropenic patients was reported by a number of investigators to be efficacious and comparable with each.

With the availability of cefamandole, with better activity against *E. coli*, *Enterobacter* spp., and *Serratia marcescens*, double β-lactam regimens were studied further (66). Cefamandole in combination with carbenicillin was comparable with cefamandole plus tobramycin as empiric therapy of infections in neutropenic patients. The two regimens of moxalactam plus ticarcillin and moxalactam plus tobramycin were equally effective for the initial treatment of infections in patients with neutropenia. The in vitro activity and pharmacokinetics of moxalactam plus piperacillin compared favorably with that of moxalactam plus amikacin (67). The two combinations were also equally efficacious for treatment of infections in neutropenic patients. In addition, significantly lower rates of both nephrotoxicity and ototoxicity were noted in the group receiving moxalactam plus piperacillin.

A review of published studies suggests that double β-lactam regimens are comparable in efficacy with aminoglycoside-containing β-lactam regimens and avoid the potential of nephrotoxicity and ototoxicity. Of concern in recent years has been the emergence of resistant gram-positive organisms as major pathogens in neutropenic patients. Neither double β-lactam nor β-lactam–aminoglycoside combinations provide adequate coverage against these organisms.

β-Lactams Plus Vancomycin With or Without Aminoglycosides

The role of vancomycin in empiric therapy of infections in neutropenic patients is not now entirely clear. The most debatable issue is whether to add vancomycin to the initial regimen or add it once the causative organism has been identified (54). Ceftazidime plus vancomycin was shown to be effective and safe for empiric therapy in neutropenic patients. However, the study did not include a regimen without vancomycin. The addition of vancomycin to ticarcillin–clavulanic acid was shown to reduce the morbidity from gram-positive infections when compared with the same regimen without vancomycin (55). A subsequent study revealed that only 15% of the febrile episodes in neutropenic patients required vancomycin in the initial empiric regimen (43). The authors suggested that the addition of vancomycin to the primary antibiotic regimens for febrile episodes in neutropenic patients would represent an overuse of an expensive and important antimicrobial agent. A more recent study, however, concluded that the combination of vancomycin ticarcillin, and amikacin is more effective than ticarcillin–clavulanate plus amikacin as empiric therapy, especially in clinical settings in which gram-positive bacteremias are a serious problem (68). The study showed a 15% failure rate with a combination of vancomycin, ticarcillin, and amikacin, compared with 38% failure rate in the group receiving ticarcillin–clavulanate and amikacin.

Monotherapy

Single-agent empiric therapy of infections in neutropenic infections may be safe and feasible under certain circumstances. The choice of antibiotic employed becomes of paramount importance in monotherapy. Most of the recent reported studies have employed third-generation cephalosporins, (cefoperazone, ceftazidime), ticarcillin–clavulanate, or imipenem. Ceftazidime alone has been as effective as ceftazidime plus tobramycin in the treatment of gram-negative bacillary infections, but was not adequate therapy for gram-positive infections (42). A prospective randomized study comparing ceftazidime alone with the combination of cephalothin, gentamicin–carbenicillin concluded that single-agent therapy is a safe alternative to standard combination antibiotic therapy (43). However, many of the patients in both groups required subsequent modifications in their therapy. No modification to either regimen was necessary for successful therapy of 78% of episodes of unexplained fever, but modification of initial therapy was required for all documented infections irrespective of the initial regimen.

Imipenem–cilastatin was evaluated for treatment of febrile episodes in cancer patients, most of whom were neutropenic (47). The overall response rate was comparable with results with β-lactam plus aminoglycoside, double β-lactam, and β-lactam plus vancomycin regimens. Similar results were obtained with ticarcillin–clavulanate as a single agent (48).

Although about 20 studies have demonstrated support for this approach, caution must be exercised because of differences in study designs, wide range of response definitions, small patient numbers, and small numbers of documented infections. However, the simplicity of administration, lower incidence of side effects, and possible lower cost are the major advantages of monotherapy.

The two important potential disadvantages with single-agent therapy are an increased risk of resistance emerging during therapy and a greater likelihood of superinfection by resistant organisms. The important factors to be taken into consideration for monotherapy are (1) the constant changes in the organisms that predominate as cause of infection; (2) the emergence of *Staph. epidermidis, C. jeikeium,* and enterococci as relatively common pathogens in some institutions; (3) an increase in the incidence of gram-negative bacilli other than *Klebsiella* spp., *E. coli,* and *P. aeruginosa* as causes of infection and their relative resistance to commonly used antibiotics; and (4) the microbial flora of the institution.

Effect of Dosing Schedules of Antibiotics on Empiric Therapy in Neutropenic Patients

The complexities of infection make it difficult to design studies that will conclusively demonstrate whether or not the schedule of antibiotic administration is an important consideration. Most of the available data suggest that the schedule of antibiotic administration is important in neutropenic patients (69). The important reasons for this observation are (1) the lack of inflammatory response in neutropenic patients makes antibiotics virtually the sole means of antibacterial activity; (2) intermittent schedules of antibiotic administration result in intervals between doses when serum concentrations are suboptimal; (3) rapid recovery of gram-negative bacilli after exposure to some antibiotics; (4) animal data indicating suboptimal response in the presence of inadequate serum antibiotic concentrations; and (5) clinical studies in neutropenic patients suggesting that continuous aminoglycoside infusion therapy is superior. A study on the comparison of standard versus pharmacokinetically adjusted amikacin dosing in neutropenic patients showed that it is difficult to achieve specifically defined serum concentrations, even with sophisticated pharmacokinetic dosing, and such techniques cannot be substituted for serum levels. However, appropriate serum levels could be established more reliably by using pharmacokinetically adjusted dosage schedules.

The response rates to ticarcillin were much better when dosages of 3.5 g every 4 hours were used, compared with 5 g every 6 hours, suggesting the importance of dosage schedule in the administration of β-lactam antibiotics (70). Cefamandole, given by continuous infusion, was shown to have better efficacy than when given by intermittent infusion (66), particularly for the therapy of gram-negative infections in patients with persistent severe neutropenia.

Definition of Response and Duration of Antimicrobial Therapy in Neutropenic Patients

The appropriate duration of therapy in a febrile neutropenic patient when no infectious source or agent is identified remains debatable. In the first study addressing this issue during 81 febrile episodes, 76 cancer patients with neutropenia were randomly allocated to continue or discontinue antibiotics 4 days after initiation of carbenicillin and cephalothin therapy, if no infection had been demonstrated (71). This study indicated that antibiotics can be discontinued after 7 days if the patient responds to initial empiric therapy and no specific infection can be documented, but earlier cessation may be hazardous, especially if the neutrophil count has not recovered. However, for patients not responding after the initial 3–4 days of therapy, modification of therapy is usually indicated. The modification most commonly involves the addition of empiric antifungal therapy. Some investigators have suggested that once antibiotic therapy has been initiated, it should be continued until the neutrophil count has recovered, even though that may be long after the infection has responded. A less expensive and equally effective approach would be to change to oral prophylaxis with trimethoprim–sulfamethoxazole or a quinolone once the infection has been treated successfully.

Role of Granulocyte Transfusions

Although early clinical trials suggested that granulocyte transfusions are useful for controlling infection in neutropenic patients who do not respond to antibiotic therapy (72), the availability of more effective antibiotic regimens has reduced the use of this therapeutic modality. The usefulness of white blood cell transfusions is limited by (1) the short half-life of these cells, (2) the requirement for histocompatible donors for effective increments in recipient's granulocyte counts, (3) the need for daily transfusions of large numbers of granulocytes (0.5×10^{10} to 3×10^{10} per transfusion for 3–4 days), and (4) the risk of rapid migration of granulocytes to the lungs, causing hypoxemia in patients with pneumonia. However, white cell transfusions remain a useful addition to antibiotics in a subset of neutropenic patients who fail to respond to appropriate therapy. Current indications for granulocyte transfusions include the clinical setting of (1) neutropenia of fewer than 100 neutrophils/μL, (2) a documented bacterial infection (especially gram-negative infection), (3) remote likelihood of bone marrow recovery within 4–7 days after the onset of infection, and (4) failure to respond despite 48–72 hours of optimal antibiotic therapy. Under these circumstances, granulocyte transfusions improve the rate of survival from the infectious episode (73). The use of prophylactic granulocyte transfusions has shown no beneficial effect.

Conclusions Concerning Initial Therapy for Fever in Neutropenic Patients

Basic principles of antibiotic therapy for infections in neutropenic patients have been established and should be observed:

1. Institution of prompt antibiotic therapy for suspected infections in neutropenic patients is of critical importance.
2. Response to effective antimicrobial therapy is related to the recovery of the neutrophil count during the infectious episode.
3. Aminoglycosides as single agents are ineffective in neutropenic patients.
4. High serum bactericidal concentrations are essential for any antimicrobial agent to constitute effective therapy.
5. β-Lactams alone or in combination form the cornerstone of antimicrobial therapy in neutropenic patients.
6. The introduction of new, more potent, and broader-spectrum β-lactams has made regimens available that spare the potential nephrotoxicity and ototoxicity related to aminoglycosides.
7. Aztreonam, a β-lactam agent, immunologically unrelated to other agents, can be given safely to patients with serious hypersensitivity reactions to other β-lactams.
8. In neutropenic patients, not responding to antimicrobial therapy, granulocyte transfusions should be considered and can be lifesaving.

Antifungal Therapy

Polyenes

Amphotericin B was the first broad-spectrum parenteral agent that provided curative therapy for systemic mycoses. It is a polyene macrolide antibiotic produced by the actinomycete, *Streptomyces nodosus*. Amphotericin B attaches to ergosterol in fungal cell membranes and interferes with their steric integrity, leading to osmotic leak of intracellular potassium and extracellular sodium. The considerable toxicity of amphotericin B is explained by the cross-reactivity between its attraction to ergosterol in fungal membranes and to cholesterol in mammalian cell membranes. Another effect that has been recently appreciated is related to fungal cell damage caused by amphotericin B auto-oxidation, which is responsible for fungal cell death (74). Whether or not this oxidative damage contributes to the toxicity of amphotericin B for mammalian cells is not known.

Resistance to amphotericin B appears to be caused by loss or substitution of ergosterol from the fungal cell membrane and has been described in rare mutants of *Candida* spp. Tolerance to amphotericin B has recently been described for *C. parapsilosis*. Isolates of *C. lusitaniae,* an emerging opportunistic pathogen in immunocompromised hosts, and *Pseudoallescheria boydii* are generally resistant to amphotericin B. Amphotericin B is the drug of choice for endemic mycoses (such as histoplasmosis, blastomycosis, and coccidioidomycosis) and for aspergillosis, candidiasis, cryptococcosis, and zygomycosis.

The usual dosage for candidiasis is 0.5–0.6 mg/kg per day. The appropriate duration of therapy has not been determined. The resolution of infection depends on recovery of the patient's neutrophil count, and almost no patients with persistent neutropenia have responded to therapy. In those patients who respond as their neutrophil count recovers, it is recommended that therapy be continued for at least 2 weeks after resolution of all signs and symptoms of infection. There are limited data suggesting that the addition of flucytosine to amphotericin B improves its efficacy against *Candida* spp. (especially *C. tropicalis*).

For infections caused by *Aspergillus* spp. and *Zygomycetes* (mucormycosis) in neutropenic patients, the dosage of amphotericin B should be escalated rapidly to 1 mg/kg per day until renal impairment requires change to an every-other-day schedule. Surgical excision of infected tissue should be considered when feasible. There is anecdotal data suggesting that combining amphotericin B with flucytosine may enhance its efficacy. As with systemic candidiasis, resolution of infection in neutropenic patients is rarely, if ever, achieved unless the neutrophil count recovers.

The pharmacokinetics of amphotericin B have not been well characterized and the standard dosage, schedule, and duration of therapy have not been defined. The mean peak serum concentration is about 1 μg/mL after 30 mg is administered intravenously over several hours and about 2 μg/mL after 50 mg is administered. Serum concentrations do not appear to increase with increasing doses over 50 mg. The average steady-state concentration of the drug in plasma is about 0.5 μg/mL. The initial serum half-life is about 24 hours, and the terminal half-life is 15 days. There is no close correlation between the dose administered and the serum concentration. The trough concentrations with the every-other-day schedule usually are similar to those achieved with the daily dosage schedule. The drug does not penetrate the blood–brain barrier adequately. A major portion of the drug is bound to tissues and released slowly. The highest concentration of amphotericin B are detected in the liver, and substantial concentrations are also detected in the spleen, kidney, and lung.

The major excretory pathway of amphotericin B remains unknown. About 3–13% appears in the urine within 24 hours after a single dose and 40% after 7 days. Only 2–5% can be detected in the urine following multiple doses. Low levels can be detected in the urine for at least 7 weeks after cessation of therapy. Reduced renal function has little effect on the serum concentration because the fraction of the drug excreted in urine is so low. The drug is not removed during dialysis procedures.

The toxicities of amphotericin B frequently dictate the dose and schedule of drug administration, rather than the response to therapy. Amphotericin B cause acute toxicities that may be idiosyncratic or dose-related, as well as chronic toxicities. Idiosyncratic reactions include flushing, anaphylactic shock, acute liver failure, thrombocytopenia, vertigo, generalized pain, grand mal seizures, ventricular fibrillation and cardiac arrest, rash, and hearing loss. Fever and chills occur in virtually all patients. Headache occurs in 45% of patients, anorexia in 50%, and vomiting in 20%.

Amphotericin B suppresses production of red blood cells, possibly by reducing erythropoietin production, and causes a normocytic normochromic anemia. The anemia occurs early during treatment, then stabilizes, and transfusions usually are not required. Nephrotoxicity is the most serious side effect of amphotericin B therapy, and virtually every patient develops some manifestation of renal damage. The usual side effects include urinary abnormalities, hyposthenuria, azotemia, hypokalemia, renal tubular acidosis, and nephrocalcinosis. Approximately 90% of patients develop an increase in blood urea nitrogen or creatinine. There is no correlation between the degree of azotemia and the total dose of amphotericin B administered. Renal tubular acidosis with renal potassium loss may result in hypokalemia, which can be minimized by supplemental alkali and potassium administration.

Flucytosine

Flucytosine (5-fluorocytosine) is a synthetic fluorinated pyramidine that is taken into the fungal cell with the aid of the enzyme cytosine permease. It is deaminated to form 5-fluorouracil and also converted to form fluorodeoxyuridine. 5-Fluorouracil is incorporated into RNA and, thus, interferes with RNA and protein synthesis. Fluorodeoxyuridine monophosphate inhibits thymidylate synthetase and DNA synthesis. Mammalian cells do not convert large amounts of flucytosine to 5-fluorouracil, hence, its selective toxicity against fungi.

The spectrum of fungal agents susceptible to flucytosine is narrow and includes *Cryptococcus neoformans, Candida* spp., and some strains of *Sporothrix* spp. and *Aspergillus* spp. Resistance to flucytosine may occur at any enzymatic step, including cytosine penetration into the fungal cell, deamination, uridine monophosphate, pyrophosphorylase, and enhancement of the de novo synthesis of pyrimidines. About 5–10% of isolates of *C. neoformans* and *Candida* spp. are inherently resistant to flucytosine, and at least 5% of susceptible organisms develop resistance during therapy. Flucytosine should not be used alone because of the problems of inherent and acquired resistance. Because of synergistic interaction between flucytosine and amphotericin B, the combination is used for therapy of cryptococcosis and candidiasis. Sporadic reports suggest that the combination may be beneficial against aspergillosis. The use of flucytosine in treating fungal infections in patients with hematological malignancies is restricted because it may interfere with bone marrow recovery in patients receiving myelosuppressive therapy.

Side effects have been reported in 5–22% of the patients, despite careful adjustment of flucytosine dose for renal failure (75). Side effects usually involve the bone marrow, liver, and gastrointestinal tract. Myelotoxicity, manifested by anemia, is the most difficult to manage and is more likely to occur if the serum concentration exceeds 100 μg/mL. Presumably, this toxicity is due to conversion of flucytosine to 5-fluorouracil in the gastrointestinal tract. The most common gastrointestinal toxicities are nausea, vomiting, and diarrhea. Hepatic toxicities consist of elevated serum transaminases and alkaline phosphatase that are reversible. Because the drug is excreted primarily in the urine, dosage must be adjusted according to renal function.

Azole Antifungal Agents

Several substituted azole compounds with substantial antifungal activity have been synthesized in the last two decades. The mechanism of action of these compounds is the inhibition of cytochrome P-450 enzymes (14α-sterol demethylase) of fungal cells and to a lesser degree of mammalian cells. This effect leads to inhibition of ergosterol synthesis, which alters cell membrane fluidity and permeability. Other target sites for these drugs may be involved and may contribute to resistance to azoles in addition to lack of sensitivity of 14α-sterol demethylase (76). Clotrimazole, econazole, and miconazole were the first three azoles reported to be suitable for human use. All three have a broad spectrum of antifungal activity in vitro. Clotrimazole and econazole are, however, utilized only as topical agents for dermatophytosis and cutaneous and mucocutaneous candidiasis because of their side effects.

Miconazole, the first azole derivative to be administered intravenously, has broad-spectrum activity against virtually all pathogenic fungi, except *Aspergillus* spp. and *Zygomycetes*. It is considered the drug of choice for infections caused by *Pseudoallescheria boydii*. Its use for other susceptible fungi should be restricted to patients who fail to respond or cannot be given amphotericin B and cannot be given oral ketoconazole.

The side effects that have been reported with miconazole are local phlebitis, pruritus, rash, nausea and vomiting, fever, and chills. About 45% of patients develop a transient normocytic or microcytic anemia. As many as 30% develop thrombocytosis, although thrombocytopenia also has been reported. Hyponatremia, hyperlipidemia, and increased serum triglycerides, with or without elevated serum cholesterol levels, occur during therapy. These side effects do not appear to be dose-related and resolve when the drug is discontinued. Transient tachycardia, cardiac arrhythmias, anaphylaxis, cardiac arrest, and respiratory arrest have occurred occasionally. These side effects have been attributed to the use of too concentrated preparations or too rapid infusion of drug.

Ketoconazole

Ketoconazole is a synthetic imidazole compound related to miconazole that is active against most pathogenic fungi, except many isolates of *C. tropicalis,*

Aspergillus spp. and *Zygomycetes*. Ketoconazole is available only as an oral preparation and requires a normal intragastric pH for absorption. Hence, the drug is not effective in patients receiving antacids or H_2 blockers. Of special concern are the observations of lower mean peak serum concentrations in neutropenic patients and in bone marrow transplant recipients. The drug penetrates the blood–brain barrier very poorly. It is metabolized in the liver by degradation of the imidazole ring, and the inactive metabolites are excreted in the bile. About 15% of ketoconazole is excreted in the urine, but only a small amount as active drug.

Ketoconazole is an effective alternative to amphotericin B for treatment of immunocompetent individuals with uncomplicated histoplasmosis, blastomycosis, mucocutaneous candidiasis, and coccidioidomycosis. A comparative study of amphotericin B and ketoconazole for therapy of presumed or proved fungal infections in neutropenic cancer patients showed the two agents were equally effective overall (77). Neither agent was effective against disseminated candidiasis or aspergillan infections. Also, none of the *C. tropicalis* infections treated with ketoconazole responded.

Anorexia, nausea, and vomiting occur in 3–10% of patients. Abdominal pain and pruritus without rash occur in 1–2% of patients. There have been rare cases of anaphylaxis following the first dose of ketoconazole. Hepatic toxicity has been observed in about 1–14% of patients and usually consists of transient elevation of serum transaminases and alkaline phosphatase levels, which return to normal upon cessation of therapy. Severe hepatic toxicity appears to be due to hypersensitivity and is characterized histopathologically by enlarged portal tracts, with infiltration by mononuclear cells and sporadic areas of necrosis. Rare cases of fatal diffuse hepatic necrosis have been reported.

Ketoconazole depresses serum testosterone concentrations, resulting in increased estradiol/testosterone ratios within 6 weeks of therapy. About 5% of males develop bilateral gynecomastia that may or may not persist until therapy is discontinued. Ketoconazole has a direct effect on steroidogenesis by the adrenal gland in humans, leading to impaired cortisol responses to corticotropin and mildly symptomatic hypoadrenalism. A case of frank adrenal crisis secondary to high-dose ketoconazole therapy was recently reported (78). Concomitant administration with cyclosporine increases the serum concentration of cyclosporine, presumably because of interference with hepatic metabolism. Ketoconazole may also enhance the anticoagulant effect of coumarin-type drugs.

Triazoles

The triazoles represent the second generation of azole derivatives. Itraconazole is a systemic antifungal triazole with a markedly increased spectrum and increased potency. It is more active than ketoconazole in vitro against *Histoplasma capsulatum, Blastomyces dermatitidis, Cryptococcus neoformans, Aspergillus* spp., and demataceous fungi (79). Although the number of patients evaluated is small, itraconazole has been shown to be effective and well-tolerated in histoplasmosis, coccidioidomycosis, and aspergillosis.

Fluconazole is available as intravenous and oral preparations and has the advantages of excellent cerebrospinal fluid penetration, prolonged serum half-life, and excretion primarily by the kidney. The spectrum of antifungal activity is, however, narrower than that of itraconazole. Clinical studies in cryptococcal meningitis using fluconazole as primary therapy as well as after failure of amphotericin B has shown fluconazole to be highly effective (79). Fluconazole is also excellent in the treatment of thrush in AIDS patients. Preliminary studies have suggested that fluconazole may be effective in the treatment of candidiasis in neutropenic patients. The toxicities of fluconazole, like itraconazole, are lower than those of ketoconazole.

Liposomal Amphotericin B

In an effort to target amphotericin B to the lesions and to decrease its toxicity, liposomal preparations have been studied in the last few years. The enhancement of therapeutic index is related to the lack of susceptibility of mammalian cells to the actions of amphotericin B in a liposomal form, and a substantial reduction of toxicity has been demonstrated in patients receiving liposomal amphotericin B. Two independent investigators have confirmed the efficacy of liposomal amphotericin B in patients with aspergillosis and candidiasis (79). The most significant responses were seen in hepatosplenic candidiasis because most of the patients had failed to respond to amphotericin B therapy. Doses up to 7 mg/kg can be given, with significantly reduced toxicity.

Role of Empiric Antifungal Therapy

Suppression of normal commensal organisms in the gastrointestinal tract by broad-spectrum antibiotics may contribute to fungal colonization of the mouth, bowel, skin, and bladder. Greater success in the treatment of bacterial infection in neutropenic patients and improved supportive care result in longer survival, thereby increasing the period at risk for development of fungal infections in these patients. The practice of using indwelling vascular catheters has been associated with an increased frequency of fungemia, especially among patients receiving total parenteral nutrition.

A major obstacle to the successful management of fungal infections in neutropenic patients is the difficulty in establishing a diagnosis. Fever is most often the only clinical sign of infection in these patients, and fungal infection may be considered clinically, but confirmed only at autopsy examination. In the past, fewer than 30% of patients with fungal infections received antifungal therapy. Consequently, empiric administration of amphotericin B to neutropenic patients with fever unresponsive to antibacterial antibiotics has become an accepted practice.

Only two randomized studies have examined the role of amphotericin B in empiric therapy of neutropenic patients (80). In one study, 38% of neutropenic patients with persistent fever, in whom combination antibacterial therapy was discontinued after 1 week, developed infection, primarily with bacterial pathogens. The same percentage (38%) of patients continued on combination therapy developed infection, most of which were caused by fungal pathogens. In contrast, only 10% of the patients who received empiric amphotericin B developed subsequent fungal infection. In a second study, patients were assigned to continued antibacterial antibiotics, with or without amphotericin B. The subsequent response rates of 60% and 37%, respectively, were significantly different, although the mortality rates were similar (17% versus 22%). Empiric antifungal therapy is clearly indicated for some patients and incidence of toxicity can be minimized by treating only those patients at greatest risk of acquiring a fungal infection.

Antiviral Therapy

During the past decade, substantial progress has been made in antiviral chemotherapy. Herpesviruses constitute the most important viral pathogens in patients with hematologic malignancies, especially those receiving bone marrow transplants. Early studies suggested possible efficacy of the nucleoside analogues, idoxuridine and cytarabine (cytosine arabinoside), but their unacceptable toxicities prevented their use in systemic viral infections. The spectrum of activity of antiviral agents available for clinical use is shown in Table 5.

Vidarabine (Adenine Arabinoside; ara-A)

Vidarabine, is an analogue of adenine deoxyriboside which has in vitro antiviral activity against herpes simplex viruses (HSV), varicella–zoster (VZV), and Epstein–Barr virus. Vidarabine inhibits the in vitro replication of acyclovir-resistant HSV strains and acyclovir-resistant VZV strains. The mechanism of antiviral activity of vidarabine is not completely understood. It is phosphorylated by cellular enzymes to the triphosphate derivative, which competitively inhibits

Table 5 Spectrum of Antiviral Agents Used in Patients with Hematological Malignancy

Organism	Vidarabine	Acyclovir	Ganciclovir
Herpes simplex virus	++	+++	+++
Varicella–zoster virus	++	+++	+++
Cytomegalovirus	Variable	Variable	+++
Epstein-Barr virus	+	+	+

HSV DNA polymerase activity. Cellular DNA polymerase is inhibited to a lesser extent. Vidarabine triphosphate is incorporated into both cellular and viral DNA and acts as a chain terminator for newly synthesized HSV nucleic acid.

The primary route of clearance is renal and most of the drug is excreted as its metabolite ara-hypoxanthine. In patients with renal insufficiency, plasma ara-hypoxanthine concentrations are increased and may be associated with neurological or other side effects.

Vidarabine has been used extensively in patients with disseminated herpes simplex infection, especially those with encephalitis. Vidarabine is also effective in immunocompromised individuals with chickenpox and localized or disseminated herpes zoster infections. For mucocutaneous herpes simplex infections, benefit from vidarabine therapy was shown to be limited to patients over 40 years of age. Clinically, modest reductions in the duration of pain, fever, and shedding of HSV type 1 were observed in vidarabine recipients.

The most common dose-related side effects are anorexia, nausea, vomiting, and weight loss. At higher dosages (20 mg/kg per day) vidarabine is associated with megaloblastic anemia, leukopenia, and thrombocytopenia. Infusion-related thrombophlebitis, hypokalemia, rash, and the syndrome of inappropriate secretion of antidiuretic hormones have been described. The neurotoxic side effects of vidarabine include pain syndromes, tremor, myoclonus, ataxis, disorientation, depression, aphasia, hallucinations, and rarely coma or seizures (81).

Acyclovir (Acycloguanosine)

Acyclovir is the prototype of a group of antiviral agents that are converted to active metabolites only in virus-infected cells by the virus-specific enzyme thymidine kinase (TK). The virus-specific TK readily phosphorylates acyclovir, forming acyclovir monophosphate (ACV-MP), which is further phosphorylated to acyclovir diphosphate (ACV-DP) and acyclovir triphosphate (ACV-TP) by cellular enzymes. Acyclovir triphosphate is a potent inhibitor of viral DNA polymerase, but exhibits for less inhibition of cellular DNA polymerases. Acyclovir resistance in herpes viruses is due to selection of mutants that lack thymidine kinase, have a kinase with altered substrate specificity, or have a DNA polymerase with altered substrate specificity.

Both oral and intravenous acyclovir prophylaxis are effective in suppressing HSV infection in bone marrow transplant recipients. Short-term acyclovir suppression should be considered in severely immunocompromised patients with a history or serologic evidence of past HSV infection who undergo bone marrow transplantation or induction chemotherapy. The use of topical acyclovir should be limited to patients with external lesions only. Randomized, controlled, double-blind studies have demonstrated that acyclovir is the most effective antiviral compound currently available for prevention or treatment of herpes simplex virus infections in patients with hematological malignancies (82). Acyclovir was demonstrated to be clearly superior to vidarabine for treatment of VZV infection in bone marrow transplant recipients and patients with hematological malignancies. Acyclovir is also preferred when there is a high risk of cardiorespiratory failure secondary to the large volume of fluid required for vidarabine infusion.

The toxicity of acyclovir is generally thought to be less than that of vidarabine. Phlebitis can occur at thc infusion site. Uncommon side effects include rash, diaphoresis, hematuria, hypotension, headache, and nausea. Encephalopathic changes characterized by lethargy, obtundation, tremors, confusion, hallucination, delerium, seizures, or coma occur in approximately 1% of patients. Administration of intrathecal methotrexate or interferon may predispose to these side effects.

Reversible renal dysfunction occurs in approximately 5% of patients treated with intravenous acyclovir, 5 mg/kg every 8 hours. Bolus infusion, dehydration, high doses, and preexisting renal insufficiency appear to predispose to renal toxicity.

Ganciclovir (Dihydroxypropoxymethylguanine;DHPG)

Ganciclovir is a nucleoside analogue that has excellent in vitro activity against the herpes group of viruses, including cytomegalovirus. Ganciclovir is phosphorylated initially by virus thymidine kinase, followed by phosphorylation to triphosphate by cellular enzymes. Ganciclovir is an effective treatment for cytomegalovirus infections in patients with AIDS or following organ transplantation. Cytomegaloviral retinitis and enteritis have a high response rate to ganciclovir, although recurrences are common after discontinuation of therapy. Cytomegaloviral pneumonitis has been studied, but no clear-cut recommendations are possible from the available data. Two recent studies with small groups of patients have shown that ganciclovir combined with high-dose intravenous immune globulin, significantly altered the outcome of patients with CMV pneumonia after allogeneic bone marrow transplantation (83), and was superior to results obtained with ganciclovir or intravenous immunoglobulin alone.

Role of Modalities to Accelerate Bone Marrow Recovery

Earlier studies with immunoregulatory reagents, such as lithium chloride, proved disappointing in shortening the period of granulocytopenia in patients with leukemia. The recent availability of recombinant cytokines, including granulocyte–monocyte colony-stimulating factor (GM-CSF) and granulocyte colony-stimulating factor (G-CSF) have provided new therapeutic opportunities. Evaluation of these factors in large groups of patients is currently underway in a number of institutions. By reducing the duration of granulocytopenia, the colony-stimulating factors may shorten the duration of antibiotic therapy and reduce the incidence of infections and, especially, superinfections caused by resistant bacteria and fungi.

PROPHYLAXIS OF INFECTIONS IN PATIENTS WITH HEMATOLOGICAL MALIGNANCY

Infection prophylaxis is an important consideration in the care of patients with hematological malignancies. The earliest attempt to prophylaxis was the use of protected environment plus prophylactic antibiotics. The original objective of prophylactic programs was to provide the patient with the maximal protection possible against microbial contamination. To achieve this goal, a program was developed that incorporated reverse isolation, filtered air, application of topical antibiotics to body orifices, special bathing procedures, "sterile" food, and nonabsorbable broad-spectrum antibiotics designed to sterilize the oropharynx and gastrointestinal tract. The development of laminar airflow rooms made patient isolation more practical. High-efficiency air filters remove 99.95% of all particulate matter. Microbial contamination of laminar airflow rooms is substantially less than in regular rooms. The results of initial studies done in patients with acute leukemia demonstrated fewer infections and infectious deaths than in control patients. Several prospective randomized studies have confirmed that protected environment–prophylactic antibiotic programs reduce the risk of infection in patients with hematological malignancies (84). Such programs do not necessarily add to the long-term survival in these patients, which is ultimately related to effective therapy of the underlying malignancy. This type of program has also been effective in bone marrow transplant recipients by preventing infections, graft-versus-host disease, and pulmonary complications.

Antibacterial Prophylaxis

The success of oral antimicrobial regimens in preventing bacterial infections in neutropenic patients is dependent on many variables. The important identifiable factors are degree and duration of neutropenia, type of underlying malignancy, the selection of antimicrobial agents and their spectrum of activity, the type and intensity of chemotherapy, the definition of an infectious complication, the criteria used to define success of prophylactic regimens, and patient compliance (85). When trimethoprim–sulfamethoxazole was demonstrated to be effective in preventing pneumocystis pneumonia in susceptible children, a concomitant reduction in bacterial infections was also observed. A multitude of studies conducted subsequently using trimethoprim–sulfamethoxazole alone or in combination with other agents have given conflicting results for the efficacy and relative safety of this approach. The availability of oral quinolones has renewed enthusiasm for antibacterial prophylaxis in neutropenic patients. Oral norfloxacin prophylaxis during granulocytopenia has been effective in reducing the frequency of aerobic gram-negative infections and in preventing the emergence of multidrug-resistant pathogens. A recent study comparing oral ciprofloxacin with trimethoprim–sulfamethoxazole plus colistin showed ciprofloxacin to be highly effective in preventing gram-negative infections. Ciprofloxacin prevented colonization with resistant gram-negative bacilli, whereas trimethoprim–sulfamethoxazole plus colistin was less effective. Ciprofloxacin was tolerated much better than trimethoprim–sulfamethoxazole plus colistin (86).

The most important drawback of antibacterial prophylaxis with nonabsorbable or systemic antibiotics is the emergence of resistant organisms. The trials of nonabsorbable antibiotics, such as neomycin, bacitracin, kanamycin, polymixin B, and gentamicin, have shown conflicting results on the emergence of resistance. In some studies the susceptibility of emerging or persisting gram-negative bacilli, such as *E. coli, Klebsiella* spp., *Enterobacter* spp., and *Proteus mirabilis* was clearly decreased in patients receiving these antibiotics. In one study, 69% of organism isolated from placebo-treated patients were sensitive to trimethoprim–sulfamethoxazole, compared with 24% in trimethoprim–sulfamethoxazole-treated patients. Although this has not yet been a problem with quinolones, it is likely to be observed in the future with more extensive use.

Immunization

Passive Immunization and Role of Immunoglobulin Therapy

The adjunctive use of immunoglobulins in the therapy of patients with hematological malignancies was first evaluated as early as 1964 (87). The study failed to demonstrate a beneficial effect of immunoglobulins during febrile episodes in patients with acute leukemia. The availability of hyperimmune sera, polyclonal intravenous, immunoglobulins, monoclonal antibodies, and the demonstration of antibody-dependent cell-mediated cytotoxicity (ADCC) against infectious agents have reactivated the interest in passive immunotherapy.

Interaction between immunoglobulins and antibiotics has been studied recently. Synergistic activity between acylureidopenicillins and IgG was demonstrated in experimental animals. In addition to stimulating phagocytosis nonspecifically, this effect is attributed to inactivation of β-lactamase activity by specific antibodies against β-lactamases. Immunoglobulin G was noted to potentiate the effects of both tobramycin and azlocillin in the treatment of *P. aeruginosa* septicemia in neutropenic mice. The protection afforded by immunoglobulins results, in part, from neutralization of exotoxin A, which is an important virulence factor in the pathogenesis of *P. aeruginosa* infection. Hyperimmune IgG preparation was effective for treatment of experimental *P. aeruginosa* pneumonia.

The use of an antiserum directed against core endotoxin antigens resulted in a significant reduction in death and increased recovery from shock complicating gram-negative sepsis. However, the protective effect was less impressive in cancer and neutropenic patients (88). Patients with acute leukemia have lower levels of antibody to the core glycolipid of *Enterobacteriaceae* than patients without cancer. The antibody levels fall in patients receiving cytotoxic therapy, and patients developing gram-negative bacteremias have lower levels of antibody than patients in whom infection does not develop.

The use of newer intravenous immunoglobulins in patients with multiple myeloma and chronic lymphocytic leukemia has had beneficial effects in lowering the incidence and severity of infections (89). The usual regimen employed is 400 mg/kg of body weight every 3–4 weeks. Bone marrow transplant recipients in the postengraftment period also have deficiency of humoral immune defense mechanisms. Various immunoglobulin preparations have been used in these patients, primarily for prophylaxis and therapy of cytomegalovirus infections. These studies suggested that administration of intravenous immunoglobulins may be an effective method to decrease the incidence of septicemias, other than those caused by coagulase-negative staphylococci (90).

Postexposure prophylaxis using varicella–zoster immune globulin is recommended for all susceptible patients younger than 15 years of age and in adults and adolescents with hematological malignancies, on an individual basis.

Active Immunization

Live vaccines should be avoided in patients with hematological malignancies because of the potential of unrestricted proliferation. Killed vaccines and component vaccines are safe for these patients. The potential benefit of active immunization in these patients remains doubtful. Various immunogenic preparations of *P. aeruginosa,* including heptavalent lipopolysaccharide and O-specific side chains of *P. aeruginosa* lipopolysaccharide have failed to provide significant protection against serious infections caused by this organism (91). Patients who died of bacteremia were markedly neutropenic and deficient in type-specific opsonic antibodies against their infecting strains, and patients with pseudomonal pneumonia also had low or unmeasurable levels of antibodies against their infecting organism. A high incidence of untoward reactions, including high fevers, intense swelling and local pain, and generalized malaise, were noted in many recipients.

Children with cancer who are not receiving chemotherapy achieve significant antibody titers to influenza vaccine with the same frequency as normal children. The preponderance of evidence suggests that primary immunization with influenza virus vaccine often is not immunogenic in patients with hematological malignancies who are receiving chemotherapy. It is recommended that patients with hematological malignancies should receive influenza immunization between chemotherapy courses (92). The optimal time for immunization is 1 month after chemotherapy and when peripheral white blood counts are higher than 100/μL.

The increased risk of overwhelming infections with *Strep. pneumoniae* in patients with Hodgkin's disease after splenectomy has resulted in prophylaxis with pneumococcal vaccine and prophylactic penicillin. In untreated patients in all stages of Hodgkin's disease, the polyvalent pneumococcal vaccine will stimulate significant antibody responses. Polyvalent pneumococcal polysaccharide immunization in Hodgkin's disease patients after the start or completion of immunosuppressive therapy has shown inadequate antibody responses. Patients receiving chemotherapy will respond slightly better if chemotherapy and immunization are not administered concurrently (93), with chemotherapy given more than 10 days after immunization. Similar observations have been made with *Haemophilus influenzae* type B and meningococcal group C vaccines (94). Booster immunization of all three vaccines given fewer than 10 days before to 12 months after chemotherapy also failed to elicit an antibody increase. The available data suggest that polyvalent pneumococcal vaccine should be administered to all patients with Hodgkin's disease, preferably before or after splenectomy, but before specific immunosuppressive therapy is started.

A live attenuated varicella vaccine is now available. The early studies in children with acute leukemia in remission have shown seroresponses in 90% of recipients, without any severe adverse effects (95). Compromised vaccine recipients must be chosen carefully and should possess some degree of demonstrable cellular immune responsiveness. They should not be receiving aggressive chemotherapy at the time of immunization. Maintenance chemotherapy should not be given a week before or a week after vaccination. The vaccines are infectious and transmission can occur to other susceptible individuals. The vaccine virus establishes latent infection, with the potential of reactivation and development of typical zoster infection. The studies so far have shown the incidence of zoster among vaccinees similar to that of naturally infected persons and may actually be low.

CONCLUSIONS

Considerable progress has been made in the management of many of the infections occurring in patients with hematological malignancies. The majority of pyogenic bacterial infections can be treated successfully. Therapy is now available for some viral infections, but cytomegalic inclusion disease remains a therapeutic challenge. Systemic fungal infection remains the most serious threat to these patients. Hopefully, in the near future, better methods for diagnosis and treatment of these infections will be discovered.

REFERENCES

1. Sickles EA, Greene WH, Wiernik PH: Clinical presentations of infection in granulocytopenic patients. *Arch Intern Med* 1975;135:715.
2. Chessells JM, Leiper AD: Infection during remission induction in childhood leukemia. *Arch Dis Child* 1980;55:18–23.

3. Peter G, Pizzo P, Robichaud K, et al: Possible protective effect of circulating antibodies to the shared core glycolipid of *Enterobacteriaceae* in children with malignancy. *Pediatr Res* 1979;13:466.
4. Simone JV, Holland E, Johnson W: Fatalities during remission of childhood leukemia. *Blood* 1972;39:759.
5. Breitfield V, Hashida Y, Sherman FE, et al: Fatal measles infection in children with leukemia. *Lab Invest* 1973;28:279.
6. Pizzo PA, Ladisch S, Simon RM, et al: Increasing incidence of gram-positive sepsis in cancer patients. *Med Pediatr Oncol* 1978;5:241–244.
7. Wade JC, Schimpff SC, Newman KA, Wiernik PH: *Staphylococcus epidermidis:* An increasing cause of infection in patients with granulocytopenia. *Ann Intern Med* 1982;97:503–508.
8. Pizzo PA, Ladisch S, Witebsky FG: alpha-hemolytic streptococci: Clinical significance in the cancer patient. *Med Pediatr Oncol* 1978;4:367–370.
9. Stamm WE, Tompkins LS, Wagner KF, et al: Infection due to *Corynebacterium* species in marrow transplant patients. *Ann Intern Med* 1979;91:167–173.
10. Anaissie EJ, Bodey GP, Rinaldi MG: Emerging fungal pathogens. *Eur J Clin Microbiol Infect Dis* 1989;8:323–330.
11. Holland J: Chronic lymphocyte leukemia. In *Cancer Medicine,* 2nd ed. Philadelphia, Lea & Febiger, 1982, p. 1462.
12. Janckila AJ, Wallace JH, Yam LT: Generalized monocyte deficiency in leukemic reticuloendotheliosis. *Scand J Haematol* 1982;29:153–160.
13. Hersh EM, Quesada J, Keating MJ, et al: Host defense factors and prognosis in hairy cell leukemia. *Leuk Res* 1982;6:625–637.
14. Golomb, HM, Hadad LJ: Infectious complications in 127 patients with hairy cell leukemia. *Am J Hematol* 1984;16:393–401.
15. Salata RA, King RE, Gose F, Pearson RD: *Listeria monocytogenes* cerebritis, bacteremia, and cutaneous lesions complicating hairy cell leukemia. *Am J Med* 1986;81:1068–1072.
16. Joshi J, Schimpff SC: Infections in patients with lymphoma and myeloma. In, *Principles and Practice of Infectious Diseases,* 2nd ed. New York, John Wiley & Sons, 1985, pp 1658–1662.
17. Schimpff SC, Serpick A, Stoler B, et al: Varicella–zoster infection in patients with cancer. *Ann Intern Med* 1972;76:241.
18. Feld R, Bodey GP: Infections in patients with malignant lymphoma treated with combination chemotherapy. *Cancer* 1977;39:1018–1025.
19. Broder S, Humphrey R, Durm M, et al: Impaired synthesis of polyclonal (nonparaprotein) immunoglobulins by circulating lymphocytes from patients with multiple myeloma. *N Engl J Med* 1975;293:887–892.
20. Espersen F, Birgens HS, Hertz JB, Drivsholm V: Current patterns of bacterial infection in myelomatosis. *Eur J Infect Dis* 1984;16:169–173.
21. Kapadia SB: Multiple myeloma: A clinicopathological study of 62 corresponding autopsy cases. *Medicine* 1980;5:380.
22. Dreizen S, McCredie KB, Dicke KA, Zander AR, Peters LJ: Oral complications of bone marrow transplantation. *Postgrad Med* 1979;66:87–193.

23. Kurzrock R, Zander A, Vellekoop L, et al: Mycobacterial pulmonary infections after allogeneic bone marrow transplantation. *Am J Med* 1984;77:35–40.
24. Hersh EM, Bodey GP, Nies BA, Freireich EJ: Causes of death in acute leukemia: A ten year study of 414 patients from 1954–1963. *JAMA* 1965;193:105–109.
25. Bodey GP, Rodriguez V, Luce JK: Carbenicillin therapy of gram-negative bacilli infections. *Am J Med Sci* 1969;257:408–414.
26. Estey EH, Keating MJ, McCredie KB, et al: Causes of initial remission induction failure in acute myelogenous leukemia. *Blood* 1982;60:309–315.
27. Dosik GM, Luna M, Valdievieso M, et al: Necrotizing colitis in patients with cancer. *Am J Med* 1979;67:646.
28. Schimpff SC, Wiernik PH, Block JB: Rectal abscesses in cancer patients. *Lancet* 1972;2:844.
29. Bodey GP: Epidemiological studies of *Pseudomonas* species in patients with leukemia. *Am J Med Sci* 1970;260:82.
30. Han T, Sokal JE, Neter E: Salmonellosis in disseminated malignant diseases—a seven year review (1959–1965). *N Engl J Med* 1967;276:1945.
31. Louria DB, Henselee T, Armstrong D, et al: Listeriosis complicating malignant disease. *Ann Intern Med* 1967;67:261.
32. Murray JF, Feingold SM, Froman S, Will DW: The changing spectrum of nocardiosis. *Ann Rev Resp Dis* 1961;83:315.
33. Bodey GP, Fainstein V: Systemic candidiasis. In, Bodey GP, Fainstein V (eds): *Candidiasis*. New York, Raven Press, 1985, pp. 135–168.
34. Maksymiuk AW, Thongprasert S, Hopfer R, et al: Systemic candidiasis in cancer patients. In, Bodey GP (ed): *Candidiasis: A Growing Concern. Am J Med* 1984;77(suppl 4D):20–27.
35. Haron E, Feld R, Tuffnell P, et al: Hepatic candidiasis: An increasing problem in immunocompromised patients. *Am J Med* 1987;83:17–26.
36. Young RC, Bennett JE, Vogel CL, et al: Aspergillosis. The spectrum of the disease in 98 patients. *Medicine* 1970;49:147.
37. Zimmerman IE, Rappoport H: Occurrence of cryptococcosis in patients with malignant disease of reticuloendothelial system. *Am J Clin Pathol* 1954;24:1050.
38. Schimpff S, Serpick A, Stoler B, et al: Varicella–zoster infection in patients with cancer. *Ann Intern Med* 1972;76:241–254.
39. Vietzke WM, Gelderman AH, Grimley PM, Valsamis MP: Toxoplasmosis complicating malignancy: Experience at the National Cancer Institute. *Cancer* 1968;21:816.
40. Bodey GP, Whitecar JP, Middleman E, Rodriguez V: Carbenicillin therapy for pseudomonas infections. *JAMA* 1971;218:62–66.
41. Pizzo PA, Thaler M, Hathorn J, et al: New beta-lactam antibiotics in granulocytopenic patients: New options and new questions. *Am J Med* 1985;79(suppl 2A):75–82.
42. Fainstein V, Bodey GP, Elting L, et al: A randomized study of ceftazidime compared to ceftazidime and tobramycin for the treatment of infections in cancer patient. *J Antimicrob Chemother* 1983;(suppl A): 101–110.
43. Pizzo PA, Hathorn JW, Hiemenz J, et al: A randomized trial comparing ceftazidime

alone with combination antibiotic therapy in cancer patients with fever and neutropenia. *N Engl J Med* 1986;315:552–558.
44. Barza M: Imipenem: First of a new class of beta-lactam antibiotics. *Ann Intern Med* 1985;103:552–560.
45. Quinn JP, Studemeister AE, DiVincenzo CA, Lerner SA: Resistance to imipenem in *Pseudomonas aeruginosa:* Clinical experience and biochemical mechanisms. *Rev Infect Dis* 1988;10:892–898.
46. Calandra GP, Hesney M, Brown KR: Imipenem/cilastatin therapy of serious infections: A U.S. multicenter noncomparative trial. *Clin Ther* 1985;7:225–238.
47. Bodey GP, Elting L, Jones P, et al: Imipenem/cilastatin therapy of infections in cancer patients. *Cancer* 1987;60:255–262.
48. Fainstein V, Bodey GP: Single-agent therapy of infections in neutropenic cancer patients. *Am J Med* 1985;79:83–88.
49. Bodey GP, Middleman E, Umsawadi T, Rodriguez V: Infections in cancer patients: Results with gentamicin sulfate therapy. *Cancer* 1972;29:1697–1701.
50. Keating MJ, Bodey GP, Valdivieso M, Rodriguez V: A randomized comparative trial of three aminoglycosides—comparison of continuous infusions of gentamicin, amikacin and sisomicin combined with carbenicillin in the treatment of infections in neutropenic patients with malignancies. *Medicine* 1979;58:159–170.
51. Smith GM, Leyland MJ, Farrell ID, Geddes AM: A clinical, microbiological and pharmacokinetic study of ciprofloxacin plus vancomycin as initial therapy of febrile episodes in neutropenic patients. *J Antimicrob Chemother* 1988;21:647–655.
52. Chan CC, Oppenheim BA, Anderson H, et al: Randomized trial comparing ciprofloxacin plus netilmicin versus piperacillin plus netilmicin for empiric treatment of fever in neutropenic patients. *Antimicrob Agents Chemother* 1989;33:87–91.
53. Farber BF, Moellering RC: Retrospective study of the toxicity of preparations of vancomycin for 1974 to 1981. *Antimicrob Agents Chemother* 1983;23:138–141.
54. Schimpff SC: Empiric antibiotic therapy for granulocytopenic cancer patients. *Am J Med* 1986;80(suppl 5C):13–20.
55. Karp JE, Dick JD, Angelopulos C, et al: Empiric use of vancomycin during prolonged treatment-induced granulocytopenia. *Am J Med* 1986;81:237–242.
56. Bauernfeind A, Petermuller C: In vitro activity of teichomycin A2 in comparison with penicillin and vancomycin against gram-positive cocci. *Eur J Clin Microbiol* 1982;1:278–280.
57. Greenwood D: Microbiological properties of teicoplanin. *J Antimicrob Chemother* 1988;22(suppl A):1–13.
58. Neu, HC, Labthavikul P: In vitro activity of teichomycin compared with those of other antibiotics. *Antimicrob Agents Chemother* 1983;24:425–428.
59. Schaison GS, Arlet G, Leverger G, et al: *Infection Due to Coagulase-Negative Staphylococci in Neutropenic Children: Historical Aspects and New Trends in Therapy*. London, Royal Society of Medicine Services, 1989, pp 35–44.
60. Del Favero A, Menichetti F, Guerciolini R, et al: Prospective randomized clinical trial of teicoplanin for empiric combined antibiotic therapy in febrile, granulocytopenic acute leukemia patients. *Antimicrob Agents Chemother* 1987;31:1126–1129.

61. Pizzo PA, Ladisch S, Simon RM, et al: Increasing incidence of gram-positive sepsis in cancer patients. *Med Pediatr Oncol* 1978;5:241–244.
62. Bodey GP: Synergy: Should it determine antibiotic selection in neutropenic patients. *Arch Intern Med* 1985;145:1964–1965.
63. The European Organization for Research on Treatment of Cancer International Antimicrobial Therapy Project Group: Three antibiotic regimens in the treatment of infection in febrile granulocytopenic patients with cancer. *J Infect Dis* 1978;137:14–29.
64. Love LJ, Schimpff SC, Hahn DM, et al: Randomized trial of empiric antibiotic therapy with ticarcillin in combination with gentamicin, amikacin or netilmicin in febrile patients with granulocytopenia and cancer. *Am J Med* 1979;66:603–610.
65. Middleman EA, Watanabe A, Kaizer H, Bodey GP: Antibiotic combinations for infections in neutropenic patients. Evaluation of carbenicillin plus either cephalothin or kanamycin. *Cancer* 1972;30:573–579.
66. Bodey GP, Ketchel SJ, Rodriquez V: A randomized study of carbenicillin plus cefamandole or tobramycin in the treatment of febrile episodes in cancer patients. *Am J Med* 1979;67:608–616.
67. Drusano GL, DeJongh C, Newman K, et al: Moxalactam and piperacillin: A study of in vitro characteristics and pharmacokinetics in cancer patients. *Infection* 1988;13:20–26.
68. Shenep J, Hughes WT, Roberson PK, et al: Vancomycin, ticarcillin and amikacin compared with ticarcillin–clavulanate and amikacin in the empirical treatment of febrile, neutropenic children with cancer. *N Engl J Med* 1988;319:1053–1057.
69. Bodey GP: Continuous infusion antibiotic therapy for neutropenic patients. In, Lokich J (eds). *Cancer Chemotherapy by Infusion*. Chicago, Precept Press, 1987, pp 569–87.
70. Rodriguez V, Bodey GP, Horikoshi N, et al: Ticarcillin therapy of infections. *Antimicrob Agents Chemother* 1973;4:427–431.
71. Rodriguez V, Burgess M, Bodey GP: Management of fever of unknown origin in patients with neoplasms and neutropenia. *Cancer* 1973;32:1007–1012.
72. Alavi JB, Root RK, Djerassi I, et al: Leukocyte transfusions in acute leukemia. *N Eng J Med* 1977;296:706–711.
73. DiNubile MJ: Therapeutic role of granulocyte transfusions. *Rev Infect Dis* 1985;7:232–243.
74. Sokol-Anderson ML, Brajtburg J, Medoff G: Amphotericin B-induced oxidative damage and killing of *Candida albicans*. *J Infect Dis* 1986;154:76
75. Stamm AM, Diasio RB, Dismukes WE, et al: Toxicity of amphotericin B plus flucytosine in 194 patients with cryptococcal meningitis. *Am J Med* 1987;83:236.
76. Espinel-Ingroff A, Shadomy S: In vitro and in vivo evaluation of antifungal agents. *Eur J Clin Microbiol Infect Dis* 1989;8:352–361.
77. Fainstein V, Bodey GP, Elting L, et al: Amphotericin B or ketoconazole therapy of fungal infections in neutropenic cancer patients. *Antimicrob Agents Chemother* 1987;31:11–15.
78. Khosla S, Wolfson JS, Demerjian Z, Godine JE: Adrenal crisis in the setting of high-dose ketoconazole therapy. *Arch Intern Med* 1989;149:802–804.

79. Graybill JR: Therapeutic agents: The long and short of antifungal therapy. *Infect Dis Clin North Am* 1988;2:805.
80. Klastersky J: Concept of empiric therapy with antibiotic combinations. Indications and limits. *Am J Med* 1986;80(suppl 5C):2–12.
81. Hayden FG, Douglas G Jr: Antiviral agents. In, *Principles and Practice of Infectious Diseases,* 2nd ed., New York, John Wiley & Sons, 1985, pp 270–286.
82. Saral R: Management of mucocutaneous herpes simplex virus infections in immunocompromised patients. *Am J Med* 1988;85(suppl 2A):57–61.
83. Emanuel D, Cunningham I, Jules-Elyssee K, et al: Cytomegalovirus pneumonia after bone marrow transplantation successfully treated with the combination of ganciclovir and high-dose intravenous immune globulin. *Ann Intern Med* 1988;15:777–782.
84. Bodey GP, Rodriguez V, Cabanillas F, Freireich EJ: Protected environment–prophylactic antibiotic program for malignant lymphoma: Randomized trial during remission induction chemotherapy. *Am J Med* 1979;66:74–81.
85. Kovatch AL, Wald ER, Albo VC, et al: Oral trimethoprim/sulfamethoxazole for prevention of bacterial infection during the induction phase of cancer chemotherapy in children. *Pediatrics* 1985;76:754.
86. Dekker AW, Rozenberg-Arska M, Verhoef J: Infection prophylaxis in acute leukemia. A comparison of ciprofloxacin with trimethoprim–sulfamethaxazole and colistin. *Ann Intern Med* 1987;106:7–12.
87. Bodey GP, Nies BA, Mohberg NR, Freireich EJ: Use of gamma globulin in infection in acute leukemia patients. *JAMA* 1964;190:1099–1102.
88. Ziegler EJ, McCutchan JA, Fierer S, et al: Successful treatment of gram-negative bacteremia and shock with human antiserum to a UDP-GAL epimerase-deficient mutant *Escherichia coli. N Engl J Med* 1982;307:1225–1230.
89. Stiehm ER, Achida E, Kim KS, et al: Intravenous immunoglobulins as therapeutic agents. *Ann Intern Med* 1987;107:367–382.
90. Sullivan KM: Immunoglobulin therapy in bone marrow transplantation. *Am J Med* 1987;83(suppl 4A):34–45.
91. Young LS: Immunoprophylaxis and serotherapy of bacterial infections. *Am J Med* 1984;76:664–671.
92. Ortbals DW, Liebhaber H, Presant CA, et al: Influenza immunization of adult patients with malignant diseases. *Ann Intern Med* 1977;87:552–557.
93. Shildt RA, Boyd JF, McCracken JD, et al: Antibody response to pneumococcal vaccine in patients with solid tumors and lymphomas. *Med Pediatr Oncol* 1983;11:305–309.
94. Siber GR, Gorham C, Martin P, et al: Antibody response to pretreatment immunization and post-treatment boosting with bacterial polysaccharide vaccines in patients with Hodgkin's disease. *Ann Intern Med* 1986;104:467–475.
95. Konno T, Yamaguchi Y, Minegisii M, et al: A clinical trial of live attenuated varicella vaccine (Biken) in children with malignant diseases. *Biken J* 1984;27:73–75.

Index